D1368659

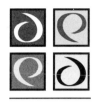

Comprehensive Rehabilitation Nursing

Jill B. Derstine, EdD, RN
Professor and Chair
Department of Nursing
College of Allied Health Professions
Temple University
Philadelphia, Pennsylvania

Shirlee Drayton Hargrove, PhD, RN, FNP, CS, CRRN
Assistant Professor of Nursing and Director, Family Nurse
  Practitioner Program
School of Nursing
Widener University
Chester, Pennsylvania

W.B. SAUNDERS COMPANY
A Harcourt Health Sciences Company
Philadelphia   London   New York   St. Louis   Sydney   Toronto

W.B. SAUNDERS COMPANY
A Harcourt Health Sciences Company

The Curtis Center
Independence Square West
Philadelphia, Pennsylvania 19106

RT 120
R4
C652
2001

Library of Congress Cataloging-in-Publication Data

Comprehensive rehabilitation nursing / [edited by] Jill B. Derstine, Shirlee Drayton Hargrove.—1st ed.

p. cm.

ISBN 0–7216–6977–8

1. Rehabilitation nursing.   I. Derstine, Jill B.   II. Hargrove, Shirlee Drayton.
   [DNLM: 1. Rehabilitation Nursing.   WY 150.5 C737 2000]

RT120.R4 C652 2000   610.73'6 21—dc21   99-040815

NOTICE

Nursing is an ever-changing field. Standard safety precautions must be followed, but as new research and clinical experience broaden our knowledge, changes in treatment and drug therapy may become necessary and appropriate. Readers are advised to check the most current product information provided by the manufacturer of each drug to be administered to verify the recommended dose, the method and duration of administration, and the contraindications. It is the responsibility of the treating physician, relying on experience and knowledge of the patient, to determine dosages and the best treatment for each individual patient. Neither the publisher nor the editor assumes any responsibility for any injury and/or damage to persons or property arising from this publication.

THE PUBLISHER

Vice President, Nursing Editorial Director: Sally Schrefer
Acquisitions Editor: Thomas Eoyang
Editorial Assistant: Adrienne Simon
Manuscript Editor: Amy Norwitz
Production Manager: Pete Faber
Illustration Specialist: Bob Quinn
Book Designer: Ellen Zanolle

COMPREHENSIVE REHABILITATION NURSING   ISBN 0–7216–6977–8

Last digit is the print number: 9   8   7   6   5   4   3   2   1

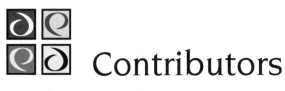# Contributors

Joanne Baggerly, MS, RN, CRRN, CNRN
Argosy Health Resource Associate, Pembroke, Massachusetts
Nursing Management of the Patient with Head Trauma

Mary P. Brassell, RN, BS, MA, CRRN
Rehabilitation Manager, BAYADA NURSES, Moorestown, New Jersey
Nursing Management of the Patient with Rheumatoid Arthritis

Helen Carmine, CRNP, MSN, CRRN
Administrative Director, Orthomedical Division, Bryn Mawr Rehabilitation/Jefferson Health Systems, Malvern, Pennsylvania
Sexuality

Susan Christie, BS, BE
Supervisor, Assistive Technology Center, Bryn Mawr Rehabilitation/Jefferson Health System, Malvern, Pennsylvania
Assistive Devices

Susan L. Dean-Baar, PhD, RN, CRRN, FAAN
Associate Dean for Academic Affairs, School of Nursing, University of Wisconsin, Milwaukee, Wisconsin
Health Policy and Legislation in Rehabilitation

Jill B. Derstine, EdD, RN
Professor and Chair, Department of Nursing, College of Allied Health Professions, Temple University, Philadelphia, Pennsylvania
Definition and Philosophy of Rehabilitation Nursing: History and Scope Including Chronicity and Disability; Theories and Models in Rehabilitation Nursing; Rehabilitation Nursing in Vietnam: A Prototype for Bringing Rehabilitation Nursing to a Third World Nation

Kristen L. Easton, MS, RN, CRRN-A, CS
Assistant Professor of Nursing, Valparaiso University; Community Health Education Director, Porter Memorial Hospital, Valparaiso, Indiana
Gerontological Rehabilitation Nursing

Patricia A. Edwards, BS, MA, EdD, CNAA
Nurse Educator, Regents College, Albany, New York
Pediatric Rehabilitation Nursing

Janet M. Farahmand, BSN, MSN, EdD
Associate Professor of Nursing, Neumann College, Division of Nursing, Aston, Pennsylvania
Cognition

Catharine Farnan, RN, MS, CRRN, ONC
Clinical Nurse Specialist, Comprehensive Acute Rehabilitation Unit, Thomas Jefferson University Hospital, Philadelphia, Pennsylvania
Elimination

Guy W. Fried, MD
Clinical Assistant Professor, Thomas Jefferson University Medical College, and Medical Director of Outpatient Services and Attending Physician, Magee Rehabilitation Hospital, Philadelphia, Pennsylvania
Elimination; Immobility

Karen Mandzak Fried, RN, MSN, CRRN, CCM
Adjunct Clinical Instructor, Thomas Jefferson University, College of Allied Health Professions; Rehabilitation Services Coordinator, Thomas Jefferson University Hospital, Department of Rehabilitation Medicine, Philadelphia, Pennsylvania
Elimination; Immobility

Shirlee Drayton Hargrove, PhD, RN, FNP, CS, CRRN
Assistant Professor of Nursing and Director, Family Nurse Practitioner Program, School of Nursing, Widener University, Chester, Pennsylvania
Definition and Philosophy of Rehabilitation Nursing: History and Scope Including Chronicity and Disability; Theories and Models in Rehabilitation Nursing; Ethics in Rehabilitation Nursing

Judith A. Hines, RN, MSN
Adjunct Faculty, Wilmington College, Wilmington, Delaware; Coordinator of Orthopedic Joint Replacement Center, Shore Health System/Memorial Hospital of Easton, Easton, Maryland
Case Management: A Client-Focused Service; Assistive Devices

Mary Jean Kotch, MSN, CRRN-A
Rehabilitation Clinical Nurse Specialist, Kaiser
    Foundation Rehabilitation Center, Vallejo,
    California
*Nursing Management of the Patient with an
    Orthopedic Disorder*

Nancy Le, RN, C, MS, CNRN
Neurology Nurse Practitioner, Braintree Hospital
    Rehabilitation Network, Braintree,
    Massachusetts
*Nursing Management of the Patient with Head
    Trauma*

Dianne Mahoney, RN, MS, CRRN
Director of Nurses, Transitional Care Unit,
    Carney Hospital, Dorchester, Massachusetts
*Nursing Management of the Patient with Spinal Cord
    Injury*

Barbara A. Marte, RN
Senior Vice President for Marketing and Best
    Practice, Lutheran Affiliated Services,
    Cranberry Township, Pennsylvania
Health Care Financing and Reimbursement

Sheila O'Shea Melli, EdD, RN
Assistant Professor–Adjunct, Teachers College,
    Columbia University—Programs in Nursing
    Education, New York, New York; and St.
    Peter's College, Department of Nursing, Jersey
    City, New Jersey
*Teaching and Learning: Educative Roles in
    Rehabilitation Nursing*

Christine L. Nagy, RN, BSN, CRRN, RNC
Director of Home Health, Community Health
    Partners, Lorrain, Ohio
Community-Focused Rehabilitation Nursing

Audrey Nelson, PhD, RN
Adjunct Faculty, College of Nursing, College of
    Public Health, University of South Florida;
    Research Scientist, James A. Haley VAMC,
    Tampa, Florida
Research in Rehabilitation Nursing

Diana M. L. Newman, RN, EdD
Associate Professor, Department of Nursing,
    Neumann College, Aston, Pennsylvania
Self-Care

Marie O'Toole, EdD, RN, FAAN
Program Coordinator and Director of Camden
    Services Graduate Program, Rutgers
    University, Camden, New Jersey
The Rehabilitation Team

Dolores S. Patrinos, RN, MA
Assistant Professor of Nursing, College of
    Applied Health Professions, Temple
    University, Philadelphia, Pennsylvania
Culturally Competent Rehabilitation Care

Cynthia Phelan, MS, RN
Nurse Manager, Beth Israel Deaconess Medical
    Center, Boston, Massachusetts
Cardiopulmonary Rehabilitation

Patricia Quigley, PhD, RN
Faculty, Graduate and Undergraduate, College of
    Nursing, University of Phoenix, Tampa
    Campus; Visiting Faculty, College of Nursing,
    University of South Florida; Rehabilitation
    Clinical Nurse Specialist, CARF Accredited
    Rehabilitation Programs, James A. Haley
    Veterans' Hospital, Tampa, Florida
Functional Assessment

Patricia S. Regojo, MSN
Nurse Manager, Temple University Hospital Burn
    Unit, Philadelphia, Pennsylvania
A Holistic Approach to Burn Rehabilitation

Sheila M. Sparks, DNSc, RN, CS
Associate Chair for Academics and Associate
    Professor, Division of Nursing, Shenandoah
    University, Winchester, Virginia
Skin Integrity

Neva White, RN, MSN, CRNP
Regional Director of Community Health, Thomas
    Jefferson University Health Systems,
    Philadelphia, Pennsylvania
Culturally Competent Rehabilitation Care

Judy Winterhalter, DNSc, RN, CS
Professor, Graduate Nursing Program, School of
    Nursing, Gwynedd-Mercy College, Gwynedd
    Valley, Pennsylvania; Psychotherapist, North
    Penn Counseling Center, Lansdale,
    Pennsylvania
*Family Dynamics; Psychosocial Issues for the Person
    with Chronic Illness or Disability*

Jean H. Woods, PhD, RN, CS
Professor Emeritus, Temple University; Private
    Practice, Philadelphia, Pennsylvania
Ethics in Rehabilitation Nursing

Corinne Wright, MSPT
Assistant Professor of Physical Therapy,
    Neumann College, Aston, Pennsylvania
A Holistic Approach to Burn Rehabilitation

Michelle Young-Stevenson, RN, MS, CRRN
Director of Nursing, Transitional Care Unit,
    Chestnut Hill Hospital, Philadelphia,
    Pennsylvania
Nursing Management of the Patient with Amputation

Nancy M. Youngblood, PhD, CRNP, FNP
Assistant Professor and Director of Adult and
    Family Nurse Practitioner Programs, LaSalle
    University, School of Nursing, Philadelphia,
    Pennsylvania
*Nursing Management of the Patient with a
    Cerebrovascular Accident*

Preface

The practice of rehabilitation nursing has changed rapidly during the past decade. In response to the changing health-care system, sicker patients are discharged more quickly. Scientific advances in the care of disabled and chronically ill patients have created new bodies of knowledge essential to rehabilitation nursing. During this period of the advancement of rehabilitation nursing, there has been a dearth of comprehensive literature addressing the essential issues in the field. This book provides a knowledge base that will contribute to the advancement of practice. It furnishes rehabilitation nurses here and abroad with a reference applicable to both education and clinical settings.

The authors have designed this book to cover the basic aspects of rehabilitation nursing, including basic concepts, nursing approaches to several common rehabilitation categories, and issues pertinent to rehabilitation nursing today. Throughout the book and in special chapters, we have emphasized culturally competent care and care of patients in the community.

Comprehensive Rehabilitation Nursing is designed to be used as a reference for graduate and undergraduate students and nurses in a multitude of settings, that is, in rehabilitation units, clinics, long-term care, and community settings. Each chapter dealing with a clinical entity covers the care of the patient from the rehabilitative stage in the hospital to the community setting. The practicing rehabilitation nurse can easily use the book when caring for a patient with a specific disorder. It is also easily referenced when information on a specific nursing approach such as elimination or functional assessment is sought.

The book's four sections provide resources for practicing rehabilitation nurses at all levels. Part I covers philosophy, a brief history, ethics, conceptual foundations, the interdisciplinary team, teaching, and learning and includes the two theme chapters: community-focused rehabilitation and culturally competent care. Part II examines rehabilitation nursing management applicable to any group of patients. These are concepts essential in several areas of rehabilitation nursing practice and have been associated with rehabilitation nursing for the past two or three decades. In Part III we have selected several common conditions or diagnoses associated with rehabilitation patients in chapters focusing on the rehabilitative nursing care of the patient with each specific disorder. Such organization guides the practicing rehabilitation nurse to easily find the information pertaining to a patient with a specific diagnosis or condition. Part IV examines evolving issues such as health care financing, international rehabilitation nursing, which is just developing, and rehabilitation nursing research, which is coming into its own. These chapters are written by nationally known experts in the field.

The editors and contributors thank all the professional associates and personal friends who have directly helped in preparing this manuscript.

Jill B. Derstine
Shirlee Drayton Hargrove

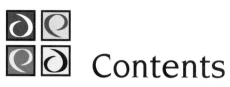

Contents

PART I

General Concepts in Rehabilitation Nursing

Definition and Philosophy of Rehabilitation Nursing: History and Scope Including Chronicity and Disability

Shirlee Drayton Hargrove and Jill B. Derstine

This chapter provides an overview of the definition of rehabilitation nursing and its historical highlights, philosophical foundations, guiding principles, and key concepts. The role of the nurse as a member of the rehabilitation team is discussed.

REHABILITATION NURSING DEFINED

Rehabilitation nursing has been defined as "the diagnosis and treatment of human responses of individuals and groups to actual or potential health problems stemming from altered functional ability and altered lifestyle" (American Nurses Association & Association of Rehabilitation Nurses, 1988, p.4). Rehabilitation nursing is a specialty practice area within the scope of professional nursing practice (American Nurses Association & Association of Rehabilitation Nurses, 1988, p. 4). Professional standards for rehabilitation nursing guide nursing practice and have been outlined by the profession. Rehabilitation nursing is a dynamic process designed to facilitate the highest level of function of the client in the environment. The *functional capacity* of a disabled individual reflects the extent to which the person can engage in dynamic interaction with the environment (Fig. 1–1). As specialists, rehabilitation nurses facilitate the maintenance and restoration of functional abilities. The Association of Rehabilitation Nurses has offered standards for rehabilitation specialty practice. Standards and professional behaviors are outlined to guide nursing practice and have been extended to include advanced clinical practice rehabilitation nursing (Association of Rehabilitation Nurses, 1994, 1996) (Tables 1–1 and 1–2).

REHABILITATION NURSES AND THE METAPARADIGM

The disabled person is viewed in a holistic manner as an interactive open system with the capacity for self-regulation. The needs and behaviors of the disabled individual and family, which reflect personal characteristics including abilities and roles, must be carefully considered during the assessment process. As a member of the family social system, the client interacts with the environment to meet physical, psychological, social, emotional, and spiritual needs; the rehabilitation nurse alters and structures that environment so that the highest level of function can be achieved.

The nurse provides care, education, and support to the client and family. Nursing care is focused on assisting disabled individuals, their families, and their communities in the development of the client's self-care skills. In addition to being an advocate for the client, family, and community, the rehabilitation nurse provides coordinated and essential interventions designed to facilitate the disabled person's adaptation to new roles and to the environment.

HISTORICAL HIGHLIGHTS

In the United States, the field of rehabilitation is linked to and has received the greatest impetus from wars. Dr. Simon Baruch, a Confederate Army surgeon, was a pioneer in physical medicine. He used physical agents such as heat, cold, water, electricity, radiation, and massage to treat impaired joints and muscles. Vocational rehabilitation for the veterans of World War I was provided by law in 1918. State legislation for rehabilitation of the disa-

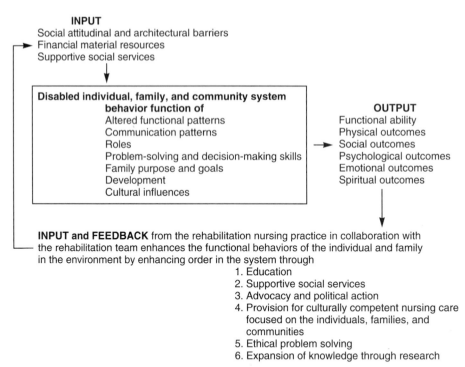

FIGURE 1–1
Dynamic interaction of the individual/family/environmental systems.

bled was preceded by the efforts of the Red Cross Institute for Crippled and Disabled Men. The Federal Rehabilitation Act of 1920 required that the state boards of vocational rehabilitation administer rehabilitation programs. Appropriations were not adequate, and progress was slow and irregular among the various states. By 1921, 123,000 disabled American soldiers who returned from war were served by this board. In 1922, the American Rehabilitation Committee was founded, and in 1927 it began to publish *The Rehabilitation Review*. This journal was devoted to the restoration and employment of disabled persons. The Social Security Act of 1935 contained a provision that increased federal appropriations to states and funded additional vocational programs (Terry, Benz, Mereness, & Kleffner, 1961).

Rehabilitation principles were employed as far back as Florence Nightingale's time. In *Notes on Nursing: What It Is and What It Is Not*, Nightingale (1859) documented that allowing the patients to do for themselves was an important nursing intervention. However, between World War I and World War II, physical medicine as a specialty expanded through the development of specialized centers for poliomyelitis. Sister Elizabeth Kenny, a nurse, is recognized for her use of muscle manipula-

tion during this time (Mumma, 1987, p. 8). Simultaneously, there was a growing recognition of societal responsibility for the needs of disabled children that resulted in the development of specialized programs and hospitals for this segment of society.

The 1940s saw significant growth in the field. During World War II, the field of physical medicine underwent greater development aided by the efforts of Dr. Howard A. Rusk. Rusk introduced psychosocial treatment and vocational training to the Air Force convalescent centers. His efforts resulted in many patients' returning to full-time and part-time employment after being bedridden for years (Terry et al., 1961). In 1943, Bernard Baruch organized the Baruch Committee on Physical Medicine as a memorial to his father, Dr. Simon Baruch. He appealed to President Franklin Roosevelt to develop comprehensive rehabilitation programs that would provide for the needs of disabled veterans. By 1945, there were eight spinal cord injury units in the United States. The rehabilitation medical specialty became firmly established, and by 1946, physiatrists were being trained in rehabilitation medicine. -

Rehabilitation nursing emerged formally as insurance companies hired nurses to complete comprehensive assessments of injured

TABLE 1–1 ■ STANDARDS AND SCOPE OF REHABILITATION NURSING PRACTICE

Standards of Care

Standard I. Assessment
   The rehabilitation nurse collects client health data
Standard II. Diagnosis
   The rehabilitation nurse analyzes the assessment data when determining diagnoses
Standard III. Outcome identification
   The rehabilitation nurse identifies expected outcomes individualized to the client
Standard IV. Planning
   The rehabilitation nurse develops a plan of care that prescribes interventions to attain expected outcomes
Standard V. Implementation
   The rehabilitation nurse implements the interventions identified in the plan of care
Standard VI. Evaluation
   The rehabilitation nurse evaluates the client's progress toward attainment of outcomes

Standards of Professional Performance

Standard I. Quality of care
   The rehabilitation nurse systematically evaluates the quality and effectiveness of rehabilitation nursing practice
Standard II. Performance appraisal
   The rehabilitation nurse evaluates his or her own nursing practice in relation to professional practice standards and
   relevant statutes and regulations
Standard III. Education
   The rehabilitation nurse acquires and maintains current knowledge in nursing practice
standard IV. Collegiality
   The rehabilitation nurse contributes to the professional development of peers, colleagues, and others
Standard V. Ethics
   The rehabilitation nurse's decisions and actions on behalf of clients are determined in an ethical manner
Standard VI. Collaboration
   The rehabilitation nurse collaborates with the client, significant others, and health care providers in providing client care
Standard VII. Research
   The rehabilitation nurse uses research findings in practice
Standard VIII. Utilization
   The rehabilitation nurse considers factors related to safety, effectiveness, and cost in planning and delivering client care

Reprinted from Association of Rehabilitation Nurses. (1994). *Standards and scope of rehabilitation nursing practice* (3rd ed.). Skokie, IL: Author, with permission of the Association of Rehabilitation Nurses, 4700 W. Lake Avenue, Glenview, IL 60025-1485. Copyright © 1994.

clients for insurance purposes. As the medical specialty developed, the formal nursing specialty and a few graduate programs emerged. These programs prepared advanced rehabilitation nurses. These early programs focused on presenting a broad background of rehabilitation techniques and emphasized the importance of the nurse as an active participant on the rehabilitation team. The content of these early programs included technical skills such as active and passive exercise, crutch walking, and bowel and bladder training. Advanced rehabilitation nursing education also included psychosocial content that fostered respect for individual differences, patient choice, and inclusion in the direction of self-care activities. "It would be extremely valuable if she [the nurse] could have additional training in physical and occupational therapy," wrote Terry et al. in 1961. Often the graduates of these programs were employed

in nursing schools, integrating rehabilitation techniques into the curriculum, which at that time was usually heavily weighted with medical-surgical content.

The emergence of rehabilitation nursing can also be credited to those individuals who were visionary, who had interest in the specialty, and who directed their efforts to formally establish and maintain the field. These pioneers included Alice Morrissey, author of the first textbook in the field, *Rehabilitation Nursing;* Lena Plaisted, the founder of the first graduate program in rehabilitation nursing; Harriet Lane, the first nurse hired by Liberty Mutual Insurance Company to coordinate client rehabilitation programs; and Mary A. Mikulic, one of the first clinical specialist employed by the Veterans Administration (McCourt, 1993). These outstanding individuals were among those who helped to launch the specialty of rehabilitation nursing.

TABLE 1–2 ▪ SCOPE AND STANDARDS OF ADVANCED CLINICAL PRACTICE IN REHABILITATION NURSING

Standards of Care

Standard I. Assessment
   The advanced practice nurse in rehabilitation collects comprehensive client health data
Standard II. Diagnosis
   The advanced practice nurse in rehabilitation critically analyzes the assessment data in determining diagnoses for clients with chronic illness or disability
Standard III. Outcome identification
   The advanced practice nurse in rehabilitation identifies expected outcomes derived from the assessment data and diagnoses and individualizes expected outcomes with clients who have chronic illness or disability and with the health care team when appropriate
Standard IV. Planning
   The advanced practice nurse in rehabilitation participates in the development of a comprehensive plan of care with the client and significant others that includes interventions and treatments to attain expected outcomes
Standard V. Implementation
   The advanced practice nurse in rehabilitation prescribes, orders, and implements interventions and treatments for the plan of care
   a. Case management/coordination of care
   b. Consultation
   c. Health promotion, health maintenance, and health teaching
   d. Prescriptive authority and treatment
   e. Referral
Standard VI. Evaluation
   The advanced practice nurse in rehabilitation evaluates the client's progress in attaining expected outcomes

Standards of Professional Performance

Standard I. Quality of care
   The advanced practice nurse in rehabilitation develops criteria for and evaluates the quality of care and effectiveness of advanced practice nursing
Standard II. Self-Evaluation
   The advanced practice nurse in rehabilitation continuously evaluates his or her own nursing practice in relation to professional practice standards and relevant statutes and regulations and is accountable to the public and to the profession for providing competent clinical care
Standard III. Education
   The advanced practice nurse in rehabilitation acquires and maintains current knowledge and skills in the specialty practice area of rehabilitation nursing
Standard IV. Leadership
   The advanced practice nurse in rehabilitation serves as a leader, effective team member, and role model in the professional development of peers, colleagues, and others
Standard V. Ethics
   The advanced practice nurse in rehabilitation integrates ethical principles and norms in all areas of practice
Standard VI. Interdisciplinary process
   The advanced practice nurse in rehabilitation promotes an interdisciplinary process in providing care for the client
Standard VII. Research
   The advanced practice nurse in rehabilitation uses research to discover, examine, and evaluate knowledge, theories, and creative approaches to health care for persons with chronic illness and disability

REHABILITATION PHILOSOPHY

The rehabilitation nurse employs education-supportive strategies based on rehabilitation philosophy, goals, and key concepts. Rehabilitation comes from the medieval Latin term *rehabilitare*, meaning "to restore to a former rank," and the late Latin term *habilitare*, meaning "to enable." There is a range of definitions of rehabilitation in the literature; however, Hickey (1986, p. 179) offers an appropriate and widely used definition of rehabilitation: "Rehabilitation is a dynamic process in which the person is aided in achieving optimum physical, emotional, psychosocial, and vocational potential in order to maintain dignity and self respect in a life that is as self fulfilling as possible." The National Council on Rehabilitation's 1994 definition states that "rehabilitation is the restoration of the handicapped to the fullest physical, mental, social, vocational, economic usefulness of which they are capable" (cited in Wright, 1983, p. 3). The Commission on Accreditation of Rehabilitation Facilities (CARF) defines rehabilitation as "the process of providing, in a coordinated manner, those comprehensive services deemed appropriate to the needs of a person with a disability in a program designed to achieve objectives of improved health, welfare, and the realization of the person's maximal physical, social, psychological and vocational potential for useful and productive activity" (CARF, 1991, p. 138).

Rehabilitation is a negentropic process that involves effort by the client, family, and health care provider. The clients are aided toward expanded freedom to mobilize resources on their own behalf. An optimal level of function is achieved through recognition of the uniqueness and wholeness of the individual.

GOALS OF REHABILITATION

Maximizing Potential

A major goal of rehabilitation is to restore and maintain maximal wellness and health. Goals for care provided to disabled individuals, their families, and their communities are designed to achieve the highest potential level of physical, psychological, social, and spiritual function. Maximum potential is achieved in agreement with important environmental influences—such as financial and human resources. The rehabilitation practitioner recognizes the uniqueness of the individual as a living open system with the potential for wellness.

Learning

Learning is a major goal of rehabilitation. The rehabilitation nurse facilitates learning through the employment of educational principles, needs assessment, and strategies. Educational strategies designed to achieve learning should be active, collaborative, highly participatory, and individualized. The rehabilitation nurse seeks to understand client and family attitudes and beliefs that influence learning and the maintenance of learned behaviors. These ethically sound and culturally competent strategies are designed to assist clients and their families to adjust to disability. The goals are that the client and family will be able to adjust to the limitation, direct the client's own care, mobilize resources on the client's own behalf, and become knowledgeable consumers of care.

Ability

A major goal and theme of rehabilitation is to focus on the client's *ability*. The rehabilitation practitioner recognizes and respects the adaptive capacity in the living organism. People are viewed as self-regulating, with an enormous capacity to cope with change. The rehabilitation client is viewed as self-motivated, capable of decision making, and capable of achieving necessary results.

Quality of Life

Rehabilitation practice is designed to enhance the quality of life for individuals, families and communities. Quality of life is a personal phenomenon that is defined by the individual's self-image, viewpoint, position, and attitudes concerning life. The rehabilitation nurse seeks to promote a quality of life that meets the client's definition of dignity and promotes self-respect and self-reliance. The quality of life is influenced by several interrelated factors such as personal and family purpose and goals, functional abilities, social supports, communication skills, activities of daily living, cognition, problem-solving and decision-making skills, pain and comfort, economic resources, and basic human requisites—food, shelter, and safety. The rehabilitation nurse considers these factors during the assessment of needs, establishment of goals, and development of intervention strategies.

Family-Centered Care

Rehabilitation is a family-centered process. The disabled individual who is part of a family is viewed as a subsystem of a living dynamic system with group core processes, needs, expectations, and roles. Rehabilitation nurses recognize that families must be equipped with knowledge and skills to support a disabled member. The purpose and goals of the individual and the family system must be clarified and/or established early in the process. The education-supportive family system approach to assessment, intervention, and evaluation of care facilitates optimal wellness and improves the quality of family life.

Wellness

Wellness is not simply the absence of symptoms but incorporates soundness of body, mind, and spirit (World Health Organization, 1948, 1986). Wellness is a dynamic process that integrates physical capabilities, psychosocial development, spirituality, and the environment. In contrast to health — the state of complete physical, mental, and social well-being, not merely the absence of disease — wellness can be achieved without complete physical well-being. The wellness orientation is fundamental to rehabilitation nursing practice. Rehabilitation nursing specialty practice achieves wellness by taking actions to reduce functional limitations. Interventions are designed to restore, maintain, and promote healthy lifestyles for disabled individuals.

Culturally Competent Care

Recipients of rehabilitation nursing care represent populations with diverse values, ethnicities, history, and social backgrounds. The rehabilitation nurse respects individual differences and individualizes care with appreciation for cultural diversity. Culturally competent care in rehabilitation reflects sensitivity to individuality and respect for beliefs, values, and customs of disabled individuals. The rehabilitation nurse respects individual needs, is a leader, and acts as a cultural broker who intervenes and assists the client to negotiate the often-unfamiliar and culturally different health care delivery systems and unfamiliar environments in the context of a disability.

Community Reintegration

Community reintegration is a major goal and central theme in rehabilitation nursing. The rehabilitation process is designed to assist the disabled individual to view impairment and functional limitations as challenges instead of as situations that "handicap" and threaten their ability to care for themselves. Disabled individuals are helped to reintegrate into society as productive citizens.

KEY CONCEPT: PHASES OF REHABILITATION

Nagi (1965) established a framework to guide understanding of the impact of functional limitations (Table 1–3). The phases of rehabilitation include the disease–organ impairment, person-disability, and societal-handicap phases. During the disease–organ impairment phase of rehabilitation, the limitations result from psychological or physical disease or injury that causes impairment of an organ. The person-disability phase results from functional limitation and the loss of the person's ability to perform activities of daily living and self-care. The societal-handicap phase results from the inability of the person to interact effectively in the environment. A client with a cerebrovascular accident has impairment due to ischemia of the brain at the organ level. The individual may sustain a hemiplegia resulting in functional limitations and deficits in self-maintenance management. The lack of a wheelchair-accessible environment

TABLE 1–3 ■ PHASES OF REHABILITATION AND RELATED CONCEPTS AS OUTLINED BY NAGI IN 1965

Phase	Definition
Disease–organ impairment	Any loss or abnormality of psychological or physiological structure or function
Person-disability (functional)	Any restriction or deficit resulting from an impairment of the ability to perform an activity in a manner or within the range considered normal for a human being
Societal-handicap	A disadvantage for a given individual, resulting from an impairment or a disability, that limits or prevents the fulfillment of a role that is normal for that individual

From Nagi, S. Z. (1965). Some conceptual issues in disability and rehabilitation. In M. B. Sussman (Ed.), *Sociology and rehabilitation* (pp. 100–113). Washington, DC: American Sociological Association.

TABLE 1–4 ■ COMPARISON OF TYPES OF REHABILITATION TEAMS

	Multidisciplinary	Interdisciplinary	Transdisciplinary
Goals	Discipline defined Isolated Imposed within a discipline	Cross-discipline defined Communally interdependently structured	Mutual goals Transcend disciplines
Decision making	Made by each discipline separately Confirmed by physician	Made within disciplines Made across disciplines through consensus	Mutual decision making Transcends disciplines
Roles	Structured with discipline-specific clear boundaries	Shared tasks	Mutual roles Need- and skills-defined roles

can limit the individual's ability to perform important life functions such as taking public transportation to get to work. An individual becomes handicapped by the failure of society to ensure ease of interaction between the person and the environment.

KEY CONCEPT: THE REHABILITATION TEAM—PURPOSES AND FUNCTIONS

The rehabilitation team comprises the client, physician, nurse, occupational therapist, physical therapist, speech therapist, social worker, and vocational counselor. The client is the most important member of the team. However, the rehabilitation team can be viewed from a community focus and might include people from churches, organizations, and neighbors who engage in roles designed to assist clients and families to meet goals.

The three major types of teams are multidisciplinary, interdisciplinary, and transdisciplinary teams (Table 1–4). The *multidiscipli-nary* team comprises members who are responsible for particular areas. During a client care conference, the multidisciplinary team member establishes section goals such as the client's nursing goals or the client's physical therapy goals. The *interdisciplinary* team may represent many disciplines but has common goals. The client care conference in an interdisciplinary team usually reflects negotiation about what goals to focus on. Interdisciplinary team functioning can be time-consuming because this type of team requires greater collaboration and communication. In the *transdisciplinary* team, there is a high degree of interaction among the disciplines, and roles and boundaries of functioning are less defined. The nurse might perform physical activities that are traditionally thought of as physical therapy and occupational therapy roles in this type of team.

The nurse is an integral part of any effectively functioning rehabilitation team. Successful rehabilitation teams work in collaboration to meet client and family goals (Table 1–5). Successful teams possess strong commu-

TABLE 1–5 ■ SUCCESSFUL VERSUS UNSUCCESSFUL REHABILITATION TEAMS

	Successful	Unsuccessful
Communication	Is free, respectful, two-way Includes acceptance and expression of ideas and feelings	Is restricted, one-way, offensive
Trust	Is achieved through dependability, follow-through, mutual respect	Is not achieved because participants are dubious
Goals	Are accomplished Are set with inclusion of patient, are mutually constructed Are clarified and clear	Are set with exclusion of team members Are unilateral Are competitive Are unclear Are imposed
Decision making	Involves patient Is done by seeking consensus	Is unilaterally made by highest authority
Clarification of roles	Is clear	Is unclear, territorial
Conflict management	Resolves	Is ignored, suppressed

nication and decision-making skills. Trust, mutual respect, and clear goals are important characteristics of high-performance teams. Decision making should be achieved by consensus, but in a rehabilitation process the client's decisions are highly respected. The nurse's skills include communicating warm regard and respect for the client's feelings. The nurse clarifies the ideas of the client and family and incorporates these in a jointly developed plan of care. These communication strategies are designed to promote client and family independence by fostering problem solving and mobilizing resources for their own behalf. The nurse inquires to ascertain the client's and family's needs, desires, and concerns through the use of questions and clarification and by providing answers. Successful teams engage in two-way communication.

Education is the primary role of the rehabilitation nurse. The nurse must consult with other disciplines, coordinate care and services, advocate for clients' rights, and provide direct care. The nurse's role is to coach the client and family, not to direct. Rehabilitation nursing specialty practice promotes independence in disabled clients and their families by assisting them to identify adaptive resources and to adjust their lifestyle to meet self-care requirements. The nurse informs and instructs but avoids fostering dependency. Instead, the client and the family are encouraged to formulate logical executable decisions, goals, and plans.

SUMMARY

Rehabilitation nursing is a specialty in nursing based on strong socially conscious historical tradition, nursing standards, rehabilitation philosophy, goals, and key concepts. The nurse provides education and supportive care to diverse populations of disabled individuals in collaboration with the family and the rehabilitation team members. The goals of rehabilitation nursing include assisting individuals and groups to achieve their maximal potential and teaching those with functional limitations how to effectively use residual abilities after a disability.

REFERENCES

American Nurses Association & Association of Rehabilitation Nurses. (1988). *Rehabilitation nursing. Scope of practice: Process and outcome criteria for selected diagnoses.* Kansas City, MO: Authors.

Association of Rehabilitation Nurses. (1994). *Standards and scope of rehabilitation nursing practice* (3rd ed.). Skokie, IL: Author.

Association of Rehabilitation Nurses. (1996). *Scope and standards of advanced clinical practice in rehabilitation nursing* (3rd ed.). Skokie, IL: Author.

Commission on Accreditation of Rehabilitation Facilities. 1991. *Standards manual for organizations serving people with disabilities.* Tucson, AZ: Author.

Hickey, J. V. (1986). *The clinical practice of neurological and neuroscience nursing* (2nd ed.). Philadelphia: J. B. Lippincott.

McCourt, A. (Ed.). (1993). *The specialty practice of rehabilitation nursing, core curriculum* (3rd ed.). Skokie, IL: Rehabilitation Nursing Foundation.

Mumma, C. M. (Ed.). (1987). *Rehabilitation nursing: Concepts and practice—A core curriculum* (2nd ed.). St. Louis: C. V. Mosby.

Nagi, S. Z. (1965). Some conceptual issues in disability and rehabilitation. In M. B. Sussman (Ed.), *Sociology and rehabilitation* (pp. 100–113). Washington, DC: American Sociological Association.

Nightingale, F. (1859). *Notes on nursing: What it is and what it is not.* London: Harrison & Sons.

Terry, F. J., Benz, G. S., Mereness, D., & Kleffner, F. K. (1961). *Principles and techniques of rehabilitation nursing* (2nd ed.). St. Louis: C. V. Mosby.

World Health Organization. (1948). Constitution. In Basic Documents. Geneva: Author.

World Health Organization. (1986). *World Health Organization report on concepts and principles of health promotion.* Geneva: Author.

Wright, B. (1983). *Physical disability: A psychosocial approach* (2nd ed.). New York: Harper & Row.

CHAPTER 2

Theories and Models in Rehabilitation Nursing

Shirlee Drayton Hargrove and Jill B. Derstine

Rehabilitation nursing is based on a broad range of theoretical concepts, constructs, principles, propositions, and assumptions that provide the guiding framework for clinical practice. These frameworks organize knowledge for nursing clinical practice, education, and research. Theories and conceptual models explicate abstract ideas. Theories are defined as constellations of integrated concepts that present a view of phenomena (Burns & Grove, 1995). Concepts are defined as terms that abstractly describe and name an object or phenomenon, thus providing it with a separate identity or meaning (Burns & Grove, 1995). Models are more abstract than theories and explain assumptions. Models also comprise a set of integrated concepts, constructs, and propositions. Nursing models address the metaparadigm phenomena of person, environment, health, and nursing (Fawcett, 1995). This chapter highlights various theories and models that have influenced and guided rehabilitation specialty practice. These frameworks are derived from the social sciences, nursing, and rehabilitation science.

SOCIAL SCIENCE THEORIES

Field Theory

Field theory was documented in the writing of Kirk Lewin. In 1946, Lewin wrote several classic papers in field theory in social science. These theoretical papers established the foundations for the translation of phenomena into concepts. Lewin introduced the importance of examining systems of concepts and is most noted for his definition of the *field*. Lewin proposed that the field that must be dealt with is the *life space*. The life space comprises the person (P) and the environment (E) in which an individual or a group exists. Behavior (B) is viewed as a function of the person in the environment; thus, $B = f(P.E)$ (Fig. 2–1). Interdependence is a basic exertion of field theory. Lewin believed that a set of interrelated facts could be best conceptually noted with the mathematical concepts of space and the dynamic concepts of tension and force (Cartwright, 1951). These basic ideas provide the foundation for systems theory and change theory. The rehabilitation

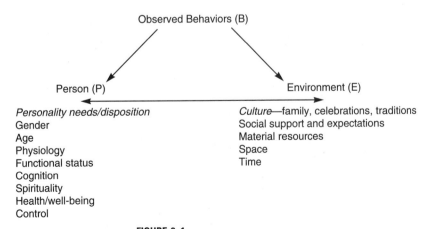

FIGURE 2–1
Field theory life space; $B = f(P.E)$.

nurse performs assessments of the person in relationship to the environment. A disabled client's self-care behavior is a function of personal factors such as knowledge, decision making, and physical limitations as well as environmental factors such as materials resources. Field theory, systems theory, and change theory have enhanced our understanding of disability and provided explanations for the development of rehabilitation practice, concepts, and principles.

Systems Theory

L. von Bertalanffy (1950) has been credited with early conceptualizations of systems theory. His classic paper published in 1950 entitled "The Theory of Open Systems in Physics and Biology" provided a framework for *system thinking*. Lewin also wrote of systems in the 1930s and 1940s. Lewin wrote of persons as a whole system in 1946. A system is an organized constellation of interdependent elements (Cartwright, 1951). Living systems are defined as open systems that are receptive to external influences from the environment.

The organization of a system reflects the degree of the system's complexity (Fig. 2–2). Subsystems are the elements that support the parent system's purposes. The suprasystem is larger than the sum of the parts. Systems have boundaries, purposes, and goals. Boundaries provide borders that separate systems from other systems. These boundaries have differing degrees of permeability or openness. The purpose of the system reflects the reason a system exists, and it is related to an environmental expectation. The goal of a system is the targets set by the system, and goals guide the system to meet its purposes or expectations.

Systems have dynamic processes (Bertalanffy, 1950) (Table 2–1). A system receives input such as material and energy resources from the environment that sustains the system's steady state. If a system does not receive the necessary inputs from the environment, then the system terminates or dies. A system transforms and performs its work or role through the process of throughput. The system then exports outputs to the environment. These outputs are designed to meet the system's purpose. Feedback informs the system if targets and purposes are met. If a living system lacks adequate input and throughput, core processes fail. The system deteriorates and undergoes a process of entropy in which the system dies due to a lack of energy to perform its purpose or work. However, living systems strive for order, complexity, and growth in a process called *negentropy*.

Classic Change Theory

While assisting disabled individuals to accommodate to a change in functional ability, the rehabilitation nurse must employ planned change strategies to assist with adaptation.

Lewin (1951) identified changing as a three-step process commonly called *force-field analysis*. This theoretical framework has frequently been employed to guide specialty practice. According to Lewin, successful change includes three aspects: *unfreezing (L1)* if necessary from the present level; *moving (L2)* to the new level; and *refreezing (L3)* to the new level (Fig. 2–3). These levels are determined by a force field. When working with disabled clients and their families, the nurse must carefully assess needs. Conceptually during an assessment, the nurse begins the

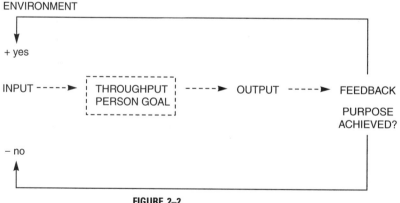

FIGURE 2–2
Key components of a system.

TABLE 2–1 ■ QUALITIES OF SYSTEMS

Input	Materials and resource energy going into system.
	Example: Family providing care. Patient education.
Throughput	Internal processes to meet system goals and purposes.
	Example: Client active in self-care.
Output	Product of system functioning.
	Example: Independence in activities of daily living.
Feedback	Output return to the system, feeding information to system about system functioning.
	Examples: Negative feedback, client having incontinent episodes. Positive feedback, client directing own care.
Steady-state homeostasis	Stabilization of transformation processes.
	Example: Client meeting goals of rehabilitation program.
Entropy	System energy decline, death, or disorganization of processes.
	Example: Client with decubitus ulcer.
Negentropy	System growth and increasing complexity.
	Example: Disabled client with gainful employment.
Equifinality	System achievement of same outcome from different points.
	Example: Employing two different exercise therapies that achieve similar results.
Specialization	System becoming more elaborate and more complex with growth and steady state.
Goal	Target set by system.
	Example: Client obtaining independence in activities of daily living.
Purpose	Reason the system exists and functions.
	Example: Individual commitments and objectives.

unfreezing process by slowing down to observe the client/family system dynamics. Restraining forces such as limited financial resources and a lack of family support may present barriers to change. Driving forces such as community/family support systems and individual resilience propel the change forward. The nurse then moves by developing strategies such as physical, educational, and supportive care interventions. Once goals are achieved, new behaviors can be maintained through the refreezing process. Goals are achieved when the new force field is relatively secure against change. However, there is an ongoing evaluation process to determine if the client/family system goals are met and maintained.

Theory of Self-Efficacy

Bandura (1977) developed a theoretical framework to guide the assessment of the individual's ability to promote health and reduce risk. The key concept in this theory is self-efficacy. According to Bandura, individuals have varied abilities to mobilize skills and resources. When faced with a stressful situation such as a new disability, some individuals can adapt by reorganizing cognitive, social, and behavioral skills as a function of their degree of self-efficacy. However, individuals who are less resilient are less able to mobilize cognitive, social, and behavioral skills. According to Bandura, these individuals have lower-degree self-efficacy. The rehabilitation nurse functions primarily in an educative supportive role to enhance the client's self-efficacy and thereby promote wellness.

Theory of Hardiness

Based on research on stressful life events, Kobasa (1979) formulated the theory of hardiness. The unitary key concept of hardiness comprises three dimensions: *commitment, challenge,* and *control.* The individual with high hardiness is committed to the truth and importance of individually defined purpose. A hardy person views threats as an opportunity for growth and change and feels a high degree of self-determination and self-control over life situations. A hardy healthy personality reduces stress and protects health. The hardy disabled person draws from a repertoire of coping skills to respond to stress. The

Unfreezing (L1) - - - - - -➤   *Moving (L2)* - - - - - - ➤   *Refreezing (L3)*

1. Data collection
2. Assessment of factors that facilitate and/or resist change

1. Planning strategies
2. Execution of interventions

1. Maintenance
2. Evaluation/renewal

FIGURE 2–3
Steps in the process of planned change.

rehabilitation nurse assists clients to develop logical executable plans and to engage in self-care.

Theory of Locus of Control

A fundamental rehabilitation goal is that the clients participate in the plan of care, have decision-making power, and direct self-care. Rehabilitation nursing interventions are grounded in these basic premises and have been influenced by the theory of locus of control. According to Rotter, Seeman, and Liverant (1962), individuals develop a generalized attitude, belief, or expectancy regarding the causal relationship between one's own behavior and the consequences of one's own behavior. There is a contingency relationship between behavior and wellness outcomes (Fig. 2–4). If the individual has a history of experiences in which the individual perceives that it is the person's own behaviors that directly influence outcomes, the person is said to have an internal locus of control. In contrast, if the individual has a history of experiences in which outcomes are perceived as the result of chance and external influencing forces, the person is said to have an external locus of control.

Health Belief Model

The health belief model was influenced by Lewinian thinking—behavior is a function of the person and the environment: $B = f(P.E)$. The model was further developed to explain health promotion and risk reduction behaviors. However, this model has been used by rehabilitation nurses as a framework to understand and employ disability prevention strategies. According to the health belief model, the individual must perceive the relative risk of the disability. This perception is influenced by modifying factors that are a function of (1) demographic factors such as age and gender, (2) social/psychological variables such as cultural beliefs, and (3) knowledge about a disability, risk reduction, and relative risk (Becker, 1974). The individual's perception is also influenced by cues to action such as safety education and health promotion/risk reduction publications and public media. The likelihood that an individual will take action to engage in rehabilitation restorative interventions is a function of a perceived threat of injury. The individual must also appreciate the relative benefits of engaging in restorative and healthy behaviors. Barriers such as basic resources to purchase protective gear to prevent injury can affect the likelihood of action.

CONCEPTUAL THEORIES AND MODELS IN NURSING

Dorothea Orems's Self-Care Model

Dorothea Orem developed the self-care model initially while a nurse educator at Catholic University in the 1950s (Fawcett, 1995). This model has had a major influence on rehabilitation nursing. The basic ideas are very aligned to fundamental rehabilitation principles and practices. The key concept of the model is self-care. *Self-care* is defined by Orem (1991) as the practice of activities that individuals initiate and perform on their own behalf in maintaining life, health, and well-being. The basic assumption of this model is that human beings have the capacity to take actions to meet their own self-care requirements. According to the model, clients can benefit from nursing care when their universal self-care requirements, developmental self-care requisites, health deviation self-care requisites, and health limitations produce self-care deficits (needs) that exceed their self-care agency (ability). The person is viewed as an embodied agent and organism who is capable of engaging in deliberate action. The environment is depicted as being external to the person. Orem defines *health* as the state of soundness and wholeness of human structures and of bodily and human functioning. She defines *nursing* as human service, helping service, and a creative effort of one human being to help another being.

The nurse functions in a wholly compensatory, partly compensatory, and/or supportive-educative nursing agency system. As a wholly compensatory system, the rehabilitation nurse provides total physical care and advocates for a client. When clients are inca-

Contingency Relationship

Behavior ——————————— Outcome

PERCEPTION

Internal LOC	Individual behavior influences outcomes
External LOC	External forces influence outcomes

FIGURE 2–4
Theory of locus of control (LOC).

pable of meeting their own self-care needs or have limited function, the nurse functions as a partially compensatory system to meet needs that the clients cannot meet on their own behalf. The educative-supportive role is the primary role of the rehabilitation nurse. In the educative-supportive role, the nurse assists the client to perform as a self-care agency by providing care for self or directing others in care delivery.

Myra Levine's Conservation Model

Myra E. Levine presented the early formulations of her model in 1966 in an article entitled "Adaptation and Assessment." Levine defines *adaptation* as the process by which individuals maintain their wholeness or integrity (Fawcett, 1995). She defines *health* as successful adaptation to change (Levine, 1991). The key concepts of the model are the principles of energy, structural integrity, personal integrity, and social integrity conservation (Fawcett, 1995). The client is viewed as being a unified whole in constant interaction with the environment. The goal of the client is to strive to maintain integrity. The goal of nursing in general and rehabilitation nursing in particular is to promote wellness. The principles of conservation serve as a framework to guide nursing interventions. Rehabilitation nursing has traditionally focused on the proper disbursement and conservation of energy. Intervention strategies are developed to support healing and functional recovery.

Sister Callista Roy's Adaptation Model

Sister Callista Roy introduced the basic assumptions and underpinnings of her conceptual model in 1970 in an article entitled "Adaptation: A Conceptual Framework for Nursing" (Fawcett, 1995). Since that time, she has further developed the ideas in the model, and they have had tremendous utility for education, research, and nursing practice. Adaptation to changing needs and changing environmental stimuli is a key concept in Roy's model (Riehl & Roy, 1980). The focus of nursing is the client, who is in constant interaction with the environment. Health is achieved when the client adapts and interacts effectively with the environment. Nursing works to maintain integrity and correct adaptive problems in four modes—basic physiological needs, self-concept, role mastery, and interdependence. Roy's model is consistent with re-

habilitation principles. The assumptions of the model clearly promote mutual respect between the client and the nurse as well as the active participation of the client in care.

Imogene King's Open System Model

Imogene King developed her model of nursing in the early 1960s, when nursing was striving to achieve acceptance as a science. King (1981) views the nursing process as functioning within a social system. Human beings are viewed as social, sentient, rational, reacting, perceiving, controlling, purposeful, action-oriented, and time-oriented beings. According to King, nursing is concerned with human beings and dynamic interacting systems—an individual personal system, a group interpersonal system, and society as the social system. King's ideas are consistent with rehabilitation nursing principles. As individuals grow and develop they experience change in structure and function of their bodies over time that influence their perception of self to start with (King, 1981).

Martha Rogers's Theory of Unitary Man

Martha Rogers (Fig. 2–5) firmly believed that there has to be a body of knowledge that is specific to and unique to nursing (Fawcett, 1995). Out of this belief and under the influ-

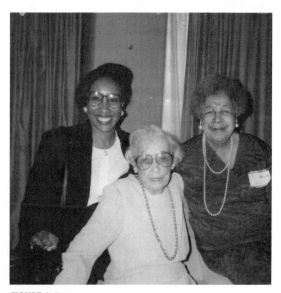

FIGURE 2–5
Dr. Drayton Hargrove (left), Dr. Martha Rogers (center), and Dr. Mary Elizabeth Carnegie (right).

ence of the social science theories, systems thinking, and homeodynamics, Rogers developed her theory. Rogers (1970) formulated her initial ideas in her book entitled *An Introduction to the Theoretical Basis of Nursing*. Rogers viewed the human as a three-dimensional negentropic energy field and unified whole that is greater than the sum of its parts. Unitary man is in constant interaction and exchanging energy with the environment. Unitary man develops through (1) reciprocity between the human field and the environment, (2) synchrony of the human field at specified points and time, (3) helicy due to continuous innovative change, and (4) resonancy of changing wave patterns between the human field and the environment (Rogers, 1980). Nursing care promotes symphonic interaction between human fields and the environment. Rogers's theoretical formulations emphasize the interaction of unitary man and provide a framework for rehabilitation nursing to promote growth, order, and change after a client sustains a disability.

Betty Neuman's Systems Model

Betty Neuman's model, developed in 1972, is a comprehensive, holistic view of all clients including individuals, groups, communities, and society. Although a nursing model, it is appropriate for other health professionals, including physical therapists. The model is based on open systems thinking (Fawcett, 1995). Neuman (Fig. 2–6) views the person as a unique, holistic system with the major components of stressors and reaction to stressors. When the actual or potential stressors are identified, nursing interventions are directed at reducing the stress on the system at three levels: primary prevention (health promotion), secondary prevention (reducing symptoms), or tertiary prevention (reconstitution and rehabilitation). Intervention can be introduced at any point on the health continuum. Nursing goals are directed at strengthening lines of resistance and defense that surround the basic core structure of the client. The client is seen as a series of concentric rings with lines of resistance at the center (representing internal factors defending against stressors), normal lines of defense (normal wellness or steady state), and a flexible line of defense (acting as a buffer). The process of nursing is concerned with strengthening these lines of resistance and defense. Neuman's model emphasizes nursing assessment of physiological, psychological, socio-

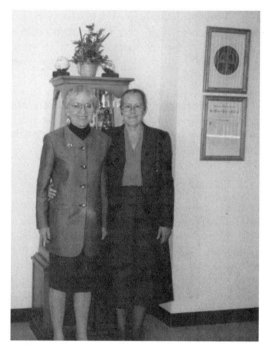

FIGURE 2–6
Dr. Jill B. Derstine (left) and Dr. Betty Neuman (right).

cultural, developmental, and spiritual variables of each client as interventions are implemented.

The Neuman system model is particularly well suited to rehabilitation nursing because of the emphasis on maximizing potential and prevention (Derstine, 1992, p. 1).

Psychosocial Rehabilitation Theories

Beatrice Wright (1983) extensively studied disabled persons, looking at values and value-laden behavior related to disability. Rehabilitation nurses, families, and social contacts of disabled persons can benefit from this classic work. Wright's concept of spread, first introduced by Tamara Dembo in 1956, refers to "the power of a single characteristic to evoke inferences about a single person" (Wright, 1983, p. 32). The classic example of this is the situation in which one set of subjects was asked to identify characteristics about a picture of a man in a wheelchair and the other set of subjects was shown the same picture with the wheelchair blocked out. It was felt that the person in the wheelchair was more conscientious, felt inferior, was a better friend, was more religious, liked parties less, and was more unhappy than the one with the wheelchair blocked out. In spread, the inference can be positive or negative; however, this concept is often recognized when persons with a disabling condition are treated as if they possess other negative attributes. The rehabilitation nurse who incorporates this concept into practice augments the assessment process (Derstine, 1992, p. 4).

Wright's work provides an excellent foundation for the rehabilitation practitioner of today. The co-management theory proposed that the client and practitioner actively participate in goal setting, treatment, and evaluation of care, resulting in increased motivation for the client. This concept is still appropriate in the managed care–dominated health system of the present.

Constantia Safilio Rothschild (1970), in an earlier classic publication, found that there is a relationship between self-concept, values, and emotions attached to a disability. This author examined disability at three analytical levels: personality, social system, and culture. She examined how different types of disabilities affect the disabled person's self-concept, the interpersonal relations between disabled persons and others, the relationship of the social system of the disabled with other social systems, and the cultural and psychological basis of discrimination and prejudice. Her discussion on returning to work and the fate of rehabilitated persons after they leave the rehabilitation facility provides valuable insight into some of the problems seen with rehabilitation clients today.

SUMMARY

Rehabilitation nursing practice has been influenced by a broad range of theories and models. These abstractions, assumptions, constructs, propositions, and interrelationships guide practice. Models and theories organize the psychosocial, cultural, emotional, spiritual, and physical variables that are influenced by disability. The rehabilitation nurse employs theories and models to understand the impact of a disability on the person and to guide nursing care, client education, and the validation of knowledge.

REFERENCES

Bandura, A. (1977). *Social learning theory.* Englewood Cliffs, NJ: Prentice-Hall.

Becker, M. H. (1974). *The health belief model and personal health behavior.* Thore, NJ: Charles B. Slack.

Bertalanffy, L. von (1950). The theory of open systems in physics and biology. *Science, 111,* 23–28.

Burns, N., & Grove, S. K. (1995). *Understanding nursing research.* Philadelphia: W. B. Saunders.

Cartwright, D. (1951). *Field theory in social science.* London: Dorsey Press.

Derstine, J. (1992). Rehabilitation: Umbrella for healthcare. *Holistic Nursing Practice, 6*(2).

Fawcett, J. (1995). *Analysis and evaluation of conceptual models of nursing.* Philadelphia: F. A. Davis.

King, I. M. (1981). *A theory for nursing: Concepts, process, and systems.* New York: Wiley.

Kobasa, S. C. (1979). Stressful life events, personality and health: An inquiry into hardiness. *Journal of Personality and Social Psychology, 37,* 1–11.

Levine, M. E. (1991). The conservation principles: A model for health. In K. M. Schaefer & J. P. Pond (Eds.), *Levine's conservation model: A framework for nursing practice* (pp. 1–11). Philadelphia: F. A. Davis.

Lewin, K. (1951). Behavior and development as a function of the total situation (1946). In D. Cartwright (Ed.), *Field theory in social science* (pp. 238–303). London: Dorsey Press.

Neuman, B. (1989). *The Neuman systems model* (2nd ed.). Norwalk, CT: Appleton & Lange.

Orem, D. E. (1991). *Nursing: Concepts of practice* (2nd ed.). New York: McGraw-Hill.

Riehl, J. P., & Roy, C. (1980). Conceptual models in nursing practice (2nd ed.). New York: Appleton-Century-Crofts.

Rogers, M. E. (1970). *An introduction to theoretical basis of nursing.* Philadelphia, F. A. Davis.

Rogers, M. E. (1980). *Science of unitary man. Tape 1, Unitary man and his world: A paradigm for nursing.* New York: Media for Nursing.

Rothschild, C. S. (1970). The society and social psychology of disability. Washington, DC: University Press of America.

Rotter, J. E., Seeman, M., & Liverant, S. (1962). Internal vs. external locus of control reinforcement: A major variable in behavior study. In N. F. Washburne (Ed.), *Decisions, values and groups.* New York: Macmillan.

Wright, B. (1983). Physical disability: A psychosocial approach (2nd ed). New York: Harper & Row.

CHAPTER 3

Case Management: A Client-Focused Service

Judith A. Hines

Case management can be described as a complex set of activities that are designed to coordinate client care services and manage the resources that are pertinent to the optimal outcome of an individual's health care (Merrill, 1985). Various measurement tools are available to assist the case manager in monitoring client outcomes. Providers of case management service include, but are not limited to, acute care and rehabilitation hospitals, corporations, public and private insurance companies, managed care organizations, independent case management companies, and government-sponsored programs.

In recent years, the delivery of our health care system has changed and has new dimensions. The major catalyst is cost containment, which has resulted in substantial changes in physicians' practices, nursing practices, institutional reimbursement, and clients' access to services. In client care services, the paradigm has shifted from the hospital to the community. Managed care, which can be defined as a cost-containment process, is creating this shift in services. Therefore, there is a need to consider a new approach to the continuum of care services. For the purpose of this chapter, *continuum of care service* is defined as prevention, wellness, acute care, rehabilitation, subacute long-term care, and hospice care (Fig. 3–1).

Zander (1988) states that "managed care and case management are clinical systems for the strategic management of clients through a continuum of care which is driven by cost, quality and outcomes." As managed care continues to emerge as the dominant structure in health care, so will the structure and the process of nursing case management respond with the evolution of new case management models. New programs will evolve to balance the delivery and cost of care to achieve desired outcomes. Today, rehabilitation nurse case management services provide the coordination of care for high-risk clients and those

with chronic illnesses. Now more than ever, management means providing a supportive link between hospitalization and community care within an integrated system of care (American Nurses Association, 1988).

The Case Management Society of America has defined case management as "a collaborative process which assesses, plans, implements, coordinates, monitors and evaluates optimum services to meet an individual's health needs through communication and available resources to promote quality cost effective outcomes."

Smith, Danforth, and Owens (1994) state that case management merges all plans into a collaborative blueprint based on mutual goals from a multidisciplinary team that is client focused. The blueprints or measurement tools that are essential to guide the clinical management of all client care services are called *clinical practice guidelines*. Tools can take the form of

- Protocols
- Algorithms
- Critical pathways
- Care maps
- Variance analysis
- Risk assessment
- Outcome measures

They are intended to identify the important aspects of a client's care for a particular diagnosis. Definitions of these tools as published by the Institute of Medicine are as follows:

- Critical pathways are tools used to plan, deliver, monitor, document, and concurrently review the care provided by multiple disciplines. Many of these tools are designed in calendar format with milestones and interventions that are considered the norms and/or standards for industry (Fig. 3–2)
- Variance analysis is the deviation of actual

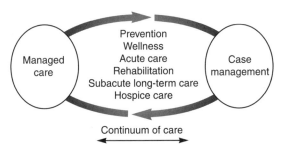

FIGURE 3–1
Continuum of care.

outcomes from a predetermined norm, standard rate, goal, threshold, or expected outcome.

- Protocols/algorithms are defined as practice guidelines that bring the best medical evidence or course of treatment defined by expert opinion and on occasion scientific research. All or a portion of the client's care may be managed according to a protocol/algorithm (Table 3–1).
- Risk assessment means identifying and managing disease risk before it turns into illness.
- Outcome measures/tools are value mea-

sures that may include disease-free years, functional life span extenuation, and improved physiological and psychosocial functioning (Strassner, 1996).

Overall, the nurse case manager and physician should co-lead to manage and monitor a client's disease process over time with outcomes or variances documented.

In summary, these tools can provide

- A structure for case management models through a continuum of care
- A system that integrates the input of all health care disciplines
- Improvement of the use of resources
- Enhancement of the quality of patient care
- A benchmark for cost-effective patient-focused health care

HISTORICAL PERSPECTIVE

A review of literature on the history of case management services suggests that they started at the turn of the 20th century, when the services were used to manage public health programs. The concept of case management services emerged after World War II.

Text continued on page 26

TABLE 3–1 ■ ORAL ANTICOAGULANT (WARFARIN) PROTOCOL OF THE MEMORIAL HOSPITAL AT EASTON, MD., INC., CLINICAL PHARMACY SERVICES

Indications

In any medical condition in which anticoagulant therapy is medically indicated and supported by literature, including, but not limited to

Atrial fibrillation
Cardiac ventricular thrombus
Maintenance of patency of native vessels following thrombolytics
Maintenance of patency of native/prosthetic revascularization
Prophylactic therapy following orthopedic joint replacement
Prosthetic mechanical cardiac valves
Pulmonary embolism
Selected cardiomyopathies
Thrombotic arterial events
Thrombotic cerebral vascular events
Transient ischemic attacks
Venous thrombosis

Initiation

The protocol will be initiated only upon the receipt of an order originating from a physician for warfarin/oral anticoagulation.

Procedure

1. The chart and/or medical record will be reviewed and various patient parameters, along with the treatment diagnosis, will be obtained. Specific parameters to be obtained include the following:

a) Patient history, including previous anticoagulation, and the presence of potential risk factors, which are to include
  Recent surgery
  Age >65 yr
  Presence of trauma
  Intramuscular injections
  Peptic ulcer disease
  Malignancy
  Severe hypertension (diastolic pressures >100)
  Potential bleeding sites (lumbar puncture, biopsy site, intra-arterial puncture)
b) History of allergy
c) Vital signs, height, weight, and age
d) Complete blood count and platelet count
e) Serum electrolytes and BUN
f) Bilirubin, alkaline phosphatase, LDH, SGOT, SGPT, and/or 12/60
g) Concurrent disease states
h) Concurrent pharmacotherapy
i) Potential drug interaction
j) Baseline anticoagulation parameters (prothrombin time, INR, aPTT)

2. If there are any concerns with the use of warfarin, the primary physician will be contacted before the protocol is initiated.

Table continued on following page

TABLE 3–1 ■ ORAL ANTICOAGULANT (WARFARIN) PROTOCOL OF THE MEMORIAL HOSPITAL AT EASTON, MD., INC., CLINICAL PHARMACY SERVICES *Continued*

3. If no laboratory data are available and none have been ordered, the pharmacist may order a battery of tests appropriate for the assessment of renal and hepatic function, coagulation status, and a complete blood count for baseline evaluation and toxicity monitoring.

4. Based upon the chart review, the patient assessment, and the clinical conditions present, the dose of warfarin will be ordered dependent upon the clinical condition being treated, the risk factors present, and the status of the patient. In all cases, the regimen selected is to be appropriate for the clinical indication present and will be prescribed in an attempt to maintain an INR in the range recommended for the condition under therapy.

5. The pharmacist may repeat laboratory tests appropriate for the determination of the patient response, to include, as necessary prothrombin times/INR, hepatic and renal function, and serum levels of concurrent medications (when available) known to be affected by warfarin therapy in situations in which literature support exists, suggesting (1) there may be an increased risk of toxicity and/or (2) response is known to be highly variable and reliance on expected outcome data may be invalid.

6. The prothrombin time/INR will be ordered on a daily basis until there is a suggestion of stability, and then at intervals deemed appropriate for monitoring therapy.

7. The therapeutic range for the prothrombin time/INR will be determined by current literature recommendations. In general, the INR will be maintained between 2 and 3 for all indications, except in cases in which there are mechanical cardiac valves, or evidence suggestive of recurrent emboli from a cardiac source. Other possible exceptions are in orthopedic procedures where the agent is being given prophylactically and in selected high-risk patients, and these conditions will be treated on an individualized basis.

8. Patient education will be instituted in all cases in which the patient is to be discharged from the hospital on warfarin. This education will be in conjunction with Nursing Services efforts and will utilize both oral and written techniques.

9. The protocol must be discontinued by a physician's order. In cases in which continued therapy is determined to be potentially detrimental to the patient outcome secondary to either suspected or proven drug toxicity, the pharmacist may order therapy suspended until the physician can be contacted and a decision as to the course of action can be made.

10. A flow sheet will be filled out and filed in the pharmacy protocol book, where daily progress notes, adverse reactions, and patient outcome will be recorded by the Clinical Pharmacy Services, based on daily observation and evaluation of the response to therapy. If indicated, assessment of the evaluation process and recommendations concerning therapy will be left in the progress note section of the patient's medical record.

Dosage

1. After evaluation of the patient parameters, risk factors present, and clinical condition being treated, select an appropriate dosage.

   Usual dosage range: 2.5 to 7.5 mg

2. If there is no history of warfarin therapy immediately preceding (defined as therapy within 7 days) and the ordering of the protocol and baseline coagulation parameters are known, the selected regimen is to be ordered daily for two (2) days and a prothrombin time/INR is to be ordered the morning of the third day.

3. If there is no history obtainable, if there is a positive history of prothrombin time prior therapy, or if no baseline values are available, the selected regimen can still be ordered, but either an INR should be obtained before the initiation of therapy, or there should be an assessment of the prothrombin time/INR within twenty-four (24) hours of the start of the protocol.

4. Dosage selection after the return of the initial prothrombin time remains empirical due to the multiplicity of factors known to affect the response; however, the following may be used as a guide (providing at least two [2] doses of warfarin have been given):

<13 sec	5 to 10 mg
≥13 ≤14.5 sec	2.5 to 7.5 mg
≥14.6 ≤16 sec	1.0 to 4 mg
>16.1 sec	Omit dose to 2 mg

   Note that recent literature suggests that elderly patients will have an INR between 2 and 3 on an average dose of 4 to 5 mg warfarin daily.

5. Prothrombin times/INR should be obtained on a daily basis until there is some suggestion of a plateau in the response (usually within 5 to 7 days, providing no complicating factors are present). After apparent stabilization, the prothrombin time/INR should be ordered on an as-needed basis, with gradual increases in the time span between evaluations if there is continued stability in the result.

6. Heparin–Warfarin Conversion

   It has been suggested that warfarin therapy (when indicated) be initiated as soon as feasible during heparin therapy, providing a 72- to 120-hour overlap in anticoagulation therapy, allowing for some estimation of warfarin requirements while attaining an INR in the range recommended. Early administration of warfarin should decrease the duration of heparin therapy, thereby reducing potential adverse effects while also potentially reducing the length of hospitalization.

   It is known that heparin will have a modest effect on the prothrombin time, and this effect increases as the intensity of anticoagulation is increased. The converse is also true, with the aPTT being affected once the prothrombin time nears an INR of 1.5 to 2.

   The procedure for dosing remains the same as noted in 1–5 above.

Abbreviations: aPTT, activated partial thromboplastin time; BUN, blood urea nitrogen; INR, International Normalized Ratio; LbH, lactate dehydrogenase; SGOT, serum glutamic-oxaloacetic transaminase (aspartate transaminase); SGPT, serum glutamic-pyruvic transaminase (alanine transaminase); 12/60, complete blood count and chemistry profile.
Courtesy of Memorial Hospital at Easton, MD, Inc.

THE MEMORIAL HOSPITAL AT EASTON, MD., INC.
TOTAL JOINT REPLACEMENT (TJR) CRITICAL PATHWAY

DRG: TJR 209
Repair Fx. Hip 210, 211

Adm. Date: _____
LOS: 5 days

Patient Problem	Preop.	DOS	Postop. Day 1	Postop. Day 2	Postop. Day 3	Postop. Day 4	Postdischarge
				Goals			
1. Pain	Assess understanding of pain and use of PCA. Assess present pain control measures.	In RR pain control is sufficient for respiratory care. Pt states pain is adequately controlled via PCA protocol.	Pt has adequate control of pain with PCA.	Pt experiences adequate pain control with PO meds. ⟶			
2. Loss of function, mobility, and/or strength	Assess: 1. Strength and ROM of upper and lower extremities. 2. Gait 3. Preop. OT evaluation	Pt's joints are supported through proper positioning. Wt. bearing as ordered.	Pt participates in exercise program by being OOB × 2, completing isometrics × 4 and PROM to 60° flexion. Walk >5' with assist.	Pt demonstrates ability to walk/crutch walk with assist, assisted knee flexion and extension. PROM to 70° flexion. Pt can verbalize proper positioning techniques to protect operated joints. PROM to 80°.	Pt demonstrates ability to walk >40' with assistance and participates in OT evaluation and instructions in joint protection principles. Pt participates in elevation activities. Pt displays independent transfers and bed mobility.	Pt demonstrates ability to walk >60' on level/elevated surface. Pt demonstrates independence in ADL using alternative methods. PROM 0–90°.	Pt continues to maintain independence in ADLs. ⟶
3. Postoperative home care placement needs	Evaluate present • Living arrangements • Support services • Family ability			Pt participates in home equipment need evaluation.	Pt supports plan for outpatient or home PT.	Pt and family agree to home equipment orders.	Necessary home equipment in use.
4. Knowledge deficit of postop. care	Pt can state postop. expectations for PT PCA LOS Resp. care Pt can describe disease process and its effect on hip/knee and the purpose of TJR in relation to physical status.	Pt can identify PCA as means of pain control. Patient demonstrates proper positioning (towel roll under ankle), leg exercises of nonaffected limb, and C + DB in appropriate manner.	Pt can demonstrate safe joint protection principles for ADL and exercise. Pt demonstrates home exercise program.	Pt demonstrates proper incisional care.	Pt verbalizes need for antibiotic prophylaxis Pt identifies reasons to call MD after discharge	⟶ ⟶ ⟶	

Illustration continued on following page

THE MEMORIAL HOSPITAL AT EASTON, MD., INC.
TOTAL JOINT REPLACEMENT (TJR) CRITICAL PATHWAY *Continued*

DRG: TJR 209
Repair Fx. Hip 210, 211

Adm. Date: _____
LOS: 5 days

Patient Problem	Preop.	DOS	Postop. Day 1	Postop. Day 2	Postop. Day 3	Postop. Day 4	Postdischarge
				Goals			
5. Possible postop. medical complications A. Respiratory		Pt displays adequate resp. excursion postop. Pt participates in activated pulmonary hygiene protocol to reduce postop. pulmonary complications.	Pt actively participates in pulmonary hygiene protocol.	Pt exhibits clearing BS.	Pt demonstrates clear BS, temp. 39.5° × 24 hr and will C + DB unassisted.		+
B. Interruption of normal elimination		Maintain ortho. bladder protocol.		Pt regains usual bowel and bladder functioning. ————→			
C. Deep vein thrombosis		Warfarin (Coumadin) protocol per Pharm D. ————→	Pt participates in measures to prevent DVT, i.e., leg exercises and mobilization plan. ————→				
				Plan			
Consults	Old records to SDS. Social work. PT-TKR/THR protocol. Medical consult.	Respiratory therapy for pulmonary hygiene protocol. Medical consult. Activate PT/OT TKR/THR protocol. Pharm D. for warfarin protocol.	OT TKR/THR protocol.				

Tests	Chest x-ray >60 yr. EKG >40 yr. CBC, 6/60, UA. T&C—2 units PRBCs. Coagulation profile. Autologous blood donation.	X-ray hip/knee in PACU.	H&H 8 AM. Notify MD if HCT ≤28. $\longrightarrow$	Evaluate urine culture results. Notify MD if positive.
Assessment	Ext. pulses. Resp. assess. CV. NMS.	Baseline VS and postop. q1h × 4. Pulses in extremity. Respiratory assessment q4h. Neuro./circ. assessment q4h. I&O related to blood loss and fluid replacement. Record output and replace as per wound drainage and reinfusion system protocol.	VS q4h—notify MD if temp. >39.5°C. Evaluate PO intake to adjust IV fluids. D/C I&O when IV fluids D/C'd.	Assess wound. VS bid unless febrile, then temp. q4h WA. $\longrightarrow$ Assess wound q day. $\longrightarrow$ Neuro. and circ. assessment q shift.
	Initiate FIM evaluation.	FIM evaluation complete.	FIM reevaluation.	Follow-up FIM evaluation by phone.
Activity	PT-TKR/THR protocol. No crossed ankle. Towel roll under ankle. Ankle pumps. Pillow between knees. Bed rest, up to commode prn.	Institute PT. TKR/THR protocol bid. CPM 0–60° flexion, rate 1–2. 8°/day (TKR). Bedside commode. Transfer with walker. Ambulation × 2 with assist → Assisted straight leg raises. CPM 0–70° flexion (TKR). Initiation OT TKR/THR protocol.	Bed mobility shower. Car transfer. Curb and stair training. CPM 0– 90° flexion (TKR).	Independent bed mobility transfer and ambulate level and unlevel surface. Active straight leg raises.

Illustration continued on following page

THE MEMORIAL HOSPITAL AT EASTON, MD., INC.
TOTAL JOINT REPLACEMENT (TJR) CRITICAL PATHWAY *Continued*

DRG: TJR 209
Repair Fx. Hip 210, 211

Adm. Date: _____
LOS: 5 days

Patient Problem	Preop.	DOS	Postop. Day 1	Postop. Day 2	Postop. Day 3	Postop. Day 4	Postdischarge
Treatments	Shave prep. male patients. Preop. IV fluids started per anesthesia protocol. Insert Foley preop. Obtain urine culture when cath. is inserted.	Postop. IV orders. C + DB q 2–4h. Incentive spirometry × 72°. Reinfuse 1 unit autologous blood in RR and 1 unit autologous blood in evening unless autoinfusion device is being used according to procedure.	Foley removed if patient is active. Wound drainage system removed if less than 50 mL drainage in 8h.	Dressing removed. Opsite on incision. Change opsite prn.	D/C incentive spirometry.		
Medications	D/C NSAIDS 10 days before scheduled OR.	Am meds. per preop. protocol. Antibiotics intraop. Postop med. orders as per order sheet.	D/C IV fluids if PO intake is adequate. KVO IV for PCA.	Initiate ortho bowel routine. D/C PCA. D/C IV line. PO pain medication.			
Nutrition	NPO after MN	Preop: If surgery after 12 noon, may have cl. liq. breakfast	Postop. high-fiber diet as tol.				
Discharge planning	Social work evaluation. Provide patient with area resource material.	Notify social work	Evaluation of home equipment needs. Home equipment prescription written.	Discharge outpatient PT orders 3 ×/wk for 2 wk.	Review home care follow-up prescribed on warfarin protocol.	Discharge/transfer PT review of home instructions PT discharge status report to accompany pt.	

					Follow-up phone call with FIM evaluation.
Teaching	Participation in preop. joint replacement classes.	Routine postop teaching to include PCA, leg exercise of nonaffected side, C+DB, and positioning. Postop PT/protocol. Institute joint protection and bed positioning teaching.	PT teaching record criteria 1–9. Daily assessment of patient learning specific to teaching record criteria.	PT instructs Pt in home exercise program. View warfarin protocol video.	PT teaching records # 10, 11, 12. Home care instructions. Pharmacy med. instruction.
Psychosocial		Significant other identified, advance directives reviewed. Family teaching and support about periop. period.	Encourage Pt toward self-care activities.	Encourage Pt and family to discuss discharge plans.	Information given regarding postop joint replacement support group. Review joint replacement support group information.

INITIALS	SIGNATURE/TITLE	DATE	TIME	INITIALS	SIGNATURE/TITLE	DATE	TIME

FORM #141860 (12/95)   PHYSICIAN SIGNATURE: _____

FIGURE 3–2

The Memorial Hospital at Easton, MD, Inc., Total Joint Replacement (TJR) Critical Pathway. DRG, diagnosis-related group; TJR, total joint replacement; fx, fractured; adm, admitted; LOS, length of stay; preop., preoperative; DOS, day of surgery; postop., postoperative; PCA, patient-controlled analgesia; RR, recovery room; Pt, patient; PO, oral; meds., medications; ROM, range of motion; OT, occupational therapy; wt, weight; OOB, out of bed; PROM, passive range of motion; ADL, activity of daily living; PT, physical therapy; resp., respiratory; C+DB, cough and deep breath; MD, physician; BS, breath sounds; temp., temperature; Pharm D., doctorate of pharmacy; DVT, deep vein thrombosis; SDS, same-day surgery; ortho, orthopedic; TKR, total knee replacement; THR, total hip replacement; EKG, electrocardiogram; CBC, complete blood count; UA, urinalysis; T&C, type and cross-match; PRBC, packed red blood cells; PACU, postanesthetic care unit; H&H, hematocrit and hemoglobin; HcT, hematocrit; ext, extremity; resp. assess., respiratory assessment; CV, cardiovascular; N-M-S, neurological motor sensory; FIM, functional independence measure; VS, vital signs; neuro, neurological; circ., circulatory; I&O, intake and output, IV, intravenous; D/C, discontinue; WA, when awake; CPM, continuous passive motion; prep., skin preparation; cath., catheter; OpSite, transparent dressing; NSAID, nonsteroidal anti-inflammatory drug; OR, operating room; AM, morning; med., medication; introp, interoperatively; KVO, keep vein open; NPO, nothing by mouth; MN, midnight; cl. liq, clear liquid; tol, tolerated; periop, perioperative. (Courtesy of Memorial Hospital at Easton, MD, Inc.)

The purpose was to manage the mental health services by coordinating the psychiatric care of veterans, who would ultimately connect with a social worker and reenter community settings.

The expanded role of the professional nurse as a case manager evolved in the 1960s with the insurance nurse. In the following decade, private rehabilitation firms began to surface in which entrepreneurial rehabilitation nurse case managers marketed their skills in clinical liability issues as related to providing a specific standard of care to a patient based upon the diagnoses; financial issues; business management; short- and long-term disability; automobile liability; accident and health insurance; workers' compensation; and catastrophic cases.

During the 1960s, the growth of the nation's health care industry surged because of the government's role in Medicare and Medicaid programs. The government became the single largest payer for health care when it shaped these two programs. A prospective payment system led the way to health maintenance organizations and capitation systems. It was at this time that case management models were introduced within the acute care delivery system because of the advent of a prospective payment system and diagnosis-related groups. The focus of the case manager was on appropriate admission, appropriate diagnosis, and aggressive discharge planning.

Rehabilitation case management was introduced in the 1980s along with case management in oncology and psychiatric and mental health services. The traditional rehabilitation case management model gradually evolved into a comprehensive service that included an interdisciplinary team. This model emphasized a client's development of skills and identified the support that a disabled client would need to become an integral part of society (McBride, 1992).

Parallel with the role of the rehabilitation case manager, the role of both the internal and the external case managers became strong. The functions of these case managers can traditionally be described as to assess the client's needs, develop a service plan, monitor the services, and evaluate the client's progress. Internal case managers for hospitals, government agencies, insurance carriers, self-insurers, and health care programs for employees developed their own case management staff. They developed detailed clinical and financial monitoring systems so that the case manager could compare a client's progress with established expectations for clinical outcomes and resource utilization.

External case managers specific for third-party payers are independent managers or consultants. This group of case managers provides active case management on behalf of a reimbursement agency. These services are coordinated in a cost-efficient manner; the manager is described by Knollmueller (1984) as a "broker of services." Insurance carriers have always had a vested interest in decreasing liability and the costs of health care for their policy holders. It is the external case manager's challenge to maximize services within the limit of the insurance policy and reimbursement constraints. Traditionally, the roles and responsibilities of all case managers were to wear several hats, including those of discharge planner and utilization review. The goal was to facilitate all the aspects of a client's stay, including testing, teaching, discharge planning, and communicating with the appropriate outside agency. There is a prediction that over the next 5 years every nurse will need to have a working knowledge of case management.

ROLES OF REHABILITATION CASE MANAGERS

Case management models have been used in rehabilitation settings in various forms based on the rehabilitation facilities' structure and operation. The concept of case management for rehabilitation settings is consistent in that the model targets its service toward the population that is identified as high risk and high cost and includes those clients whose complex medical needs require more comprehensive health care services and multiple services and procedures. These clients can generate the highest costs to meet their identified needs.

The goal of the rehabilitation nurse case manager is to plan for the coordination of care from admission through discharge and to promote self-care and enhance the quality of life to include physical, cognitive, psychological, and functional well-being. The goals are client focused and are achieved through the appropriate selection and utilization of services in the most cost-effective manner.

The rehabilitation nursing professional has taken the lead in its case management model by acting as the gatekeeper who advocates for a client's personalized health care needs over a continuum of service. Case management models for both acute and subacute rehabilitation settings have created a new nurse practitioner who initiates the precertification screening before the appropriate level of services can be offered to clinically manage, educate, and provide discharge planning and utilization management skills to a caseload of clients.

Today's case manager must be well organized and straightforward, work well in a team, and facilitate communication and collaboration while advocating for what is clinically best for the clients and the support system.

HEALTH CARE ORGANIZATION OF THE 1990s

Health care systems have changed their way of conducting business and are primarily driven by health maintenance organizations, preferred provider organizations, and other managed care providers. The patient population in acute care has changed. Acute care hospitals are experiencing an increase in admissions in an aging population with chronic illnesses and in a population with an increase in substance abuse and problems such as acquired immunodeficiency syndrome; this has translated into multiple medical diagnoses and multisystem failure. There are supporting data that chronic care is the largest and fastest-growing segment of health care (Bringewatt, 1995).

The health care industry is in the midst of profound change, much of which is due to an uneven balance in the delivery of care and the cost of care. There is a paradigm shift from competitive fees for service to an integration of capitation.

The old paradigm focuses on inpatient care, and the hospital is the "hub"; the paradigm involves managing costs, a reduced length of hospital stay, physician entrepreneurs, profit centers, solo physician practices, and superspecialists to treat the sick. The new paradigm involves ambulatory services, regionalized tertiary services, physician business partners, group practices, primary care, and the promotion of health and wellness (Cochrane, 1995).

According to the Integrated Health Care Report (Cochrane, 1995), within the new paradigm, payers are asking all providers for cost savings and value in the following forms:

- A shift to a lower-cost setting
- A reduced length of the hospital stay
- High-tech capabilities in a lower-cost setting

- Effective patient management
- Outcomes that are clinically sound and cost-effective
- Patient satisfaction
- Responsiveness to treatment based upon diagnosis
- Ongoing communication

The new paradigm shift has not yet begun to implement an aggressive system for the utilization of resources for the identification and management of the rehabilitation client (high-risk population). A model for rehabilitation case management can now more than ever be properly defined as a systematic approach to an identified suitable patient population with the opportunity to provide coordinated care and to assess and choose treatment options.

EVOLUTION OF THE NEW ROLE OF CASE MANAGEMENT

Models are moving from event, episodic, or illness models that incorporate the business of nursing and health care with the delivery of quality patient care to the continuum of care model. A specific case management model definition depends on the discipline, the employer, and the setting in which case management is being implemented. However, the primary goal of most models focuses on prevention, primary care, and disease management (Murer, 1996). From a business standpoint, case management is currently provided to only a small percentage of the population that is insured, such as those with chronic illnesses.

A new model on the horizon that will target this population is called *disease state management*. In this model there are methods to identify the at-risk population, and early case management is applied to this population. The model provides case management over the continuum of care from prevention to management of the chronic disease and its comorbidities (Johnson, 1996). The model also includes a focus on the client and consumer as a self-advocate, one who makes informed choices that result in improved compliance. In order for self-advocacy to occur, the consumer's health care must include education regarding prevention and wellness strategies. Ideally, the clients are educated throughout the process to manage their wellness and become self-advocates (Paone, 1995; Smith, 1995). Disease state management models provide an integrated approach to managing.

Health and chronic disease across the continuum, including management in the community as long as the community services impact positively on the cost and outcomes.

The *virtual health management model for health care* uses a lifetime case manager who works with the primary care physician in promoting the treatment and management of chronic disease throughout the client's lifetime (Meyer, 1996). The integrated delivery of this case management model meets the dictate of managed care risk contracts in which a health care system shares the risk for an assigned number of lives and is responsible for providing all the health care for those lives. Strategic management of costs and quality patient care outcomes as well as the most appropriate level of care drive this case management model (Beckley, 1995). These newer case management models are moving case management to a new entry point, the community. There is a changing focus on prevention, which includes preparing and educating the clients/consumers to their role as self-advocates.

Because of high costs in our changing health care system, case management models and their specialized services may be limited to clients who are receiving the most complex service. In models in which case managers manage this population, the caseload may be large; therefore, the nurse case manager must be efficient and use resources wisely. Clinical practice guidelines and analogous tools are essential to better identify the at-risk population and assist the case manager in prioritizing clients' needs through their continuum of health care needs and services.

REHABILITATION CASE MANAGEMENT—STANDARDS AND FUNCTIONS

Standards of practice for case management, which follow the nursing process, were published by the Case Management Society of America in October 1995. This framework is used to discuss rehabilitation case management functions emphasizing the ability to individualize the process and achieve clinical quality associated with good economic outcomes.

There are several components of case management that are common to all models; these include patient identification, assessment, planning, implementation, coordination, and evaluation of the delivery of service through a continuum of care (Fig. 3–3).

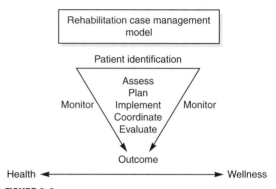

FIGURE 3–3
Key components of case management.

Patient Identification

The first step in the process is to identify those clients who realistically require rehabilitation case management services. Clinical guidelines such as clinical pathways or care maps may be available to the case manager to identify clients who require case management services. These clients may have deviated from their diagnostic pathway.

In a rehabilitation setting, most clients benefit from case management services, considering that they suffer some impairment such as physical or cognitive limitations, an alteration in their environment, or changes in their family role or employment capabilities. Certain catastrophic and chronic illnesses may require different intensities of service depending on the clients' previous health history and wellness care and alterations of their physical and mental status. When the client has been identified by a case manager because of medical, functional, psychological, or social problems, the client is triaged to the most appropriate level of care. The primary goal is access to services across the continuum to achieve the most functional outcomes for the client. If the case manager is the internal case manager for the rehabilitation facility, responsibilities may include precertification, a utilization review, an appeal of insurance denial, and possibly arrangements for out-of-contract benefits. In today's health care arena, the case manager is often the advocate for the client to the third-party payer for the most cost-effective care to achieve maximal benefits.

Assessment

Using a holistic approach, the case manager performs a comprehensive assessment using the client's history, current health status, treatment plan, prognosis, social and environmental support, financial resources, insurance benefits, and disposition options, keeping in mind the client's and family's goals and educational needs.

- Case managers are in a unique position because they play a pivotal role in identifying what is important to the client and the family and act as the client's advocate within the treatment team.
- Many clients in rehabilitation are cared for in accordance with tools such as critical pathways and/or protocols. However, those clients who progress and meet desired outcomes as communicated by the multidisciplinary team may not need the advanced assessment skills and services of a case manager. The effectiveness of the case manager's service can be focused on planning and coordinating the care for those clients who require advanced assessment skills and services to meet a desired outcome. Because the assessment of the client and family is an ongoing process, current and potential clinical problems as well as discharge planning problems can be identified through ongoing assessment of the following:
    - The client's rehabilitation potential
    - The educational needs of the client and family regarding rehabilitation and its ongoing process
    - Whether the client can return to the previous level of function and residence
    - Activities of daily living
    - The level at which the client will return to the previous environment
    - The accessibility and adaptability of the client's residence
    - The insurance company's goals and benefits, making sure they match the client's long- and short-term goals
    - What is acceptable within the client's social and cultural roles

Planning and Resource Identification

The case manager plans and identifies current, short-term, and long-term needs and reviews options as to where, when, and how the client's needs can be addressed (Case Management Society of America, 1995). Planning includes appropriate treatment goals and time frames that may or may not be established through a clinical pathway or other tool. For example, the plan of care might include methods of achieving wellness, prevention, and restorative strategies to educate both the client and the family to the components of care. Barriers to achieving goals and/or wellness may not be found within the plan of care; hence, reasonable goals must be identified to meet the needs of the client, the family, and the payer. For example, if it is acceptable for a spouse to provide hands-on care such as feeding the client, then independence in feeding may not be a necessary goal. On the other hand, if a spouse does not find bathing the client socially acceptable, bathing then becomes a primary goal and the case manager assists the client in identifying alternative resources to meet this functional need. Another example is the client with a significant physical impairment whose goal is employment, and in order to get to work on time, the client may need assistance with morning dressing and grooming tasks. In this situation, the case manager must be knowledgeable about the available services in the community and identify the external resources and related costs. The case manager plans and utilizes resources available to the client within the realm of cost containment. In addition, the case manager monitors compliance with overutilization or underutilization of services within the scope of an individual's insurance benefits. The physician and case manager generally co-lead the client's plan of care. The case manager may take the process a step further by advocating for the client and the treatment team in planning alternatives to overcome varied obstacles in a client's ability to achieve successful outcomes. The treatment plan is adjusted and reviewed for its completeness to meet the holistic needs of the client. In today's health care arena, the client's insurance company and/or its external case manager is essential to acceptance of the plan. It is reasonable to presume that with the evolving health care system the case manager balances the treatment plan and resource allocation for cost and quality (Strassner, 1996).

Implementation and Coordination

The implementation and coordination of a plan include planning for discharge, which can be constantly evolving, as is the assessment, evaluation, and reevaluation of the client's progress. The multidisciplinary team implements the plan while the rehabilitation nurse–client relationship is refined through ongoing communication. The dynamics of the team and the client's involvement in evaluating progress and achievement of goals promote a positive outcome. In the inpatient rehabilitation setting, the case manager may also be the client's care manager and is usually the leader of the rehabilitation team as is recommended by the Certifying Association of Rehabilitation Facilities. The direct care manager ensures that recommendations including discharge plans are identified by the rehabilitation team and are incorporated into the plan of care. Discharge plans must focus on the most appropriate level of care. If appropriate, the case manager anticipates the client's discharge needs for reentry into the community and assists the client in preparing the home environment for discharge. Often, home evaluations are recommended and implemented as part of the plan. When postdis charge services are required, the case man ager assists the client and family to investigate their resources including options for services from the current facility. The client and family should be empowered to choose the most cost-efficient quality services to meet the continuum of care needs. If the client needs alternative living arrangements, the case manager provides information and education regarding available services so that early and appropriate referrals can be made to an identified level of care.

In many organizations, case managers are beginning to use clinical practice guidelines to concurrently monitor an acceptable standard of care for a client's specific diagnosis. This may be monitored in tandem with the client's specific treatment plans. If tools such as clinical pathways, care pathways, standards of care, and protocols are available, they are most often used to document treatment plans for the more common medical and rehabilitation diagnoses. These tools promote a "gold standard" in consistency, completeness, and quality in providing care and service in addition to preventing repetition and unnecessary care. Many health maintenance organizations or managed care organizations often look for the use of these tools when negotiating contracts with providers. Accordingly, these tools may assist in identifying those clients who require case management and assign a case manager only to those clients who deviate from the clinical pathway.

Information systems, computers, and appropriate software packages are becoming essential to case managers because they provide the support to concurrently coordinate and navigate the payer process, reimbursement codes, variance tracking, outcomes, and quality measurement. For example, information systems have the ability to recognize an individual client's disease process, comorbidity, and deviations from the clinical pathway. Inconsistencies are called *variances,* and these variances are outcome monitors that have the potential to justify the client's quality of service and cost issues. Ideally, a clinical pathway encompasses all health care providers in preadmission, hospital interventions, and postdischarge plans. The providers document the expected plan of care for a specific diagnosis with specific outcomes based on a time line. There are no standard formats for case management clinical pathways, but the inclusion of a time line and outcomes should be fundamental (Daus, 1996). It is essential that physicians accept the development and use of these pathways. For example, if a necessary treatment or test was not ordered but is included in the standard pathway, the team members do not have to wait for physician initiation. The case manager also attempts early intervention to prevent client and internal health care variances. Part of coordination means identifying areas in need of additional interventions to prevent complications and promote anticipated or better outcomes. Because of improvements in technology and tools, case managers are now better prepared to recognize those clients who vary from the demonstrated standard of care and can monitor variances for a particular client population or diagnosis as well as the analysis of variances for the use of services. They can recommend altered interventions when a case is catastrophic with many variances from the plan of care. Requests are made for cost projections and cost analysis of current and future care, as well as life care planning to determine care and cost projections over a client's anticipated life span.

The ultimate goal is to implement and coordinate cost, quality, and positive movement toward achievement of the client's clinical goals and continuum of care service. The internal case manager reviews the documentation to determine that services are appropriate for the client's level of care. The external case manager, insurance companies, other payer sources, referrals, and primary care sources then review verbal and/or written communication.

In summary, case managers are responsible for the implementation and coordination of a process to monitor, manage, and document the quality of care and services through clinical outcome tools and/or a client's deviations from the acceptable standard of care. When the process is in place, it determines if the goals of the care plan are being accomplished to meet the needs of the client, family, and payer and are still achievable within the limitations of the client's disease state (Case Management Society of America, 1995). It is projected that long-term case management outcome data will be collected universally to benchmark achievements and validate the result as the quality of cost-effective care. Variance tracking can justify the role of the case managers who ensure the evaluation of risk by recognizing and providing treatment strategies for potential disease states before they turn into episodes of illness (Strassner, 1996).

Evaluation and Outcomes

The case manager evaluates the client's progress within the treatment plan, the products used, and the appropriateness of the plan of care. Evaluation is accomplished through concurrent and periodical review of the client's progress toward the achievement of goals. The plan of care is always in motion toward the achievement of goals in addition to being modified to assist the client in moving toward an acceptable outcome. Client satisfaction and compliance with the treatment program are critical to the evaluation process. Team conferences are held with the client, family, and team members to alter the treatment plan or to modify the goals if the previous goals were unachievable.

The case manager can educate the client and family to the concept of adjustment and adaptation to altered goals. To put closure to the current level of care and recognize that it is unattainable is often difficult for the client and family. Yet it is important to move to the next level of care without delay.

An outcome monitor such as cost containment is ineffective in case management. The best approach in the case management process uses identified goals and the achievement of goals, and then a final report of cost-benefit analysis is prepared that incorporates the goals achieved with the cost-effectiveness of care. Long-term care outcomes are determined by the case manager; follow-up with the client after discharge is another measure.

Generally accepted measures are

- The frequency of reentry into the acute care system
- The function at home compared with the functional level at the time of discharge

The forms of services used are

- Subjective and objective data regarding the wellness
- Positive changes in the client's overall care
- The quality and cost-effectiveness of the referral service

The case manager may collect and analyze data for particular diagnoses, patient populations, physicians, or specialties. The Functional Independence Measure is an objective measure of the client's functional outcomes and is a widely accepted assessment tool in the rehabilitation field. It is readily integrated into a measure of cost-effectiveness when costs are compared with changes in Functional Independence Measure scores. Other outcome systems used by case managers today are the Joint Commission on Accreditation of Healthcare Organization's indicators, the Rapid Disability Rating scale, and the short form '36 Medical Outcomes Measures (Strassner, 1996).

To meet the challenge of case management in the 21st century, outcome monitoring is becoming part of the management of clients. National recognition and the acceptance of clinical practice standards are primarily due to their potential role in benchmarking and improving care. Case managers must continue to monitor their value in terms of quality and outcomes in this emerging health care market. The case manager must produce results for a variety of customers, patients, physicians, providers, and payers. The value and anticipated results of case management may be different for each of these consumers. Case management results focused on quality care, cost containment, access to care, and satisfaction should meet most consumer needs (Mullahy, 1995; St. Coeur, 1995)

The case manager participates in facility/agency/quality assurance activities and ensures that the case management process is evaluated for timely and appropriate services. Overall outcomes are continually evaluated to improve case management services. The case manager is responsible for the identification of and adherence to changes in federal and state regulations, health care policy, and reimbursement guidelines.

REGULATORY, ETHICAL, AND LEGAL IMPLICATIONS

The entry into case management is controversial, with disagreement over whether registered nurses or other health care professionals should be accepted into the profession. The American Nurses Association recommends a bachelor of science degree in nursing and 1 year of clinical experience (American Nurses Association, 1988). The Case Management Society of America recommends professional licensure, a bachelor of health and human service degree, 24 months of clinical experience, and case manager certification (Case Management Society of America, 1995). There is also discussion of whether the case manager should be at an advanced practice level with a master of science degree in nursing. The role requires current clinical knowledge in the specialty areas of the rehabilitation process and rehabilitation techniques. One needs to be knowledgeable about the health care system including discharge planning, external community resources, and appropriate utilization of health care services. Essential are effective written and verbal communication skills and an ability to look at the whole person, not just the disease process. The case manager requires skill in assertiveness, advocacy, creativity, collaboration, negotiation, flexibility, leadership, and conflict resolution (Strassner, 1996).

Certification in the manager's nursing area of expertise and in case management is highly recommended but not a nationally established standard for working as a case manager. The Case Management Society of America regulates case management certification. Legally, the case manager must practice within the scope of the health care profession in which the manager is licensed as well as the Standards of Practice for Case Management. The courts have yet to sufficiently test the Standards of Practice for Case Management. Case managers may be held liable if they breach their obligations to make a reasonable decision because they did not act on something or there was an omission and that act or omission caused harm or injury to the patient. The courts also have determined that the provider has a legal and ethical obligation to provide care whether or not the provider is reimbursed. Professional case managers can protect themselves by following the clinical guidelines for care, monitoring the protocols, and documenting the plan of care and the response to care according to the policy and procedures of each institution (Hogue, 1995).

It must be remembered that treatment must be verified by a physician's order according to the medical staff approval process for protocols and algorithms. Client confidentiality, the cost of treatment, the release of information from institutions, durable powers of attorney, and advance medical directives are paramount legal features of the case manager's practice. The case manager works within the guidelines of the Americans with Disabilities Act and workers' compensation laws. The case manager should be involved in promoting legislation that assists the client in obtaining health care and be aware of legislation that adversely affects health care delivery and reimbursement (Case Management Society of America, 1995).

Ethically, the case manager treats the client and all consumers with dignity and respect. Confidentiality and the judicious sharing of information are respected in all aspects of case management. The case manager educates the clients in their rights and assists as an advocate in helping them exercise these rights. Resource utilization is an area of ethical controversy within today's case management arena. This is of particular concern in the areas of precertification reimbursement, utilization review, and the evolving Managed Care Organization's issues of access to care, denials, and ethics, with which the case manager deals on a daily basis.

RESEARCH

With the nationwide advancement of managed care and risk assignment to health care providers, documentation of clinical outcomes is valuable in providing the appropriate level of client-focused care. Case management needs to validate its practice with consistent research data such as outcomes and other measurement tools used in a client's plan of care. A commitment to evaluating, validating, and communicating research findings with other case managers is important to advanced practice. The business of health care continues to emerge while the cost of health care continues to climb. The focus on outcomes can only assist the case manager to document the value added. The nationally recognized Standardization of Clinical Guidelines including clinical pathways is based on scientific research and will assist in the development of case management models across the continuum of the care delivery system.

REFERENCES

American Nurses Association. (1988). *Nursing case management*. Washington, DC: American Nurses Publishing.

Beckley, N. J. (1995). Case management and integrated delivery. *Case Review, 1*(2), 25–30.

Bringewatt, R. (1995). You have not yet begun to integrate. *Health Systems Review, 28*(5):50–54.

Case Management Society of America. (1995). Standards of practice for case management. Centered care. *The Journal of Care Management, 1*(4), 7–12.

Cochrane, J. D. (1995). Will reengineering save us all? Integrated Health Care Report, p. 1: Adaptation printed in *Health Trends, 7*(12), Oct 1995.

Daus, C. (1996). Following the steps of efficiency. *Case Review, 2*(l), 41–46.

Hogue, E. (1995). Are case managers liable? *The Journal of Care Management, 1*(2), 35–38, 53.

Johnson, S. K. (1986). The state of disease management. *Case Review, 2*(4), 51–59.

Knollmueller, R. N. (1984). Funding home care in climate of cost containment. *Public Health Nursing, 1*(1), 16–22.

McBride S. M. (1992). Rehabilitation case managers: Ahead of their time. *Holistic Nursing Practice, 6*(2), 67–75.

Merrill, J. (1985). Defining case management. *Business and Health, 2*(8), 5–9.

Meyer, L. C. (1996). It's about time—Virtual health management. *The Case Manager, 7*(2), 53–60, 62, 64.

Mullahy, C. M. (1995). Establishing a value for your services. *Continuing Care, 14*(8), 20–21, 24.

Murer, M. (1996). Case management challenges. *Integrated Health System, 15*(3), 14–30.

Paone, D. L. (1995). Care across the continuum. *Case Review, 1*(2), 11–12.

Smith, D. S. (1995). Standard of practice for case management. The importance of practice standard. *Journal of Case Management, 1*(3), 6–7, 9, 12, 15, 16.

Smith, G. B., Danforth, D. A., Owens, P. J. (1994). Role restructuring: Nurse, case manager, and educator. *Nursing Administration Quarterly, 19*(1), 21–32.

St. Coeur, M. (1995). Care management guidelines. *Case Review, 1*(2), 46–47.

Strassner, L. F. (1996). Evaluating critical pathways. *Continuing Care, 15*(4), 24–26, 28–33.

Zander, K. (1988). Nursing case management: Resolving the DRG paradox. *Nursing Clinics of North America, 23*(3), 503–520.

BIBLIOGRAPHY

Chimner, N. E., Easterling, A. (1993). Collaborative practice through nursing. Case management. *Rehabilitation Nursing, 18*(4), 226–230.

Good, C. J. (1995). Impact of a CareMap® and case management on patient satisfaction and staff satisfaction, collaboration, and autonomy. *Nursing Economics, 13*(6), 337–348.

Guinan, J. K. (1993). Facility based case management—Its role in rehabilitation nursing. *Rehabilitation Nursing, 18*(4), 253–256.

Hale, C. (1995). Research issues in case management. *Nursing Standard, 26*(9), 29–32.

Lee, S. (1996). New trends in disease management. *Continuing Care, 15*(7), 37–39.

Leigh, B. (1993). Case management in a health maintenance organization: Improving quality of care. *AAOHN Journal, 41*(4), 170–173.

Murer, C. G. (1996). Creating common knowledge. The role of case management is the nucleus of effective negotiation. *Rehabilitation Management, 9*(4), 62–63, 66.

Nicolaysen, L. (1996). More than just. . . . *Continuing Care, 15*(3), 22–25.

Ward, M. D., & Rieve, J. (1995). Disease management: Case management's return to patient centered care. *The Journal of Care Management, 1*(4), 7–12.

Welsenfels, B. (1996). The case management law forum. *The Case Manager, 7*(1), 51–57.

CHAPTER 4

The Rehabilitation Team

Marie O'Toole

The *health care team* is a term that is frequently used when describing the wide range of practitioners who deliver health services. The *rehabilitation team* is a specialized version of a health care team whose members collaborate with each other to establish a plan and goals for the achievement of a client's maximal potential. This chapter describes the evolution of the rehabilitation team, the function of the contemporary rehabilitation team, and the unique composition and roles of some of the typical members of the rehabilitation team.

EVOLUTION AND HISTORY OF THE REHABILITATION TEAM

A team of health care providers was first highlighted in the literature in 1922 as a mechanism to avoid compartmentalization of expertise. The early reports related to interdisciplinary teams focused on child guidance and health care professionals organizing to address mental health issues.

After World War I, a great deal of attention was focused on soldiers recovering from both mental and physical disabilities. A pioneer in rehabilitation wrote that "one of our principal aims is to create morale and to provide early opportunity for the coordination of all hospital efforts toward returning the patient to community life and economic usefulness" (Slagle, 1927, p. 128). Two years later, the first academic department of physical medicine in the United States was founded at Temple University in Philadelphia, Pennsylvania. This department offered lectures for future physicians, physical therapists, and nurses and emphasized the measurement of the effects of physical agents (Opitz, Folz, Gelfman, & Peters, 1997). This established a strong base for the development of the interdisciplinary rehabilitation team.

The scope of rehabilitation services expanded dramatically in 1943, when longstanding programs in vocational rehabilitation were expanded to medical rehabilitation beyond guidance and vocational training.

The need to address a patient from a holistic focus was a major impetus to the development of the team and was articulated in 1951 by Whitehouse (1951). At that time, three assumptions that remain true to this day were identified. The first assumption concerned the nature of the human organism as a dynamic, interacting, and integrated whole. The second assumption noted the importance of the need for treatments to be dynamic and to keep pace with the changing person's needs. The third assumption identified teamwork as the interacting partnership of professionals specializing in these needs and dealing with the person as a whole as a valid method for meeting these requirements.

Lydia E. Hall, the first rehabilitation nurse inducted into the American Nurses Association's Hall of Fame, advanced the team concept by her insistence that staff from all disciplines make notations on the same patient progress notes. A revolutionary concept in the 1960s, it is one that emphasized the importance of every member of the team's sharing experiences and knowledge. It is interesting to note that in a time when many nursing professionals were focused on the team nursing philosophy, with a variety of unlicensed personnel directed by the registered professional nurse, Hall's rehabilitation team included only professional nurses who established a one-to-one patient relationship (Loose, 1994).

Throughout the 1970s, the concept of the rehabilitation team emphasized the meetings of the team that planned for rehabilitation in the inpatient setting; however, members of the contemporary rehabilitation team are much more flexible in their enactment of team functions (Rehabilitation Outlook, 1996). Howard Rusk, M.D., a visionary leader in the development of modern rehabilitation, acknowledged that there must be specialized rehabilitation centers utilizing the team approach. Also noted was the fact that the paucity of funds, equipment, and specialized professional staff created a situation in which there would never be an adequate number of centers for all patients requiring services (Rusk, 1977). The indispensable element for the rehabilitation team was considered to be the desire on the part of all team members to cooperate and to elicit cooperation. The current health care environment is certainly one that requires the judicious allocation of the resources of the team.

The successful rehabilitation of a patient depends on the collaboration and cooperation of a large number of people with a common, client-focused goal. The team approach to rehabilitation is rooted in the belief that rehabilitation is a complex process. The skills and expertise of a wide variety of individuals are required to ensure a successful outcome for the patient and the family. The assumption is that a team is more effective, is better coordinated, and provides better-quality services for the recipients of care (Ducanis & Golin, 1979). Utilization of the team concept allows a group of people, working together, to identify critical issues and communicate effectively. Current research on the effectiveness of coordinated teams in a variety of disciplines and specialties continues to support the assumption that the team approach is both enduring and efficient (Felten, Cady, Metzler, & Burton, 1997; Houston & Fleschler, 1997; Simpson & Garrity, 1997).

FUNCTIONS OF THE REHABILITATION TEAM

The dynamic nature of the health care system profoundly affects the rehabilitation team and its function. A rehabilitation team at the start of the 21st century may communicate via videoconferencing, fax, and e-mail. Interdisciplinary teaching records and documentation can be maintained in a computerized format. The sites for care delivery are varied. The contemporary rehabilitation team is rarely viewed exclusively as a group of health care professionals gathered around a conference table planning for a lengthy hospital stay in a specialized rehabilitation hospital as it might have been in the past. However, the team clearly continues to work together for the benefit of the patient.

The rehabilitation team represents a client-oriented group of professionals focused on enhancing outcomes for individuals and families facing the challenges presented by a disability. Although a wide variety of memberships and team configurations exists, the rehabilitation team remains an important and unified force. Collaboration has always been one of the hallmarks of the rehabilitation team and an element in the coordination and successful implementation of a comprehensive rehabilitation program. An important principle supporting the team concept is the notion that a team accomplishes goals by using the individual strengths of each member, which can only be done by using the spirit of collaboration.

The rehabilitation team plays a critical role in the determination of appropriate services to ensure maximal functional outcomes and the highest quality of life possible. In order to use resources for the maximal benefit of the recipient of care, services must be matched to needs. This requires a thorough assessment of clients before admission to a program, with a careful matching of the most suitable level of care and attention to the unique contributions of each member of the team. An effective rehabilitation team functions not only within a specific organization but also between organizations to support the long-term needs of the patient.

The sites of activity for the rehabilitation team include rehabilitation facilities or centers that specialize in the long-term issues facing individuals and families dealing with a disability. It is often this setting that people envision when they speak of rehabilitation. However, the rehabilitation team also plays a major role in skilled nursing facilities, whose numbers have increased dramatically over the past 25 years. Another growing area in which the team functions is community health agencies, which include public and home health nursing services, visiting nurse associations, clinics, and nursing centers. It is not unreasonable to note that the rehabilitation team functions in whatever setting the situation and location of the patient and the patient's family mandate.

The functions or tasks of the contemporary rehabilitation team include, but are not limited to, (1) establishing realistic goals with the client and family, (2) ensuring continuity of care and coordination of available resources, and (3) serving as a mechanism to evaluate the progress of the patient and the quality of care. The complexity of achieving these goals supports the rehabilitation team concept whose overriding concern is for the well-being of the consumer of the team's services.

The clients in rehabilitation represent individuals from birth to death with a variety of impairments resulting from any number of physical or psychological causes. Management of the client is complex because all aspects of the client's life must be considered in both the evaluation and the treatment if the goals are to be achieved. Although it is important to address health care concerns, the rehabilitation team must also concern itself with all the resources and services needed throughout the life span. The rehabilitation team has always been concerned with the care of the "whole" person. Moreover, the family and the community are considered integral to the successful rehabilitation of the person. A team that functions effectively coordinates the rehabilitation plan in a way that avoids fragmentation and emphasizes coordination.

COMPOSITION AND ROLES OF THE TEAM

A distinctive feature of the rehabilitation team has always been that there is no set composition of the team. The needs of the client determine the team composition and to a great extent the magnitude of the role played by most of the individual team members. The client is, however, the most important member of the rehabilitation team and is an active participant in formulating the plan and goals. Other members of the rehabilitation team may include the nurse; the physician; physical, occupational, speech, and recreational therapists; social workers; case managers; dietitians; vocational counselors; and the psychologist. This list is not by any means exhaustive. Other professionals are added when the plans and goals developed with the client indicate a need for additional expertise.

Role overlap has consistently been identified as a barrier to the effective functioning of rehabilitation teams, as has a lack of understanding among professionals. It has also been noted that interdisciplinary cohesion and integration are enhanced when an understanding of unique professional values is present within the context of the rehabilitation team. Some specific members of the rehabilitation team and their roles are identified as follows.

Rehabilitation Nurse

The rehabilitation nurse is a registered nurse with a specialty within the profession in which many functions of nursing can be identified. These functions are applied to clients, families, and communities requiring rehabili-

tation services. The roles include, but are not limited to, teacher, facilitator, client advocate, change agent, caregiver, coordinator, counselor, consultant, and researcher.

The nurse member of the rehabilitation team has a comprehensive focus on the whole client, not just the disease process or disability that precipitated the need for rehabilitation, and has the ability to understand individual and family needs across the life span. The caregiver role for the rehabilitation nurse is important, but because the focus of rehabilitation is to help the individual or group to restore or maintain maximal health, caregiving components are usually undertaken with an emphasis on patient and family education. The intensity of the nurse-client relationship places the nurse member of the team in an excellent position to play a critical role in assisting the client and family to meet immediate and long-term needs.

In many instances, the rehabilitation nurse also fulfills the designated role of team coordinator. The rehabilitation team nurse collaborates with other members of the team, resource personnel from insurance carriers, school personnel, and home health and community agencies, as appropriate; most importantly, the nurse ensures that the client and family continue to be an integral component of the rehabilitation process. Regardless of whether the rehabilitation nurse serves as the formal team coordinator, it is his or her responsibility to guide the team in implementing the principle that the client's needs guide the rehabilitation process, and that to do this successfully the client should be viewed as a member of a family and a larger community.

The Association of Rehabilitation Nurses has developed standards for rehabilitation nursing in collaboration with the American Nurses Association that identify specific functions of the rehabilitation nurse. It also administers certification examinations for rehabilitation nursing. The rehabilitation nurse who has met the requirements for certification at a basic level may use the designation *certified rehabilitation registered nurse* (CRRN). The nurse in an advanced practice role meeting the requirements for certification uses the designation *certified rehabilitation registered nurse–advanced* (CRRN-A). Although all nurses can certainly use rehabilitation principles in their practice, not all nurses are rehabilitation nurses.

The Association of Rehabilitation Nurses has identified basic knowledge and skills that

TABLE 4-1 ■ BASIC NURSING ACTIVITIES IN REHABILITATION

All professional nurses practicing rehabilitation nursing should possess the basic knowledge and skills that enable them to do the following:

- Establish an effective relationship with the client and significant other(s) to facilitate the development of a plan of care.
- Collect appropriate assessment data for each rehabilitation client; determine significant problems; establish appropriate nursing diagnoses; and set goals and identify outcomes that reflect an understanding of the impact of the disability or chronic illness on the planning, delivery, and evaluation of care within the limit of available economic resources.
- Coordinate and collaborate with the interdisciplinary team in assessing, planning, implementing, and evaluating the individual's care, rehabilitation program, progress toward goals, and related rehabilitation activities.
- Demonstrate knowledge of the profound and prolonged impact of disability and chronic illness on an individual's developmental, physical, social, emotional, spiritual, economic, vocational, and leisure status.
- Employ clinical assessment skills as the basis for sound judgment and decisions regarding the client's actual and potential health problems.
- Use the standards of rehabilitation nursing practice and the nursing process to improve the quality of care for rehabilitation clients.
- Modify assessment and management strategies based on a consideration of the physical, functional, cultural, social, economic, and spiritual dimensions of human responses to actual and potential health problems.
- Participate with clients, families, and other health professionals in collaborative decision making that reflects the understanding that care should be culturally sensitive, ethical, legal, informed, compassionate, and humane.
- Develop a discharge and/or transition plan in collaboration with the client and family that provides for continuity of care and has a goal of continued progress toward outcomes that are desirable to, affordable for, and potentially achievable by the client.
- Maintain communication with and/or make referrals to appropriate institutions and community agencies involved in the delivery of rehabilitative care.
- Apply research findings in practice decisions, identify problems for research, and, when appropriate, participate in the nursing research process.
- Educate clients, their significant others, and payers about the knowledge and skills that promote adaptation to disability and chronic illness.

From Association of Rehabilitation Nurses. (1994). *Standards and scope of rehabilitation nursing practice* (3rd ed.). Glenview, IL: Author. Copyright 1994. With permission of The Association of Rehabilitation Nurses, 4700 W. Lake Avenue, Glenview, IL 60025-1485.

all nurses practicing rehabilitation nursing should possess. They are identified in Table 4–1.

Rehabilitation nurses prepared at the master's level and beyond build on the basic skills and knowledge and also place an emphasis on research and leadership. The Association of Rehabilitation Nurses has also identified the activities for the advanced practice identified in Table 4–2.

Case Manager

The case manager is a relatively new member of the rehabilitation team. The goals of case managers are to assist individuals and families affected by catastrophic illness and/or disability to optimize services and outcomes in a cost-efficient manner.

The case manager typically develops a formal, written, comprehensive needs assessment that usually includes a formal review of evaluations performed by other members of the rehabilitation team. The case manager then assists the client and service provider in planning and program development that meet the needs identified and prioritized in the assessment. Monitoring is incorporated into the case manager's plan and is often

TABLE 4-2 ■ ACTIVITIES OF ADVANCED PRACTICE NURSES IN REHABILITATION

Advanced practice nurses in rehabilitation work with individuals, families, and communities to assess health needs; develop diagnoses; plan, implement, and manage care; and evaluate outcomes of care. Advanced practice nurses in rehabilitation are involved in activities aimed at

- Assisting clients to regain, maintain, or improve their functional and self-care abilities
- Advocating for care that promotes health and wellness for individuals with chronic illness or disability and that prevents additional disabilities
- Obtaining appropriate health, legal, social, vocational, and community services
- Evaluating programs (including those related to environmental monitoring and public policy) for individuals, families, and communities at risk
- Providing leadership and contributing to the advancement of rehabilitation nursing, rehabilitation, and nursing.

From Rehabilitation Nursing Foundation. (1996). *Standards and scope of rehabilitation nursing practice.* Glenview, IL: Author. Copyright 1996. With permission of The Association of Rehabilitation Nurses, 4700 W. Lake Avenue, Glenview, IL 60025-1485.

done collaboratively with other health care providers on the rehabilitation team. The case manager helps to determine not only if modifications to a plan are needed but also if a change of service provider may be required.

The case manager is often the member of the team who maintains regular contact with the client and family through home and telephone visits, site visits to schools and other educational facilities, the workplace, and institutional settings. The roles and functions of the case manager vary depending on the practice setting. Case managers may be employed in an institutional setting, or, as is increasingly the case, they may work in the insurance industry.

Physiatrist

The physiatrist is a physician who specializes in medical or physical rehabilitation, diagnosing and managing medical problems associated with disease, disability, and functional impairments. Frank Krusen, M.D., first coined the word *physiatrist* in 1938 to describe the small group of physicians who were dedicated to the combination of physical medicine and medical therapeutics to treat neurological and musculoskeletal disorders. The term *physiatry* is derived from the Greek words *physikos*, which means "natural," and *iatreia*, which signifies the "art of healing." The physical agents prescribed by the physiatrist include exercise, heat, massage, biofeedback, electrical stimulation, and diathermy.

Formal education for physiatry began in 1926 at Northwestern University Medical School, and physiatry was first recognized as a medical specialty in 1947. The major organizations for physiatrists include the American Academy of Physical Medicine and Rehabilitation, the American Board of Physical Medicine and Rehabilitation, and the American Congress of Rehabilitation Medicine.

The physiatrist is in an excellent position to bridge any gaps that may exist among medical issues and rehabilitation efforts. The guiding principle for the physiatrist, like that of other members of the rehabilitation team, is that treatment involves the whole person and addresses the physical, emotional, and social needs that must be satisfied to successfully restore the patient's quality of life to its maximal potential.

Primary or Consulting Physician

An accurate diagnosis and effective early treatment during the acute phases of an illness or impairment have a profound effect on issues affecting rehabilitation outcomes. Thus, the primary physician is often the first member of the rehabilitation team to encounter the patient and manage care in a way that complements the total rehabilitation plan. Relevant referrals and the prevention of complications position the individual and family in a manner that allows optimal rehabilitation. The primary physician plays an important role in the appropriate and timely placement in inpatient, outpatient, and home health care facilities to ensure the highest functional outcome.

The primary physician, if other than the physiatrist during the rehabilitation phase of an illness, is responsible for the medical and/or surgical management of the person. This physician is often used as a consultant to the team.

Physical Therapist

The physical therapist is a health care professional who evaluates and treats people with health care problems resulting from injury or disease (American Physical Therapy Association, 1999). Modern physical therapy began during World War I when the U.S. Surgeon General's Office established the Division of Special Hospitals and Physical Reconstruction that included as an integral part of the rehabilitation program the services of "reconstruction aides," now known as physical therapists. The first professional association was formed in 1921 and known as the American Women's Physical Therapeutic Association, which has evolved over the years to the present American Physical Therapy Association.

Physical therapists perform a number of functions that include, but are not limited to, assessing joint motion, muscle strength and endurance, the function of the heart and lungs, and performance of activities of daily living. Activities with which the physical therapist is frequently involved include mobility activities such as transfers, locomotion, and the development and execution of exercise programs designed to prevent deconditioning. Modalities that may be employed by the physical therapist also include hydrotherapy, electrotherapy, and massage.

The physical therapist, too, is guided in practice by principles that include a concern for the physical, psychological, and socioeconomic welfare of the clients with whom they work.

Occupational Therapist

The occupational therapist is also involved in the increase or restoration of muscle strength, coordination, and mobility through the use of therapeutic activities. World War I provided the impetus for the modern conception of occupational therapy, although the use of work as a treatment for mental patients was systematized in the late 19th century. The National Society for the Promotion of Occupational Therapy was established in 1925 and was the forerunner of the American Occupational Therapy Association.

The occupational therapist focuses on functional activities and other forms of work with the goal of restoring endurance, safety, and self-sufficiency. The occupational therapist not only restores independence in activities of daily living but also uses these skills to meet cognitive and psychosocial needs of clients. For example, teaching a client how to cook safely not only enhances independent living skills but is an excellent tool to teach safety needs and to allow the client to practice the interpersonal skills needed to communicate effectively. The responsibilities of the occupational therapist include all the activities needed to help the client accomplish commitments of daily life such as caring for home and family, as well as gainful employment and a meaningful education. The occupational therapist provides valuable expertise in the selection of adaptive equipment and assistive technologies.

Professional Occupations in Therapy and Assessment

Recreational therapists contribute to the improved functioning and independence of the client through pleasant and rewarding avocational activities in a safe, controlled environment. Recreation and other activities can be prescribed as treatment interventions for persons whose functional abilities are impaired due to physical, mental, emotional, and/or social conditions. The therapeutic activities of the recreational therapist facilitate the development of creativity, cooperation, and social interaction that enhances self-esteem and improves overall functional activities.

Other professional occupations in therapy include the art therapist, athletic therapist, dance therapist, and music therapist. These specialized therapists use the techniques identified in their title to aid in the treatment of both mental and physical disabilities and to initiate, design, and implement unique therapy programs to enhance physical and mental well-being.

Psychologist

The emotional adjustment of a person, the family, and the multiple communities of which the person is a member is critical to the successful adaptation of the individual undergoing rehabilitation. Psychological variables have a profound impact on the expression of a medical disability and may determine the extent to which the disability has an impact on functional adaptation (Trexler & Fordyce, 1996). Subspecialties within the field of rehabilitation psychology include chronic pain management, inpatient rehabilitation, vocational and industrial rehabilitation, and brain injury rehabilitation.

The psychological assessment of a person undergoing rehabilitation is a comprehensive effort to identify those factors that affect rehabilitation and the outcomes in impairment and disability. Psychological tests are usually administered and scored by the psychologists, but the assessment must incorporate feedback from all members of the team in order to arrive at a valid clinical interpretation. Psychological goals and interventions should be congruent with and support the goals of the entire team.

Psychological interventions of the team are generally divided into two categories, maximizing general rehabilitation progress and teaching specific skills to facilitate psychosocial adjustment (Trexler & Fordyce, 1996). The psychologist often enacts the role of consultant to the team as consistent, meaningful interventions are identified to enhance psychosocial adjustment.

Additionally, the psychologist plays an important role in maintaining the mental health of colleagues on the team. The rehabilitation team must care for itself if it is to be successful in caring for others, and the psychologist can recognize stressors that can interfere with the proper functioning of the team.

Mental health needs may also be addressed by a psychiatrist. As a physician, the psychiatrist may also prescribe medications as an adjunct to other treatments.

Speech-Language Pathologist

The diagnosis and treatment of individuals of all ages with communication problems falls within the domain of practice for the speech-language pathologist. They are specialists in human communication, its development, and its disorders (Malone, 1997). Certified speech-language pathologists have a master's or doctoral degree from an accredited program and pass a national examination to receive a certificate of clinical competence from the American Speech-Language-Hearing Association. Speech-language pathologists work cooperatively with the rehabilitation team to develop a treatment plan individualized for clients experiencing communication and/or swallowing disorders. Common types of speech-language disorders that are addressed by the speech-language pathologist include those that result in receptive and expressive aphasia including cognitive communication disorders that occur after brain injury or stroke, and dysphagia or swallowing disorders that occur as a result of illness, surgery, stroke, or injury. Treatment may involve direct individual or group therapy or indirect treatment in coordination with various health care professionals on the rehabilitation team.

This member of the rehabilitation team typically works in a wide variety of settings to address the communication needs of clients. These settings include, but are not limited to, schools, hospitals, rehabilitation centers, specialized institutions, clinics, and private practice environments.

Social Worker

Social workers focus on psychosocial problems of patients and their families and emphasize interactions among families, groups, organizations, and communities (Heiss, 1997). The social worker enacts a unique helping role within the rehabilitation team by possessing an in-depth knowledge of social welfare policies and federal policies and entitlements. It falls within the social worker's domain of practice to evaluate the impact of these policies on the social problems of clients and families with disabilities. Social workers in rehabilitation settings frequently provide invaluable support to the team through their assistance with long-term living arrangements and referrals to coordinating agencies. The social worker also plays an important role in client and family counseling. Support groups are often established and maintained by the social worker.

SUMMARY

The rehabilitation team as a whole, as well as many other individuals, identifies important issues in collaboration with the client and family and communicates interpersonally as well as with institutions and agencies needed to achieve goals. The rehabilitation team is a powerful coalition capable of planning, managing, and evaluating strategies designed to enhance human performance on many levels.

REFERENCES

American Physical Therapy Association. *APTA background sheet 1999*. Alexandria, VA: Author. (1999).

Ducanis, A. J., & Golin, A. K. (1979). *The interdisciplinary health care team*. Rockville, MD: Aspen.

Felten, S., Cady, N., Metzler, M. H., & Burton, S. (1997). Implementation of collaborative practice through interdisciplinary rounds on a general surgery service. *Nursing Case Management, 2*, 122–126.

Heiss, W. (1997). Window on social work. In M. O'Toole (Ed.), *The Miller-Keane encyclopedia & dictionary of medicine, nursing, & allied health* (p. 1499). Philadelphia: W. B. Saunders.

Houston, S., & Fleschler, R. (1997). Outcomes management in women's health. *Journal of Obstetric, Gynecologic & Neonatal Nursing, 26*, 342–350.

Loose, V. (1994). Lydia E. Hall: Rehabilitation nursing pioneer in the ANA Hall of Fame. *Rehabilitation Nursing, 19*, 174–176.

Malone, R. L. (1997). Window on speech-language pathologists. In M. O'Toole (Ed.), *The Miller-Keane encyclopedia & dictionary of medicine, nursing, & allied health* (p. 1509). Philadelphia: W. B. Saunders.

Opitz, J. L., Folz, T. J., Gelfman, R., & Peters, D. J. (1997). The history of physical medicine and rehabilitation as recorded in the diary of Dr. Frank Krusen: Part 1. *Archives of Physical Medicine & Rehabilitation, 78*, 422–445.

Rehabilitation Outlook. (1996).

Rusk, H. A. (1977). *Rehabilitation medicine*. St. Louis: C. V. Mosby.

Simpson, K. P., & Garrity, E. R. (1997). Perioperative management in lung transplantation. *Clinics in Chest Medicine, 18*, 277–284.

Slagle, E. C. (1927). To organize an "O.T." department. *Occupational Therapy and Rehabilitation, 6*, 125–130.

Trexler, L. E., & Fordyce, D. J. (1996). In R. Braddom (Ed.), *Physical Medicine and Rehabilitation* (pp. 66–81). Philadelphia: W. B. Saunders.

Whitehouse, F. A. (1951). Teamwork—A democracy of professions. *Exceptional Children, 18*, 5–52.

CHAPTER 5

Health Policy and Legislation in Rehabilitation

Susan Dean-Baar

Nursing has great potential for influencing health policy at all levels. Policy can be viewed as a purposive course of action to address a problem or matter of concern; it starts by getting a problem on the policy agenda and continues through evaluating the effectiveness of an adopted policy in achieving the outcome (Anderson, 1975). Health policy has been defined as dealing with the problems and issues concerning the organization, delivery, and financing of health care from the level of the patient-provider encounter to society as a whole, as well as those issues affecting public health, provider education, and biomedical research (Calkins, Fernandopulle, & Marino, 1995). Policy decisions are made at a variety of levels from the agency, organization, or institution that employs a nurse to local, state, and federal governments. Health policy is important for nurses to understand because policy decisions made at any level will affect the professional practice of nursing. Policy decisions are the product of a process that is influenced by the values and interests of the parties involved.

The development of health policy can be viewed as a four-phase process that includes problem identification and issue recognition, policy formulation, policy implementation, and policy evaluation (Cohen & Milburn, 1986). Nurses are in a key position to influence health policy at all phases (Stimpson & Hanley, 1991). Nurses bring a perspective that advocates that individuals be active consumers and participants in health care. In rehabilitation, nurses, perhaps more so than in any other discipline, are in a position to influence policymaking because of our role in overseeing and coordinating all aspects of care (Sherwen, 1992). Our holistic, realistic approach provides us with expert knowledge in creating solutions to complex problems. Unfortunately, nurses have been limited in their ability to influence policy because of a lack of

access to information and decision makers (Murphy, 1991). Nurses need to increase their participation as members of decision-making committees in health care institutions and organizations and at the local, state, and federal levels of government. From these positions, nurses are able to communicate a nursing perspective to influence policy decisions made formally or informally and at any organizational or governmental level. To do this effectively, nurses need to acquire political competence, which includes the ability to mobilize the support of important constituencies, develop relationships, and educate professional colleagues, legislators, clients, and the public at large (Thomas & Shelton, 1994).

This chapter focuses on health policy in rehabilitation and includes a discussion of the major issues confronting the organization, delivery, and financing of rehabilitation services and the major legislation that has impacted the field of rehabilitation. In discussing health care policy and rehabilitation, it is helpful to remember Dunn's (1981) conceptualization of policy analysis as having three interrelated elements: policies, stakeholders, and the environment. Policies are decisions about how resources are allocated and used. Stakeholders are persons or groups who have vested interests in policies whether as influencers or as those affected by the policy change. The environment is the context, including history, current events, values, beliefs, and biases within which policies evolve (Miller & Russell, 1992).

HEALTH POLICY AND REHABILITATION

The field of rehabilitation serves individuals with disabilities and chronic illnesses. This is a population that has historically been underserved and ignored in many areas of society. Public policy has addressed the needs of this population to varied degrees during the 20th century. Today health care policy is frequently debated with respect to the issues of access, cost, and quality. These discussions are always influenced by a set of values. It is helpful to preface a discussion of health care policy and rehabilitation with a look at the values that are particularly evident in this area.

Ethical Principles and Rehabilitation Health Policy

Much of social and health care policy is influenced by the values within the ethical principles of beneficence, autonomy, and justice. Rubin and Millard (1991) present a very thoughtful analysis of the imbalance that appears to exist between the principles of beneficence and autonomy in regard to American public policy on disability. Beneficence-driven programs include income programs such as Social Security Disability Insurance (SSDI), which can reinforce dependency and provide disincentives to being gainfully employed. Vocational rehabilitation and independent living are examples of autonomy-driven programs that have consistently been funded at much lower levels than the beneficence-driven programs. This inequity in funding reflects a major philosophical conflict. Among the major difficulties are the structural and attitudinal barriers that pervade society. These barriers have prevented persons with disabilities from having fair opportunity to acquire the services that would maximize autonomy. Fair opportunity under the principle of justice requires that no individual be denied benefits generally available to others allowing full participation in all aspects of society and community life. Fair opportunity is what allows the financial support of services to address the needs of a portion of society so that people with disabilities may realistically participate more fully in society. The passage of the Americans with Disabilities Act (ADA) in 1990 has made strides in eliminating some of the structural barriers. Attention now needs to turn to eliminating attitudinal barriers so that individuals with disabilities are seen as capable of making contributions to society.

A societal attitude of this type would support the allocation of sufficient funds to programs that support autonomy more than beneficence. This approach is not as simple as it may appear. The reality is that there are not unlimited resources to support programs that strive for maximal improvement without any consideration of cost. One of the major policy

issues confronting rehabilitation may be how financial constraints are determined and which values guide those discussions. Resources, economic and others, are increasingly allocated based on the likelihood of making a meaningful contribution to the attainment of a desired outcome. Rehabilitation services provided in a traditional fee-for-service environment focused on assisting an individual with a disability to his or her highest potential without regard to cost. With the financing of health care changing, this is no longer the prevailing approach.

Banja and Johnston (1994) use persons with traumatic brain injury as a paradigm of a particularly vulnerable population in rehabilitation change. As outcomes are increasingly used to determine what rehabilitation services will be provided, there are at least three ways that the use of various outcome measures can impede a rehabilitation client's progress. First is when length of stay is used as the predominant outcome measure. In this situation, when an individual has reached a predetermined length of stay, services are terminated regardless of the individual's progress toward individualized goals for maximal functional ability. Second is the determination that only "basic" therapies are necessary in rehabilitation. In providing rehabilitation for many individuals with traumatic brain injury, these basic services may be suboptimal and impede the ability to achieve realistic functional goals. The third way that using outcomes may impede the provision of appropriate care is in situations in which a provider's level of reimbursement is higher if referrals for specialized care are not made or when a payer decides that a certain outcome is not worth paying for at all. In both these cases, the individual may receive no rehabilitation services. Again the issue of justice is raised, in this case not from a perspective of federal policy but from the perspective of the payer and provider of rehabilitation services. What will be the differences if rehabilitation is viewed as an entitlement for all citizens or as a service that is provided only to the extent of the individual's insurance coverage? What outcomes will merit the allocation of resources? How will a projected outcome be determined to be "good enough"? These are fundamental questions related to access, cost, and quality.

Access, Cost, and Quality

Symington (1994) identified seven mega-trends that are shaping the future of persons with disabilities. They are the changing demography of disability, the emancipation of persons with disability, a policy shift from isolation to segregation to integration, the rising costs of health and social services, changes in service delivery (from center-based to community-based to a comprehensive continuum), empowerment through assistive technology, and the shift from empiricism to applied science. These changes are all related to developing issues about access, cost, and the quality of all health care services, including rehabilitation.

Access. Access to health care is one of the major areas of debate in health care policy today. Access is not synonymous with availability. Access is the ability to acquire timely and appropriate health care services. Access is a major issue for those who are either uninsured or underinsured. The uninsured are those without coverage in either a private health insurance plan or a public program such as Medicaid or Medicare. In addition, it is estimated that as many as 40 million of those with some form of private insurance coverage are underinsured. Underinsured is defined by the Pepper Commission (1990) as being at risk of spending more than 10% of one's annual income for health care in the event of serious illness. The primary problem confronted by individuals with disabilities is not access to health insurance in general but rather access to adequate coverage that meets their specific needs (Batavia, 1993). One study found that 23% of persons with disabilities spent more than 10% of family income on out-of-pocket health care expenses compared with 3% of persons who did not have disabilities. Persons with disabilities spent nearly four times as much out of pocket as persons who did not have disabilities, yet they were almost twice as likely to have family incomes less than 200% of the poverty level (Alecxih, Corea, & Kennell, 1995).

This is only one view of the access issue. Another view is that of the individual with a disability and the strategies that person is forced to use to obtain or keep any health insurance at all. The barriers to adequate and affordable health insurance include high premiums, cancellations because of use, preexisting condition exclusions, and exclusion or limited coverage of specific services. In addition, many individuals are locked into their present employment for fear of losing insurance benefits if they switch jobs. Insurance underwriting and cost-containment practices can have a devastating effect on individuals

with a disability (Kinney & Steinmetz, 1994). Other problems that an individual with a chronic illness or disability may experience that affect access to care are a lack of coordination of services, transportation barriers, and inconvenient clinic hours and long waiting periods (Callahan & David, 1995).

Cost. Closely related to access are issues of cost. Health care spending accounts for more than 13% of the gross domestic product and continues to grow at a rate that exceeds growth in the rest of the economy. Although the proportion of individuals with disabilities in the overall population is small (2% in 1987), they account for a disproportionate amount of the health care expenditures (13% in 1987). The portion of expenditures within government health programs (Medicare and Medicaid) for persons with disabilities is substantial. For instance, Medicare covered 71.6% of rehabilitation patients from a 1990–1991 sample of facilities reporting data to the Uniform Data System (UDS) for Medical Rehabilitation (Stineman et al., 1994). An analysis of the 1987 National Medical Expenditure Survey found that expenditures for persons with disabilities were more than six times the level of those for persons without disabilities. Per capita health expenditures for persons with disabilities were more than four times higher than for those without disabilities. The largest single source of out-of-pocket expenditures for persons with disabilities was home- and community-based services (Alecxih et al., 1995). Health care cost-containment efforts, especially those directed at government health care programs, can have more profound effects on the population of individuals with disabilities than on other beneficiaries. Rehabilitation professionals in partnership with individuals in the population we serve will have to be vigilant in our monitoring of proposed cost-containment policies to ensure that access to needed services is not compromised in an effort to control costs.

Quality. The quality of care is the third discussion point in many debates about health care policy. How can the quality of care be maintained in an era of cost containment? What is quality care? How can an acceptable level of quality be determined? Two areas receiving considerable attention in this discussion are patient outcomes and clinical practice guidelines. The emphasis on outcomes is based on the increasing need to look at the effectiveness of care. A growing body of evidence shows that there is considerable variation in clinical decision making and health care delivery, resulting in differences in patient outcomes. Clinical practice guidelines are developed to control unnecessary variations in practice.

Patient Outcomes. Outcomes are patient focused and not discipline specific. In order to evaluate and improve the effectiveness of nursing care, it is necessary to identify which patient outcomes are most sensitive to intervention by professional nursing. Nursing's attention to patient outcomes is not a new phenomenon. Florence Nightingale spent much of her energy evaluating the linkages between intervention and outcomes with her statistics on mortality and morbidity in the Crimean War.

Many definitions of outcomes can be found in the literature. Outcome can be broadly defined as the end result of a treatment or intervention. Using outcomes as a measure of the quality of care provided requires an understanding of the complexity within outcomes. Four areas need to be considered (Lang & Marek, 1990). (1) What will the end-result outcome measure? Is it death, quality of life, symptom control such as continence, or cost? (2) When does the end point occur? Immediately after the treatment or intervention? Or, in the case of rehabilitation interventions, is it several months or years later? (3) What is the treatment or intervention? Is it a type of care delivery like case management or a specific intervention like bladder training? (4) What is the problem, diagnosis, or population for which the treatment or intervention is done and to which the outcome is related? Inherent within this is the need to recognize what patient or population characteristics will influence outcomes. Understanding the answers to these questions is important when using outcomes data in any phase of policy development.

The National Center for Medical Rehabilitation Research and the Agency for Health Care Policy and Research cosponsored a 1994 conference that resulted in an agenda for medical rehabilitation outcomes research. Included in the discussions were recommendations regarding philosophical issues, strategies and design issues, measurement of disability and handicap, and measurement of the quality of life and of health status in medical rehabilitation outcomes studies. Recommendations were also developed for specific disabling conditions including nervous system, cardiovascular, musculoskeletal, early development, and aging-related conditions

(Fuhrer, 1995). Research that furthers this agenda will assist in policy development addressing the organization, delivery, and financing of health services for individuals with chronic illnesses and disabilities. The ability to understand and apply outcomes research is a critical skill necessary for all rehabilitation professionals in order to improve the lives of persons with disabilities (Johnston & Granger, 1994).

One of the tools that will assist in the accomplishment of rehabilitation outcomes studies will be the development of and access to large clinical and administrative databases (Lange & Jacox, 1993). One example within the field of rehabilitation in which large databases are being used to explore the intersection of quality and cost issues in rehabilitation is the analysis of payment for outpatient services (Buchanan, Rumpel, & Hoenig, 1996) and several proposals for payment of inpatient rehabilitation on the basis of function-related groups (Harada, Sofaer, & Kominski, 1993; Stineman et al., 1994). Although large databases have great potential for worthwhile applications as discussed, there is a need to remain aware of potential limitations inherent within them. These limitations include questions about the reliability and validity of the data across hundreds of individuals entering it, the issue of missing data, and the inconsistency of the inclusion of structure, process, and outcomes data within the same data set.

Clinical Practice Guidelines. Clinical practice guidelines are being developed to identify and decrease unnecessary variability in practice and to assist practitioner and consumer decision making to improve the quality of care provided. Guidelines are systematically developed statements that convert science-based knowledge into specific clinical recommendations. The Agency for Health Care Policy and Research (AHCPR) devoted considerable resources to the development of multidisciplinary guidelines (Agency for Health Care Policy and Research, 1993), including several with direct application to rehabilitation in the areas of urinary incontinence, poststroke rehabilitation, and low back pain. The policy agency has described how to translate clinical practice guidelines into evaluation tools and how to use those tools to evaluate the quality of care provided (Agency for Health Care Policy and Research, 1995a, 1995b). Recommendations from nationally developed practice guidelines influence policy at many levels. They have the potential to influence access to services regulated by state and federal health care programs. Recommendations within practice guidelines about specific interventions may end up included in regulations about what services will be covered and in what frequency or duration. Practice guidelines also influence policy within individual health care institutions or agencies when they are used as a basis for the development of clinical pathways or algorithms used by practitioners within that agency.

LEGISLATION

Legislation is one way that policy is codified and enacted. The field of rehabilitation has been heavily influenced by several key policy initiatives that have come from legislation (Verville, 1988; Watson, 1979, 1988). A historical review shows that early legislation that affects rehabilitation unites rehabilitation services with gainful employment and return to work. This is seen in the Social Security Act of 1935, which included income assistance to blind persons, services to crippled children, funds to strengthen vocational rehabilitation, and regulations to universalize workers' compensation. Beginning in the 1940s there has been legislation that has a direct impact on the provision of rehabilitation services. The Barden-LaFollete Act (Pub. L. No. 78-113) passed in 1943 expanded vocational rehabilitation coverage to include medical rehabilitation services. The Veterans Bureau was also created through the Disabled Veterans Rehabilitation Act passed in 1943. This legislation authorized medical and other rehabilitation services for disabled veterans.

Present support for physical medicine and rehabilitation research and training programs funded by the federal government can be traced to the 1950s, when major revisions were made to the Vocational Rehabilitation Act (1954). The 1956 Amendments to the Social Security Act protected benefits for covered workers who became disabled through the authorization of the SSDI program.

The enactment of the Medicare and Medicaid legislation in 1965 had a tremendous impact on rehabilitation. Although established predominantly to provide coverage for episodic, inpatient acute care, it did include rehabilitation in the definition of services covered for both programs. Medicaid, designed to provide medical care to poor or medically indigent persons, has also become the major source of public funding for nursing home care. The 1965 Older Americans Act (OAA) provided supportive services to foster the independence of individuals older than 60

years to remain in their homes and community. Rehabilitation services were not specifically included in the original legislation, but changes in the 1992 reauthorization of the Older Americans Act did include limited references to rehabilitation services of age-related diseases and chronic disabling conditions (Torres-Gil & Wray, 1993).

The 1970s saw some of the most significant legislation affecting rehabilitation. The Rehabilitation Act of 1973 (Pub. L. No. 93-112) impacted both social and health-related areas of life and is viewed as one of the major pieces of civil rights legislation for individuals with disabilities. This legislation addressed employment, education, and the use of public facilities including transportation for individuals with disabilities. It also emphasized services to individuals with severe disabilities and created a federal program to support model spinal cord injury systems of care. The 1978 Amendments to the Rehabilitation Act of 1973 (Pub. L. No. 95-602) included Title VII, which created the Comprehensive Services for Independent Living program, a program intended to provide a variety of services to assist individuals with severe disabilities to live as independently as possible. The 1978 amendments also created the National Institute on Rehabilitation Research within the Department of Health, Education, and Welfare (now the National Institute on Disability and Rehabilitation Research in the Department of Education). Another event in the 1970s with an impact on rehabilitation was the creation of the Supplemental Security Income (SSI) program, which was included in the Social Security Amendments of 1972 (Pub. L. No. 92-602).

Legislation affecting rehabilitation continued into the 1980s; however, none of the legislation passed during this decade was as significant as that passed in the 1970s or that would be passed in the 1990s. The Surface Transportation Act (Pub. L. No. 97-424) provided tax incentives for the removal of barriers for those who were not required to do so by the Rehabilitation Act of 1973. Further amendments to the Rehabilitation Act of 1973 were passed in 1984 (Pub. L. No. 98-221) and 1986 (Pub. L. No. 99-506). Both pieces of legislation offered further clarification in areas of definition and emphasis for funding. The 1984 amendments were most significant for the modification made in the definition of "severely disabled" to include those 16 years or older. The 1986 amendments emphasized the rehabilitation needs of Native Americans, expanded the influence of the National Council on the Handicapped, and provided funding for rehabilitation engineering (Watson, 1988).

Two major pieces of legislation affecting rehabilitation were passed in 1990. The Americans with Disabilities Act (Pub. L. No. 101-336), signed into law on July 26, 1990, is landmark legislation that provides all Americans with disabilities equal opportunity and access in the areas of employment, state and local government services, transportation, public accommodation, and telephone services to that offered to the general public (Craven & Gleason, 1995). This legislation is believed by many to be the most far-reaching civil rights law ever enacted. The Americans with Disabilities Act included five titles: I, Employment; II, Public Services; III, Public Accommodations and Services Operated by Public Entities; IV, Telecommunications; and V, Miscellaneous Provisions. Title I prohibits discrimination by employers with more than 15 employees. It requires that "reasonable accommodations" be made unless "undue hardship" exists. The act defines reasonable accommodations to include: "(A) making existing facilities used by employees readily accessible to and usable by individuals with disabilities; and (B) job restructuring, part time or modified work schedules, reassignment to a vacant position, acquisition or modification of equipment or devices, appropriate adjustment or modifications of examinations, training materials or policies, the provision of qualified readers or interpreters and other similar accommodations" (Americans with Disabilities Act, Title I, Section 101[9]). Undue hardship means an action requiring significant difficulty or expense. This title prohibits discrimination in the job application procedure, hiring, advancement, or discharge of employees, employee compensation, job training, and other terms, conditions, and privileges of employment. It requires that pre-employment physical examinations not take place until after a job has been offered and that medical information cannot be kept in personnel files and must be treated as confidential. This title also provides protection to those who have successfully completed a drug or alcohol rehabilitation program.

Title II provides for access to public services and programs including public transportation. It requires that public entities that operate fixed route systems purchase buses that are accessible and provide complimentary paratransit or other special transportation services. Requirements for rapid, light,

and Amtrak rail systems to become accessible are also included in this title.

Title III addresses access to public accommodations and services operated by private entities. The act specifically names over 50 types of private entities including places of lodging, restaurants, bars, theaters, stadiums, convention centers, retail stores and shopping centers, museums, schools, social service establishments, recreation facilities, and service establishments such as laundromats, banks, gas stations, hospitals, and health care provider offices. Included in Title III are expectations regarding new construction and the alteration of existing places of public accommodation and commercial facilities as well as transportation provided by privately owned companies whose primary business is transporting people.

Title IV ensures that all Americans have access to the same communication services. It requires that carriers engaged in interstate communication by wire or radio provide special telecommunication relay devices to enable individuals with speech and hearing impairments to communicate on a level functionally equivalent to that of individuals without impairment.

The other important legislation that was passed is found in the National Institutes of Health Amendments of 1990 (Pub. L. No. 101-613). This legislation established the National Center for Medical Rehabilitation Research within the National Institute of Child Health and Human Development at the National Institutes of Health. The National Center for Medical Rehabilitation Research was created to support multidisciplinary medical rehabilitation research and research training; the development of orthotic and prosthetic devices; dissemination of health information; and other programs with respect to the rehabilitation of individuals with physical disabilities from diseases or disorders of the neurological, musculoskeletal, cardiovascular, pulmonary, or other physiological systems.

Much of the legislation previously described affected adults with disabilities. There has also been considerable legislation focusing specifically on children and including services and programs for children with disabilities (Hoeman & Repetto, 1992; Oberg, Bryant, & Bach, 1994). One of the earliest pieces of legislation that funded Crippled Children's Services was the Sheppard-Towner Maternity and Infancy Protection Act of 1921. Title V of the Social Security Act of 1935 established a federal-state system of services for crippled children. The Maternal and Child Health and Mental Retardation Planning Amendments of 1963 revised and expanded Title V. Included were the needs of young people with or at risk for chronic and disabling conditions. Six Title V programs were consolidated in the Omnibus Budget Reconciliation Act of 1981 (Pub. L. No. 97-35). One of the effects of this consolidation was an increase in the disparities in Medicaid eligibility between the Aid to Families with Dependent Children and Supplemental Security Income populations. These disparities were eventually addressed in legislation beginning in 1984.

There is also educational legislation that has had a direct impact on rehabilitation services for children. The Education of All Handicapped Children Act of 1975 (Pub. L. No. 94-142) amended to the Individuals with Disabilities Education Act (IDEA) established education as a right for all children between the ages of 5 and 17 years. This legislation provided for private school education at public expense if a child cannot be served in a public school setting. It also requires Individual Education Plans (IEPs) that delineate specific learning goals and objectives. Services include medical evaluation, psychological services, counseling, occupational therapy, physical therapy, speech pathology, audiology, and recreational therapy. Extension of these services to infants and toddlers with special needs was enacted with the 1986 Amendments (Pub. L. No. 99-457).

SUMMARY

Rehabilitation nursing has much to contribute to the area of health policy for individuals with chronic illnesses and disability. An understanding of access, cost, and quality can improve the ability of rehabilitation nurses to influence the development of health policy that will find the right balance between the principles of beneficence and autonomy. This, coupled with an appreciation of the legislative history of policy that has affected the field of rehabilitation, provides a context for evaluating present and future policy discussions. The future will continue to focus on the questions of access, cost, and quality. It appears likely that there will continue to be discussion about the appropriate roles of state and federal programs, including what services will be included in these programs and how those services will be paid for. Rehabilitation services were exempted from the changes in financing of Medicare-covered services ushered in by the diagnosis-related group (DRG) prospective-payment system. It is very unlikely that this exemption will continue for much longer. Changes in financing of rehabilitation services have the potential to affect quality and access. It is also very likely that there will be an increase in the discussion about the appropriate interface between public and private initiatives. This has recently been seen in legislation aimed at dictating minimal lengths of stay after the birth of a child or after a mastectomy for individuals covered by private insurance. With the advances in genetics, what role will legislation have in developing policy about private insurance coverage for individuals found to be genetically at risk for a chronic condition? Will legislation protect individuals from being dropped by private insurance companies because of results of genetic testing? The future is likely to provide different challenges, problems, and issues requiring the development of new and different health policy solutions. Understanding the role that policy and legislation has played in rehabilitation will allow rehabilitation nurses to become more effective participants in the various health policy arenas.

REFERENCES

Agency for Health Care Policy and Research. (1993). *Clinical practice guideline development* (AHCPR Pub. No. 93-0023). Rockville, MD: Author.

Agency for Health Care Policy and Research. (1995a). *Using clinical practice guidelines to evaluate quality of care: Vol. 1, Issues* (AHCPR Pub. No. 95-0045). Rockville, MD: Author.

Agency for Health Care Policy and Research. (1995b). *Using clinical practice guidelines to evaluate quality of care: Vol. 2, Methodology* (AHCPR Pub. No. 95-0046). Rockville, MD: Author.

Alecxih, L. M. B., Corea, J, & Kennell D. L. (1995). Implications of health care financing, delivery, and benefit design for persons with disabilities. In J. M. Weiner, S. B. Clauser, D. L. Kennell (Eds.), *Persons with disabilities: Issues in health care financing and service delivery* (p. 95). Washington, DC: The Brookings Institution.

Anderson, J. (1975). *Public policy making.* New York, NY: Praeger.

Banja, J., & Johnston, M. V. (1994). Ethical perspectives and social policy. *Archives of Physical Medicine and Rehabilitation, 75,* SC19–SC26.

Batavia, A. I. (1993). Health care reform and people with disabilities. *Health Affairs, 12(1),* 40–57.

Buchanan, J. L., Rumpel, J. D., & Hoenig, H. (1996). Charges for outpatient rehabilitation: Growth and differences in provider types. *Archives of Physical Medicine and Rehabilitation, 77,* 320–328.

Calkins, D., Fernandopulle, R. J., & Marino, B. S. (1995). *Health care policy.* Cambridge, MA: Blackwell Science.

Callahan, T. L., & David, R. (1995). Access. In D. Calkins,

R. J. Fernandopulle, & B. S. Marino (Eds.), *Health care policy* (p. 173). Cambridge, MA: Blackwell Science.

Cohen, W., & Milburn, L. (1986). What every nurse should know about political action. *Nursing and Health Care, 7,* 295–297.

Craven, G. T. A., & Gleason, C. A. (1995). Public policy and rehabilitation nursing. In S. Hoeman (Ed.), *Rehabilitation nursing* (p. 61). St. Louis, C. V. Mosby.

Dunn, W. N. (1981). *Public policy analysis.* Englewood Cliffs, NJ: Prentice-Hall.

Fuhrer, M. J. (1995). Conference report: An agenda for medical rehabilitation outcomes research. *Journal of Allied Health, 24,* 79–87.

Harada, N., Sofaer, S., & Kominski, G. (1993). Functional status outcomes in rehabilitation: Implications for prospective payment. *Medical Care, 31,* 345–357.

Hoeman, S. P., & Repetto, M. A. (1992). Legislation and children with special needs from 1903–1990. *Western Journal of Nursing Research, 14,* 102–105.

Johnston, M. V., & Granger, C. V. (1994). Outcomes research in medical rehabilitation. *American Journal of Physical Medicine & Rehabilitation, 73,* 296–303.

Kinney, E. D., & Steinmetz, S. K. (1994). Notes from the insurance underground: How the chronically ill cope. *Journal of Health Politics, Policy and Law, 19,* 633–642.

Lang, N., & Marek, K. (1990). The classification of patient outcomes. *Journal of Professional Nursing, 6,* 158–163.

Lange, L. L., & Jacox, A. (1993). Using large data bases in nursing and health policy research. *Journal of Professional Nursing, 9,* 204–211.

Miller, A. M., & Russell, K. M. (1992). Public policy analysis for registered nurses in a baccalaureate curriculum. *Nursing Connections, 5(4),* 17–24.

Murphy, N. J. (1991). Nursing leadership in health policy decision making. *Nursing Outlook, 40,* 158–161.

Oberg, C. N., Bryant, N. A., & Bach, M. L. (1994). Ethics, values, and policy decisions for children with disabilities: What are the costs of political correctness? *Journal of School Health, 64,* 223–228.

Pepper Commission (U.S. Bipartisan Commission on Comprehensive Health Care). (1990). *A call for action: Final report* (101st Cong., 2d sess. S. Rept. 113).

Rubin, S. E., & Millard, R. P. (1991). Ethical principles and American public policy on disability. *Journal of Rehabilitation 57(1),* 13–16.

Sherwen, L. N. (1992). Rehabilitation: The prototype for holistic health policy formation. *Holistic Nursing Practice, 6(2),* 84–89.

Stimpson, M., & Hanley, B. (1991). Nurse policy analyst. *Nursing and Health Care, 12,* 10–15.

Stineman, M. G., Escarce, J., Goin, J. E., Hamilton, B. B., Granger, C. V., & Williams, S. V. (1994). A case-mix classification system for medical rehabilitation. *Medical Care, 32,* 366–379.

Symington, D. C. (1994). Megatrends in rehabilitation: A Canadian perspective. *International Journal of Rehabilitation Research, 17,* 1–14.

Thomas, P. A., & Shelton, C. R. (1994). Teaching students to become active in public policy. *Public Health Nursing, 11,* 75–79.

Torres-Gil, F. M., & Wray, L. A. (1993). Funding and policies affecting geriatric rehabilitation. *Clinics in Geriatric Medicine, 9,* 831–840.

Verville, R. E. (1988). Fifty years of federal legislation and programs affecting PM&R. *Archives of Physical Medicine and Rehabilitation 69* (Special issue), 64–68.

Watson, P. G. (1979). Rehabilitation legislation of the seventies and the severely disabled. *ARN Journal, 4,* 4–6, 8–11.

Watson, P. G. (1988). Rehabilitation legislation of the 1980's: Implications for nurses as healthcare providers. *Rehabilitation Nursing, 13,* 136–141.

CHAPTER 6

Ethics in Rehabilitation Nursing

Shirlee Drayton Hargrove and Jean H. Woods

Rehabilitation nurses are committed to providing high-quality care to disabled individuals. Nursing interventions are designed to enhance the quality of life and to ensure respect for human dignity. On a daily basis, rehabilitation nurses encounter ethical dilemmas in patient care. These ethical dilemmas tend to have equally undesirable alternatives, involve divergent choices between potential courses of action, and have far-reaching implications for the patient, family, society, and health care providers.

The Standards of Professional Performance outlined in *Standards and Scope of Rehabilitation Practice* (Association of Rehabilitation Nurses, 1994) clearly state that the rehabilitation nurse's decisions and actions on behalf of the patient must be made and performed in an ethical manner. The guiding decision-making frameworks for solving ethical dilemmas often reside in ethical theories and principles in the Code for Nurses (American Nurses Association, 1985) and in moral obligations that translate into standards for nursing practice. When the rehabilitation nurse decides on a method or approach to ethical problem solving, the experiences, feelings, values, and cultural beliefs of the patient and family are considered and respected. This chapter provides an overview of ethical theories and principles; values clarification; religion and ethics; the ethics of managed care; patient rights; and patient advocacy.

THEORIES OF ETHICS

Definition

Ethics is the study of the human conduct, moral character, and motives inherent in deliberate human actions (Davis & Aroskar, 1983; Hamilton, 1992). Ethics is not an exact science, and ethical problem-solving processes do not yield a set of universal right actions. However, guided by ethical theories and principles, the nurse uses systematic decision-making processes to ascertain that

moral actions are undertaken on behalf of the patient, family, and community. Ethical theories provide the foundation for understanding dilemmas and the basis for problem solving and decision making (Brillhart, 1995).

Early Western Theories

Greek philosophers such as Socrates, Plato, and Aristotle explored the tenets that influence conduct and behaviors (Davis & Aroskar, 1983). The Socratic method of teaching through questions and answers continues to influence ethical problem solving today. Socrates believed that it was important to examine life and that it was good for human beings to discuss virtues. The Athenian philosopher Plato, a student of Socrates, recorded dialogues in which many dilemmas were debated. Plato wrote of truth, virtue, and the performance of truth. Later, Aristotle, a student of Plato, developed a deductive approach to understanding everyday problems. These early philosophers were among those who influenced modern ethical theories. Several of their theories influence rehabilitation nursing practice today.

MODERN ETHICAL PRINCIPLES

Two efficacious modern ethical problem-solving models are derived from the moral philosophies of Immanuel Kant, Jeremy Bentham, John Stuart Mills, and others. The *deontological* formalism espoused by Kant (Fig. 6–1) provides a duty-based orientation to ethical decision making (Yeo, 1991). Kant believed that actions were "good" if they could be applied universally regardless of the circumstances. He espoused a categorical imperative that humanity should always be treated as an end and never as a means. From a deontological perspective, certain actions are inherently wrong regardless of the outcome of the deed (Aiken & Catalano, 1994). Brillhart (1995, p. 45) outlined the underlying themes of deontological ethics as follows:

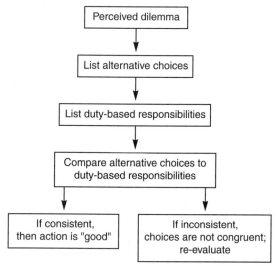

FIGURE 6–1
Deontology: A decision-making and problem-solving approach.

Rules are the basis for action.
A rule is good regardless of the result.
Rules represent intrinsic good.
Results help discover which rule applies.

Utilitarianism (Fig. 6–2) was espoused by Jeremy Bentham and John Stuart Mills. It provides a greatest-good orientation to ethics. From a utilitarian perspective, one acts best by making choices that produce the greatest good and the least harm for the greatest number of persons. Utilitarianism adds a majority,

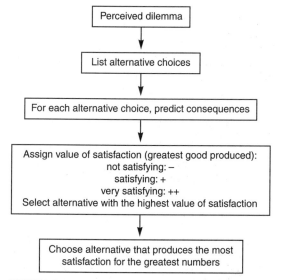

FIGURE 6–2
Utilitarianism: A decision-making and problem-solving approach.

democratic philosophy to decision making. The rehabilitation nurse with limited time might be forced to set priorities in care delivery and employ the utilitarian principle.

CODES AND PRINCIPLES

Standards of professional practice may be followed to guide nursing action in ethical dilemmas. The nurse must take steps to formally analyze situations. Nursing actions on behalf of disabled individuals and families must be consistent with guiding ethical theories and professional nursing principles as outlined in the American Nurses Association Code for Nurses with Interpretive Statements (Table 6–1). These statements guide the ethical conduct of the rehabilitation nurse. The nurse must be aware of the boundaries in the therapeutic patient-nurse relationship. There-

TABLE 6–1 ■ AMERICAN NURSES ASSOCIATION CODE FOR NURSES

1. The nurse provides services with respect for human dignity and the uniqueness of the client, *unrestricted* by considerations of social or economic status, personal attributes, or the nature of health problems.
2. The nurse safeguards the client's right to privacy by judiciously protecting information of a confidential nature.
3. The nurse acts to safeguard the client and the public when health care and safety are affected by the incompetent, unethical, or illegal practice of any person.
4. The nurse assumes responsibility and accountability for individual nursing judgments and actions.
5. The nurse maintains competence in nursing.
6. The nurse exercises informed judgment and uses individual competence and qualifications as criteria in seeking consultation, accepting responsibilities, and delegating nursing activities to others.
7. The nurse participates in activities that contribute to the ongoing development of the profession's body of knowledge.
8. The nurse participates in the profession's efforts to implement and improve standards of nursing.
9. The nurse participates in the profession's efforts to establish and maintain conditions of employment conductive to high-quality nursing care.
10. The nurse participates in the profession's effort to protect the public from misinformation and misrepresentation and to maintain the integrity of nursing.
11. The nurse collaborates with members of the health professions and other citizens in promoting community and national efforts to meet the health needs of the public.

From American Nurses Association. (1985). *Code for nurses with interpretive statements* (p. 1). Washington, DC: Author. Reprinted with permission from American Nurses Association. Copyright 1985, American Nurses Publishing, American Nurses Foundation/American Nurses Association, 600 Maryland Avenue, SW, Suite 100W, Washington, DC 20024-2571.

fore, the rehabilitation nurse must have either in-depth knowledge of ethical theories, principles, codes, rules, and the meaning of decision making among cultural groups, or access to a mentoring relationship that will offer assistance in formulating solutions.

Ethical principles of the rehabilitation nurse help to guide nursing practice behavior in regard to the patient, family, and society. Ethical principles are fundamental standards of judgment. They are not rules about what to do; rather, they describe relationships or the nature of things. Thus, ethical principles give rise to values. Values, in turn, point out obligations, and the obligations for the rehabilitation nurse include truthfulness, confidentiality, respect for privacy, and fidelity (trust). The following tenets of conduct and behaviors are among the most prominent principles guiding nursing practice (Davis & Aroskar, 1983).

Autonomy

The rehabilitation nurse respects the patient's right to information, right to choose to make decisions based on the information provided, and informed right to refuse treatment. Autonomy does not negate the interdependent nature of human beings with other human beings and the environment. The rehabilitation nurse supports patients' choices while being careful to avoid patients' risks to themselves and others.

Autonomy is exemplified in the management of a 65-year-old man who has recently sustained a mild right cerebrovascular accident: He requires minimal to moderate assistance with washing, dressing, and eating. His daughter plans to take him to her home. The rehabilitation team agrees that the patient could use someone in the home to assist him in his activities of daily living. The patient insists on returning to his own home with a part-time aide, thereby exercising his right of autonomy.

Beneficence

Beneficence is the duty to act in a manner with the intent to do good. Beneficence is exemplified in the following management of a 16-year-old male spinal cord–injured patient who refuses to allow the nurses to perform passive range-of-motion exercises: A nurse develops an educational plan for the patient with the goal of increasing the patient's knowledge of the critical importance of maintaining mobility after injury through range-of-motion exercises. The nursing intervention is influenced by the principle of beneficence.

Nonmaleficence

Nonmaleficence is the intent to avoid doing harm. The principle of nonmaleficence underlies many themes in the literature on health system reform. Health professionals are ethically mandated to refrain from overt or covert actions that impose harm (Hamilton, 1992). However, ethical difficulties emerge as a consequence of actions; unintended harm may occur. Concepts such as fair access, free choice, privacy, economics, paternalism, and equality may mask harmful effects on economically disadvantaged persons and at-risk, vulnerable communities.

Nonmaleficence is exemplified in the handling of a 16-year-old amputee patient who makes a remark with sexual overtones to the nurse in front of three other male patients: The nurse is embarrassed and angry. Although she is very upset, she leaves the room and states that she will discuss the concern with the patient later. The nurse waits to discuss the situation with the patient when the patient is alone. The nurse exercises the principle of nonmaleficence—the intent is to address the patient's inappropriate behaviors without embarrassment or insult to the patient's self-esteem.

Justice

Justice means to engage in fair practices. An example of justice is the following management of a patient who complains that his call is never answered when he rings for the nurse: The patient states that he observes the nurses spending time with the patient in the next room. The nurse discusses the patient's concern and agrees that they do spend extra time with the patient in the next room because the patient has many care needs. The nurses agree to make every attempt to reduce the patient's wait for the call to promote fair access. The nurses are employing the principle of justice in this situation.

Veracity

Veracity means to tell the truth. Veracity is exemplified in the following management of a C5 complete spinal cord–injured patient who asks the nurse if he will walk again: The nurse responds that no one really knows for sure, but it is likely that he may not walk. The nurse has also exemplified the principles of autonomy and nonmaleficence.

Utility

Utility is the intent to achieve the greatest good. Utility is exemplified by a rehabilitation nurse who has a very large assignment on an evening shift: She decides to spend a large portion of her evening delivering the discharge instructions for a patient who is scheduled for an early discharge in the morning. The nurse is aware that there were several morning patient admissions to the unit. Several patients who enjoy an evening bath have not received a bath, and she schedules them for an early morning bath before therapy. The nurse decides to ask the night nurses to set up a bath for one of her patients before leaving in the morning. The nurse has exercised the principle of utility based on her intent to achieve the greatest good.

Fidelity

Fidelity is the execution of duties and obligations. The rehabilitation nurse carries out duties and obligations to avoid injury to patients or breach of duty. Fidelity is exemplified by the rehabilitation nurse who spends numerous hours in the preparation of a teaching plan for the patient and future family caregivers. The plan is a nursing duty designed to maintain patient safety.

VALUES CLARIFICATION AND ETHICAL ANALYSIS PROCESS

Moral and ethical decision making begins with a clarification of basic values. Morals reflect standards of what is right versus what is wrong. Although values mirror what is important to a given way of life, ethics reflect our personal, professional, and cultural-societal-religious values. These basic values provide a guiding framework to how problems are solved, goals are set, and decisions are made. When faced with an ethical dilemma, the rehabilitation nurse must first assess her or his own personal cultural differences and values to attempt to clarify them in relationship to the dilemma. Values clarification is critical in determining the best ethical principle needed for decision making in situations in which no alternative choice seems acceptable.

Values and Ethical Principles

Values, morals, ethics, human rights, and legal frameworks are highly interrelated yet often noncomplementary. A patient may hold a value, such as the idea that life is not worth living after a devastating disability, whereas Western medical philosophy, codes of professional nursing, and the law would not guide the rehabilitation nurse to assist suicide. The rehabilitation nurse uses values for the protection of human rights.

The encounters of the rehabilitation nurse with clients are guided by the value system brought with the nurse. These systems of values and behavior relate to the ethical orientation of the nurse. Values clarification can help the nurse to recognize and establish a working philosophy that promotes quality of life, satisfaction, and integrity and to resolve some of the problems related to personal and professional identity. Values develop gradually as a person matures. A person forms value sets to be used in various roles and relationships of life. Value sets can be expanded and integrated into a relatively stable value system that is applied habitually. This habitual way of judging and acting is what constitutes integrity. The professional nurse exhibits a commitment to values and priorities that ranks above self-interest and strives to achieve high standards of performance.

Values Clarification Process

Values clarification is the process of personal decision making about morals and values. It is the process of focusing and organizing personal moral commitments and priorities, based on the need to clarify one's notions of right and wrong and systems of valued behaviors. This entails a process of gaining new insight through exposure to new information and different world views that are not consistent with the present value system, analyzing inconsistencies, and refining and redefining values and beliefs.

Nurses should be able to answer the question "What is important to me?" Value systems are concepts that are formed as a result of life experiences with family, friends, culture, education, work, and relaxation. The word *value* has positive connotations because it denotes worth or significance. Yet values also relate to negative characteristics. If nurses value honesty, then it follows that nurses do not value dishonesty. People are likely to hold strong values in their religious beliefs, family ties, sexual preferences, attitudes toward other ethnic groups, and sex role beliefs.

During the values clarification process, the individual is allowed to explore and rediscover personal values. The rehabilitation nurse must engage a process of self-exploration by assessing, exploring, and determining what the patient's personal values are and what priority they hold in the decision-making processes. The focus is placed on the process of valuing, not on the individual's value system. Raths, Harmin, and Simmons (1979) identified three steps in the process that can be applied to rehabilitation nursing practice:

■ *Choosing:* The rehabilitation nurse chooses freely from several alternatives and gives careful consideration to the consequences attending to each alternative after making the choice.
■ *Prizing:* The rehabilitation nurse is happy with the choice and is willing to voice to others the choice made.
■ *Acting:* The rehabilitation nurse puts the choice into action and is able to use the choice in other situations.

ETHICS OF MANAGED CARE

In the current managed care climate of health care delivery, there are many times when the rehabilitation nurse encounters patient problems in which there is a need for services and equipment but resources are too limited and rehabilitation services cannot be obtained. Disabled individuals are often represented among the ranks of uninsured, underinsured, and underserved populations. Patients are discharged from hospitals earlier than ever before. Many never receive the benefits of rehabilitation services. Rehabilitation practitioners and consumers face a major challenge in their attempts to ensure access to necessary services for disabled populations while ensuring minimal cost.

Priester (1992) and Reifsnider (1992) describe the problem of distributive justice. The conflict centers around whose care should receive the highest priority. Health care resources are scarce. Therefore, not every citizen may be able to obtain all the health care services that are available, desired, and needed. Is it morally preferable to distribute resources unevenly, with more benefits going to those people who can afford the best services? Human needs should be more prominent in solving this ethical dilemma. Because

the health of the population is so poor in underserved communities, it will take a multiplicity of services to elevate the health of the disadvantaged to a level equal to that of more affluent communities (Drayton-Hargrove & Woods, 1995).

In the process of attempting to do good, decision makers must confront the ethical effect of their determination of what constitutes a decent minimum of health care services. Conflicts emerge in defining the minimal standard and its universality. Stevens (1992) questioned who should determine the definition of *basic services*. Offering the less fortunate "basic" health services while the advantaged members of this society have access to higher technology and better services would exacerbate class, race, and gender stratification (Stevens, 1992, p. 243). Clarification of what constitutes the decent minimum is further complicated by the vague and undefined language that has been used to describe the scope of coverage. Common ambiguous phrases employed in the health care reform debate of the 1990s included "standard packages of health care," "health care for everyone," "basic packages," "fair access," and "universal access." All these terms are vague and subject to misrepresentation or misinterpretation by health care insurers and the medical community in general. Rehabilitation nurses employed in managed care systems are faced with ensuring efficiency and lower cost for the organizations that hire them while attempting to advocate for all the services that a disabled patient needs.

In addition to the ethical issues inherent in a managed care system, the nurse must consider the ethics of environmental systems. Many patients successfully go through inpatient rehabilitation programs after a disability, only to face environmental and social-attitudinal barriers that discriminate and inhibit successful integration into society and thereby limit their quality of life. Although the value of reintegration into society is articulated, disabled individuals continue to find difficulty accessing resources that are desired and needed. The rehabilitation nurse must engage in an advocacy role to ensure equality and fair access to health care resources.

RELIGION AND ETHICAL DECISION MAKING

Many religious teachings clearly outline moral concerns and influence values and decision-making processes. Understanding the central beliefs, rituals, and practices of various common religions may be helpful for the rehabilitation nurse (Table 6–2). These religious beliefs often influence one's spirituality. The duty to do good and avoid harm is clearly outlined in most religions. The Ten Commandments outlined in the Old Testament of the Bible describe humanity's duties to God and to other people. King Solomon's dilemma of the parenting of a baby by two women who both swore motherhood gives an early example of a decision-making process. King Solomon employed a decision based on cultural, religious, and value principles by suggesting that he would cut the baby in half. Knowing the women's value system, King Solomon knew that the mother would rather give up the child than see the child die. The rehabilitation nurse must consider religious and spiritual beliefs when employing the ethical analysis process.

PROFESSIONAL CODE OF ETHICS

The rehabilitation nurse considers professional tenets and patient rights when employing ethical decision-making and problem-solving models. The rehabilitation nurse ascertains that patients' rights are respected. The American Nurses Association long ago established codes of ethics to guide nurses' actions. These documents reflect nurses' duties to the patient and to the profession. Therefore, the rehabilitation nurse must have knowledge of professional ethical codes and patients' rights (see Table 6–1).

PATIENTS' RIGHTS AND ADVOCACY

The rehabilitation nurse is morally obligated to advocate for disabled individuals in particular. This advocacy role includes providing institutional standards and guidelines for practice, working collaboratively with interdisciplinary teams on institutional ethics committees, and working with legislative policy makers at the local, state, and national level. Even in an economically constrained era, policy makers must be continually reminded of the need for high-quality restorative care.

The disabled individual may express a loss of will to engage in activities of daily living after a devastating injury. The nurse must weigh the rights of the patient to choose and to determine an acceptable-level quality of life while simultaneously providing encouragement and balancing the obligations to do good and to avoid harm. The patient's expressed wishes and values must be honored whenever possible. In the advocacy role, the rehabilitation nurses provide education for patients related to rights. The American Hospital Association (1992) has developed A Patient's Bill of Rights to further and clearly outline expected obligations to patients (Table 6–3). Ethical legal documents and actions have further outlined the rights of patients in health care systems (Table 6–4).

AVOIDANCE OF HARM: NEGLIGENCE AND ABUSE TO PATIENTS

The rehabilitation nurse engages in actions that are designed to promote the quality of life of disabled clients. The nurse reports to the appropriate authority cases of actual or suspected abuse. When ethical dilemmas surface, the nurse presents issues to the interdisciplinary team and/or the institutional ethics committee for joint deliberations, problem solving, and decision making. The nurse is responsible to know the state mandates, rec-

---

TABLE 6–2 ■ RELIGIOUS BELIEF SYSTEMS

Protestantism: Protestants are believers in the Holy Trinity and followers of Jesus Christ. They follow congregational policy and the reformed tradition in worship and believe in individual freedom, in the separation of church and state, and in the baptism of voluntary, conscious believers. They are influenced by a set of values. Protestant ethics include ideas of strict compliance to law and the desirability of work, thrift, competition, and a profit motive in life.

Catholicism: Catholics are believers in the Holy Trinity and followers of Jesus Christ. They follow the ancient undivided Christian church and believe in the intercession of saints.

Judaism: Jews follow a religion based on the teachings of Moses and the prophets of the Old Testament, in the oneness of God, that the Messiah is yet to come, and observance of Jewish rules, tradition, and culture as a part of the religion.

Islam: Moslems are followers of the Islamic tradition, the teachings of prophet Mohammed, and the of the Holy Koran. They are believers in submission under the will of Allah, God.

Buddhism: Buddhists follow a religion based on the teaching of Gautama Buddha that teaches that right living enables the individual to obtain nirvana, a condition in which the soul can live outside the body and is free from all desire and pain.

Confucianism: Confucianists follow a system based on the teachings of Confucius that teaches virtues—respect of parents and ancestors; kindness; faithfulness; intelligence; and proper behavior.

TABLE 6-3 ■ AMERICAN HOSPITAL ASSOCIATION: A PATIENT'S BILL OF RIGHTS*

1. The patient has the right to considerate and respectful care.
2. The patient has the right to and is encouraged to obtain from physicians and other direct caregivers relevant, current, and understandable information concerning diagnosis, treatment, and prognosis.

   Except in emergencies when the patient lacks decision-making capacity and the need for treatment is urgent, the patient is entitled to the opportunity to discuss and request information related to the specific procedures and/or treatments, the risks involved, the possible length of recuperation, and the medically reasonable alternatives and their accompanying risks and benefits.

   Patients have the right to know the identity of physicians, nurses, and others involved in their care, as well as when those involved are students, residents, or other trainees. The patient also has the right to know the immediate and long-term financial implications of treatment choices, insofar as they are known.
3. The patient has the right to make decisions about the plan of care prior to and during the course of treatment and to refuse a recommended treatment or plan of care to the extent permitted by law and hospital policy and to be informed of the medical consequences of this action. In case of such refusal, the patient is entitled to other appropriate care and services that the hospital provides or transfer to another hospital. The hospital should notify patients of any policy that might affect patient choice within the institution.
4. The patient has the right to have an advance directive (such as a living will, health care proxy, or durable power of attorney for health care) concerning treatment or designating a surrogate decision maker with the expectation that the hospital will honor the intent of that directive to the extent permitted by law and hospital policy.

   Health care institutions must advise patients of their rights under state law and hospital policy to make informed medical choices, ask if the patient has an advance directive, and include that information in patient records. The patient has the right to timely information about hospital policy that may limit its ability to implement fully a legally valid advance directive.
5. The patient has the right to every consideration of privacy. Case discussion, consultation, examination, and treatment should be conducted so as to protect each patient's privacy.
6. The patient has the right to expect that all communications and records pertaining to his/her care will be treated as confidential by the hospital, except in cases such as suspected abuse and public health hazards when reporting is permitted or required by law. The patient has the right to expect that the hospital will emphasize the confidentiality of this information when it releases it to any other parties entitled to review information in these records.
7. The patient has the right to review the records pertaining to his/her medical care and to have the information explained or interpreted as necessary, except when restricted by law.
8. The patient has the right to expect that, within its capacity and policies, a hospital will make reasonable response to the request of a patient for appropriate and medically indicated care and services. The hospital must provide evaluation, service, and/or referral as indicated by the urgency of the case. When medically appropriate and legally permissible, or when a patient has so requested, a patient may be transferred to another facility. The institution to which the patient is to be transferred must first have accepted the patient for transfer. The patient must also have the benefit of complete information and explanation concerning the need for, risks, benefits, and alternatives to such a transfer.
9. The patient has the right to ask (about) and be informed of the existence of business relationships among the hospital, educational institutions, other health care providers, or payers that may influence the patient's treatment and care.
10. The patient has the right to consent to or decline to participate in proposed research studies or human experimentation affecting care and treatment or requiring direct patient involvement, and to have those studies fully explained prior to consent. A patient who declines to participate in research or experimentation is entitled to the most effective care that the hospital can otherwise provide.
11. The patient has the right to expect reasonable continuity of care when appropriate and to be informed by physicians and other caregivers of available and realistic patient care options when hospital care is no longer appropriate.
12. The patient has the right to be informed of hospital policies and practices that relate to patient care, treatment, and responsibilities. The patient has the right to be informed of available resources for resolving disputes, grievances, and conflicts, such as ethics committees, patient representatives, or other mechanisms available in the institution. The patient has the right to be informed of the hospital's charges for services and available payment methods.

*These rights can be exercised on the patient's behalf by a designated surrogate or proxy decision maker if the patient lacks decision-making capacity, is legally incompetent, or is a minor.

A Patient's Bill of Rights was first adopted by the American Hospital Association (AHA) in 1973. This revision was approved by the AHA Board of Trustees on October 21, 1992.

American Hospital Association. (1992). *A patient's bill of rights* [management advisory] (pp. 1–2). Chicago: Reprinted with permission of the American Hospital Association, copyright 1992.

ognize indicators of abuse or negligence, and attain knowledge of proper reporting mechanisms. In rehabilitation settings, the nurse often has the opportunity to work with families and assesses caregiver strain and frustration, substance abuse, and lack of knowledge. Early recognition of at-risk families can lead to facilitation of education and support.

TABLE 6–4 ■ SELECTED ETHICAL LEGAL PATIENT RIGHTS

The Patient Self-Determination Act: This law was passed by Congress in December 1991 to ensure that patients understand the right to consent and to make choices. Institutions are required to inquire if a patient has an advance directive and provide patients with the necessary information if needed.

Right to Die: This right is to decide medical treatment and decline services. This right is derive from common law, the U.S. Constitution, Amendment XIV, due process, and informed-consent laws.

Living Will: In response to the Patient Self-Determination Act, many states have passed living will laws. The living will becomes effective when a person becomes incompetent, has a terminal condition, or is permanently unconscious.

Durable Power of Attorney: This power is given by a competent person before becoming incapacitated to another competent person to act on the first person's behalf in cases in which the person cannot act on his or her own behalf.

Guardianship: This is a legal relationship involving a court-appointed person (guardian) to act on the behalf of another who cannot function independently (the ward).

Informed Consent: This consent involves the right to be notified and knowledgeable of treatment or inquiry performed and to give permission for the same.

Advance Directives: This document states an individual's preference and instructions to guide medical treatment in case the person becomes incapacitated in the future.

SUMMARY

The rehabilitation nurse employs ethical decision-making processes on a daily basis. The professional actions of the nurse are guided by morals, principles, and values, and an ethical decision-making framework is employed.

Professional codes and standards outline the nurse's duty to the patient and the profession. The nurse must engage in an ongoing process of values clarification and ethical analysis to explore and refine value systems. The rehabilitation nurse respects the values and ethical decision-making process of patients while employing the highest level of professional conduct in patient care.

REFERENCES

Aiken, T. D., & Catalano, J. T. (1994). *Legal, ethical and practice issues in nursing.* Philadelphia, PA: F. A. Davis.

American Hospital Association. (1992). *A patient's bill of rights.* Chicago, IL: Author.

American Nurses Association. (1985). *Code for nurses with interpretive statements.* Washington, DC: ANF/ANA.

Association of Rehabilitation Nurses. (1994). *Standards and scope of rehabilitation nursing practice* (3rd ed.). Skokie, IL: Author.

Brillhart, B.(1995). Ethics in rehabilitation nursing. *Rehabilitation Nursing, 20,* 44–47.

Drayton-Hargrove, S., & Woods, J. H. (1995). Ethical analysis of health care reform: Implications for diverse communities. *The ABNF Journal, 6,* 99–103.

Davis, A., & Aroskar, M. (1983). Ethical dilemmas and nursing practice. Norwalk, CT: Appleton & Lange.

Hamilton, P. M. (1992). *Realities of contemporary nursing.* Connecticut: Addison-Wesley Nursing.

Priester, R. (1992). A value framework for health system reform. *Health Affairs, 11,* 85–107.

Raths, L. E., Harmin, M., & Simmons S. B. (1979). *Values and teaching* (2nd ed.). Columbus, Ohio: Charles E. Merrill.

Reifsnider, E. (1992). Restructuring the American health care system: An analysis of nursing's agenda for health care reform. *Nurse Practitioner, 17,* 65–75.

Stevens, P. E. (1992). Equitable access to health care: Continuing the dialogue. *Scholarly Inquiry for Nursing Practice, 6(3),* 241–246.

Yeo, M. (1991). Concepts and cases in nursing ethics. Peterborough, Ontario, Canada: Broadview Press.

CHAPTER 7

Community-Focused Rehabilitation Nursing

Christine L. Nagy

COMMUNITY-BASED PRACTICE

The basic ingredients that made early community-based care or home care a cornerstone in American health care were still the foundations for community- or home-based nursing care in the 1990s and will be in the future. Once overshadowed by the centralization of patient care in the acute hospital setting, community or home care has stepped into a place of collaboration and cooperative health care with hospitals and nursing homes and is even branching out as a viable contender in today's health care reform arena.

Historical Overview

Home health nursing began in 1888 with the work of Lillian Wald and Lavinia Dock (pioneers in public health and American nursing), who made home visits out of a New York City mission and eventually started the Henry Street Settlement House (Zerwekh, 1992). From these humble beginnings of caring for and teaching hygienic practices to the "sick poor" at home grew the home health care and community-based agencies of today, which have provided care to millions of clients and have grown into a multimillion dollar industry that is recognized as a valuable health care system resource.

The basic ingredients of home nursing practiced in the 1800s remain the same for a home care nurse today. Because of changes in public needs, new developments in medicine and technology, and changes in the nuclear family structure, home visits in the present day are conducted in an entirely different world from that of our nursing pioneers.

There are four basic ingredients in community-based care. The first is the finding that patients overwhelmingly prefer to go home with qualified services than to remain within an acute care setting. The second ingredient is the unchanging direction of home nursing focus. Home care continues to focus on the relief of pain and suffering and education to prevent further discomfort. Added to this focus are today's concepts of restorative and rehabilitative care, which assist patients to function at their highest or most optimal levels and within their levels of physical limitation. The third basic ingredient is the goal that patients remain as the focus of all aspects of their health care and rehabilitation. The fourth and final ingredient is the provision of quality care and patient education that will promote independence and cost-effective health care practices in the home, as well as optimal health maintenance.

Dollars and "Sense"

The cost-effectiveness of home- or community-based health care is widely documented. In chronic obstructive pulmonary disease patients, a home respiratory/pulmonary rehabilitation program proved to be beneficial in the improvement in health status and in quality of life of 38 patients after their hospital discharge (American Journal of Nursing, 1995). In another study, a cardiac rehabilitation home program provided improved customer satisfaction while providing quality and cost-effective care and an enhanced patient quality of life (Green & Lydon, 1995). There is no question that patients recover from illness or injury much quicker in their own environment. Patients are also able to prevent infection and save money by using "clean" techniques instead of specific "sterile" techniques for home wound and catheter maintenance. Another way home care patients benefit is by decreased exposure to nosocomial infections. These hospital-acquired infections can be costly and take extensive time and staff effort to treat.

The evolution of the specialty practice of home- or community-based care from those early Henry Street Settlement days has reached a point where today the home is recognized as the preferred site for the provision of health and sickness care. In the July 28, 1993, issue of *Advance Data*, the U.S. Department of Health and Human Services Public Health Service defines home health care as "care provided to individuals in their places of residence for the purpose of promoting, maintaining, or restoring health, or for maximizing the level of independence while minimizing the effects of disability and illness, including terminal illness." It also defines the 8000 agencies in the 1992 National Home and Hospice Survey as "hospitals without walls" because "advances in technology allow dozens of complex illnesses once treated almost exclusively in the hospital to be treated at home."

The October 29, 1993, edition of *Morbidity and Mortality Weekly Report* includes a report called "Home Health and Hospice Care—United States, 1992" (Morbidity and Mortality Weekly Report, 1993). This article reports that an estimated 9.5 million persons in the United States have difficulty performing basic life activities because of mental or physical health conditions. It further states that "in recent years, an increasing range of home-care services, including home health care and hospice care, have been created for persons requiring long-term care, and access to such care programs has been increased through public programs such as Medicare and Medicaid." The results of this survey show that an estimated 1,237,100 patients received home health care during 1992 and that the most frequent diagnoses were diseases of the heart (12%), diabetes mellitus (8%), arthropathies and related disorders (6%), malignancies (6%), cerebrovascular accident or disease (6%), essential hypertension (4%), and fractures (4%). The remaining patients were grouped into mental or behavioral disorders, other musculoskeletal disorders, and nonspecific secondary or tertiary diagnoses.

These insights into the home health care industry lead us to consider the large impact home health practitioners can have on the future of health care reform. Home health care agencies provide a major segment of acute care in the United States. Although long-term care as well as preventive care is a critical part of the business of the home care industry, acute care is the current strength of the business, both in the number of patient visits and in reimbursement dollars. Complex high-technology procedures are managed safely by patients and caregivers in their homes with assistance from skilled home health care professionals. This is accomplished not only with a significantly lower rate of infections and hospital readmission but also at a lower cost than in the hospital or nursing home setting.

As a result, hospitals currently have reduced their lengths of stay by 35 to 50%. The patient census has fallen to about 60% in most hospitals, and home health care providers have effectively replaced one-third to one-half of the hospital beds in America. Therefore, it is imperative that home- or community-based care be a prominent player in any future health care reform activity.

Health care reform must balance all forms of care with the right of all Americans to coverage. These basic benefits should include skilled home care, home hospice care, and home restorative or rehabilitative care as an alternative to institutionalized care. Community health care professionals are concerned with public and nongovernmental decisions that shape the health care services and delivery system and affect access to care. Community health care professionals have special concerns related to adequate standards of living, appropriate and available health care, and social services for the underserved and at-risk populations. They work toward environmental management and preservation of community resources and empowerment of community members (Smith & Maurer, 1995).

Wellness, prevention, and restorative activities will be the cornerstone on which the future health care delivery system will rest. A continuum of care should be available across the life span, beginning with a system of preventive and follow-up care for all ages that culminates in long-term care for elderly persons. Despite the fact that 14 to 15% of the gross national product is spent on health care, and in 1996, national health care expenditures mushroomed to an astounding $1008 trillion, home care represents only 3.7% of this total amount (Fig. 7–1), but it remains the fastest-growing segment of the health care market.

The number of home care agencies operating in the United States has increased more than 200% since 1986, and home health care revenues have increased from $1 billion to over $20 billion over the past three decades (National Association for Home Care, 1992). Yet the United States, which offers the best health care in the world with state-of-the-art equipment and medical facilities, as well as advanced education and well-trained profes-

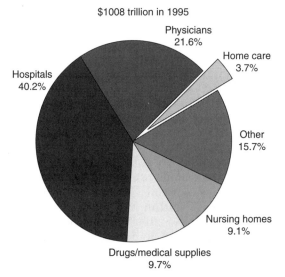

FIGURE 7–1
National health care expenditures in 1995. (Data from Office of National Health Statistics and National Association for Home Care. [1996]. *Basic statistics about home-care—1996.* Washington, DC: Author.)

sionals, is in a health care crisis of major proportions, and the crisis is representative of what the citizens are lacking. Millions of Americans are denied access to the full spectrum of medical services because there is not enough available funding. An estimated 42 million people, or one in seven, are uninsured, and 25 million are underinsured (Saucier, 1991).

More than 3 million children between the ages of 1 and 19 years suffer from chronic illness and require long-term care (O'Conner, Vander Platts, & Betz, 1992). The number of individuals needing long-term care is expected to rise with the increase in the elderly population and with continued improvements in medical technology that can save the lives of premature infants and lengthen the lives of persons with chronic disease. Our elected officials need to understand that home- and community-based care promise a new, cost-effective, quality-based future for health care.

Home care professionals must prepare themselves and their organizations for the responsibilities expected of them in their expanded roles as major providers of health care. Providers must be attuned to changes taking place at the local and state levels and continue to advocate for a cost-effective, quality health care delivery system. It is imperative that we look for solutions within our own agencies and communities while working for larger reforms at the national level. Fund-raising efforts to subsidize current programs or to expand the scope of current services are one way to respond to consumer needs. Instead of our setting up barriers to home care services, those services should be encouraged and ways found to provide them as efficiently as possible (Deets, 1995).

Present and Future

Health care reform is resulting in a myriad of changes in the current health care delivery system. Hospital mergers, buyouts, and acquisitions; managed care; and acute care facility closings are common. Acute hospital stays are shorter, and patients are being discharged much sooner than ever before. The acuteness of patients' conditions is higher now in the home setting, and patients are left with increased knowledge deficits in all areas of their health regimen. Hospitals are challenged by the goal to educate patients about how to care for themselves at home before discharge. As a result, the transition from the hospital to the home is sometimes very difficult and frightening for patients and their families.

In addition, advances in medical technology and knowledge have enabled health care professionals to provide an ever-widening array of multidisciplinary services and procedures in the same setting. With increasing hospital and insurance costs, more patient care is given in alternative care settings, and the number one community setting is the patient's home. But if community-based health care is to survive into the 21st century and beyond, a positive image with emphasis on quality and cost-effectiveness needs to be implemented and supported. Home health care providers will be expected to "do more with less," meaning less time, money, equipment, and insurance reimbursement and fewer medical supplies and resources. Home care providers will be expected to be more innovative and creative with patient care and treatment modalities. They will be required to continuously show a need for skilled services for a patient as well as progression toward medical and rehabilitative goals.

Quality home health care will embrace the concept of total client care: physical, psychological, spiritual, cultural, social, and economic well-being. More importantly, the skilled services required to help a patient achieve optimal functional levels of self-care, independence, and health recovery from illness or impairment will focus on rehabilitation or restorative concepts. And last but not least, home caregivers must provide less tangible elements of care such as compassion, patience, understanding, and emotional support.

ROLE OF THE HOME CAREGIVER

As more and more services shift from institutions and into community-based care, it is important to note that 80% of these health-related care-giving tasks are performed by a home care professional, friend, or family member (Blaines & Oglesby, 1992). Perhaps no role is more demanding than being a caregiver to someone who is seriously or chronically ill. Similarly, being ill or disabled enough to be dependent on a family home caregiver is an equally difficult situation that most persons hope never to face. By incorporating family and friends into the patient's care and rehabilitation program, home health care professionals are able to provide quality care in a comfortable as well as familiar recovery setting. Patients become more involved in their self-care activities because they choose when to eat, sleep, bathe, toilet themselves, and, within reason, take medications and exercise. These basic daily living activities are not dictated to them. They have some control over their health care and treatment decisions, and this ultimately promotes increased patient compliance and self-care independence.

It is estimated that 95% of home health care patients today have some rehabilitation need (Avillion & Scott, 1995). Rehabilitative services in home health care represent the essence of what home health care professionals strive for every day. They assist the client and the family or caregiver to maximize the patient's potential and quality of life within the limitations of the patient's disease or disability process. Furthermore, rehabilitation is by nature interdisciplinary and depends on the efforts of each home health care rehabilitation team member to help the patient to achieve mutual rehabilitation goals for optimal independence. This concept again reflects the essence of home health care in general as well as the purposeful inclusion of all persons who interact with the home care client on a daily basis.

Home health care professionals caring for people in their homes—whether nurses, aides, physical therapists, occupational thera-pists, or speech-language pathologists—are challenged by patients with multisystem dysfunction, multiple diagnoses, and complex disabilities. The rehabilitation team approach is imperative to meet these patients' needs successfully. The keys to the successful delivery of rehabilitative services are teamwork, collaboration, efficiency, patience, motivation, and ongoing education and patient or caregiver feedback.

The home health care team's therapeutic function and framework should be consistent with the purpose of maximizing the individual's potential within the environment in which the person is functioning. The rehabilitation goals should be mutually defined and have a patient-centered focus. The unique characteristic of rehabilitation is helping a person to achieve the highest functional level for which that person is capable. This philosophy of rehabilitation and its team approach necessitates the involvement of different home health care disciplines working together and offering their individual levels of expertise to achieve a positive outcome. The blending of these professional disciplines requires common values, collaboration, trust, frequent communication, and confidence in each other as well as compassion and respect for the patient and the home caregiver.

ASSESSMENT OF THE REHABILITATION CLIENT AND THE COMMUNITY SETTING

Between 34 and 43 million people in the United States have significant chronic disabilities (U.S. Department of Health and Human Services, 1990), and the number continues to grow each year. Of these people with disabilities, approximately 70% are unable to perform or have some limitation in their average daily living activities (play, school, work, self-care). The others are limited in their ability to perform nonmajor activities such as driving or climbing stairs.

Disabilities have a variety of causes and are not evenly distributed among the population. Although disability occurs in people of all ages, disability rates increase with age, and disability rates are higher among poor and elderly persons (U.S. Department of Health and Human Services, 1990).

Many terms are used to describe people who live with disabilities. To establish a common frame of reference, several terms are defined in Table 7–1.

TABLE 7–1 ■ DEFINITION OF TERMS

Chronic illness	The presence, accumulation, or latency of irreversible disease states or impairments that involve the total human environment. Chronic illnesses have different implications for different people and are never completely cured or prevented.
Impairment	The residual limitation resulting from disease, injury, or a congenital defect.
Functional limitation	The result of an impairment; refers to the loss of the ability to perform self-care tasks and fulfill usual social roles and normal activities.
Disability	The inability to perform some key life functioning. This term is often used interchangeably with *functional limitation.*
Handicap	The interaction of a person with a disability with the environment.

Modified from Dittmar, S. (1989). Scope of rehabilitation. In S. Dittmar (Ed.). *Rehabilitation nursing process and application* (p. 7). St. Louis: Mosby–Year Book.

The most important determinant of the extent of an individual's degree of disability is the person's environment. Disabilities may be handicapping in one situation but not in another.

The environment has a critical impact on the successful rehabilitation of a home health care patient. Environmental conditions and their influences must be coped with as patients learn to reintegrate themselves into the community. Physical barriers such as steps, curbs, public transportation, doorways, and the patient's immediate living space may significantly impede independent functioning. The psychosocial components or myths regarding individuals with disabilities can also inhibit or decrease a patient's motivation during the rehabilitation process. Community health care professionals must help to alleviate the fear in the community regarding disabled individuals and the apprehension some feel about allowing people with physical or emotional disabilities to live their lives to their fullest in relationships, recreation, and work.

Community health care professionals seek to prevent and decrease sources of handicaps, such as stereotyping, architectural barriers, and discrimination from others who fail to accommodate the needs of persons with chronic or temporary disabilities. Such interventions are all part of community-based rehabilitation.

REHABILITATION PROCESS IN COMMUNITY-BASED PRACTICE

Rehabilitation may be defined as a dynamic process that helps a disabled person to achieve optimal physical, emotional, psychological, social, or vocational potential in order to maintain dignity, self-respect, independence, and self-fulfillment (Hickey, 1992).

The general premise of rehabilitation fits nicely in the community setting because its objectives reach well beyond the individual needs of the patient. The focus includes successful community reintegration; continued access to health care; the availability of physical and interpersonal resources; safety; psychosocial and cultural concerns; and the promotion of a barrier-free environment for all persons with disabilities. The major focus of rehabilitation continues to be education, not only education for the patient and family but also ongoing education for all health care professionals, as well as reinforcement of wellness ideas in the general public.

Society has fostered the myth that individuals with disabilities must be cared for and should not or cannot live independently. The 1988 Fair Housing Amendments attempted to increase the access of individuals with disabilities to more housing opportunities (U.S. Department of Education, 1988). Since passage of these amendments, a variety of living arrangements have been made available for individuals with disabilities and their families, based on their income, functional status, and existing support systems. Examples of community living arrangements include nursing homes; group homes; transitional living; senior and disabled citizen housing; independent-living apartments; assisted-living apartments; and a variety of support services within the community that assist individuals to find a suitable living situation that is comfortable and safe and meets their specific needs.

Community health care nurses work with patients and their families or caregivers in a variety of settings. Schools, workplaces, clinics, and homes are the most popular settings. Medicare pays for inpatient rehabilitation and home health care services for elderly persons and other disabled individuals, regardless of age, who receive Social Security disability benefits. Rehabilitation services under Medicaid vary by state. Many private insurers and health maintenance organizations have insti-

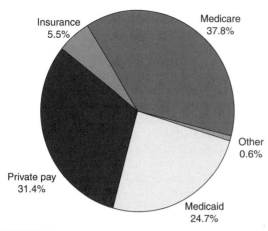

FIGURE 7–2
Payment sources for home care in 1996. (Data from National Health Statistics and National Association for Home Care. [1996]. *Basic statistics about homecare—1996.* Washington, DC: Author.)

tuted strict case management guidelines to control health care costs for those with severe disabilities (Ross, 1992) (Fig. 7–2).

REIMBURSEMENT FOR COMMUNITY-BASED SERVICES

Most community-based and home health care agencies are Medicare certified, and the majority of patients receive Medicare reimbursement for home health care services received. Home health care services that are eligible for Medicare reimbursement must be medically necessary, of a skilled nature, intermittent, and delivered to a home-bound beneficiary in his or her place of residence under a plan of treatment established by a physician. In addition, the total home care plan must be reviewed by the physician at least every 60 days. Medicare will not provide home health care coverage for custodial care or home-maker/chore-type services.

Primary qualifying services for Medicare reimbursement of home health care are skilled nursing, physical therapy, and speech therapy. If the patient is in need of at least one of these, the services of a home health aide or an occupational therapist, medical social work services, and medical supplies and equipment may also be provided in accordance with the physician's plan of treatment.

For an agency to be reimbursed by Medicare for services provided to clients, it must be Medicare certified, and this certification or accreditation means that an agency meets the conditions of participation, which include rules, standards, regulations, and specific criteria established by the federal government and stipulate what is defined as a minimal standard for patient safety and quality of care. A community agency that is accredited seeks to demonstrate to consumers that it far exceeds the minimal standards for a quality patient operation and has achieved a standard of excellence that is superior to that of its nonaccredited competitors in the community home health care marketplace.

There are two accreditation programs for home health agencies throughout the United States: the Community Health Accreditation Program, administered through the National League for Nursing (Mitchell, 1992), and the Home Care Accreditation Program of the Joint Commission on Accreditation of Healthcare Organizations (Rooney & Biere, 1992). Both programs require the agency to conduct a thorough self-evaluation and report of the agency and its protocols and procedures. An unannounced, on-site inspection and survey is also conducted by peer reviewers. On the basis of a successful survey outcome, the accrediting agency, either the Community Health Accreditation Program or the Joint Commission on Accreditation of Healthcare Organizations, makes a determination as to whether the agency will or will not be accredited.

In 1981, as a result of the Omnibus Reconciliation Act, home- and community-based care waivers were made available to individual states under their respective Medicaid programs. These waivers allow matching federal dollars for reimbursement of services not normally covered under the Medicaid program. The services provided must be adequate to meet the patient's home health care needs and must cost less than institutionalization. Fortunately, unless a patient becomes seriously ill at home, or the existing primary caregiver can no longer care for the patient safely or adequately in the home setting, Medicare programs can cover the majority of patient home care expenses, but this may not be the case in the future. Community-based agencies must be prepared for capitation of home health care costs, increased scrutiny of Medicare spending dollars, and compliance with interim payment systems enforced by the federal government and as described in the 1997 Balanced Budget Act.

Impact of the Balanced Budget Act and Home Health Services

On August 5, 1997, the Balanced Budget Act (BBA) was signed into law; it subsequently transformed the entire arena of home- and community-based care. Inappropriate use of services has been an identified problem for the Medicare program, and the goal of the BBA is to balance the federal budget and maintain solvency of the Medicare program until 2010. The BBA poses challenges to home care providers as well as the beneficiaries. Home care service providers have been forced to alter their previous modes of delivery of service and not only be cost-effective but also deliver quality care in a limited-visit environment. The Congressional Budget Office estimates that the BBA will reduce Medicare home care expenditures by $16.2 billion over a 5-year period.

Home care is reimbursed under Medicare Part A and Part B. However, as there are currently no coverage limitations on the number of visits under Part A, the majority of home care claims are reimbursed from Part A. Medicare Part A is funded by the Medicare Trust Fund. Medicare Part B is funded by a premium share paid by the beneficiary and the general treasury. The BBA mandates many changes in the overall arena of home care. Not only does the BBA restructure the reimbursement aspect of home care services, but it also mandates changes in the structure and delivery of these services.

There are several other changes that are affecting home care as mandated by the BBA. Medicare reimbursement now requires that all Medicare-certified agencies wishing to care for Medicare beneficiaries have a surety bond in place, be subject to formal policies on audits, and comply with protocols clearly defining part-time, intermittent care for delivery to strictly homebound patients. Another change is the exclusion of venipuncture as a qualifying skilled service, although a new legislative bill has been proposed that would halt this exclusion.

Reimbursement for home care services is based on an episodic prospective payment system that became effective on October 1, 1999. The process of determining the prospective payment system is very broad, with the intent of decreasing Medicare costs another 15%. Until the prospective payment system is in place, an interim payment system (IPS) has been established, and it is this system that currently has home care agencies extremely concerned. IPS reimburses home health care providers the lesser of (1) their actual, allowable costs, (2) the per-visit cost limit (which has been reduced from 112% to 105% of the

national median), or (3) a per-beneficiary annual limit.

Both the new per-visit cost limits and the per-beneficiary annual limit are applied in the aggregate. The IPS has been in effect for home care cost-reporting periods since October 1, 1997.

The new per-visit cost limits have been published by the Health Care Financing Administration (HCFA) *Federal Register.* These new limits reflect a reduction of approximately 20%. HCFA has estimated that about 65% of all home care agencies will have costs that exceed limits, whereas the National Association for Home Care estimates that this figure is more likely to be closer to 75%. It is also estimated that 30 to 40% of previously Medicare-certified home care agencies will not be able to meet the surety bond requirements and therefore will be forced to discharge or not admit Medicare patients. Most of those same agencies may also be forced out of business owing to financial losses.

The new IPS as it currently stands will not reimburse agencies at an adequate level to continue to provide the care their patients need. Many agencies will have to limit the services they provide, which in turn could affect patient accessibility to services. Home care agencies find themselves attempting to drastically cut costs per visit and costs per patient. These cost-containment measures can be done only by controlling the overall number of visits provided to patients. These visits and limitations pertain to all disciplines involved in the patient's care at home.

Another real concern with IPS is for the beneficiaries. The patients who need the most care are the first to be examined for reduced services and possible discharge. As reimbursement decreases, home care agencies will be discouraged from accepting patients who have high needs or are chronically or critically ill. These patients are at risk to be denied or lose necessary care.

Medicare recipients make up the majority of home health care patients, and with the burden of care falling onto the families and personal caregivers of home care patients, families will find themselves financially, physically, and emotionally strained to meet these new care needs. Critics of the IPS are also quick to point out that although home care is slated to take 14% of the Medicare cuts, it makes up only about 9% of the overall Medicare budget.

Fortunately, home health care agencies,

community-based service organizations, medical professionals, legal specialists, and the general public are beginning to band together to advocate strongly for patients' rights in regard to provision of home care services. Agencies will not be allowed to abandon care or refuse necessary services to a client in need unless there is a very specific and legitimate reason that those services could not be reasonably or safely performed in the home setting.

Home health care agencies will need to look at their current patient census and begin to work more efficiently and cost-effectively. They will need to develop protocols for future admissions, quality assurance, care planning, and the coordination of patient services without jeopardizing the quality of care. Finally, they will need to collaborate as a team, invoking the services and expertise of all home health care professionals in a variety of community settings to achieve the highest positive outcome measurements possible.

PROVISION OF COMMUNITY-BASED SERVICES

There are many types of community home health care agencies. In the early days of home health care, most services were delivered by a traditional visiting nurse performing only a small number of basic medical-surgical–type interventions. In some parts of the country, this continues to be true; however, in most of the country, a variety of agencies provide a multitude of different home health care services to meet the needs of a variety of patients. The majority of home health care agencies are categorized as official, proprietary, and hospital-based agencies.

Official or public agencies are supported by tax dollars and are given power through statutes enacted by legislation. Examples are state and local health departments with a nursing division. Traditional public health nursing (care of the sick poor, care of the sick homeless, and preventive care) also falls into this category. There has been a gradual decline in the services of this type of agency, mainly owing to decreased federal funding and a lack of qualified personnel.

Many community health agencies are governed by a volunteer board of directors and are supported primarily with nontax funds such as donations and endowments and third-party-payer reimbursement. They are considered to be mainly community based because of the wide range of services provided throughout a large geographical area. These agencies are nonprofit and therefore tax-exempt. The nonprofit status implies that the accrued profit goes back into the daily operative functioning of the agency. Two examples of voluntary agencies are the Visiting Nurse Association and the United Way.

Private agencies can be either for profit or not for profit. These agencies are governed by a board of directors or by the agency's owner. The majority of private community agencies are proprietary, which simply means they make a profit on the home care they provide. Proprietary agencies make up the largest group of home health care agencies in this country. These companies are not tax-exempt, and there is no requirement that the profits go back into the agency operations.

Hospital-based agencies began in large numbers during the 1980s to maintain clients within their health care system, provide a more comprehensive program of health care services, provide continuity of care, and increase hospital stability and revenue. The majority of patient referrals come directly from the hospital or hospital physician staff.

Home care aide agencies provide only paraprofessional services to clients, such as homemaking, companionship, or custodial care. These agencies are privately owned and operated and receive direct payment from the patient or private insurance company.

Certified hospice care agencies receive certification from the federal government as Medicare hospice providers. Hospice home care has grown as a result of a trend toward providing terminal care in the comfort of a patient's home. Some hospices are freestanding and others are part of a larger organization such as the Visiting Nurse Association. Reimbursement comes from Medicare, a private insurance company, or the patient.

Community home health care agencies have the ability to serve a variety of client needs. Services currently range from the traditional skilled nursing tasks of wound management, infusion therapy, diabetic teaching, and cardiopulmonary functional monitoring to pediatric and geriatric programs, maternal-child assistance, ventilator-dependency, and cardiac and pulmonary home rehabilitation programs to spinal cord injury and ortho/neuro rehabilitation with the specific intervention of a home health care therapist. Home health care professionals also deal with chronic pain management and a variety of musculoskeletal disorders.

REHABILITATION NURSE IN THE COMMUNITY SETTING

"Rehabilitation nursing is the diagnosis and treatment of human responses of individuals and groups to actual or potential health problems stemming from altered functional ability and related altered lifestyle" (American Nurses Association & Association of Rehabilitation Nurses [ANA & ARN], 1988). Community health nurses who provide rehabilitation must be skilled in providing comfort and therapy, promoting adjustment and coping, supporting adaptive capabilities, and promoting achievable independence and meaning to life (ANA & ARN, 1988).

Conditions necessitating rehabilitation in the home are numerous. By the year 2030, 55 million Americans, or nearly one person in five, will be older than 65 years. The elderly population is the fastest-growing age group in this country (National Association for Home Care, 1996). Persons in this age group and those who are disabled as a result of a chronic illness currently make up the majority of patients requiring rehabilitation services (Avillion & Mirgon, 1989). Long-term disabilities such as arthritis, atherosclerosis, and osteoporosis are very common among older patients requiring home rehabilitation. Sudden or critical illnesses such as heart attacks and strokes, which often leave the patient with long-term residual effects in mobility, self-care, elimination, thought processes, and speech, can be devastating.

The residual effects of a traumatic injury such as traumatic brain injury, spinal cord injury, amputation, or multiple fractures often require the patient to learn and adapt to many changes in lifestyle, and often the patient will deal with chronic pain and discomfort for the rest of his or her life. Mobility, the ability to work, sexual identity, self-concept, and self-worth are always affected in these patients. Wound healing and infection are a constant threat. Financial hardship due to an inability to work and/or inadequate health insurance coverage may also be present.

Many areas must be assessed to facilitate community reintegration for rehabilitation patients with disabilities of all degrees. The extent of community services the individual requires must be determined. It is imperative to establish the amount of care required for the patient and to establish who will be assisting the patient in the home setting. The home health care professional and more specifically the rehabilitation nurse will be responsible for teaching the appropriate and safe physical care of the patient and for referral for any other resources to which the patient may be entitled.

Psychosocial issues are important as well. The patient, in order to complete a successful course of rehabilitation, must remain positive and motivated to achieve the highest functional level possible. The patient's educational and vocational interests should be explored. Family or spousal roles will have to be altered and adapted too. Sexuality issues may also need to be addressed. The nurse must also be well versed in areas of cultural sensitivity in a variety of settings. Acknowledgment of and respect toward particular cultural or religious practices must also be components of all aspects of home care and treatment to fully meet the needs of the client in the client's community reintegration.

Cultural Sensitivity in Community-Based Nursing

As Spruhan (1996) suggests, "Culture affects all areas of the home health clients' life, including their beliefs about health and illness. Home care nurses must consider the clients' cultural values in planning effective and culturally competent nursing care." And further, "Getting in touch with one's own heritage helps nurses to understand and appreciate the cultures of others."

According to Rempusheski (1989), culture can be defined as "the communal life view of a particular group, including its beliefs, rituals, symbols, language and dietary practices." Such beliefs can and are passed from generation to generation with great pride and respect. Other components of culture include education, communication style, time and personal space issues, personal family rituals, and beliefs about health and illness (Niederhauser, 1989).

The home health care nurse must have a basic understanding of the client's beliefs about health and illness because this can have a significant impact on the client's compliance with the home care program. It is important for the nurse to provide home health care interventions that do not embarrass or intimidate the client or family. The nurse should respect the use of certain folk or home remedies and incorporate their use into the home plan of treatment whenever possible. The client's refusal of certain home care interventions should be respected and alternatives to care offered as applicable.

Cultural and spiritual assessments should be performed as part of the initial home admission visit. The home health care nurse should use culture-specific teaching materials whenever possible as well as gain assistance from specific cultural or religious community agencies to assist with any psychosocial or socioeconomic needs that may arise.

As the home health rehabilitation patient adapts within and continues to modify his or her own environment, the home health care professional must continually assess the patient's health problems and community reintegration needs. Table 7–2 lists guidelines for assessing health problems and barriers for persons with disabilities in the community. Access to reasonable health care; the availability of physical and interpersonal resources; safety; psychosocial concerns; and the promotion of a barrier-free environment are essential for patient well-being (see Table 7–2).

In summary, to be an effective community health care professional, one must use all available resources to benefit the patient and ultimately achieve specific rehabilitation goals and promote patient health and wellness.

Resources

Many times, clients need services not provided by the primary home caregiver or even the primary home health care agency. Home health care rehabilitation professionals and case managers must be knowledgeable about the many community resources available to meet the needs of the patients in their homes. Simply defined, a community resource is any agency, organization, program, or individual that delivers a service to the residents in the community (Nuzzo-Milone, 1995). Sources of information can easily be obtained from any local telephone directory or a directory of organizations and services sponsored in a specific city or geographical area. The United Way can be useful in assisting home health care providers and the clients that they serve to locate the specific type of assistance that is needed. It is also strongly encouraged that each home health care agency, as part of its initial staff orientation program, provide a listing of area-specific community resources for individual home health care professionals to use in the field and keep handy as a personal reference. Table 7–3 lists some national resources that may also provide useful information regarding home and community-based patient health care.

It is also encouraged that home health care and rehabilitation professionals seek out the assistance of their own professional organizations for further information on available resources. An encyclopedia of associations is available, as well as a U.S. government manual (1988) by the Office of the Federal Register of the National Archives and Records Administration. This is a very thorough listing of government agencies and state and locally sponsored community organizations.

Community Nursing Interventions With the Rehabilitation Client

The goal of community-based or home rehabilitation is to move patients to a point of optimal physical functional ability and increase the patients' health, well-being, and quality of life within the limitations imposed by their current health or disability status. Dittmar (1989, p. 6) stated that the goal of rehabilitation is to "facilitate the movement of individuals toward independence while helping them satisfy their needs. Therefore the approach is holistic, caring, and optimistic."

Additionally, the home health care agency has a responsibility to (1) provide care that meets the needs of the patient, as ordered by the physician; (2) coordinate the care provided by all home health care professionals involved in the case, so that all are working toward common medical as well as rehabilitative goals; (3) ensure that the patient and the primary home caregiver agree about the established goals, treatment plan, and home health care guidelines; and (4) ensure that the care provided meets eligibility criteria for reimbursement of services as appropriate.

The responsibilities of the community health nurse in rehabilitation are varied and challenging. Rehabilitation nurses in the community have an expertise derived from a variety of areas and a variety of traditional nursing roles. Dealing with patients in the home setting and assisting them to adapt and modify their everyday living routine are challenging and sometimes frustrating. Nurses need to remain flexible and creative in their home care interventions.

The rehabilitation or restorative nurse in the community takes on the multiple roles of caregiver, client advocate, team leader, educator, consultant, and case manager.

TABLE 7–2 ■ GUIDELINES FOR ASSESSING COMMUNITY REINTEGRATION NEEDS OF PERSONS WITH DISABILITIES

Access to Health Care

Are health care facilities architecturally accessible?

Does the client have access to either private or public transportation that may be used by a person with his or her specific disability?

Are needed health care programs available? (Substance abuse treatment programs may not be accessible or available.)

Are health care programs financially accessible?

Are negative attitudes on the part of the client, family, or health care professionals prohibiting adequate health care? (Feelings regarding sexuality or employment capability may have a major impact on community reintegration.)

Does the client want to promote his or her own wellness?

Availability of Community Resources

Are community resources financially, attitudinally, and architecturally accessible?

Are the sources used credible?

Do the client and/or family know how to locate resources? This may be a particular problem in a rural area where resources and transportation may be limited.

The telephone book may be a valuable resource for locating community resources. Do the client and/or family have the necessary reading and verbal skills to use this method?

Has the rehabilitation team investigated community resources available in the client's environment, and has the team notified both the client and the resources?

Does the health care professional make it a point to network with key community resource personnel?

Safety

Has the home been assessed for potential safety problems?

Do the client and/or family know how to assess workplaces, schools, and recreational areas for potential problems?

Does the client have a plan in the event he or she must summon help? (For example, how will a person with a communication disorder report an emergency situation over the telephone?)

Has crime prevention been addressed? An individual using a wheelchair may be especially vulnerable to street crime.

Psychosocial Issues

What role changes have taken place as a result of the client's disability?

What are the financial resources, and what effects do they have on wellness?

If the person with a disability requires assistance with activities of daily living, are other members of the family unit feeling neglected by the caregiver?

Is the caregiver given a chance to grieve? Is the caregiver devoting all of his or her energy to the person with the disability and is the caregiver in danger of compromising his or her own wellness?

Has the family been assessed for adequate coping skills?

Are the cultural and spiritual needs of the client and family being addressed?

Does the client have emotional as well as physical support systems?

Are the developmental tasks of the client and family being addressed?

Promotion of a Barrier-Free Environment

What attitudinal barriers exist in the client's environment?

Are there feelings that individuals with disabilities cannot adequately work, attend school, or enjoy leisure activities?

How is the client's sexuality viewed by him- or herself and others?

Does the client have a negative outlook? Does he or she avoid interpersonal relationships or refuse to maintain wellness, look for a job, attend school, or interact with the health care system?

Is there adequate housing for individuals with disabilities?

Is there barrier-free public and/or private transportation?

If the client requires 24-hour caregivers, how are these persons located, evaluated, and trained?

Are the client's place of worship, school, work setting, and shopping facilities accessible?

What advocacy groups exist in the community? What barriers to these groups exist?

Do health care providers have feelings that negatively influence their ability to provide adequate care for the disabled?

Are there cultural or religious barriers that need to be incorporated into the home care program?

Have the client and/or family been taught to plan ahead when going to a new setting for the first time? Are schools, restaurants, and stores assessed before attending?

What provisions are available for travel and vacations?

Adapted from Smith, C., & Maurer, F. (Eds.). (1995). *Community health nursing: Theory and practice.* Philadelphia: W.B. Saunders.

TABLE 7–3 ■ NATIONAL AND REHABILITATION HOME CARE RESOURCES

Alzheimer's Disease and Related Disorders Association, Inc.
919 N. Michigan Avenue, Suite 1000
Chicago, IL 60611
(800) 272-3900

American Association of Neuroscience Nurses
224 N. Des Plaines
Chicago, IL 60661
(312) 993-0043

American Association of Retired Persons
1909 K Street NW
Washington, DC 20049
(202) 872-4700

American Association of Spinal Cord Injury Nurses
75-20 Astoria Boulevard
Jackson Heights, NY 11370
(718) 803-3782

The American Cancer Society
1599 Clifford Road NE
Atlanta, GA 30329
(800) 227-2345

American Diabetic Association
430 N. Michigan Avenue
Chicago, IL 60611
(312) 899-0046

American Foundation for the Blind, Inc.
15 W. 16th Street
New York, NY 10011
(212) 620-2000

American Health Care Association
1202 L Street NW
Washington, DC 20005
(202) 842-4444

American Heart Association
7320 Greenville Avenue
Dallas, TX 75231
(214) 373-6300

American Lung Association
1740 Broadway
New York, NY 10019
(212) 315-8700

American Nurses Association
600 Maryland Avenue SW
Washington, DC 20024
(202) 554-4444

American Public Health Association
1015 15th Street NW
Washington, DC 20005
(202) 789-5600

Arthritis Foundation
1314 Spring Street NW
Atlanta, GA 30309
(404) 872-7100

Association of Rehabilitation Nurses
5700 Old Orchard Road
Skokie, IL 60077
(708) 966-3433

Clearinghouse on Health Indexes
National Center for Health Statistics Center
Division of Epidemiology and Health Promotion
3700 East-West Highway, Room 2-27
Hyattsville, MD 20782
(301) 436-7035

Commission on Accreditation of Rehabilitation Facilities
101 N. Wilmot Road, Suite 500
Tucson, AZ 85711
(602) 748-1212

Department of Housing and Urban Development
HUD Building
Washington, DC 20410
(202) 755-5720

Information for Individuals with Disabilities Hotline
(617) 727-5540

Joint Commission on Accreditation of Healthcare
  Organizations
One Renaissance Boulevard
Oakbrook Terrace, IL 60181
(708) 916-5600

National Amputation Foundation
12-45 150th Street
Whitestone, NY 11357
(718) 767-0596

TABLE 7–3 ■ NATIONAL AND REHABILITATION HOME CARE RESOURCES *Continued*

National Association for Hearing and Speech Action Line
(800) 638-8255

National Association for Home Care
519 C Street NE
Washington, DC 20005
(202) 547-7424

National Clearinghouse for Mental Health Information
5600 Fishers Lane
Rockville, MD 20857
(301) 443-4517

National Council on Child Abuse and Family Violence
1155 Connecticut Ave NW, Suite 400
Washington, DC 20013
(800) 222-2000

National Diabetes Information Clearinghouse
Box NDIC, 9000 Rockville Pike
Bethesda, MD 20892
(301) 468-2162

National Head Injury Foundation
1776 Massachusetts Ave NW
Washington, DC 20036
(202) 296-6443

National Hearing Aid Helpline
(800) 521-5247

National League for Nursing
Community Health Accreditation Program
350 Hudson Street
New York, NY 10014
(800) 669-1657

National Multiple Sclerosis Society
205 East 42nd Street
New York, NY 10017
(212) 986-3240

National Nurses Society on Addictions
5700 Old Orchard Road
Skokie, IL 60077
(708) 966-5010

The National Osteoporosis Foundation
2100 M Street NW, Suite 602
Washington, DC 20037
(202) 223-2226

National Rehabilitation Information Center
8455 Colesville Road, Suite 935
Silver Spring, MD 20910
(800) 346-2742

National Stroke Association
300 East Hamden Avenue Suite 240
Englewood, CO 80110
(303) 762-9922

Occupational Safety and Health Administration
Office of Public and Consumer Affairs
U.S. Department of Labor
200 Constitution Avenue NW
Washington, DC 20210
(202) 523-8148

The Parkinson's Disease Foundation
Columbia–Presbyterian Medical Center
650 West 168th Street
New York, NY 10032
(800) 457-6676

Public Health Service AIDS Information Hotline
(800) 342-AIDS

U.S. Department of Health & Human Services
330 C Street SW
Washington, DC 20201
(202) 205-8611

U.S. Public Health Service
200 Independence Avenue SW
Washington, DC 20201
(202) 245-7694

Visiting Nurse Association of America
3801 East Florida Avenue, Suite 900
Denver, CO 80210
(303) 629-8622

The role of caregiver is always first and foremost. A nurse must promote positive home medical management techniques, environmental safety, and preventive rehabilitation nursing interventions to ensure that clients reach their maximal functional capabilities and to avoid further disability and prevent medical or physical complications.

The rehabilitation nurse serves as an advocate for the client and the family and acts as an agency for change to empower the client and the family to evaluate options and plan outcomes. This requires that clients and families work as partners or team members with home health care professionals to accomplish mutually established rehabilitation goals.

Rehabilitation nurses further serve as team builders or leaders among professional colleagues and collaborate among various home health care disciplines. They serve as educators, consultants, and rehabilitation case managers and utilize all rehabilitation disciplines to achieve the patient's outcome goals.

Rehabilitation nurses monitor compliance with home exercise programs or rehabilitation programs initiated in either an acute care setting or another rehabilitation facility, an outpatient program, or a long-term care program.

Rehabilitation nurses encourage patient participation in home rehabilitation in conjunction with a physical, occupational, or speech therapist, or in a program already established by one of these health care professionals. They train and supervise home health aides in patient-specific therapy plans for follow-through in the home.

Utilization of the Restorative Nurse in the Community Setting

For those community or home health care agencies that are unable to adequately meet the rehabilitative needs of their clients in the home because of a shortage of qualified professional therapy staff, the development and utilization of restorative nursing services is a sensible but often overlooked alternative in the community setting.

Restorative nursing, as defined by the HCFA, "includes exercises, transfer training, carrying out of restorative or rehabilitative programs ordered by a physician. This may or may not be already established by a physical therapist" (Medical Home Health Agency Manual, 1989).

The definition further describes specific functions of the home restorative nurse in the forms of education and training of a client to perform activities of daily living (ADLs), which include bathing, toileting, eating, grooming, dressing, and functional communication, either independently or with directed assistance of a caregiver. These functions include the proper use of assistive and adaptive devices for ADLs and mobility; safety in transfer techniques in a variety of situations; proper body alignment and bed mobility; prosthesis care and gait training; proper and safe use of braces, splints, and orthoses; and associated daily skin integrity maintenance.

It is the restorative or rehabilitative nurse who is most qualified to conduct the home health program admission visit and to design the subsequent plan of treatment. The data obtained by the nurse during the admission visit form the initial prediction of the client's rehabilitation goal potential. In addition, the restorative or rehabilitative nurse understands the importance of the rehabilitation interdisciplinary team approach and is able to make appropriate referrals for skilled therapy services quickly and accurately.

It would prove to be beneficial for the home client to have restorative services instituted from day one of the home health program to prevent further deconditioned status and to promote optimal functioning and independence in self-care. The strict professional boundaries of rehabilitation training—for example, that physical therapists work only on activities that involve gait and transfer training; occupational therapists work only on tub transfers, ADLs, and kitchen skills; and registered home health care nurses work only on the assessment of medical and rehabilitative needs and then make the necessary referrals to other disciplines—need to be reviewed and eliminated.

Professionals from all home health care disciplines should work together toward common rehabilitation goals, care planning, evaluation of interventions, and outcome measurements for client satisfaction. They should enforce safe home management with each and every home care visit, and it should be every rehabilitation team member's responsibility to promote wellness, independence, and safety in all aspects of the home health program.

Every effort should be made to encourage and support the client's decision to return to and remain independent in the community and home. The restorative nurse can assist with and facilitate patient independence by making proper recommendations about the immediate environment. Adapting the home to the patient's specific limitations due to illness, injury, or disability can be challenging and costly, so any modifications to the home should be carefully planned for safety, accessibility, and necessity. All areas, inside and outside the home, should be examined. Specific areas on which to focus safety modification and energy conservation are in the bathroom and the kitchen, primarily because these rooms are where the majority of ADLs are performed.

Furniture in the home should be sturdy, easily cleaned, and arranged in a way that will not present an obstacle to patient mobility. Hallways should be well lit and wide enough to accommodate whatever assistive or adaptive devices are needed, and suggestions for adaptation or alternative interventions initiated. All loose rugs should be removed, and carpet edges should be securely tacked in place. Handrails should be placed at all stairways, in bathrooms near the commode and tub or shower, and at all main home entry decks or ramps.

The patient should be encouraged to keep properly functioning fire extinguishers and smoke detectors in the home and to keep a list of important numbers prominently displayed near the main telephone.

All home health care professionals should instruct the patient, the caregivers, and any other family members in the home to devise a safety evacuation route in case of fire or other emergency so that access to safety can be achieved.

Community Home Health Case Management

The goal of rehabilitation nursing is "to assist the individual with disability and chronic illness in the restoration and maintenance of maximal health" (ANA & ARN, 1988). For the rehabilitation patient in the home, effective health management is critical to achieve and maintain the patient's optimal physical functional level, increase the patient's self-esteem and emotional control, promote wellness and self-care independence, avoid further functional impairment or injury, and basically increase the patient's overall quality of life.

In order to accomplish this, the home health rehabilitation nurse must develop and implement a plan of treatment designed especially for the individual patient, based on the patient's functional and emotional needs (Fig. 7–3). Nurses are educated to follow the "nursing process" for care plan development and implementation. This process includes, in specific order, data collection, assessment, goal setting, planning, implementation, evaluation, and modification of goals and plans if necessary until successful completion of care and goal attainment are achieved.

After necessary data collection and thorough physical examination and assessment, the rehabilitation nurse analyzes the data by classifying and examining relationships among the subjective and objective observations. A clinical judgment or conclusions are made, and from this a nursing diagnosis is obtained.

Bonney and Rothberg (1963) define a nursing diagnosis as "an evaluation within the framework of current knowledge of the patient's condition as a total human being, including physical, physiological, and behavioral facets." More recently, Gordon (1987) stated that the three essential components for a nursing diagnosis are the health problem (P), the etiological or related factors (E), and the defining characteristics or symptoms (S). This is referred to as the PES format. Common nursing diagnoses used by rehabilitation nurses in care of individuals in the home include impaired physical mobility, self-care deficit syndrome, an alteration in the urinary or bowel elimination pattern, impaired skin integrity, knowledge deficit, potential for physical inquiry, impaired verbal communication, and decreased activity tolerance. The bottom line with a nursing diagnosis is that it reflects the patient's actual needs, and this provides the basis for care plan formulation.

Figure 7–3 is an example of an actual home rehabilitation care plan with a patient education instruction sheet. This care plan is used in a suburban, hospital-based home health care agency. The average number of skilled rehabilitation service referrals total 536 monthly at this agency. The average total number of home health patient admissions is 5880 annually.

EVALUATION OF OUTCOMES AND CLIENT SATISFACTION

Because the basic definition of rehabilitation is "the achievement of a maximum level of independent function in light of the individual's physical, cognitive, and motivational abilities and limitations" (Dittmar, 1989), the question arises of how a patient's maximal

Text continued on page 80

HOME HEALTH CARE
PATIENT SERVICE RECORD

NAME _____   CASE # _____

ADDRESS _____   PHONE _____   DATE REVIEWED _____

CARETAKER _____   Page _____

Date Identified	Prob. No.	PATIENT & FAMILY PROBLEM INDEX	Date Resol.	Date	PATIENT GOALS	Date Goals Met
		Impaired physical mobility			Vital signs will remain WNL.	
		related to musculoskeletal			Pt will receive adequate	
		impairment; as manifested			nutrition & hydration as	
		by Fx. hip, ORIF, hip or			reflected in 3-day diet Hx.	
		knee prosthesis,			Pt/Ct will identify s/sx of	
		replacement, or revision;			pain & ways to alleviate	
		orthopedic deformity,			same by D/C date.	
		rheumatoid or degenerative			Pt/Ct will comply with	
		arthritis			medication regimen as	
		Other:			ordered by MD.	
					Pt will comply with current	
					weight-bearing limitations.	
					Pt will adhere to current	
					activity restrictions.	
					Pt/Ct will identify 911/EMS	
					access and indication for	
					use by the _____ visit.	
					Pt will remain safe in the	
					home.	
					Pt will not suffer from	
					hazards of immobility or	
					''disuse syndrome.''	
					Pt will experience adequate	
					activity and mobility as	
					evidenced by progressive	
					ROM within imposed	
					limitations.	
					Pt will experience optimal	
					physical functional	
					mobility and independence	
					in ADLs within imposed	
					restriction to maintain	
ADVANCE DIRECTIVES:					health without complications.	
Yes	No	Living Will			*Surgical incision site will	
Yes	No	Power of Attorney			remain clean, dry, well-	
SPECIAL NOTES:					approximated, and without	
					impairment; Pt/Ct will	
					perform skin care properly	
					by _____ visit.	
Directions to home:						

A

FIGURE 7–3A
Sample home health care patient service records. *A,* Impaired physical mobility record.

PATIENT SERVICE RECORD

Page _____

Name _____ Physician _____ Tele.: _____

Allergies _____ Address _____

Date	Prob #	PATIENT CARE PLAN	YEAR _____
		CHN will assess vital signs for deviation q visit.	Temp.
			Pulse A/P
			Resp. rate
			BP
			Lung sounds: Ant.
			Post.
			Edema
		CHN will have Pt/Ct do 3-day nutritional assessment, forward to nutritionist, and review recommendations.	
		CHN will assess ability to participate in ADLs, mobility status, and need for assistive devices for ambulation, mobility, and self-care.	
		CHN will assess and evaluate for presence of s/sx of musculoskeletal impairment with each visit:	
		Burning/pain/swelling in joints	
		SOB/tingling/muscle, weakness/twitching	
		Decreased endurance/numbness/deterioration/paralysis	
		Gait unsteady/Homans' sign/decreased ROM/balance/poor coordination/ contractures/stiffness.	
		CHN will assess/instruct in medication compliance and understanding with each visit.	
		CHN will assess/instruct in pain tolerance and control with each visit.	
		CHN will assess/instruct Pt/Ct in activity and weight-bearing limitations.	
		CHN will instruct Pt/Ct in appropriate ROM exercises as ordered by the MD and therapist and will monitor proper use of assistive mobility devices.	
		CHN will instruct and encourage Pt/Ct to perform all ADL needs to an optimal level and will monitor proper use of assistive devices in the home.	
		CHN will refer a home health aide to assist in ADLs as needed; CHN will supervise HHA 2 weeks.	
		CHN will initiate referral to appropriate home therapy services, and will reinforce rehab team instruction each visit. CHN will attend weekly interdisciplinary care conference meeting to collaborate in PT/OT.	
		CHN will assess/instruct in proper skin care; intervene as necessary.	
		CHN will assess Pt/Ct response to teaching q visit.	
		CHN will review plan of care and goals with Pt/Ct q 3rd visit.	
		CHN will notify physician for any change in Pt's condition.	

HHA SUPV. _____

M.D. VISIT _____

RN VISIT FREQUENCY _____

PAYMENT SOURCE _____

SIGNATURE & TITLE _____

FIGURE 7–3A *Continued*

Illustration continued on following page

PATIENT EDUCATION: IMPAIRED PHYSICAL MOBILITY

I. Disease process

Pt/Ct can define "impaired physical mobility" as an inability to purposefully move within the physical environment. This includes all mobility activities, transfers, ambulation, gait pattern, and bed mobility.

II. Risk factors

 a. Decreased physical activity
 b. Limited range of motion
 c. Decreased muscle strength/control/mass
 d. Perceived inability to move
 e. Constancy of a body part in relation to gravity
 f. Medically or mechanically imposed restrictions on movement, such as casts, splints, braces, traction, monitors/ventilators/O_2 concentrators, IV access lines, or feeding tubes
 g. Commonly seen in individuals experiencing CNS disorders, neuromuscular impairment, perceptual or cognitive impairments, joint/bone disorders, pain and discomfort, generalized weakness, trauma or surgical procedures, and bedrest

III. Goals

Pt/Ct will be able to perform active and/or passive range of motion to the highest physical functional level, or within the limitations imposed by injury or situation; and will continue to participate in or direct mobility needs (with or without assistive aids or devices) to achieve physical functional independence.

IV. Expected outcomes

 a. Pt/Ct verbalizes importance of participation and independence in mobility daily
 b. Pt/Ct performs mobility activities at an optimal physical functional level
 c. Pt/Ct maintains skin integrity
 d. Pt/Ct maintains bowel and bladder management
 e. Pt/Ct maintains adequate food/fluid intake
 f. Pt/Ct performs range of motion exercises daily
 g. Pt/Ct uses safety measures to decrease potential for injury in activities
 h. Pt/Ct demonstrates safe and proper use of assistive aids or devices to facilitate ADLs or mobility independence
 i. Pt/Ct recognizes the importance of daily exercises and movement to prevent "hazards of immobility," such as contractures, infection, skin breakdown, and decreased strength and function
 j. Pt/Ct will cope more effectively with injury or disability
 k. Pt/Ct complies with rehab team education and interventions to increase self-care and mobility independence, increase self-esteem and self-worth, and promote a more positive body image

FIGURE 7–3A *Continued*

HOME HEALTH CARE
PATIENT SERVICE RECORD

NAME _____   CASE # _____

ADDRESS _____ PHONE _____ DATE REVIEWED _____

CARETAKER _____ Page _____

Date Identified	Prob. No.	PATIENT & FAMILY PROBLEM INDEX	Date Resol.	Date	PATIENT GOALS	Date Goals Met
		Self-care deficit syndrome			Vital signs will remain WNL.	
		related to neuromuscular			Pt will receive adequate	
		impairment or impaired			nutrition & hydration as	
		physical functional			reflected in 3-day diet Hx.	
		status; as manifested by			Pt will remain safe in the	
		patient's inability to			home.	
		feed, bathe, groom, dress,			Pt/Ct will identify 911/EMS	
		toilet, or make ADL needs			access and indication for	
		known.			use by the visit.	
					Pt/Ct will comply with	
					medication regimen as	
					ordered by MD.	
					Pt will be motivated to	
					participate in ADLs within	
					limits imposed by injury or	
					situation.	
					Pt will optimally perform	
					self-care for ADLs with or	
					without assistive devices	
					to achieve maximum	
					independence.	
					Pt, if not able to perform	
					ADLs, will be able to	
					appropriately direct ADL	
					care needs to a caretaker	
					without difficulty.	
					Pt will comply with rehab/	
					therapy home program at an	
					optimal level.	
					Pt will maintain adequate	
					bowel & bladder function in	
					the home.	
					Pt will be able to transfer	
					safely into a tub/shower, or	
					onto a toilet or commode.	
					Pt will show positive coping	
					skills, focusing on progress	
					in ADL independence	

ADVANCE DIRECTIVES:

Yes		No		Living Will	achieved & not on remaining
Yes		No		Power of Attorney	loss of function or physical
					disability.

SPECIAL NOTES:

Pt will respond to positive
reinforcements to encourage
continued effort in home
rehab program and ADL needs.

Directions to home:

B

FIGURE 7–3 *Continued. B,* Self-care deficit syndrome record.

Illustration continued on following page

PATIENT SERVICE RECORD   Page _____

Name _____ Physician _____ Tele.: _____

Allergies _____ Address _____

Date	Prob #	PATIENT CARE PLAN	YEAR _____
		CHN will assess vital signs for deviation q visit.	Temp.
			Pulse A/P
			Resp. rate
			BP
			Lung sounds: Ant.
			Post.
			Edema
		CHN will have Pt/Ct do 3-day nutritional assessment, forward to nutritionist, and	
		review recommendations.	
		CHN will assess Pt/Ct ability to perform ADL needs q visit, & will provide assistance	
		or supervision as needed, encouraging Pt to ask for help or instructing Ct in self-	
		care assistance when appropriate.	
		CHN will assess/instruct in proper use of assistive devices for ADLs.	
		CHN will initiate referral to appropriate home therapy services, and will	
		collaborate with the rehab team during weekly interdisciplinary care conferences	
		to maximize Pt's rehab potential.	
		CHN will refer home health aide services (if needed) to assist in ADL needs; CHN will	
		supervise HHA q 2 weeks.	
		CHN will encourage/instruct Pt/Ct in allowing time to perform ADLs at own pace, and	
		as independently as functionally possible.	
		CHN will encourage Pt to comply with rehab/therapy program and promote and instruct	
		in activities that will increase Pt's physical functional level.	
		CHN will assess/instruct in medication compliance and understanding with q visit.	
		CHN will assess/instruct in safe home maintenance and need for home modification.	
		CHN will monitor/instruct Pt's bowel & bladder functional status and ability to	
		safely transfer to toilet/commode q visit.	
		CHN will assess for psychogenic factors that may impede Pt's participation &	
		motivation in self-care activities. CHN will monitor coping skills.	
		CHN will assess Pt/Ct response to teaching q visit.	
		CHN will review plan of care and goals with Pt/Ct q 3rd visit.	
		CHN will notify physician for any change in Pt's condition.	

HHA SUPV. _____

M.D. VISIT _____

RN VISIT FREQUENCY _____

PAYMENT SOURCE _____

SIGNATURE & TITLE _____

FIGURE 7–3B *Continued*

PATIENT EDUCATION: SELF-CARE DEFICIT SYNDROME

I. Disease process

Pt/Ct can define "self-care deficit syndrome" as an inability to complete activities of daily living (ADLs); more specifically, feeding, bathing, dressing, toileting, grooming, personal hygiene, safe mobility, and transfers.

II. Risk factors

  a. Decreased range of motion

  b. Decreased circulation

  c. Potential for skin integrity impairment

  d. Decreased motivation and participation in activity

  e. Decreased feelings of self-esteem and self-worth, ineffective coping, anxiety, and depression

III. Goals

Pt/Ct will be able to perform self-care/ADLs at an optimal level, or within the limitations imposed by injury or situation; and will continue to participate in or direct care given (with or without assistive aids or devices) to achieve physical functional independence.

IV. Expected outcomes

  a. Pt/Ct verbalizes importance of participation and independence in ADL needs

  b. Pt/Ct performs self-care and mobility activities at an optimal physical functional level

  c. Pt/Ct maintains skin integrity

  d. Pt/Ct maintains bowel and bladder management

  e. Pt/Ct maintains adequate food/fluid intake

  f. Pt/Ct performs range of motion exercises daily

  g. Pt/Ct uses safety measures to decrease potential for injury in activities

  h. Pt/Ct demonstrates safe and proper use of assistive aids or devices to facilitate ADL independence

  i. Pt/Ct recognizes the importance of performing personal hygiene, bathing, and grooming activities to promote positive body image and increased self-esteem and self-worth

  j. Pt/Ct will cope more effectively with injury or disability

  k. Pt/Ct complies with rehab team education and interventions to increase self-care independence

FIGURE 7–3B *Continued*

Illustration continued on following page

SELF-HELP HINTS AND DEVICES

I. Dressing
   A. Use Velcro instead of buttons or hooks to fasten clothing.
   B. Buy clothes that are large enough to slip on easily.
   C. Wear elastic waistbands that stretch easily.
   D. Use a dressing stick to pull up pants or retrieve clothing.
   E. Wear garments that open in the front.
   F. Use elastic shoelaces or slip-on shoes to eliminate need to tie shoelaces.
II. Bathing and Hygiene
   A. Use a long-handled sponge to wash back and lower extremities.
   B. Use a shower bench if unable to sit down in the tub.
   C. Use a long shower hose to make rinsing easier.
   D. Use long-handled combs or brushes if reaching is limited.
   E. Use safety rails in the bathroom.
III. Mobility
   A. Use raised toilet seat to decrease difficulty in standing from a sitting position.
   B. Place blocks under chairs to ease standing from a sitting position.
   C. Place rails at all stairways.
   D. Use ramps instead of stairs as needed.
IV. Cooking
   A. Use microwaves. They are safe, fast, and convenient.
   B. Use a jar opener to grip a jar and open the lid.
   C. Use efficient storage.
   D. Use a food processor to conserve energy required in food preparation.
   E. Use containers that are easy to open.

F. Wear long oven mitts; they are safer than potholders.
   G. Use a cutting board with stainless steel nails to stabilize food while cutting.
   H. Use convenience or easily prepared foods.
V. Eating
   A. Use a plate guard to prevent food from slipping off the plate.
   B. Purchase large-handled utensils or use foam to make handles of utensils wider to improve the grip required for eating.
   C. If needed, purchase special elongated, curved, or swivel utensils.
   D. Use unbreakable cups with handles if your hand is unsteady.
VI. Recreation or Leisure
   A. Use card holders and card shufflers when playing cards.
   B. Purchase self-threading needles for sewing.
VII. Miscellaneous
   A. Make phone dialing easier by using a pencil.
   B. Use a clipboard to keep writing paper steady.
   C. Use a bookholder to stabilize a book you are reading.
   D. Check catalogs that carry multiple self-help devices.

REFERENCES

Lorig, K., & Fries, J. (1980). *Arthritis helpbook.* Reading, MA: Addison-Wesley.
Pedretti, L. W. (1985). *Occupational therapy: Practice skills for physical dysfunction.* St. Louis: C. V. Mosby.
Springhouse Corporation. (1987). *Patient teaching.* Springhouse, PA: Author.

C

FIGURE 7–3 *Continued*
C, Self-help hints and devices. (*C* from Avillion, A. E., & Mirgon, B. B. [1989]. *Quality assurance in rehabilitation nursing. A practical guide.* Rockville, MD: Aspen.)

functional level can be measured, and if that level is truly achieved within the time frame allotted for the rehabilitation program.

To answer this question, we need to look at the evaluation of outcomes. Evaluation is the "planned, systematic comparison of the client's health status with defined goals and objectives. It is an ongoing activity involving the patient, nurse, and other health care team members. Evaluation is used to determine if the goal established for the nursing diagnosis was accomplished by the nursing intervention" (Dittmar, 1989). Evaluation often leads to redefining the plan of treatment (or care plan) and updating mutual goals.

The critical elements to be monitored for outcome evaluation should be the patient's health and functional status before and after a home rehabilitation program; the patient's compliance with the rehabilitation program; the patient's knowledge base, information retention, and understanding; and the patient's overall program satisfaction.

As patients are discharged from acute care medical facilities, their medical needs at home are more intensive and complex than ever before. Along with these needs, patients will have special rehabilitative needs and goals to achieve in order to gain more independence at home and for community reintegration.

Because this is the case now and will be with future managed care, home health care agencies will need to develop specialty rehabilitation programs that stay within the homebound guidelines and regulations set forth by Medicare, with standards set in place that allow for home care reimbursement.

A few outcome measurements were developed in the 1990s, but no one set measurement seems to appeal to the home care community at large. The Commission on Accreditation of Rehabilitation Facilities (CARF) is the industry leader for rehabilitation standards of quality care.

Before 1996, CARF certified only organizations involved with acute care or comprehensive inpatient medical, rehabilitation, spinal cord, pain management, and brain injury programs and outpatient medical rehabilitation programs. In July 1996, CARF introduced agency certification standards for home- and community-based rehabilitation programs as well. When an organization applies for CARF certification, a strict protocol for standards and rehabilitation program evaluation is followed. A survey and on-site inspection are required, and if the organization passes, CARF's prestigious certification award is given.

CARF standards predominantly evaluate the dynamic process of quality improvement and the patient's outcome in a rehabilitation program. The rehabilitation program should evaluate the characteristics of the persons served; the effectiveness of the rehabilitation program; the efficiency of the rehabilitation program; the satisfaction of the patient; the progress of the patient; and the follow-up after discharge from the rehabilitation program. In addition, CARF requires home- and community-based programs to track the number of patients who return to an acute care or other institutional setting; those patients who remain at home or in the community; medical interventions that interrupt rehabilitation service delivery; and patients who meet discharge goals and maintain a satisfactory level of functional ability.

The Functional Independence Measure (FIM) is a seven-level scale with ratings from 1 to 7 (1 indicating total assistance or dependence, and 7 indicating complete independence). There are 18 items within six categories of ADLs that are measured: self-care, sphincter control, mobility, locomotion, communication, and social cognition (Uniform Data System for Medical Rehabilitation, 1990).

It is the hope of the users of the FIM scale that clients will progress in their rehabilitation programs from low-score levels to higher-score levels before discharge. The FIM scale is very useful in the acute rehabilitation setting; however, in the home care setting, it is difficult to utilize FIMs because of home care staff inability to evaluate the client on a daily basis, as well as possible unreliable information from the client or caregiver on the amount of assistance needed to perform ADLs.

The Rehab Without Walls program, affiliated with Olsten Kimberly Quality Care, is another example of a community rehabilitation program in which a key component of the plan of treatment is the setting of functional outcome goals. The outcome goals focus the patient's treatment on those areas of need that most directly affect the independent functioning of the client. They are characterized as "outcomes" because they are stated in a manner that predicts a level of functioning that the client will reach given the amount and type of services proposed in the treatment plan on admission.

The treatment plan is developed in a true rehabilitation team forum with the participation of all members, including the client. Once all assessments of the client are made and treatments have begun in the client's home environment, ongoing evaluation and analysis of the program and treatment plan are initiated in the form of subjective and objective data collection. These data directly reflect the client's rehabilitation progress. The seven functional areas of analysis are the level of supervision required for the client in the home or community; productive activity; identification of the living setting; ambulation independence; the mode of ambulation; independence with ADLs; and social behavior. Client satisfaction forms are sent out, and postdischarge calls are made about 1 year from the client program discharge date to measure the durability of the outcomes and program compliance.

The Rehab Without Walls program has been shown to be a positive-outcome measurement tool for those agencies that have implemented it. However, it will take more time for the majority of community-based agencies to accept this type of outcome measurement for their own use.

Cofounded by the Robert Wood Johnson Foundation and the HCFA, the Center for Health Policy Research and the Center for Health Services Research at the University of

Colorado Health Sciences Center conducted a research program targeted at developing a broad-based quality assurance, patient outcome system for home health care. This project began in 1991 with the combined efforts of Dr. Peter W. Shaughnessy and others in an effort to set a standard across the nation to measure quality and successful patient outcomes in various home health programs (Shaughnessy, 1992).

The focus of the Oasis (Standardized Outcome and Assessment Information Set) outcome measurement is looking at goal attainment in patient and instrumental ADLs; severe family and home caregiver stress; complications from poor medication compliance; poor initial assessment of patient home needs; and rehospitalization due to inadequate home care.

Quality indicator groups were also looked at in the categories of acute conditions, chronic conditions, and primary prevention and screening (Shaughnessy, 1992).

Selected information on patient assessment findings, patient functioning, patient problems, and services used (including discharge to a hospital or nursing home) was obtained at program admission and at 60-day intervals until the patient was discharged from home care. The premise of this time interval is to determine if problems exist in any portion of the patient's home care needs, thus allowing the home health agency to assist in or correct problems as applicable.

Shaughnessy published and presented his Oasis model for outcome measurements formally in 1995 as an acceptable tool for use by home health agencies, private payers, regulatory groups, and insurance companies to facilitate higher standards of quality home- and community-based care for the future (Shaughnessy & Crisler, 1995).

The National Medicare Quality Assurance and Improvement Demonstration Project describes basically three types of home patient outcomes. An end-result outcome is a change in patient health status between two or more timed points. An intermediate-result outcome is a change in patient or informal caregiver's behavior, emotions, or knowledge that can influence the patient's end-result outcomes. A utilization outcome is a type of health care utilization that reflects a typically substantial change in patient health status over time. Examples of this type of outcome are a hospital, nursing home, or emergency care admission during the home care program (Harris & Dugan, 1996). It should also be noted that these outcomes can result in positive, neutral, or negative changes that can occur as a result of home care provided or the natural progression of the disease or disability.

It is hoped that this project program will be a prototype of the national program to be implemented by Medicare. Medicare's Oasis program for home health care is supported and endorsed by HCFA, and it is expected that outcome-based quality improvement will become mandatory for Medicare certification and also as a condition of participation in home health care agency accreditation.

To date, Shaughnessy's Oasis outcome measurement tool appears to be the most accepted standard for quality care and home health outcome measurement. HCFA has not imposed this standard on any agency in the community; however, it would be a positive step for nationwide standardization of managed home health care.

The ideal model for ongoing home health rehabilitation treatment planning and evaluation of outcomes flows as follows:

1. Home rehabilitation nurse's performance of client evaluation
   a. Before acute care facility discharge to assess homegoing needs
   b. Again within 24 hours of acute care facility discharge to home to continue assessment
2. Determination of outcome goals
   a. Preferably by all professional disciplines to be involved
   b. Information presented in interdisciplinary team forum
3. Identification of barriers to achieving outcome goals
   a. Environmental, medical, psychosocial, emotional, and physical
4. Development of treatment objectives to alleviate barriers
5. Development of treatment protocols based on treatment objectives
6. Protocol implementation
7. Data collection and analysis of subjective and objective information
8. Clinical decision regarding whether criteria are met
   a. Yes—discharge patient if goals are met
   b. No—continue with plan of treatment or make changes to plan as needed and continue this flow until patient has achieved satisfactory level of functional independence

The most important program outcome of all is client satisfaction. Clients may not always achieve full independence in their reha-bilitation program; however, they may have achieved an "optimal" level of independence based on their current degree of physical or emotional ability. It is the responsibility of the home rehabilitation nurse to assist patients in understanding this concept of optimal levels of functional independence and help them to adapt to their current functional level to the best of their ability.

Client satisfaction will be achieved when clients adapt to the disability; modify their environment to make home living conducive to functioning with their disability; and safely perform their ADLs at their highest func-tional level or are able to direct their personal care needs to a caregiver appropriately and within the range of activities that they truly could not complete themselves.

SUMMARY

Rehabilitation nurses can be instrumental in performing the tasks necessary for home care clients to achieve functional independence and community reintegration. Home care nursing does and will continue to involve an array of nursing responsibilities including high-technology skills; case management of multiple medical and chronically ill patient needs; hospice care; and rehabilitative needs. As home health practice continues to change, so must the skilled service providers; stan-dards for quality improvement and evalua-tion; and outcome measurements.

Home care is an integral part of the health care delivery system. It is a less costly alterna-tive to hospital care, and it is quite reasonable to consider the home as a primary site for health care delivery, with the institutional or acute care setting as the alternative.

Nurses in home health care must be ac-tively involved in the practice, not only clini-cally but in research, continuing education activities, community and patient advocacy, and political reform.

Home care nursing is much more than physically caring for an individual or family at home; it is the dedication to and responsi-bility of being aware of and involved in changing the home care climate toward a more holistic approach in nursing practice. Basic rehabilitative principles of indepen-dence, self-care, and education are also the same as the principles that make up the back-bone of home health care nursing.

Is it any wonder that patients prefer to be in their own beds, eating their own foods, and surrounded by those who have always loved and cared for them? Is it any wonder why hundreds of nurses every year move toward some form of community- or home-based nursing practice as a way of personal job fulfillment, or getting back to the roots of why they became nurses in the first place? As health care reform continues to look toward the home health industry to pull the United States out of the current health care dilemma, hospitals are constantly downsizing staff and services, and massive medical facility closings continue to take place, whereas home health care continues to flourish and grow and seeks to make health care convenient, affordable, and available for all citizens.

REFERENCES

American Nurses Association & Association of Rehabili-tation Nurses. (1988). *Rehabilitation nursing: Scope of practice, process and outcome criteria for selected diagno-ses*. Washington, DC: American Nurses Association.

Avillion, A. E., & Mirgon, B. B. (1989). *Quality assurance in rehabilitation nursing: A practical guide*. Rockville, MD: Aspen.

Avillion, A. E, & Scott, J. B. (1995). Rehabilitation clients in the community. In C. Smith & F. Maurer (Eds.), *Community health nursing: Theory and practice*. Philadel-phia: W. B. Saunders.

Blaines, E., & Oglesby, M. (1992). The elderly as caregiv-ers of the elderly. *Holistic Nurse Practitioner, 7(4)*, 61–69.

Bonney, V., & Rothberg, J. (1963). *Nursing diagnosis and therapy: An instrument for evaluation and measurement*. New York: National League for Nursing.

Deets, H. (1995). Home care in the 21st century. *Caring, 14(9)*, 50–52.

Dittmar, S. (1989). *Rehabilitation nursing. Process and appli-cation*. St. Louis: C. V. Mosby.

Gordon, M. (1987). *Nursing diagnosis: Process and applica-tion* (2nd ed.). New York: McGraw-Hill.

Green, K., & Lydon, S. (1995). Home health cardiac reha-bilitation. *Home Health Care Nurse, 13(2)*, 29–39.

Harris, M., & Dugan, M. (1996). Understanding the Na-tional Medicare Quality Assurance and Improvement Demonstration Project, and its effect on patient out-comes measurement. *Home Health Care Nurse, 14(6)*, 463–468.

Hickey, J. (1992). *The clinical practice of neurosurgical nurs-ing*. Philadelphia: J. B. Lippincott.

Home health and hospice care—United States, 1992. (1993). *Morbidity and Mortality Weekly Report*, October 29.

Medical home health agency manual. (1989). (HIM-11. Pub. 11. 10–89, Transmittal No. 228; 04-89, Sect. 205.1, Rev. 14.15–14.16.) Washington DC: Health Care Financing Administration.

Mitchell, M. K. (1992). Nursing's legacy of leadership. *Nursing and Heath Care, 13(6)*, 295–297.

National Association for Home Care. (1992). *Basic statis-tics about home care—1992* (p. 3). Washington DC: Au-thor.

National Association for Home Care. (1996). *Basic statis-tics about homecare—1996*. Washington DC: Author.

National Home and Hospice Survey 1992. (1993). *Advance data*. Washington, DC: U.S. Department of Health and Human Services, Public Health Service.

Niederhauser, V. (1989). Healthcare of immigrant children. *Pediatric Nursing, 15*, 569–574.

Nuzzo-Milone, P. (1995). Home health care. In C. Smith & F. Maurer (Eds.), *Community health nursing: Theory and practice*. Philadelphia: W. B. Saunders.

O'Conner, P., Vander Platts, S., & Betz, C. (1992). Respite care services to caretakers of chronically ill children in California. *Journal of Pediatric Nursing, 7(4),* 269–275.

Rempusheski, V. (1989). The role of ethnicity in elder care. *Nursing Clinics of North America, 24,* 717–724.

Respiratory rehab proves its worth. (1995, March). *American Journal of Nursing,* p. 9.

Rooney, A. L., & Biere, D. M. (1992). Demonstrating excellence in home care through Joint Commission accreditation. *Journal of Nursing Administration, 22(9),* 31–36.

Ross, B. (1992). The impact of reimbursement issues on rehabilitation nursing practice and patient care. *Rehabilitation Nursing, 17(5),* 236–238.

Saucier, K. *(1991). Perspectives in family and community health (p. 161).* St. Louis: Mosby–Year Book.

Shaughnessy, P. W. (1992). *Caring, 11(3),* 44–48.

Shaughnessy, P., & Crisler, K. (1995). *Outcome based quality improvement.* Washington, DC: National Association for Home Care.

Smith, C., & Maurer, F. (Eds.), (1995). *Community health nursing: Theory and practice* (p. 22). Philadelphia: W. B. Saunders.

Spruhan, J. B. (1996). Beyond traditional nursing care: Cultural awareness and successful home health nursing. *Home Health Care Nurse, 14(6),* 445–449.

Uniform data system for medical rehabilitation. Guide for the use of the uniform data set for medical rehabilitation in the functional independence measure. (1990). Buffalo, NY: State University of New York, Buffalo.

U.S. Department of Education. (1988). Fair housing amendments.

U.S. Department of Health and Human Services. (1990). *Healthy people 2000: National health promotion and disease prevention objectives summary report.* Washington, DC: U.S. Government Printing Office.

Zerwekh, J. V. (1992). Public health nursing legacy, historical, practical. *Nursing and Health Care, 13,* 84–91.

BIBLIOGRAPHY

Carr, P. (1996). Get ready for Oasis. *Home Health Care Nurse, 14,* 61–62.

Shaughnessy, P., Crisler, K., & Schlenker, R. (1995). *Medicare's Oasis: Standardized outcome and assessment information set for home health care.* Washington, DC: National Association for Home Care.

CHAPTER 8

Culturally Competent Rehabilitation Care

Dolores S. Patrinos and Neva White

Rehabilitation nursing must be based upon the diversity in the client population it serves. The rehabilitation nurse needs to be knowledgeable and sensitive to the historical factors that shape this country's demographic profile. Historically and culturally, the republic of the United States has had an Anglo-Saxon base modified, enriched, and reconstituted by successive transfusions from other continents. Homogeneity disappeared well over a century ago, never to return. American history can be divided into a series of five racial-cultural phases. The first phase was a period of Anglo-Saxon dominance in a hierarchical society in which the elite controlled politics, and citizenship was linked to the ownership of property. The second phase was the westward expansion period of the 19th century, resulting in a more expansive definition of American democracy to include the concept of a class-mobile society, which came with the category of whiteness (Litwack, 1998). The third phase was a period of a succession of mass immigrations of non–Anglo-Saxon Euro-Americans lasting from the end of the 19th century to the first quarter of the 20th century (Lind, 1995). The fourth phase was the decades of the 1960s and 1970s, in which black Americans and, later, women and special-interest groups including antiwar demonstrators, gay men and women, elderly people, and disabled people (between 1979 and 1986) organized nationally "to demand a more equitable distribution of economic and educational resources and inclusion in the public domain of power and influence" (Schensul & Carroll, 1990, p. 339). The fifth phase was the mass immigration period of the latter part of the 20th century, which has changed the landscape of America as we witness a large immigration of people of color that continues to the present. The mix is even more diverse today, with an overwhelming number of newcomers to America coming from Latin America, Asia, and the Caribbean (Ford, 1995).

The civil rights struggles of the late 1950s and early 1960s challenged the notion of democracy. The literature of the late 1950s and early 1960s described oppressive conditions for some minority populations, such as invisibility, namelessness, alienation, and described the quest for an identity as a way of offsetting the dehumanization phenomenon, a legacy of chattel slavery (Ellison, 1970). The actor Paul Winfield described eloquently in a recent television broadcast the dilemma facing black America in 1972, when he starred in the film *Sounder*, which depicted an African-American family in rural America: "A white person wrote me and expressed her surprise that black children actually had relationships with fathers intimate enough to call their fathers 'Dad.' " The civil rights struggles challenged American democracy to extend full citizenship to black America, emphasizing inclusion and egalitarian and representative principles as set down by our founding fathers, the uniquely American promise that those coming to our shores would be clothed in dignity (Gitlin, 1995).

In the national conversation, there have been three approaches to empowerment in American society: (1) assimilation into the larger society; (2) separatism and rejection from the larger society; and (3) transformation of society into a multicultural democracy with the elimination of racism and the celebration of both differences and common membership in the larger society (Funderberg, 1994; Marable; 1996). Diversity means reclaiming "historical memory" to include those who were originally left out as if they were invisible (Ellison, 1970). "Diversity is the very ingredient that has given the United States its distinctive, vital, and ever-evolving, ever-changing mix of old and new" (Litwack, 1998). America's identity is its heterogeneity—different kinds of people in dynamic interaction have produced and continue to reshape that complex set of identities, values, and cultural products called Americans (Gitlin, 1995). The revision of American history is a human drama of multiculturalism, with different actors playing a leading role at different times.

At the new millennium, one in four Americans are members of a minority group, and Americans are still preoccupied with forging a single nation from people of remarkably diverse racial, religious, and ethnic origins with tolerance of differences based on mutual respect (Gitlin, 1995; West & Lerner, 1995). The question of the 21st century is, How do we surmount our historical obsession with practices of discrimination and categorization related to disability prejudices, agism, homophobia, sexism, racism, antisemitism, and ethnic differences? The challenge for all of us is finding a way to participate in the new world order that will be a more inclusive and tolerant society that, at the same time, will place positive value on cultural diversity while recognizing national commonalities. The majority of Americans are peoples who crossed oceans or are descendants of those who came from many countries, even when brought here in chains, to share in the American dream. Americans share the belief that the journey to a better life exists in this, our adopted country. Our national character has been, and will continue to be, shaped by our strength of the differences that have been and continue to be brought to this shore. The failure at national assimilation has left the country with competing views on how to forge a characteristically American experience that cuts across racial, ethnic, and cultural lines. The pluralistic character of American society has had a bracing impact on all institutions. The health care system mirrors the challenge to manage the diversity of the American population (Denboba, Bragdon, Epstein, Garthright & Goldman, 1998). For example, demographic data confirm that American families are varied and only rarely represent the nuclear family fantasy of the Ozzie and Harriet or the Huxtables variety as seen on television. Nurses serve single parents, families, extended families, gay and lesbian families, and non–English-speaking families. Nurses are increasingly faced with the prospect of caring for people with perspectives and lifestyles that may not represent their own (Woodruff, 1995). There is an even greater increase in the number of people over 75 years old who are living alone (Woodruff,

1995). There are presently 52,000 centenarians in America today, more than 12 times the number just 30 years ago (U.S. News & World Report, September 4, 1999. p 59). The challenge from a nursing perspective is to educate students and graduates to respond to the diversity of new patients (Stanhope, 1996).

Education continues largely to support a type of nursing practice that gives recognition and social sanction to treatments and approaches based primarily on Western biomedical health beliefs and healing practices. Basic to the traditional medical model is the emphasis on sickness as a purely biological phenomenon that implies nothing at all about the character of the person who is ill (Kleinman, 1996; MacFarquhar, 1996). Nurses are socialized to value curing and an objective approach to illness and treatment, deemphasizing cooperation, connectedness, and subjective experiences. Students are educated to seek the right answer or cause, and are rewarded for quick closure and tidy formulations. Humans are not easily accepting of informed skepticism, respect for the views of others, and subjective evidence that creates uncertainty rather than quick closure. Uncertainty carries with it giving things up and keeping open other possibilities, with the understanding that challenges can emerge to raise other options, and that the dismissal of the subjective experiences as if they were mere side effects is no longer applicable (Middlemiss & Neste-Kenny, 1994).

As nursing struggles with a genuine desire to deliver competent care to clients from multiple cultures and perspectives, the question raised is, How do we as nurses approach the notion of diversity? We believe in equal access to services as part of the fairness paradigm. Yet nursing is not always sure what an operational definition of fair access means in terms of a diverse population. What does *group differences* mean for our practice? Is being color-blind or gender-blind a positive value or does it compromise quality care when we assume that everyone is the same, that is, that black people are just like white people, or that all black people are really alike? Can health research findings on white males be generalized to the entire population? Does *fairness* mean treating people the same or choosing a yardstick appropriate to the person and group? For example, who defines what constitutes a family or a supportive network, the nurse or the client? Do we use the client's definition for therapeutic purposes or persist in imposing our definition of a family?

We are committed to offering quality care as part of the fairness paradigm but have been reluctant to let diversity influence or change individual practice or the health care delivery system in general. Therefore, when the culture-bound nurse provides care to a client from a different background, both are frequently in conflict because of unspoken, collective assumptions about the appropriate client, the appropriate network of support, appropriate treatment, and appropriate role relationships.

For rehabilitation nurses, the issue is how the discipline of nursing can deliver culturally sensitive health and nursing care services. Present models of care are modified on a continual basis as ethnic and cultural groups intersect in the society (Charlton, 1998). As systems accommodate to diversity, the interplay may also change health care practices. In this century, health care workers will do more than provide traditional services: we may see the expansion of what constitutes health practices and the healing process. What we do with diversity once we accept and admit it is the central challenge of the 21st century.

In the year 2000, minorities will constitute nearly one-fourth of the total population (Davidhizar, Dowd, & Giger, 1998). An increasingly diverse population means providing nursing care in the context of many different ethnic groups and cultures (ANA, 1992; Crow, 1993). Behaving with a multicultural perspective is imperative but difficult because of a number of barriers. This chapter will (1) identify and describe barriers to providing competent nursing care rooted in historical inequality, long-standing cultural stereotypes, and a lack of consistent dialogue across race, class, and cultural lines in order to debunk the pervasive images, (2) identify and discuss the components of the culturally competent nurse, and (3) provide a series of case studies to illustrate the complexity of delivering competent care in American society.

BARRIERS OR IMPEDIMENTS TO PROVIDING COMPETENT AND CULTURALLY SENSITIVE CARE

Visible Differences

Color is one of the most obvious characteristics on first contact between blacks, whites, and browns. It comes as the initial introduction, before a handshake or a word, before a name, an accent, an idea, a place in the hierarchy of class, or a glimpse of personality. We do not have a historical and cultural framework that provides an understanding of people who look and think differently, so the problem is solved by automatic categorizing. In our nation, differences in color trigger assumptions about an individuals' intelligence, morality, reliability, and skills (Shipley, 1997). Interpersonal encounters can also trigger anxiety, antagonism, and hatred because there is a tendency to feel negative about the "other" who either is not understood or is conditioned by society to react automatically with fear. Many times, cultural differences and the ethnic identification of the individual become obscured or suppressed in favor of racial stereotypes and labeling, rather than being appreciated as complex and coexisting realities (Funderburg, 1994).

Many expect to find others with perfect, intact bodies that accent beauty and youth. Anything less is seen as imperfection and less desirable. "The use of a wheelchair, shortness of breath, an unsteady gait, or a deficiency in hearing, seeing or speech will be perceived as more than a health problem. They may be seen as indications that the individual is less competent, less intelligent, less worthy than others, more bodily mess, and more menacing to the observer" (Saylor, 1990, p. 47). Although they make up 12 to 15% of the people of a country, the disabled are marginalized, as reflected in the absence of accurate representation in film and television, and the myths and stereotypes about disability and sexuality (Charlton, 1998). Think of the demonic crippled King Richard III (Fries, 1998).

Speech and language patterns that differ from what one is accustomed to also have negative connotations. Differences can conjure up images of inferiority or incompetency (Rainwater, 1970; Reed, 1998). In an evaluation, a student once assigned a simian quality to a faculty member from a different cultural and regional background, describing her speech and accent as "primitive."

Worldview

Worldview is the perspective from which a person views the world. It is an interpretation of an individual's reality, shaped by a set of assumptions, concepts, and premises which are assumed to be true and are usually not questioned (Crow, 1993). Culture is a flexible learning system that transforms basic biological components into meaningful thoughts and behaviors shared by its members. Culture includes such attributes as beliefs; rituals; symbols; language; communication style; time and personal space issues; family rituals; and beliefs about health and health practices (McCormick, 1987; Spruhan, 1996). A social life that isolates people by race, class, gender, and ethnicity in America is such that many of us come to institutions of higher learning from cloistered living situations in which our worldview has never been challenged. The nature of segregated communities causes us to live in exclusive groups with people with similar perspectives, so we have rarely been challenged in terms of the conventional wisdom we learned as part of the socialization process. We may be so culturally bound that we do not recognize that our perspective is only one of many (Morgan, 1990; Moses, 1990). We may not even recognize that our perspective is culturally bound. A lack of awareness and naiveté in knowledge of cultural differences can create an environment of erroneous assumptions, interpretations, and judgments when we encounter people who think and act differently. Because we have varied perspectives and experiences that make for different histories, the absolute concept of "truth" is not always scientifically discernible. Kotlowitz (1998) describes how two groups of people in the same town perceive the same incident differently. He concludes by writing, "The prism depends on which side of the river one resides on and creates wholly different explanations. . . ."

In addition to perception, worldview means we come with varied assumptions about appropriate social behavior, what constitutes problems, and where problems are to be found (Estin, 1998; Gent & Thornton, 1995; Naido, 1989). How we define problems determines what we will do about them. The tunnel vision perspective focuses one's attention on a certain set of possible solutions while neglecting others. Even when we speak of a strange or incomprehensible situation, we are really saying the person has a cognitive system that is different from our own and is therefore less comprehensible. For example, people who go to the emergency room for care and also use the local healer (*curanderos*) have a logical approach to meeting their health needs if the *curanderos* is perceived as essential in the healing process. When forced by the nurse to choose between a cultural health practice and the "right" treatment, these people may become what is called *noncompliant* or nonadherent to the prescribed regimen because the nurse is unfamiliar or unwilling to incorporate the rules of the game, that is, the culture (Grothaus, 1996). Many of the problems in the nurse-client relationship can be located in cultural differences brought to the cross-cultural interpersonal encounter. For example, even when data support that teaching the family would be more health reinforcing than teaching the individual, health workers may remain frozen in the individual-teaching mode as part of America's emphasis on individual empowerment, resulting in noise in communication and disruption in the learning process (Cuthbert-Allman & Conti, 1995). Moving beyond the intuitive, nurses will have to supplement their life experiences in a purposeful way in order to become reeducated for ethnic practice.

Prejudice, Racism, Stereotyping, Sexism, and Ethnocentrism

Nurses may set up cognitions that create barriers or interference when interacting with clients. Even when we try to articulate an agenda of multicultural care, we run immediately into the stumbling blocks of prejudice, racism, stereotyping, and ethnocentricism (Bower, 1996; Bower, 1997). Prejudice is a prejudgment that is not open to reconsideration in the light of any new particular experience because it is an emotional manifestation of deeply held beliefs about other groups. Prejudices are also preconscious cultural assumptions and habits that are systemically reinforced by the biases of the dominant culture. Prejudged attitudes and beliefs breed intolerance and hatred of others. Prejudice, and its sequela, discrimination, are devices at the heart of sexism, racism, homophobia, and classism (McGoldrick & Rohrbaugh, 1987; McGoldrick, Giordano, & Pearce 1996; Morgan, 1990).

Racism is about unequal and unearned power and privileges, a form of prejudice that has been institutionalized and pervades the actions, attitudes, and behaviors in a country. For example, before students enter the classroom, structural supports in the society lead students to have strong inclinations to believe what is intentionally confirmed for them: that those who have been excluded ought to have been and that what does not benefit them ought not to exist (Morgan, 1990; Kleinman, 1996). Marginalization by those in power is justified, endowing some with special privileges and others with less than full citizenship based on subtle policies implying inferior genes, moral shortcomings, and other self-defeating traits. Other "isms" include sexism, classism, and agism and are also about unequal power and privileges. These "isms" bequeath to us a set of deeply ingrained precepts about people derived from their being born into a particular society, group, or family. In the implementation of the nursing process, nurses who have been influenced by these beliefs are able to justify the use of paternalism as opposed to collaboration and give insufficient teaching because the patient is thought not capable of understanding (Shipley, 1997).

Stereotyping is a lack of power to see others as complex beings and therefore robs people of an independent identity and the opportunity to reach one's potential unfettered by self-limiting labels. Racial stereotypes include perceptions such as African Americans' being stupid, hypersexual, immoral, simian, and violent. Gender stereotypes in the larger society include believing that caregiving is still predominantly a woman's responsibility (Debold, Wilson, & Malave, 1993). The recent restructuring of health care that views hospitalization as managing a crisis event releases all but the most acutely ill patients in a few days with the assumption that care will be provided by family members in the home; this is an example of the assumptions made about gender and individual responsibility. As society wavers about how best to fill this gap when the family feels stressed, the emphasis is inevitably on what people are doing wrong as individuals and families. Because ways of living in families are still primarily structured by culture and gender, we need to take these factors into account when critiquing and lobbying for family-friendly policies (Campbell, 1996).

Ethnocentrism supports stereotyping because the ethnocentric standard of normalcy determines the yardstick by which all other groups are to be judged. Among Americans, there seems to be great ethnocentricism (Gent & Thornton, 1995). Rooda (1993 p. 212) reports that individuals are likely to be more positive toward their own ethnic and cultural groups than toward others. The belief in one's own superiority may lead to cultural imposition—the process of imposing one's values on others. Cultural blindness, or being culturally bound, confuses sameness with equality and goodness. The childhood egocentric worldview is that most people are "just like me" where "just like me" is positive and "unlike me" is negative (Smith, Colling, Elander, & Latham, 1993). Deconstructing myths is a difficult challenge that nurses must

undertake in order to move toward culturally sensitive care. Like a child who fearfully reads a book about a monster, only to find at the end that Grover, the friend the child loves all along, is the monster, the nurse has to look inward (Layton, 1992). We should strive for attitudes and ways of being with others that encourage intercultural appreciation and respect. We need to bring open minds and hearts, compassion, and a sense of justice, as well as intelligence, to reduce our anxieties about the otherness. Living and working in a complex world asks us to stretch our definition of American life while recognizing our commonalities. We have to learn to listen to each other more deeply, to evaluate critically our own methodologies, and to use our imaginations to create new possibilities, experimenting and perhaps never arriving at final rights or definitive wrongs.

Medical Deficit Model

The medical deficit model is a barrier because practitioners socialized in dominant norms may bring to their practice beliefs that people from different cultures are inferior, deprived, and disabled by their own experiences and knowledge (Chychula, 1990; West, 1993). Loaded categories are created distinguishing between the problematic and the nonproblematic client (compliant versus noncompliant; motivated versus lacking in motivation). Inherent in this perspective is that the clients need to change themselves or their conditions. Clients may be talked to and about, and not with. The coded descriptions prevent the nurse from asking critical questions and lead to noise in communication and failure of bonding in the nurse-client system. Many hidden cultural demands of institutional encounters must be analyzed and reflected upon because as they produce rule-governed activities that may be counterproductive to creating the healing alliance.

Culture and Poverty

The way Americans think about poverty and poor people gets in the way of investing low-income people with full citizenship. The American dream is the defining characteristic of the dominant culture (Hochschild, 1995). The dream promises that all Americans have a reasonable chance to achieve success through their own efforts and to attain virtue and fulfillment through success. Success is defined as reaching some threshold higher than the point at which one starts and is central to the American's self-image and to the national character. If success implies virtue, then failure implies sin. "Devaluing losers allows people to maintain their belief that the world is fundamentally just" (Hochschild, 1995, p. 31). In the context of the American dream, to be poor can be perceived as a moral flaw and can rob one of independent identity and full human worth. Despite persistent myths such as "They are always asking for handouts" or "They wreck the inner city," the generation of what appears to be a more or less permanent group of poor people can be traced to many factors including the economic and structural changes in society between the 1950s and the 1980s, when industrial jobs left the cities. Second-generation inner-city Puerto Ricans and others were trapped in the most vulnerable niche of a factory-based economy that was rapidly being replaced by service industries. Between 1950 and 1990, the proportion of factory jobs in New York City decreased approximately threefold. The pronounced effect of poverty is diminishing opportunity, because the real engines of opportunity, new jobs and better schools, are moving to the periphery (Wilson, 1995).

Contrary to stereotypes and beliefs, poor people survive because they do work in ways that are possible. Females supplement meager incomes and keep families surviving by babysitting neighbors' children, housekeeping for paying boarders, bartending at local clubs, working off the books as seamstresses for garment contractors, or, caught in the female dependency trap, establishing amorous relationships with men who are willing to make cash contributions to household expenses. Male income strategies include an underground economy of repairing cars on the streets, running unlicensed construction businesses, selling numbers (off-track betting), and making drug sales—cocaine and crack in the 1980s, and heroin in the 1990s. When people feel they have no place in society, the hopelessness is evidenced in such survival skills as peer pressure on teenagers not to succeed in school, which keeps them in their place; early parenting; and alienation from the larger society, including distrust of the health care system and minimal connection to health care practices such as health promotion (Humphries, 1998).

Individualism

For Americans, the highest ideal is to seize control of one's own life by refusing to be confined or manipulated by anyone else's definition of who or what one should be (Smith, Colling, Elander, & Latham, 1993, p. 206). The valuing of individuality is integral to the American character and nourishes the mind against all obstacles. It can also become an end in itself separated from social context and social consequences. Think about the female student who earns a prestigious award normally meant for males and believes that it is based on her own merit. Think about those who open up the space for her to be perceived on her own merit. Many problems are not individual problems but those of women, families, and men as a whole. Issues such as substance abuse are not an individual problem but have deeper dynamics of social alienation and marginalization. Furthermore, the traditional nursing curriculum extolling individuality, self-reliance, and self-empowerment may be off-putting, insensitive, and alien to members of many ethnic minority groups who value family and family problem solving around issues such as health. For example, when cultural assessment suggests that teaching the family would be more health reinforcing than teaching the individual, the nurse can remain frozen in the one-to-one teaching mode, leading to noise in communication and failure in health promotion activities (Grant & Sleeter, 1997).

Overgeneralization

Taking cultural differences too literally may also create barriers by overemphasizing exclusive membership in particular social groups and deemphasizing individual differences within a group. People are influenced by a multitude of other factors. Life in a particular culture is an interplay between the versions of the world that people form under its institutional sway and the versions of it that are the products of their individual history (Brunner, 1995). The variance in a group is also affected by its members' degree of acculturation to the larger society. For example, an individual can modify cultural expectations about the use and nonuse of eye contact (Narayan & Rea, 1997). Also, cultures are dynamic and change continually as they intersect with time and other groups (Lind, 1995; Woodruff, 1995). Groups exist only sometimes, and even then individuals participate only sometimes. The nurse learns how to walk a thin line between being culturally sensitive and reinforcing unfortunate stereotypes (Bredok & McDermott, 1995, p. 257).

Maintaining a degree of skepticism and openness is a stance that will serve the nurses well as they go about their interpersonal encounters.

All of these factors are barriers and are incompatible with empathy and collaboration. In addition, they prevent health providers from focusing on differences in competency and deny clients a chance to participate in their own care.

Components of Culturally Competent Nursing Practice

Nursing leaders tell us that one of the major goals of the 21st century is achieving cultural competency as part of professional nursing. Cultural competence refers to the nurse's ability to honor and respect differences and to incorporate them into our care planning. It is not something we possess, but a dynamic process in which we engage; it is a way of thinking and behaving. Cultural competence is a way of being self-aware and at the same time stepping outside one's traditional value orientation. "It is knowing who we are that provides us with some sense of limits of our understanding of others" (Bartol & Richardson, 1998, p. 76). Being culturally competent increases the likelihood of the nurse's being able to provide high-quality care (Nelson, Wood, & Nalepka, 1993). Cultural competence is a complex, multidimensional way of practicing that motivates nurses to develop the knowledge, skills, and ability necessary to care for diverse clients, families, and communities (Crow, 1993; Holtz & Wilson, 1992). Diversity relates to the differences that people present and the knowledge of such differences. Cultural diversity includes such variables as ethnicity, race, gender, sexual orientation, spirituality, religion, family style, family makeup, age, region of origin, language, physical appearance, and socioeconomic status. The development of cultural competence, along with professional practice, enables the nurse to provide services in forms consistent with the client's value system. Because people make health choices and decisions that draw on their cultural backgrounds and group affiliations, the provision of care that is consistent with the cultural parameters has been defined by American Nurses Association's Expert Panel report (1992):

> Care designed for the individual person; care based on the uniqueness of the person's cultural [values] and includes cultural norms and values; care includes empowerment

strategies to facilitate client decision making in health behavior; and care is provided with sensitivity to the cultural uniqueness of the client.

Culturally competent care requires

- Awareness and examination of one's own attitudes toward diversity
- Sensitivity and respect for differences
- Cultural knowledge
- Cultural skills
- Cross-cultural communication skills
- Cultural brokering for a client

Awareness of One's Own Attitudes Toward Diversity

We began by accepting that each of us has a cognitive system, a way of looking at the world that comes from membership in several groups, beginning with the culture and family we are born into. Cognitive systems include all those unconscious classifications, judgments, and values that trigger most of an adult's initial responses to events. Awareness of our own cultural influences, including professional socialization, sensitizes us to recognizing that people of other cultures may have the same or different beliefs and values. Self-examination is being able to take an honest look at our own beliefs, values, and interpersonal styles that arise from our own cultural upbringing. The culturally sensitive nurse is not ahistorical but is able to place herself or himself in context. Becoming connected to this historical continuity allows viewing others in the context of their connectedness. From that basis, one might be able to imagine what it means to live out the experiences of being a refugee; being black, brown, or yellow in the United States; being male; being female; and being of different sexual orientations (Brunner, 1995).

Sensitivity and Respect

For a culturally competent nurse, sensitivity means the ability to shift perspectives; to imagine and think beyond the identity associated with one's own background. Respect involves the ability to accept the client as a unique person, suspending judgment; accepting the client where and as the client is; valuing the client as an individual; and accepting the client's worldview as that person's reality. To understand well what something means requires some awareness of the alternative meanings that can be attached to the matter under scrutiny, whether one agrees with them or not (Brunner, 1995). If one can't imagine, one can't see whomever one chooses to disdain or hate or dismiss as being connected with one's fate. One can be an extremely competent nurse with a monocultural perspective if one chooses to work only with people like oneself. But in a diverse culture like America in which consensus about what needs to be known is negotiated through the day-to-day exchange of its participants, a culture-bound nurse soon becomes burned out and inept in providing competent care.

Cultural Knowledge

Along with the use of imagination and self-knowledge, nurses need some basic knowledge about the culture of the clients they serve. The nurse needs the knowledge to help understand the conversations of many kinds of people. Nurses who do not have basic cultural knowledge may have difficulty in interpreting clients' behaviors and as a consequence may develop feelings of inadequacy and helplessness (Leininger, 1991). Knowledge alone does not ensure cultural competence. Knowledge does, however, provide an opportunity for the delivery of health care that is culturally congruent with the basic beliefs of the target group and may replace myths and stereotypes.

Cultural Skills

Cultural skills are used when cultural awareness and cultural knowledge merge to meet clients' needs. When interacting, the culturally responsible nurse uses culturally sensitive interventions such as appropriate touch or nontouch during conversation, modified physical distance between self and others, and strategies to avoid cultural misunderstandings while meeting mutually agreed upon goals. An example of the respecting and valuing of culture is the nurse who assists the client to integrate cultural food and religious practices into weight reduction and diabetes management strategies.

Communication Across Cultures

Interpersonal interaction and communication in today's world are done across societal, ethnic, racial, national, generational, and gender-based barriers (Gent & Thornton, 1995). Bridging language, attitudinal, and cultural differences means (1) entering into conversation and learning from clients about their ex-

periences and the significance of these experiences for their health, and (2) giving space for viewpoints that differ from one's own. One doesn't speak just to a person; one speaks to a set of beliefs about the world (Crow, 1993). The nurse learns what is meaningful for the client through conversations that draw the nurse into the client's world (Brislin, 1993). The nurse participates in conversation with the clients in a way that makes it possible for the clients to find their own solutions. A powerful intervention is being a good conversationalist (Berg & DeJong, 1996). The practitioner's role is continually to invite clients to explore and define two matters: (1) what it is they want different in their lives (goals), and (2) what strengths and resources they can bring to bear on making these desired differences a reality.

Language is important to every group and is vital for communication. Knowledge of the formal language as well as the colloquialisms, slang, and everyday common usage of words is significant when aiming for quality care. Competent nursing care requires a culturally diverse workforce that is reflective of the community. Relying on a translator, especially someone with limited or no health care knowledge, may result in an interpretation that is not relevant for the care provider or the person seeking care. Also, translation is different from interpretation. In sharing sensitive information, a translator may complicate the situation. There is a need to expand the recruiting of multilingual nurses (Cuthbert-Allman & Conti, 1995).

Culture Brokering

In every client interaction, there are at least three cultures: The personal culture of the provider, the culture of the client, and the culture of the health care delivery system (Kavanaugh, 1993). The culture broker can be seen as a link in the process of cultural competence. The broker links the concerns of the client and those of the health care system. The culture broker may be able to represent clients or groups that are otherwise unheard by linking health institutions more effectively to culturally diverse communities and insisting on a dialogue between unresponsive mainstream institutions and cultural groups. Activities include advocating, mediating, negotiating, and intervening for the client. The broker is in a position to understand both cultures and to use knowledge to resolve or minimize problems that may have resulted from individuals in either culture not understanding the other person's culture.

Many people call the culture broker a person who is enough of an outsider and has freedom from institutional restraints to fashion an autonomous macroscopic view of a given situation (Reed, 1998). The culture broker's most powerful tools are (1) information, (2) negotiating skills, and (3) an ongoing relationship to the health care system, protecting yet connecting to the treatment desired and needed by the client in a manner that supports the client's perspective. A good nurse is passionately on the side of the patient. Support doesn't mean "I support you in everything you do," but "I will listen and help you figure out what might work best for you."

Concepts Relevant to a Working Knowledge of Diverse Cultures

The acknowledgment and valuing of cultural differences have implications in providing quality nursing care to diverse populations and represent a challenge to the competent cross-cultural nurse. Diversity should be understood as the varied perspectives and approaches that clients bring when interacting in the health care process (Thomas & Ely, 1996). They bring different, important, and competitively relevant knowledge and perspectives about how to be healthy and treat sickness. The knowledge and perspectives are providing some fresh and meaningful approaches to health care in terms of the holistic paradigm. In accordance with concepts of cultural transition, acculturation, and assimilation, the professional nurse should counteract overgeneralizations and stereotyping by attentive listening and questioning during the cultural assessment. The cultural assessment seeks to see the problem from the client's perspective and focuses on the client's understanding of the problem. Assuming without asking may lead to grossly incorrect presumptions (Spruhan, 1996, p. 448). An example is the medical concern of noncompliance. Noncompliance may be described as purposeful behavior within the context of the client's perceptual world.

Concepts relevant to understanding diverse cultures include the following:

1. *Family structure.* Ethnicity, values, and beliefs are deeply tied to the family through which they are transmitted. Family structure includes events (rites of passage, rituals), holidays, and festivities that can serve as a window into the worldview of a specific group. Nurses need to be able to identify who constitutes the family for a given client. Incompetent care can occur when the nurse defines the family in one way and the client defines the support system differently.

2. *Communication.* Communication is the first step in delivering quality health care. Because of the complexity of communication, the cross-cultural nurse has to bridge cultural and language differences. Verbal and nonverbal patterns vary from culture to culture. Culture also influences how people use space, both personal and private, and how time is perceived and used. Many times intercultural differences can impede communication when a nurse is unaware of cultural differences in the components of communication. Nurses need some knowledge of expectations for visitors, the rules for polite behavior, and the norms for verbal and nonverbal communication.

3. *Health practices.* Health practices deal with methods to prevent sickness, promote health, or prevent death. Given particular beliefs, the nurse assesses what practices are desired, expected, or not desired and what the processes involved in sustaining these practices are, as well as the type of providers used to seek help before or during periods of imbalance.

4. *Health and illness beliefs.* Beliefs instruct a culture about the meaning of health and illness, the causation of health and illness, what is labeled as problematic, and how to go about problem solving.

5. *Religious and death beliefs.* Existential questions such as the meaning of pain, suffering, and death are embedded in the culture and expressed differently by different groups. Each ethnic group has a particular view on the dying process itself. When a death is imminent, cultural or religious beliefs are brought forward in how the death is handled. Customs and rituals vary and can be a barrier between the nurse, the client, and the family if the nurse provides interventions that intimidate the integrity of a family (Spruhan, 1996).

6. *Dietary practices.* Dietary preferences are inextricably linked to culture and rituals within the culture. Knowledge about food practices and the modification of dietary practices during specific events in the culture is germane to competent nursing care.

7. *Geography.* Those who cross national borders are known as emigrants or immi-

grants. Mass emigration occurs when large numbers of people leave their country because of social, political, or religious upheavals played out by war, genocide, or threats of imprisonment. Usually, migrating people tend to cluster together in designated parts of the new country.

8. *Child rearing and childbearing practices.* These tell much about how the culture transmits values and beliefs to the next generation.

National Character

The prevailing cultural beliefs, attitudes, and values within the United States are based on the white Anglo-Saxon Protestant ethic (Table 8–1). It is this framework that many nurses are reared in or acculturated to during the socialization process in professional education. Discussion of the national character is a beginning step for nurses so that they can gain a perspective on the relativity of their professional belief system as they interact with others in a pluralistic society.

African Americans (Table 8–2). African Americans make up about 12% of the national population. Because African Americans have a history of chattel slavery, the ability to survive under all conditions is an important value and is indicated in some traditional practices such as family structure, child-rearing practices, and dietary practices. This is a heterogeneous group with much intraethnic variation.

Jewish Americans (Table 8–3). Jewish-American people are called Jews, and their faith is Judaism. Israel was founded by Jews, and its language is Hebrew, the language of the Jewish religious texts. The term *Jewish* refers to both a people and a religion, and not a race. The terms *Hebrew, Israelite,* and *Jew* have been used interchangeably. The Jewish presence in the United States extends back to the 17th century. The largest emigration from eastern Europe and Russia was between 1880 and 1920 during waves of pogroms (anti-Jewish riots and murders). Other migrations occurred in the 1930s and 1940s during the Nazi period in Europe and in the 1980s and 1990s from the former Union of Soviet Socialist Republics.

South Asians (Table 8–4). South Asians are people of a Hindu, Muslim, or Sikh tradition who come from India, Pakistan, Bangladesh, Sri Lanka, and Nepal.

Asian Americans (Table 8–5). Although Asians are often put into the same category, each group is different. For example, even within one group, such as Chinese Americans, cultural values differ according to various factors, for example, a rural or an urban background. With immigration comes acculturation with a mixture of both traditional and Western influences. Because of the risk of simplification, Asians are defined here primarily as Chinese, Japanese, Koreans, and Filipinos. There are many commonalities among these four groups in health practices, philosophies, and theories about health and illness.

Southeast Asians (Table 8–6). Southeast Asians consist of South Vietnamese, Laotians, Cambodians, and Hmong. The first wave of refugees was in 1975. They were predominantly professionals, military personnel, and government officials who had some close affiliation with the United States. The second wave in 1979 consisted of people who were uneducated and underskilled from more rural areas. Southeast Asians constitute a diverse group with many different languages and dialects.

Hispanic Americans (Table 8–7). The Hispanic (a term used by the federal government) American population is the largest minority group in the United States. The terms *Hispanic* or *Latino* are inclusive of all Spanish-speaking people (Grothaus, 1996, p. 31). The population is made up of a complex ethnic mixture of Indian, Spanish, African, and even Asian cultures and comes from different geographical, economic, and political contexts (Mexico, Puerto Rico, Cuba, and Central and South America).

Native Americans (Table 8–8). American Indians or Native Americans are the indigenous population of North America. The Bureau of Indian Affairs recognizes over 500 different tribes. They make up the smallest ethnic group in North America. There is no international language among tribes, and cultures vary as much as Irish Americans and Italian Americans.

Cultural Assessment

The culturally responsible nurse includes cultural assessment as integral to the nursing process. Following are examples of religious beliefs integral in planning culturally competent care:

1. A mother refused to let her child undergo

TABLE 8–1 ■ PREVAILING U.S. CULTURE

Geographical Pattern	Health Practices	Health/Illness Beliefs
Members live in all regions of the United States	Physician is the gateway to health and to treatment of illness Human body is divided according to specialists Members try to get the best medical care by the best physician specialist and in the best hospital possible Members use the medical model—scientific investigation and problem solving based on symptoms being diagnosed and cured by "the doctor" Members are confident in the ability of technology and science to cure disease There has been little emphasis on prevention and preventive practices until recently Recent trend within the dominant society is to use herbs, certain foods, special dietary prescriptions, and natural curative measures to gain a sense of well-being outside the boundary of modern medicine Nursing can be narrowly conceived of as carrying out medical orders	Disease process is a result of germs, microorganisms Disease creates structural and functional changes Symptoms are diagnosed and treated There is a split between mind and body Emphasis is on disease rather than illness Integration of mind and body to maintain health is a recent belief about health Emphasis on self-determination and empowerment in maintaining health is a phenomenon of the 1960s that has only recently generalized to the general public

Family Structure	Social Issues	Communication
Great value is placed on the nuclear family Family is individual-centered; members believe in the individual, self-determination, and empowerment	There is culturally prescribed aspiration for career success; as way of introduction people ask what one does as a means of giving identity Status is tied to money and success	Less value is placed on emotional expressivensss. Uninhibited display of suffering is distrusted and apt to be labeled as emotional instability Talk is valued, with discomfort for silences during conversation Patients react to pain as stoically and calmly as possible, choosing to withdraw if pain becomes intense Great value is placed on adequate space, both physically and psychologically; people who live in a small space are assumed to be poor and probably uneducated It is assumed that any honest and open communication requires eye contact Privacy during nurse-client conversation is valued as part of self-determination; family may be seen as intrusive to confidentiality Touch is valued and perceived as a gesture of warmth and caring

Dietary Practices	Religious and Death Practices	Childbearing and Child Rearing
Large amount of meat protein Generous amount of milk, butter, and dairy products	Members are usually Protestant Characteristics are optimism, rationality, belief in the future, independence, and individualism Characteristic of optimism often leads to the inability to cope with tragedy or to engage in mourning Death is perceived as a defeat rather than integral to the life process	Partner is expected to be present during the birthing experience Independence is valued; becoming an adult means leaving home, being on one's own A sign of successful rearing is independence and leaving home as a young adult

TABLE 8-2 ▪ AFRICAN-AMERICAN CULTURE

Geographical Patterns	Health Practices	Health/Illness Beliefs
Fifty percent live in the South; majority live in 11 large cities: Atlanta; Washington, D.C.; Baltimore; Jackson, Miss.; Gary, Ind.; Newark, N.J.; Detroit; Memphis; Birmingham, Ala.; Richmond, Va.; and New Orleans Members represent a large segment of the blue-collar workers Jamaicans tend to locate in New York or Miami Members constitute about 12% of the population of the United States	Evil spirit or a hex is put on person by someone; needs to be taken off by a root doctor to cast out or contain the evil May consult with a root doctor who is born with a gift for healing. Many times the root doctor is described as being born with a "veil" Folk medicine healers also include spiritualists or fortune tellers who combine reading or telling the future with herbs and special oils to ward off evil Folk practices are usually combined with Western medicine There is tendency to take medication on an as-needed basis, when there are signs of illness such as pain, headaches, etc.; medication stops when symptom disappears God remains an important source of coping and healing Prayer and touching are believed to be helpful in curing illness Process of healing is a relationship with God. When in physical and emotional pain, talk to God Some may use potions to purge the body of the "evil spirits," including sugar and turpentine, herbal drinks, and hot drinks with tea and honey Poultices may be used to treat a variety of illnesses A belly band around the abdomen of a newborn is thought to prevent umbilical hernia Garlic placed on the person or in the room is believed to rid the area of evil spirits By turning black, copper or silver bracelets are believed to protect the wearer when illness is about to occur There is a tolerant attitude toward obesity	Health is being in balance spiritually, emotionally, and physically; health hinges on leading a good Christian life, having strong faith in God and Jesus, and oneness with God Wellness is related to being productive and the absence of pain Each event, including health and illness, has socioreligious significance Illness is disharmony with nature resulting from natural or unnatural causes Natural illnesses are caused by nature's forces such as the weather conditions, bad food, or bad water Unnatural illnesses are brought about by evil forces such as hoodoo, voodoo, witchcraft, rootwork, or hexes

surgery until she came to visit and pray over the equipment and to anoint it with holy oil; then she felt it was safe to use.

2. A woman who was agitated at night became calmer after the priest sprinkled holy water throughout the apartment.

▪ CASE STUDY 8-1

Ms. Jones was a 60-year-old widowed, obese Hispanic woman who lived alone in a senior citizen high-rise apartment in the inner city. During the last 10 years she had become secluded, venturing from her apartment for only short periods after the sudden death of her two sons and an experience in which she was accosted in an attempted robbery. She fell while walking downstairs, and the fall resulted in chronic lower back pain. She was receiving home care services but was minimally cooperative with the nurse and home health aides and homemaker. She resisted getting out of bed, complained of sustained

TABLE 8–2 ■ AFRICAN-AMERICAN CULTURE *Continued*

Family Structure	Social Issues	Communication

Family has egalitarian structure, with shared economic responsibility
There are a large number of female-headed households
Close relationship may exist between adult female child and mother
Grandmother has a central role in economic contribution and child rearing
Because informal "adopting" is an accepted practice, family may include non–blood relatives; children are taken into households when a relative or neighbor dies or is unable to function as a parent for a period of time due to crises
Family system supports adult children as they meet career goals after early parenthood
	Police may be perceived as the ultimate projection of white power
	Conservative social agenda
	  1. Difficult for gays and lesbians to network
	  2. Limited support for abortions; abortions are linked to genocide
	  3. Sexual information and teaching may be linked to giving permission for sexual promiscuity
	There is disapproval of premarital sexual relations but acceptance of children: "Anyone can make one mistake"
	There is high prevalence of hypertension, diabetes mellitus, chronic illnesses, and cancer
		Members tend to be pessimistic about human relationships, especially outside the family
		Members may enter the health care system as the last resort because of historical experiences and prevalence of racism
		Establishment of trust is a paramount issue since historical experiences have made black Americans doubt they will receive fair and good treatment
		First name preceded by "Miss" as a sign of respect may be used—Miss Dolores
		Members are highly verbal: emphasis is on oral history
		Members are expressive and use body movements with speech
		Members are comfortable with close personal space
		Range of eye contact varies; one may speak without direct eye contact and then make eye contact while listening

Dietary Practices	Religious and Death Practices	Child Rearing
Diet is influenced by African ancestors, white Southerners, and Native Americans Diet was developed as a result of the resources and accommodations available to the group during slavery period; high in fat-fried food and sodium; more animal fats, less fiber, and fewer fruits and vegetables are eaten Beans and dark vegetables such as kale and collard greens are used; sometimes are overcooked, and vegetables are cooked with smoke and salty meats (less so presently) Root vegetables such as turnips, sweet potatoes, and yams are used Those African Americans who practice the Islamic faith follow the dietary practices of Islam, including eating no pork Members are averse to using foods and drinks made with dietetic sugars Grains such as rice and a corn-based grain called hominy grits are used	Church is central to community life; members believe in prayer for all situations encountered; strengths or coping come from praying and believing in God Church has served as an institution of health, education, and political activity and may function as the extended family Members express feelings openly during funeral services with visual confrontation of body and support process of embalming so body can look as good as it can for viewing and afterlife The theology of the black Baptist church is fundamentally about Jesus, perceived as a personal relationship with Jesus; people talk about a daily dialogue with Jesus who loves and is concerned Growing number of African Americans practice the Islamic faith, as discussed under South Asia	Self-reliance and education are valued There is acceptance of corporal punishment; members tend to be protective of children, and keep them away from public places in order to protect them from dangers in the society Respectfulness, obedience, conformity to rules, and good behavior are stressed In violence-ridden areas, as an attempt to keep children physically safe and away from undue influence, parents keep children off the street with limited access to peer groups outside school; as children get older, this may become increasingly futile, and parent may give up, disengage, and allow them their freedom Parents may show little affection in public domains

pain, and exhibited self-care deficits, including incontinence. The community nurse had attempted to develop plans with the daughter to help care for her mother but had come to view the daughter as insensitive and inept and had spoken to Ms. Jones about going to a nursing home where her needs would be taken care of.

Because the community nurse's relationship with Ms. Jones was deteriorating as the latter became more withdrawn and angry, a psychiatric nurse was called in for a consulta-

Text continued on page 103

TABLE 8–3 ■ JEWISH-AMERICAN CULTURE

Geographical Patterns	Health Practices	Health/Illness Beliefs
Members are found in every large city—there is greater prevalence in states of California, New York, Texas, Pennsylvania, Illinois, New Jersey, Massachusetts, Maryland, and Ohio; 49% live in the Northeast	Emphasis is on keeping mind and body clean	Body is the temple of God and must be protected from harm

Family Structure	Social Issues	Communication
Care of Jewish society is emphasized Marriage is ideal state In terms of life transitions, Jews may give particular attention to the *bar mitzvah* (for boys) or *bat mitzvah* (for girls), religious ceremonies that are rites of passage and recognition of adulthood Maximization of individual potentials is emphasized	There is historical emphasis on social justice through social action There is more of a tendency to accept or tolerate gay and lesbian lifestyles; members believe in inherent dignity and equality of all God's children Old age is a state of mind; it is believed that learning and involvement continue	Hasidic Jews do not touch women other than their wives and do not shake hands with women Modesty is valued in Orthodox circles and it involves humility Non-Hasidic Jews use touch and short spatial distance when communicating

Dietary Practices (Orthodox Households)	Religious and Death Practices	Childbearing and Child Rearing
Foods are divided into *kosher* (clean) and *treyf* (unclean) Animals are killed instantly with one stroke, and all blood is drained from animal before eating it Pork and birds of prey are unclean and not eaten; shellfish are also not eaten Milk and meat are not mixed together in cooking, serving, or eating. Utensils used to prepare foods and the plates used to serve them are separated Because glass is not absorbent, it can be used for either meat or milk Neutral foods are fish, eggs, vegetables, and fruits and may be used with either dairy or meat dishes Chicken soup is staple	Hebrew language is used for prayers Religion is practiced along a wide continuum from liberal Reform to strict Orthodox Reform Jews may not engage in any special daily practices but may still observe holidays, religious rites, and selected dietary cultural customs Orthodox Jews adhere to most religious practices Ultra-orthodox Jews such as Hasidic Jews eat no product with yeast at Passover Members observe the Sabbath from Friday sunset until Saturday sunset Orthodox women separate themselves during their menstrual periods and may not touch or sit with men until they have been to the *mikveh*, a ritual bath after their period is over	Orthodox husband may not come into the birthing room; he believes he protects wife's dignity by not viewing her genitalia; when husband is in the birthing room, wife should be fully covered, including her head Circumcision of male child is done on the 8th day after delivery A Jew by Jewish law is a child born to a Jewish mother Orthodox groups believe that children have the right to be born; when acceptance of birth control exists, there is approval of oral contraceptives and rhythm; members do not believe that barrier techniques are acceptable

TABLE 8–4 ■ SOUTH-ASIAN CULTURE

Geographical Patterns	Health Practices	Health/Illness Beliefs
Live in New York, Washington, DC, Massachusetts, Pennsylvania, Michigan, Ohio, Illinois, Texas, California	Oldest woman is considered the authority on health and healing matters Family is expected to be involved in all health care decisions Often women are reluctant to seek care because of emphasis placed on modesty and shyness about disrobing; families object to female family members' being examined by men Members may delay seeking care because of fear that a medical diagnosis may decrease marriage prospect Health problems and solutions are viewed as the concern of the entire family; husbands and fathers are the spokesmen about all family matters, including health; if the patient is the wife, she expects her husband to answer all the questions Husband's mother is perceived as the family expert on health and nutrition and is frequently consulted on these matters	Familism and fatalism influence health pattern Some believe in faith healing, and others believe illness is punishment for one's sins or actions in a previous or present life There is strong belief in fate—individual has little control over what happens

Family Structure	Social Issues	Communication
Extended family is the norm; married sons, along with their wives and children, live with their parents and are subject to parental authority Self-determination and empowerment have little value Decisions are made by the family elders or head of the household based on the good of the family; daughters, whose marriages are usually arranged by their parents, live with their in-laws Filial piety refers to the duty and obligation of the son to care for elderly parents. Perception of self is in relation to the family. A woman in the household may expect husband or other male to speak for her	Attitude is that mental illness is a major social stigma, so psychiatric symptoms are denied and usually displayed somatically Attitude toward the disabled can traditionally be negative, and expectations with respect to education and rehabilitation are low; disabled are often kept from public view; amputations may be perceived as due to sins of a previous life	It is sign of respect to leave one shoe at the door of a traditional Indian home In greeting the family, one begins by greeting the eldest male first, then other males, followed by females in sequence by age It is rude for females to make eye contact with males; this might be misinterpreted as sexual overture; women tend to draw eyes downward as a sign of respect Public touching is socially unacceptable and taboo South Asians speak in a very soft tone, but not out of shyness or uncertainty

Table continued on following page

TABLE 8–4 ■ SOUTH-ASIAN CULTURE *Continued*

Dietary Practices	Religious and Death Practices	Childbearing and Child Rearing
Members practice Ayurvedic diet system that keeps cold and hot foods in balance; for example, pregnancy is a hot state, and cold foods are prescribed Hindus do not eat meat because it involves harming living creatures Muslims do not eat pork or take intoxicating beverages	Three major religious beliefs are Hindu, Islam (Muslim), and Sikh **Hindu** Vedas is the sacred writing, and Brahman is the principle and source of the universe and the center from which all things proceed and return Karma determines one's life Reincarnation is a central belief and depends on moral behavior The goal is liberation from cycle of rebirth and redeath, and entrance into Nirvana **Islam (Muslim)** Mohammed is the prophet of Allah (God) and founder of Islam, which means submission to the will of Allah Koran (Qur'an) is the Word of God Prayer is performed five times a day, facing East to Mecca Belief is in a judgment day and life after death **Sikh** Doctrine is based on both Hindu and Islamic beliefs **Death Practices** Euthanasia and right to die are not accepted The dying person may not be told of impending death Death at home surrounded by family and friends is encouraged For Hindus, acceptance of hospice care for the dying is not automatic; depends on a variety of things For Muslims, no one can touch the body except for the family and the priest; if a man dies, a woman can not touch the body; the death of an individual is mourned by chanting loudly Ritual washing of the body is performed by family members or priest only For Hindus and Sikhs, the body is cremated; mourning is done in a loud and clear voice for all to bear witness Autopsy is acceptable if necessary	Members are taught to maintain self-control and suppress their feelings; emotional outbursts such as expression of anger or pain are discouraged and may be viewed as a sign of weakness Muslim tradition does not allow unfamiliar men to touch another man's wife without permission; husband may perceive a male nurse or physician who touches and exposes a wife during labor and delivery as violating Islamic beliefs

TABLE 8–5 ■ ASIAN-AMERICAN CULTURE

Geographical Patterns	Health and Healing Practices	Health/Illness Beliefs
Large communities are located in cities, mostly in the western part of the United States, with small groupings of inhabitants evident in almost all communities The largest Chinese community in the United States is located in New York City, and the second largest in San Francisco Seventy percent of Japanese population live in Hawaii and California Initial Japanese arrived in the West in 19th century and worked on the railroads, farms, and fishing industry; third and fourth generation have assimilated well into the dominant culture; 50% are married to non-Japanese persons	Chinese medicine encompasses meditation, nutrition, martial arts, herbology, acumassage, acupressure, moxibustion, acupuncture, and spiritual healing Acupressure, acumassage, and moxibustion apply to focal points to reestablish the balance between yin and yang Moxibustion is a procedure using a small cone consisting of dried herbs, garlic and salt; it is heated with an incense stick and placed over a site where the heat is felt; used to heal wounds, abscesses, etc. Spiritual healing is carried out by temple healers in the Chinese culture, called *espiritas* in the Filipino culture; this involves the utilization of ethereal healing by using auras and psychic energies within and surrounding the human body to heal a condition Acupuncture is the most visible demonstration of the energy system; it involves the insertion of hairlike needles into special acupuncture points on the skin; these points are located on meridian pathways of energy, *chi,* leading to the various organs of the body Herbal therapy falls into four categories of energy (cold, hot, warm, and cool), five categories of taste, and a neutral group Shiastsu is a Japanese style of massage, involving placing intense pressure to specific areas of the foot or hand to treat various ailments Martial arts and movement exercises are used to foster physical strength and internal homeostasis *T'ai chi* is exercise that relaxes the mind as well as the body Spiritual	Chinese medicine is based on the theoretical concept of energy with the emphasis on mind-body integration, health, and prevention Concept of energy is derived from the Taoist religion, which maintains that nature maintains an energy balance in humans by the dual polarities of *yin* and *yang;* yin is negative, dark, cold, and feminine; yang is positive, light, warm, and masculine Members believe that most imbalances in energy are caused by a wrong diet or by strong emotional feelings; self-restraint, healing techniques, and herbs can restore the balance Japanese health beliefs are rooted in the Shinto religion, which holds that humans are inherently good; evil is caused by outside spirits who punish humans who have succumbed to temptation; health is achieved through balance, prevention, and cleanliness

Family Structure	Social Issues	Communication
Kinship is traditionally organized around male lines; fathers, sons, and uncles are the important, recognized relationships between and among families There are strong family ties; family comes first and the individual last Daughter-in-law is submissive to the mother-in-law	For the Japanese communities, mental illness, disfiguring physical disabilities, and congenital deformities are viewed as an embarrassment and are met with isolation	Members emphasize harmony in social interactions Emphasis is on social acceptance in all human interactions; members often avoid direct expressions of conflict Filipino who disagrees may use a "go-between person" to iron out the differences *Table continued on following page*

TABLE 8–5 ■ ASIAN-AMERICAN CULTURE *Continued*

Family Structure	Social Issues	Communication
Japanese Issei (first generation immigrant)—family obligations may take precedence over own needs, including health needs Role is to nurture husband and children and care for the in-laws Age is important for prestige Obedience to parents and preservation of the family's good name are highly regarded		Members have concern about interactions not shaming the family Members may respond to suggestions in a positive manner but may not follow through, accepting input but reserving judgment for later Members generally speak in a moderate to low tone; a nurse talking loudly may be interpreted as being angry Touching should be kept to a minimum; a formal distance, which is a form of respect, should be maintained Many are uncomfortable with face-to-face communication, especially direct eye contact Nurse should be polite and formal and address client by the whole name or by the family name and title; the family name is stated first and then the given name; addressing a person by other than the family name is considered rude Members believe in social reciprocity as expressed in kind words or symbolic gifts; they may wish to reciprocate as a gesture of appreciation for services rendered; rejection of such gifts may offend

Dietary Practices	Religious and Death Practices	Childbearing and Child Rearing
Foods are classifed as *yin* (cold) and *yang* (hot); a balance between the two is important to health; chicken (yang) and melon (yin) constitute a healthy diet Yang illness may be counteracted by a yin food A Yang condition indicates an overabundance of energy—fever, parched throat, crusty nose, and watery eyes; it is treated with watercress or watermelon soup (yin) The value of food is taught to children according to what it does to keep the body healthy Chinese: mixture of meat and vegetables; rice, noodles, beans, meat choices, and tofu as a staple of the diet Japanese: Diet consists primarily of rice, vegetables, fish, pickled fruits, and little meat	Half of Japanese Americans are Christians and half are Buddhists Members have tradition of ancestor worship and believe that the spirits of dead relatives continue to dwell among them and protect their descendants; many believe that their spirits can never rest unless living descendants provide care of the grave and worship their memory Members consult spiritual healers, temple healers, or fortune healers who can visualize good and bad spirits, recall the past, and predict the future Many Filipinos are devout Catholics and have a fatalistic view of life based on the belief that God's will and supernatural forces control the entire universe	Because pregnancy and birth are said to weaken the body and are accompanied by the loss of blood (yin), a yang diet is adopted for 1 month postpartum; mother eats five to six meals a day, including rice, soups, and seven to eight eggs; a typical dish includes rice wine, chicken, and lichen; another dish is soup of pigs' feet, sweet vinegar, black beans, ginger, and hard-boiled eggs Members believe that these kinds of dishes get rid of gas, assist in the involution process of the uterus, and provide a great deal of calcium, protein, and minerals; an analysis of pigs' feet reveals they are primarily bone and marrow with high mineral and protein content; wine vinegar is believed to increase the strength of the mother, but this vinegar may also increase the bleeding time

TABLE 8–5 ■ ASIAN-AMERICAN CULTURE *Continued*

Dietary Practices	Religious and Death Practices	Childbearing and Child Rearing
Lightly cooked or "stir-fried" vegetables are often preferred by Chinese or Japanese; monosodium glutamate and soy or teriyaki sauces, all high in sodium, are frequently used in food preparation Chinese or Japanese may avoid milk because of preference or lactose intolerance and may believe icy drinks are harmful to health; prefer warm or hot drinks Chinese or Japanese practice is to have light breakfast, a large midday meal, and a light late supper; women usually serve the men and eat only after the men have finished their meals Chinese and Japanese purify themselves by fasting one day for purification	For Japanese, traditionally, the number 4 is considered unlucky because it provokes *shi*, which sounds like the word for death; therefore, the number 4 is never said or used alone; a medicine marked q.i.d. may produce noncompliance Hospice care is an acceptable form of care and dying at home for the Japanese; exhibiting fear of dying is perceived as a sign of weakness because death is considered a natural phenomenon; may not participate in prolongation of life by costly artificial means Chinese may not plan ahead for funerals because planning may bring bad luck	Fruits and vegetables are avoided during postpartum period because they are considered cold foods Members may not expose themselves to cold air and do not go outside right after bathing because cold air can enter the body Obedience to parents and preservation of the family's good name are highly regarded Members are taught to conform to a code of behavior and fulfilment of obligation; if not met, it can bring shame to the family *Save face* means going around situations that may bring conflict Self-control is important and children are taught to control their feelings Japanese: Social self develops in the context of correcting mistakes to bring oneself closer to group expectations Important to adjust to social feedback since the self in Japan means "any shared of the shared space between us"

tion to support a plan to have Ms. Jones admitted to a nursing home. The psychiatric nurse's assessment showed that Ms. Jones was profoundly depressed, suspicious, and withdrawn. During the initial visit, Ms. Jones spoke angrily about people trying to get her out of her apartment and putting her in the nursing home. She spoke lovingly of her only living child, a daughter who lived in a shelter with her children and visited several times a week, buying her some groceries and keeping her company. The psychiatric nurse explained that Ms. Jones had interpreted the discussions about nursing home placement as a loss of control of her life and her independence because she perceived that the health professionals were going to determine where and how she lived. She insisted she did not want to leave her apartment and was not cooperating with home care service workers because of her suspiciousness of them. A lot of discussion ensued, including the ethical implications of leaving her unsupervised. Was she mentally competent? Was she confused? Would she harm herself? Didn't she have a legal right to self-determination since there was no evidence of confusion, there were no grounds for identifying her as mentally in-

competent, and she had no desire to hurt herself? What about the evening hours when no one might be available? In the client's mind she was doing okay. Her priority needs were being met. She perceived removal from her environment as an imposition by others and a negative factor in the quality-of-life issue. The solution of placement in a nursing home was unacceptable to both the client and her daughter since they perceived that plan as abandonment in a community in which people talked about "taking care of their own." In addition, many poor people believe that the kind of care they will receive in a low-income nursing home will be substandard.

As a broker, the psychiatric nurse arranged a meeting of all the staff involved in Ms. Jones's care. There were several discussions pointing out ethical dilemmas. Wasn't it unethical for professionals to "allow" her to stay in her apartment when she was unable to care for herself without assistance? What about her rights in a democratic society to determine what she should do with her life? Is a person who depends on so many people to keep her at home in the position to determine what she should do? Following the

TABLE 8-6 ■ SOUTHEAST-ASIAN CULTURE

Geographical Patterns	Health Practices	Health/Illness Beliefs
	Laotian and Hmong: Balance restored through use of herbs, self-restraint, meditation, and dermabrasive procedures Health promotion includes herbal medicine and use of folk healers Dermabrasive procedures are used to alleviate symptoms such as nausea, cough, headache, sore throat, backache, and joint pain; example is cupping, in which a heat cup or glass jar is put on the skin, creating a vacuum, which causes the skin to be drawn into the cup; the heat that is generated is used to treat pain; the redness on the skin may be interpreted as child abuse by a practitioner who does not know about the practice Rubbing is done with the edge of a coin, piece of bamboo, or spoon; rubbing leaves minor bruises and is used to diagnose or release excessive air that is attributed to certain disorders	Members believe in the hot-cold theory The Hill people (Laotians and Hmong) believe that diseases are caused by the wrath of the gods because of bad conduct by an individual or family member

Family Structure	Social Issues	Communication
Extended family is the basic unit; members show respect and obligation toward older family members Family is hierarchical with clear-cut sex roles, men handling the outside world and women maintaining the family The senior male acts as head of the household, although children who speak English may represent family in the community Married women may live with in-laws Decisions are made by family elders, based on the good for the family	Members have high incidence of psychiatric and psychosomatic problems and tension headaches as part of transition to United States	Members have speech anxiety and are reluctant to speak before a group or a meeting to express view Modesty, shyness, and respect for authority are found Modesty is an issue during physical examinations Members may live in crowded quarters, socialized to require little personal space

Dietary Practices	Religious and Death Practices	Childbearing and Child Rearing
Members may fast once a week for purification	Religious beliefs and practices include Buddhism, Confucianism, and Taoist teachings Members have tradition of ancestor worship and believe that the spirits of dead relatives continue to dwell among them and protect descendants Many believe that their ancestors' spirits can never rest unless living descendants provide care of the grave and worship their memory	During pregnancy, women may take special care to avoid visiting churches that might be inhabited by evil spirits Members believe that looking at pictures of healthy children will assist in delivering a healthy baby Pregnant women may not leave the house at night because of evil spirits Members place strong emphasis on respect and obedience Much attention is paid to form or to the manner in which things are said and done, and in not losing face Social self develops in the context of correcting mistakes to bring oneself closer to group expectations Individuals are part of the interconnected social web Self-improvement hinges on repairing social failures to advance social discourse

TABLE 8–7 ■ HISPANIC-AMERICAN CULTURE

Geographical Patterns	Health Practices	Health/Illness Beliefs
Majority of the population lives in Los Angeles and San Diego, Calif.; Texas; New York; Phoenix, Ariz.; Denver; and New Mexico Large number of Puerto Ricans live in north central United States Nicaraguans and Cubans live in Miami Dominicans live in New York and New Jersey Colombians live in New York and Florida Guatemalans live in Los Angeles, and Salvadorans in Los Angeles, Washington, D.C., and Houston Mexicans live in California, Arizona, and Texas	Members use home remedies *(remedios casero)*; degree of reliance on folk practices is related to class Members consult folk healers *(curanderos* and *espiritualista)* as well as Western health professionals Curandero is consulted by family; he assesses the situation and symptoms, followed by an individualized care plan using touch, talking, herbs, etc. A hot disease is treated with cold treatments; for example, an earache is thought to be caused by cold air and is treated with heat such as hot soups and broths; a hot disease such as a kidney infection is treated with cold fluids such as juices Common herbs used to treat illnesses are garlic for fever, anorexia, bronchitis, or toothache; rose water for fever, cold sweats, or infant diarrhea; oregano for fever, dry cough, or asthma; mint for indigestion, stomach pains, or nausea; aloe for burns or sunburn *Mal de ojo* is an illness resulting from the influence of an intruder outside the family who, as a result of envy, creates imbalance by sickness; victim usually seeks out an espiritualista who had special powers while still in his mother's womb, has the ability to see the future and can institute magical protection through prayer, medals, and certain rituals If a client is being treated for infection with symptoms of diarrhea, which is considered hot, family members may be reluctant to use a hot medicine such as penicillin; the hot effect of penicillin can be neutralized by mixing with fruit juices	Members view disease as having a spiritual and social context and utilize people, artifacts, and materials to combat illnesses Members believe in hot-cold theory of four humors in the body: black bile, blood, phlegm, and yellow bile; black bile is dry and cold; blood is wet and hot; phlegm is wet and cold; yellow bile is dry and hot; disease occurs when there is excess of hot, cold, wet, or dry conditions, which upsets one of the humors Members have strong belief in magic and witchcraft; diseases are attributed to a spell or hex or poor relationships or to evil eye (mal de ojo)

Table continued on following page

principles of beneficence and nonmalificence, how does the nurse help Ms. Jones and do no harm (Brakman, 1995).

The team decided to meet with Ms. Jones and her family to implement Ms. Jones's decision. During the meeting, the group collaborated with Ms. Jones, discussing the risks and benefits of her request. When it became obvious that remaining at home was the only option Ms. Jones was willing to entertain, the group began to plan services to cover a 24-hour period. The services included morning and evening visits by home health aides to assist with activities of daily living and prepare breakfast; a daily afternoon homemaker who would prepare lunch, do laundry, and maintain the apartment; a daily Meal on Wheels; weekly shopping by the daughter, along with visits by the daughter and grandchildren; twice-a-week visits by the community health nurse to coordinate the services; a weekly visit by the psychiatric nurse to provide support to the family; occupational therapy for stimulation; transportation to visits

TABLE 8–7 ■ HISPANIC-AMERICAN CULTURE *Continued*

Family Structure	Social Issues	Communication
The family is the main focus of social identification; familism is extended to third and fourth cousins and often includes best friends; extended family provides safety and security for the individual and in turn expects loyalty Members have *compadre* system or one who will assume the parenting role should anything happen to the natural parents Older daughters and sons do as their parents suggest and live in close proximity to families of procreation Families are usually large, with five or more children; children cement the marital relationship between parents and are considered to be more important than the marital relationship Emotional intimacy is not expected; children are the center of the family Hierarchical organization is usual and the older male is in the central position and given much respect There are pronounced differences in gender roles; females may not leave home until married *Machismo* is an important value for men; term denotes aggressiveness, sexual experience, manliness, courage, and being protective of females *Marianismo* is the complementary role that implies a self-sacrificing mother, nurturer, and manager of the household	Population of Hispanic Americans is youthful, with a median age of 25 years Most Hispanics live at or below the poverty level (about 1 in 4 live below the poverty level) About 50% complete high school and 10% complete college Term *barrio* connotes a community occupied predominantly by persons of Latino birth or descent	Modesty is an important concept; disrobing for physical examination may be perceived as invasion of personal space Personal space may also include reluctance to talk about personal matters outside the family; may respond better to family discussions Talking about family planning may necessitate having the senior male of the family present; nurse needs to listen and to explore this area Members may be expressive and emotional during interactions with nurse Touch may be a strong form of expression during interactions; physical contact such as greeting with a hug is an acceptable expression of welcoming

with the primary doctor; and access to a neighbor by telephone during the night.

The depression lifted, and as Ms. Jones began to become actively involved in her own care, a physical therapist came in to assist in Ms. Jones's desire to increase her mobility and involvement in her own care. She progressed to a state in which she was able to ambulate, use a commode, and perform other activities of daily living unassisted. ■

■ **CASE STUDY 8–2**

Mr. Braxton is a 57-year-old African-American man. He had a cerebrovascular accident 1 month ago, resulting in right-sided hemiparalysis. He is ambulatory with a walker or a cane. Mr. Braxton cannot feed himself and is unable to perform many of his activities of daily living. He is a certified plumber, mar-

ried, and the father of five children aged 25 to 31 years. His wife is 53 years old and has been a homemaker for 30 years. Mr. Braxton has always lived a very independent lifestyle. He has always been the strong force that has held his family together and is having a very difficult time adjusting to his current health condition.

Mr. Braxton is very depressed and withdrawn. He has been documented as saying, "This is hopeless, and I will be a cripple forever." His family is very supportive, and each of his children takes turns accompanying him to physical therapy. His children are willing to take a more active part in his care; however, the nursing staff is having difficulty with the frequent presence of his children. At times the staff has complained that the children are getting in the way of his nursing care. His oldest son has been labeled by the nursing staff as a troublemaker. One

TABLE 8–7 ■ HISPANIC-AMERICAN CULTURE *Continued*

Dietary Practices	Religious and Death Practices	Child Rearing
Beans, rice, pork, fruit, and fleshy vegetables are the basis of the diet Foods are classified according to their effect; chili and meat are hot foods, and ice cream and fruits are cold foods; hot and cold foods are eaten according to the appropriateness to the condition of the client; cool liquids and fruit are used to combat fever During pregnancy, mothers are encouraged to avoid hot, spicy foods and to drink special teas	Religion plays a central role in family life; large percentage are Roman Catholics, but many practice other religions Members forbid mentioning the deceased's name after a mourning period of 10 days Members believe that God controls all events	There is strong emphasis on respect and obedience What is valued is how respectful and good the children are Godparents *(padrinos)* often assist in child rearing and child care Individuality and personal achievement are not valued; members value interdependence A disorder called *mal de ojo* (evil eye) may affect infants and children; members believe it occurs when a strong person looks at a child but does not touch it; symptoms are fever, weeping, rashes, vomiting, and loss of appetite; treatment can include having the person touch the infant or a ritual of passing an unbroken egg over the body of the infant then placing it under the crib to draw the fever from the child *Caidade mollera* or "fallen fontanel" is believed to be caused by the sudden removal of the mother's nipple during nursing, resulting in difficulty in sucking; symptoms are dehydration, diarrhea, vomiting, and restlessness; the treatment involves holding the infant upside down over a pail of hot water or stimulating the roof of the mouth

nurse comments during the morning report, "Be careful around his oldest son. He asks too many questions. He wants to know everything. I think he might be trying to find something to file a lawsuit over. Just cover yourself. Try not to give him too much information. Tell him the doctor will answer all of his questions in time." ■

■ CASE STUDY 8–3

Mr. Rodriquez is a 27-year-old Hispanic man, a victim of a diving accident resulting in a C6 spinal cord injury. He is a high school physics teacher who has been married for 4 months. His wife is a high school chemistry teacher. Mr. Rodriquez is slowly progressing with his injuries. He is paralyzed from his shoulders

to his feet and requires mechanical ventilation. He must have complete skilled nursing care 24 hours a day. Mr. Rodriquez and his wife live in a duplex on the second floor. There is no elevator in the building, and it is not wheelchair-accessible. Mr. Rodriquez's parents agree to take him into their house. Mr. Rodriquez has a very large family; however, most of his family and all of his wife's family live in New Mexico. Family is very important to Mr. Rodriquez. He is encouraged when his family is around him and is more active in his care. Many of his family members have come from New Mexico to be here with him. There may be as many as five to seven people visiting at one time. Mr. Rodriquez and his wife are the only two who speak conversational English.

The nurses are in the process of teaching Mr. Rodriquez's wife and mother how to care for him at home. His wife works during the

TABLE 8–8 ■ NATIVE-AMERICAN CULTURE

Geographical Patterns	Health and Healing Practices	Health/Illness Beliefs
Members are primarily concentrated in the western portion of the country; Oklahoma, Arizona, California, and New Mexico are the states with the largest populations of American Indians What formerly were nations of people are now more commonly referred to as tribes Ten most common tribes are Navajo, Cherokee, Sioux (Dakota), Chippewa, Pueblo, Lumbee, Choctaw, Houma, Apache, Iroquois, Creek	Members have healing ceremonies to restore mental, physical, and spiritual balance There may be people in a community who function as cultural brokers and assist by helping non-Indian staff to understand important cultural issues Practitioners may include the medicine man, herbalists, and diagnosticians such as the *hand tremblers* There is ritual of the diagnostician, called the hand trembler; diagnosis is made with the intervention of the deities who take over the diagnostician's hand; the trembling hand then draws a picture that interprets the cause of the illness, followed by treatment recommendations Recommendation for cure may be a series of ceremonies or a one-time treatment by the medicine man to remove the illness Religious ceremonies and tribal dances are important in preventive care to convey good and drive away evil Herbs are used in the treatment of many illnesses to cleanse the body of ill spirits or poisons; Indians used over 200 drugs made from herbs, which are now included in the Official Drug Compendium of the United States Other recommended treatments include sweats, bed rest, diet, and charms to secure protection	Spirituality is not separated from the healing process; illness results from not being in harmony with nature, the spirits of evil persons such as a witch, or violation of taboos Among medicine men, health is considered as embracing the body, the mind, and the ecological sphere of humans; treatment is to address the disequilibrium and bring person back in balance with surroundings

day and must receive her teaching in the evenings. Mr. Rodriquez's mother is having difficulty learning some of the procedure because she has difficulty with the translator. Most of the time, the translators are nonmedical people and have very little knowledge about the procedures. There is only one nurse who speaks Spanish in the entire hospital, and she works in another unit on weekends only.

Most of the medical staff believe it would be best to place Mr. Rodriquez in a nursing house where he could receive the 24-hour-a-day nursing care he needs. ■

■ CASE STUDY 8–4

Mr. Lee is a 72-year-old Asian American who was born in China and has lived in the United States for 5 years. Mr. Lee is a widower and lives with his daughter and son-in-law. He knows only a few words of English. One week ago, Mr. Lee had surgery, an open reduction and internal fixation of the left hip, which was fractured when he fell off a stepladder in his kitchen while reaching for a spice he kept high on the cabinet shelf. No one else was home at the time of his accident

TABLE 8–8 ■ NATIVE-AMERICAN CULTURE *Continued*

Family Structure	Social Issues	Communication
Extended family members are important, particularly the mother's family Family unit consists of the nuclear family and relatives such as sisters, aunts, and their female descendants Society is primarily matrilineal in nature, and grandmothers and mothers are at the center of Indian society Family may range from a single family, nuclear or extended living in a community, to large land bases called reservations on which thousands of families live Elderly persons are respected and usually have the role of keeping the rituals and instructing children and grandchildren When providing family care, it is important to note that no decision is made until the appropriate elderly woman is present; it is important for a health care worker to find the appropriate gatekeeper when solving health issues	Cirrhosis, suicide, and homicide are social issues Single-parent families are becoming more prevalent Type 2 diabetes mellitus is the third most prevalent disease affecting all American Indian tribes, with poor control and dietary compliance associated with long-term complications such as blindness and kidney failure There is increased incidence of gallbladder disease associated with popularity of commercial fast-food chicken establishments Mental illness is perceived as resulting from witches or a curse; persons may wear turquoise to ward off evil Concept of rehabilitation is relatively new because, in years past, members did not survive to an age where chronic diseases became issue Autopsy and organ transplantation are unacceptable practices to traditional Indians, and the decision to perform them may create a cultural dilemma for the family Children are welcome, and there is limited practice of birth control; the birth rate among Indians is 96% higher than the birth rate in the overall U.S. population	Because of experiences with the larger society, suspicion looms large, and the establishment of trust with anyone outside the clan takes time Concepts of autonomy and sharing in decision making may be in conflict with the tradition; asking the client questions to make a diagnosis may foster mistrust, since traditional medicine men tell people what is wrong without their having to say anything The ability of the nurse to comfortably enter into the space of silence with the client is important; nurses need to use attentive listening skills and wait for responses, which may be slow and cautious in coming since the client might perceive silence as supportive Older children are taught to be stoic and uncomplaining; they have minimal nonverbal expressions The use of touch, outside of a handshake, is a form of communication that needs to be carefully assessed since many tribes perceive touch as associated with familiarity Personal space may be greater than that of most Americans Time has little meaning or importance; events do not always start on time but rather when people gather There may be a tendency to avoid talking through conflictual issues or talking about a fatal disease or illness; this may be frustrating to a health care worker who believes that conflicts should be talked through and resolved; health care worker may be perceived as rude

Table continued on following page

so he crawled to the telephone, further damaging his left hip.

Mr. Lee's daughter feels responsible for her father's fall. She and her husband work 8 to 12 hours a day. They cannot afford a companion to stay with their father. He has no interest in senior centers or any senior activities in his community. He has only one friend, who is very ill. Mr. Lee expresses that he wants to be left alone to enjoy his life quietly.

Mr. Lee currently has many care needs. He needs assistance with his activities of daily living. He also has insulin-dependent diabetes and has very poor vision. The medical staff strongly agrees that Mr. Lee must be placed in a nursing home or have in-home 24-hour nursing supervision. His daughter and son-in-law are outraged. They will never consent to their father's being placed in a nursing home. His daughter states, "This is

TABLE 8–8 ■ NATIVE-AMERICAN CULTURE *Continued*

Dietary Practices	Religious and Death Practices	Childbearing and Child Rearing
Food is not usually associated with promoting health	In some tribes, there are ceremonial rituals to initiate such transitions as the onset of menarche, or beginning of manhood	There are many restrictive and taboo practices related to pregnancy; members are reluctant to deliver baby in hospital
Sheep are a major source of meat, and brain is considered a delicacy	Many Indians remain traditional in practice of religious activities and often need time off from work to attend these ceremonies	During delivery necklaces are worn to provide for a safe birth, birth chants may be sung, and woven belts or sashes are used to help push the baby out
Fry bread and mutton are cooked in solid fat called lard (derived from pork)	Many tribes believe that dead spirits roam the earth if the living have failed to remember them	Taboo exists about purchasing clothing until after the birth
Corn is a staple of many tribes' diet	In most tribes, the body must go into the afterlife as whole as possible, including any amputated limbs	There are many different postpartum rituals, depending on the tribe, that the nurse should know
Access to fresh fruits or vegetables is minimal; squash is common at harvest time	Cleansing ceremony is performed in order for the spirits of the deceased to restrain from assuming control of someone else's spirit; therefore, body may not be buried for a number of days	Infants are kept in cradle boards until they begin walking, with possible complication of hip dysplasia; the use of diapers has decreased the potential for hip dysplasia because diapers bind the hips in a slightly abducted position
Diet may be deficient in vitamin D because many suffer from lactose intolerance or do not drink milk or eat dark leafy vegetables.		The postcradle period ushers in tasks of weaning, toilet training, and discipline, which are frequently left to the grandmother
There may be dietary restrictions associated with ceremony rituals		With increased bottle feeding and practice of putting baby to bed with a bottle of milk or juice, dental caries are frequent, with possible loss of teeth
		Because of the social premise that no one has a right to speak for another, children may be allowed to decide if they want to take their medicine
		Twins are not looked on favorably and were frequently believed to be the work of a witch; even though this belief is much less prevalent, there can be a risk of neglect and failure to thrive

against my culture. I will not let my father waste away in a nursing home and be treated like an animal." Because Mr. Lee understands very little English, he is unclear about what his daughter and son-in-law are saying to the nurses and doctors on his behalf. He wishes they would speak in Chinese so he could understand the conversations. ■

■ **CASE STUDY 8–5**

Mr. Hickman is a 65-year-old African-American man. He had a cerebrovascular accident 2 weeks ago and has right-sided hemiparesis.

He had supported his family as a "handy man," doing home repairs by referrals from other customers. His wife is 52 years old and works as a clerk at one of the local banks. They have two children, a son 19 years old and daughter 20 years old. Their daughter attends community college, and their son works in the plumbing business with his father.

Mr. Hickman has a past medical history of severe hypertension, diagnosed 2 years ago. He was prescribed a series of behavior modifications that included dietary changes (reducing sodium and cholesterol and increasing fiber), daily exercise, and a strict medication regimen. Mr. Hickman found this treatment regimen difficult to follow. He was experiencing many negative side effects from the medication including intermittent impotence. However, he was very uncomfortable discussing his concerns with the female doctor appointed by his health maintenance organization. He also had difficulty discussing his medical condition and treatment regimen with his wife. He just didn't want to bother anyone with his problems. Mr. Hickman was experiencing difficulty with his new dietary regimen. He did not take his medication because of the side effects he experienced. He missed doctors' appointments because of his busy work schedule. He was always worried about the family's financial status because most of his savings went into building and maintaining the business.

Mr. Hickman is currently a patient in an extended rehabilitation center. He has difficulty with his activities of daily living and must use assistive devices such as a utensil cuff to hold his toothbrush, a buttonhook to fasten his shirt, and an extended brush to brush his hair. He is ambulatory with a walker. Mr. Hickman has always considered himself to be a spiritual person. He and his family attended church services regularly. Spirituality now has a greater meaning in his life. He believes that God has given him another chance at life. He states that he is now ready to make some major behavior modifications in his life. Mr. Hickman has many visitors. His church members and friends come to visit often and have a time of praise. During this time of praise, they pray and sing songs. Although none of the other patients have complained about the volume, the nurses are uncomfortable with prayer time. Mr. Hickman also prays and reads his Bible throughout the day. He often speaks about his spirituality and his renewed relationship with God. Many of the nurses do not know how to respond to Mr. Hickman when he speaks about his spirituality. ■

Discussion Questions for the Case Studies

1. How many generations has the family or individual been in America? How has it affected their health belief system?
2. What is the age, gender, and marital status of the client? With what groups does the client identify?
3. How does the individual or family define health and illness?

4. What is thought to be the cause of the illness?
5. Who determines when a family member is sick? How?
6. Who does the healing in the home culture: The medical doctor, the herbalist, the spiritualist, etc.?
7. When will each be used?
8. What are the home treatments and the nutritional remedies?
9. What does this family usually do before seeking traditional health services?
10. What has been the experience of the family with the health care system?
11. What have been the family's personal experiences, and what myths and legends have been handed down about health care resources?
12. Who are perceived as helping people? Who does the individual or family go to first when seeking help with a health problem?
13. What are the major health practices? What kind of help would be requested?
14. What are the lifestyle patterns? How do these patterns influence the health of this individual or family?
15. How does religion influence health care practices?

REFERENCES

American Nurses Association Expert Panel on Culturally Competent Health Care Report. (1992). Culturally competent health care. *Nursing Outlook, 40*, 277–283.

Andrews, M. M., & Boyle, J. S. (1995). *Transcultural concepts in nursing care.* Philadelphia: J. B. Lippincott Company.

Bartol, G. M., & Richardson, L. (1998). Using literature to create cultural competence. *Image: Journal of Nursing Scholarship, 30*, 75–79.

Berg, K. I., & DeJong, P. (1996). Solution-building conversations: Co-constructing a sense of competence with clients. *Families In Society: The Journal of Contemporary Human Services, 20*, 376–391.

Bower, B. (1996). Fighting stereotypes stigma. *Science News, 149*, 408–409.

Bower, B. (1997). My culture, my self. *Science News, 152*, 248–249.

Brakman, S.V. (1995). Filial responsibility and long term care decision making. In McCullough, L.B., & Wilson, N.I. (eds), *Long term care decisions: Ethical and conceptual dimensions.* Baltimore: John Hopkins University press.

Bredok, H., & McDermott, J. (1995). The cultural organization of teaching and learning. *Harvard Educational Review, 60*, 247–259.

Brislin, R. (1990). *Applied Cross-Cultural Psychology.* Newbury Park, California: Sage.

Brunner, J. (1995). *The culture of education.* Cambridge: Harvard University Press.

Campinha-Bacote, J., & Ferguson, S. (1991). Cultural considerations in childrearing practices: A transcultural perspective. *Journal of the National Black Nurses Association, 5,* 11–17.

Carroll, T. G. (1990). Who owns culture? *Education and Urban Society, 22,* 346–355.

Charlton, J.T. (1998). *Nothing about us without us: Disability, oppression, and empowerment.* Berkeley: University of California Press.

Charnes, L. S., & Moore, P. S. (1992). Meeting patients' spiritual needs: The Jewish perspective. *Holistic Nursing Practice, 6,* 64–72.

Chychula, N.M. (1990). The cocaine epidemic: Treatment options for cocaine dependence. *Nurse Practitioner 15,* 33–40.

Crow, K. (1993). Multiculturalism and pluralistic thought in nursing education: Native American world view and the nursing academic world view. *Journal of Nursing Education, 32,* 198–204.

Cuthbert-Allman, C., & Conti, P. A. (1995). VNA of Boston addresses cultural barriers in home-based care. *Caring Magazine, 12,* 22–25.

Davidhizar, R., Dowd, S. B., & Giger, J. N. (1998). Educating the culturally diverse health care student. *Nurse Educator, 23,* 38–42.

Davis, D. S. (1991). Dealing with real Jewish patients. *Journal of Clinical Ethics, 2,* 211–212.

Davis, R. E. (1997). Trauma and addiction experiences of African American women. *Journal of Nursing Research, 19,* 442–460.

Debold, E., Wilson, M., & Malave, I. (1993). *From betrayal to power: Mother, daughter revolution.* New York: Addison-Wesley.

Denboba, D. L., Bragdon, J. L., Epstein, L. G., Garthright, K., & Goldman, T. M. (1998). Reducing health disparities through cultural competence. *Journal of Health Education, 29,* 47–53.

DeTornyay, R. (1992). Reconsidering nursing education: The report of the Pew Health Professions Commission. *Journal of Nursing Education, 31,* 296–301.

Ellison, R. (1970). *The invisible man.* New York: Vintage International.

Estin, P. (1998). Spotting depression in Asian patients. *RN, 62,* 39–42.

Ford, M. (1995). Innovation in refugee health care. *Caring Magazine, 12,* 32–35.

Ford-Gilboe, M., & Campbell, J. (1996). The mother-headed single-parent family: A feminist critique of the nursing literature. *Nursing Outlook, 44,* 173–183.

Friedan, B. (1997). *Beyond gender: The new politics of work and family.* New York: Woodrow Wilson Center.

Fries, K. (1998). *The disability experience from the inside out.* New York: Plume.

Funderburg, F. (1994). *Black, white, and others.* New York: William Morrow and Company, Inc.

Gates, M. (1991). Transcultural comparison of hospitals and hospice as caring environments for dying patients. *Journal of Transcultural Nursing, 2,* 3–15.

Gent, R. M., & Thornton, H. B. (1995). Apples and oranges: A look at cultural diversity. *Caring Magazine, 12,* 16–20.

Gitlin, T. (1995). *The twilight of common dreams: Why America is wrecked by culture wars.* New York: Metropolitan.

Grothaus, K. L. (1996). Family dynamics and family therapy with Mexican Americans. *Journal of Psychosocial Nursing, 34,* 31–35.

Hautman, M. A., & Harrison, J. K. (1992). Health beliefs and practices in a middle-income Anglo-American neighborhood. *Advances in Nursing Science, 4,* 49–63.

Hochschild, J. L. (1995). *Facing up to the American dream.* Princeton, New Jersey: Princeton University Press.

Holtz, C., & Wilson, C. (1992). The culturally diverse

student: A model for empowerment. *Nurse Educator, 17,* 28–31.

Humphries, D. (1998). Crack mothers at 6. *Violence Against Women, 4,* 45–62.

A hundred years (1999). *U.S. News & World Report,* September 24, 1999, p. 59.

Kavanaugh, K. H. (1993). Transcultural nursing: Facing the challenges of advocacy and diversity/universality. *Journal of Transcultural Nursing, 5,* 4–13.

Kleinman, A. (1996). *Writing at the margin: Discourse between anthropology and medicine.* New York: Doubleday.

Kotlowitz, A (1998). *The other side of the river: A story of two towns, a death, and the America's dilemma.* New York: Doubleday.

Layton, M. (1992). Dying in the attic: The preservation of self in marriage. *Journal of Feminist Family Therapy, 4,* 31–51.

Leininger, M. (1991). Leninger's acculturation health care assessment tool for cultural patterns in traditional and nontradition lifeways. *Journal of Transcultural Nursing, 2,* 40–42.

Lind, M. (1995). *The next American nation: The new nationalism and the fourth American revolution.* New York: The Free Press.

Lipson, J. & Meleis, A. I. (1985). Culturally appropriate care: The case of immigrants. *Topics in Clinical Nursing, 7,* 48–56.

Litwack, L. F. (1998). *Trouble in mind: Black southerners in the age of jim crow.* New York: Knopf.

MacFarquhar, L. (1996). Suffering Subjectivity. *The Nation, 262,* 30–32.

Marable, M. (1996). *Speaking truth to power.* Boulder, Colorado: Westview Press.

McCormick, G. L. (1987). Culture and communication in the treatment planning for occupational therapy with minority patients. *Occupational Therapy in Health Care,* New York: Haworth Press, Inc.

McGoldrick, M., & Rohrbaugh, M. (1987). Researching ethnic family stereotypes. *Family Process, 26,* 89–98.

McGoldrick, M., Pearce, J. K., & Giordano, J. (1996). *Ethnicity and Family Therapy.* New York: Guilford Press.

Morgan, S. (1990). Challenging the politics of exclusion. *Education and Urban Society, 22,* 393–401.

Moses, Y. (1990). The challenge of diversity. *Education and Urban Society, 22,* 402–415.

Muecke, M. A. (1983). Caring for Southeast Asian refugee patients in the USA. *American Journal of Public Health, 73,* 431–438.

Naido, T. (1989). Health and healthcare: A Hindu perspective. *Medicine & Law, 7,* 643–647.

Narayan, M. C., & Rea, H. (1997). The South Asian client. *Home Healthcare Nurse, 15,* 461–469.

Neighbors, H. W., Musick, M. A., & Williams, D. R. (1998). *Health Education & Behavior, 25,* 759–777.

Nelson, W., Wood, S.O., & Nalepka, C.D. (1993). Development of a culturally sensitive rural practitioner. *Nurse Educator 18,* 10–12.

Parnell, L. D., & Paulanka, B. J. (1998). *Transcultural health care.* Philadelphia: F. A. Davis Company.

Premdas, K. (1995). Weathering multicultural clashes: Knowing hospice patient ethnicity. *Caring Magazine, 12,* 36–42.

Rainwater, L. (1970). *Behind ghetto walls.* Chicago: Aldine Publishing Company.

Reed, A. L. (1998). *W.E.B. DuBois and American political thought.* London: Oxford Press.

Riley, M. M. (1995). Diversity for the duration. Caring Magazine, 12, 54–56.

Romero, H. G., & Hoffman, M. J. (1995). Cross-cultural

caring positive outcomes in Hawaii. *Caring Magazine,* 12, 26–30.

Rooda, L. A. (1993). Knowledge and attitudes of nurses toward culturally different patients: Implications for nursing education. *Journal of Nursing Education, 25,* 209–213.

Ross, B., & Cobb, K. L. (1990). *Family nursing: A nursing process approach.* Redwood City, California: Addison-Wesley Nursing.

Saylor, C. R. (1990). Themanagement of stigma: Redefinition and presentation. *Holistic Nursing Practice, 5,* 45–53.

Saylor, C. R., & Taylor, T. (1993). Transformation: Nursing and cultural diversity. *Nurse Educator, 18,* 26–28.

Schensul, J. J., & Carroll, T. G. (1990). Visions of America in the 1990s and beyond: Negotiating cultural diversity and educational change. *Education and Urban Society, 22,* 339–345.

Scott, J., & Rantz, R. (1997). Managing chronically ill older people in the midst of the health care revolution. *Nursing Administration, 21,* 55–64.

Shipley, A. (1997). *A country of strangers: Blacks and whites in America.* New York: A. A. Knopf.

Smith, B. E., Colling, K., Elander, E., & Latham, C. (1993). A model for multicultural curriculum development in baccalaureate nursing education. *Journal of Nursing Education, 32,* 205–208.

Spark, S. M., & Rizzolo, M. A. (1998). Shifting images of chronic illness. *Image: Journal of Nursing Scholarship, 30,* 173–178.

Spruhan, J. B. (1996). Beyond traditional nursing care: Cultural awareness and successful home healthcare nursing. *Home Healthcare Nurse, 14,* 445–449.

Standley, F. L., & Pratt, L. H. (1989). *Conversations with James Baldwin.* Jackson Mississippi: University of Mississippi Press.

Stanhope, M. & Lancaster, J. (1996). *Community health nursing: Promoting health of aggregates, families, and individuals.* St. Louis: Mosby.

Stevens, P. E. (1995). Structural and interpersonal impact of heterosexual assumptions on lesbian health care clients. *Nursing Research, 44,* 25–30.

Thomas, D. A., and Ely, R. J. (1996). Making differences matter: A new paradigm for managing diversity. *Harvard Business Review, 56,* 79–90.

Wells, S. A. (1995). Creating a culturally competent workforce. *Caring Magazine, 12,* 50–53.

West, C. (1993). *Keeping faith.* New York: Routledge.

West, C., & Lerner, M. (1995). *Jews and blacks: Let the healing begin.* New York: G, P. Putnam's Sons.

Wilson, W.J. (1996). *When work disappears: The World of the New Urban Poor.* New York: Alfred A. Knopf.

Woodruff, L. (1995). Growing diversity in the aging population. *Caring Magazine, 12,* 4–10.

BIBLIOGRAPHY

Andrews, M. M., & Boyle, J. S. (1995). *Transcultural concepts in nursing care.* Philadelphia: J.B. Lippincott Company.

Campinha-Bacote, J., & Ferguson, S. (1991). Cultural considerations in childrearing practices: A transcultural

perspective. *Journal of the National Black Nurses Association, 5,* 11–17.

Carroll, T. G. (1990). Who owns culture? *Education and Urban Society, 22,* 346–355.

Charnes, L. S. & Moore, P. S. (1992). Meeting patients' spiritual needs: The Jewish perspective. *Holistic Nursing Practice, 6,* 64–72.

Davis, D. S. (1991). Dealing with real Jewish patients. *Journal of Clinical Ethics, 2,* 211–212.

Davis, R. E. (1997). Trauma and addiction experiences of African American women. *Journal of Nursing Research, 19,* 442–460.

De Tornyay, R. (1992). Reconsidering nursing education: The report of the Pew Health Professions Commission. *Journal of Nursing Education, 31,* 296–301.

Ford-Gilboe, M., & Campbell, J. (1996). The mother-headed single-parent family: A feminist critique of the nursing literature. *Nursing Outlook, 44,* 173–183.

Friedan, B. (1997). *Beyond gender: The new politics of work and family.* New York: Woodrow Wilson Center.

Gates, M. (1991). Transcultural comparison of hospitals and hospice as caring environments for dying patients. *Journal of Transcultural Nursing, 2,* 3–15.

Hautman, M. A., & Harrison, J. K. (1992). Health beliefs and practices in a middle-income Anglo-American neighborhood. *Advances in Nursing Science, 4,* 49–63.

Lipson, J. & Meleis, A. I. (1985). Culturally appropriate care: The case of immigrants. *Topics in Clinical Nursing, 7,* 48–56.

Muecke, M. A. (1983). Caring for Southeast Asian refugee patients in the USA. *American Journal of Public Health, 73,* 431–438.

Neighbors, H. W., Musick, M. A., & Williams, D. R. (1998). *Health Education & Behavior, 25,* 759–777.

Parnell, L. D., & Paulanka, B. J. (1998). *Transcultural health care.* Philadelphia: F. A. Davis Company.

Premdas, K. (1995). Weathering multicultural clashes: Knowing hospice patient ethnicity. *Caring Magazine, 12,* 36–42.

Riley, M. M. (1995). Diversity for the duration. *Caring Magazine, 12,* 54–56.

Romero, H. G., & Hoffman, M. J. (1995). Cross-cultural caring positive outcomes in Hawaii. *Caring Magazine, 12,* 26–30.

Saylor, C. R., & Taylor, T. (1993). Transformation: Nursing and cultural diversity. *Nurse Educator, 18,* 26–28.

Scott, J., & Rantz, R. (1997). Managing chronically ill older people in the midst of the health care revolution. *Nursing Administration, 21,* 55–64.

Spark, S. M., & Rizzolo, M. A. (1998). Shifting images of chronic illness. *Image: Journal of Nursing Scholarship, 30,* 173–178.

Standley, F. L., & Pratt, L. H. (1989). *Conversations with James Baldwin.* Jackson, Mississippi: University of Mississippi Press.

Stanhope, M., & Lancaster, J. (1996). *Community health nursing: Promoting health of aggregates, families, and individuals.* St. Louis: Mosby.

Stevens, P. E. (1995). Structural and interpersonal impact of heterosexual assumptions on lesbian health care clients. *Nursing Research, 44,* 25–30.

Wells, S. A. (1995). Creating a culturally competent workforce. *Caring Magazine, 12,* 50–53.

CHAPTER 9

Teaching and Learning: Educative Roles in Rehabilitation Nursing

Sheila O'Shea Melli

This chapter focuses on the nurse-client relationship in the complex teaching and learning process. Theories of learning, principles, and preferred styles of learning are presented to illustrate how and why people learn. Methods of teaching that have been successful in working with people with disabilities are explored. The teaching process is used as a model in preparing an inclusive, multifaceted teaching plan for a client.

BACKGROUND

Need for Client Education

The typical consumer of health care is likely active in seeking and maintaining wellness. Because resources are limited, people are being forced to assume a more responsible role in seeking better health care. The clients of health care are making decisions that will affect their daily lives, whether they are facing acute illness or preserving a certain level of functioning and health. Major changes in health payment plans have decreased lengths of stay in hospitals and other care facilities and have allotted fewer home visits by nurses. Because the client will have less contact and fewer visits with the professional nurse, there is more need than ever for the nurse to be an effective educator.

Who Is the Learner?

The *learner* is the rehabilitation client who is the focus of care. In a broader sense, the *client* is the person engaged in the health care system as part of a family, a system of friends, and/or others who play significant roles in his or her life. The family or system of friends is referred to as the client's *support system*. The community in which the person lives or works can also be included under the term *client*. This more inclusive interpretation is used when looking at who or what may be involved with and affected by this person's participation in the home, family, or job.

Rehabilitation clients may have to make changes in their lives, ranging from finding a different way to engage in a simple daily task to changes in lifestyle and self-esteem. Returning to the same environment with different abilities is especially difficult. Environment is not limited to physical surroundings but includes the person's social system, measures of comfort, and privacy, as well as distractions, noise, and other obstacles.

The rehabilitation client is part of an inclusive personal, social, and community system and is in the process of reintegrating to a complex environment. Today, clients are less likely to be discharged to home from a facility where they were engaged in a lengthy rehabilitation program. The nurse faces many challenges in providing focused, appropriate teaching for the client who is discharged directly to the home environment.

Teaching as Collaboration

Teaching is an activity to induce learning—the process by which one's knowledge or behavior is changed as a result of the experience. Because of past experiences, many see teaching as an isolated role, performed by the teacher alone; to look at teaching as a collaborative process is to recognize it as being more active and inclusive. The client is now a partner in this process and shares in decisions, goals, and preparations. This is an opportunity for the client to have a voice and take responsibility for self-care. Learning is more likely to occur and will be longer lasting when the learner is invested in the teaching process. Of course, this does not mean that the client is taking the primary responsibility or is involved in the act of teaching; rather, it means that the client is active in identifying what needs to be learned, how the client prefers to learn, and when this should be accomplished.

Acting in partnership with clients can make the challenge of teaching more complicated at first. In many ways it was easier for the nurse to be in full control—that is, to set up goals and outcomes, plan and teach the sessions according to the nurse's schedule and availability, and evaluate by objective standards. Nurses may need to reorient as they move from this traditional model to that of facilitators in sharing these responsibilities with their clients. The adjustment may be challenging in that it is a move away from something familiar, but overall, it is a more functional, less intensive project for the nurse. It is more likely that the client will reach and maintain personal goals when working in collaboration with the teacher. It is important for the nurse to be comfortable in the role of facilitator.

THEORIES OF LEARNING

Experts in education and psychology have conflicting views on the nature and process of learning. Theorists have proposed descriptions of the course of learning—the *how* and *why* of learning. No theory is perfect, and none addresses all types of learning. Overall, however, they are useful for organizing and understanding information about the learning process, in addition to providing a practical framework for assessing the consistency and effectiveness of teaching.

There are three schools of learning theory: association, cognitive, and humanistic. *Association* theories look at the way the learner reacts to changes in the external environment. The basic process in learning is the formation of a connection between a stimulus and a response. The process of the stimulus-response association is known as *conditioning*. Pavlov described conditioning in reference to a dog's salivating in response to the sight of food. He rang a bell regularly before serving a dog's food and discovered that the dog could be trained to salivate on hearing the bell, even when no food was served. The repeated pairing of the adequate stimulus (food) with a second, neutral stimulus (ringing bell) causes the dog to associate the two stimuli. Eventually, the dog responds to the

neutral stimulus in the same way as to the adequate stimulus. Pavlov termed this a *conditioned* response—there is a bond between a stimulus and a response.

Association psychologists who study the way stimuli in the environment affect observable behavior are known as *behaviorists*. Learning (or a change in behavior) is viewed as a product of reinforcement following the repetition of an act. This results in a desired or conditioned response. Behavior modification is an example of a behaviorist approach to learning. In essence, it provides rewards as a result of desired behavior. Note that behaviorist learning theories promote self-direction and require a planned and systematic learning plan. Many clients are already familiar with this approach as it has been used successfully in weight-loss and smoking-cessation programs.

In contrast to the stimulus-response theorists, *cognitive* theorists stress the organization of knowledge, need for understanding, feedback of results, and goal setting by the learner. This theory is based on the idea that instruction brings about changes in the knowledge (as opposed to behavior) of the learner. Cognitive theorists believe that the process of gaining insight is the most valuable aspect of learning. The person, viewed within the holistic, psychological environment, is engaged in the search for information in order to *make connections, answer the questions*. This approach values perceptions and feelings in learning. A problem is solved depending on the way it is perceived. Focusing on the perceptual and psychological forces within the learner's field, cognitive theory explains complex forms of learning. The theory looks at how the person solves problems, processes information, or perceives new relationships.

Cognitive theories add internal conditions to learning such as the learner's characteristics, learning processes, and learning outcomes—they focus on changes in knowledge. On the other hand, behaviorist theories are concerned with external conditions of learning such as instructional manipulations and outcome performance—they look at changes in behavior.

In contrast to behaviorist theories that concentrate on observable behavior shaped by the environment, and the cognitive approach that deals with the mental processing of information, *humanistic* theories look at learning from the perspective of the human potential for growth. It is a uniquely personal view that places responsibility on the learner to identify the learner's own problems. In doing so, the learner goes through the process of prioritizing needs, actively planning and seeking goals, and engaging in self-evaluation, thus resulting in growth and maturity. The humanistic approach incorporates affective as well as cognitive dimensions of learning. Carl Rogers and Abraham Maslow were advocates of this humanistic approach to learning. Humanism emphasizes a person's perceptions that are centered in experience and advocates freedom and responsibility to reach one's potential. Humanistic theories are concerned with significant learning that leads to personal growth and development—they holistically consider cultural, psychosocial, and spiritual factors in a person's life.

DOMAINS OF LEARNING

Benjamin Bloom classified the actions, feelings, and thoughts clients are expected to develop as a result of learning into three major types of learning—cognitive, affective, and psychomotor (Krathwhol, Bloom, & Masia, 1964). The *cognitive domain* deals with recall or recognition of knowledge and the development of intellectual skills, ranging from simple recall of material to original and creative ways of combining and synthesizing new ideas (Bloom, 1987). The *affective domain* involves learning associated with values, attitudes, feelings, and emotions. It deals with issues of acceptance or rejection that range from the simple recognition of phenomena (feelings) to the complex stage of integrating certain qualities of character and formulating a philosophy of life. *Psychomotor learning* is the acquisition of a motor skill, such as changing a dressing or learning to walk with a cane. The skill is learned and improved through practice.

Understanding the system of learning domains is helpful when planning a teaching session in that it is a way to prepare outcomes and goals that focus on the learner, not the teacher. In addition to considering the level of learning, Bloom's taxonomy of educational objectives is organized as a hierarchy, proceeding from the concrete to the complex, from lower skills to higher skills. The taxonomy is useful as a guide when the nurse and the client work together in setting goals. The client who is involved in planning at this early stage is more likely to follow through in meeting the objectives.

The terms *objectives* and *goals* are not interchangeable—an objective addresses a specific and more immediate (either short-term or long-term) client need, whereas a goal is more general. The following are examples:

- *Goal:* The client will achieve maximal daily functions in the home environment.
- *Long-term objective:* In 2 weeks, the client and "support system" will understand the need for increased mobility and the client will participate in a program of mobilization.
- *Short-term objective:* By Thursday, the client will practice and safely demonstrate the use of a walker, increasing the distance by a total of 10 to 15 feet.

A learning goal is a broad statement about the desired status of a client after teaching interventions have been carried out. It is necessary that the overall goals and objectives be realistic and attainable. Working together, the nurse and client must prioritize them, placing the more important goals and objectives first.

Several criteria should be kept in mind when writing learning objectives. They should be written clearly, in terms of client behavior that describes what the client will be able to do after meeting the objective. The behavior or knowledge content it targets must be specific. A practical approach is to start with basic concepts as a foundation for more complex ones. The behavior should be written as an observable act so that the client's progress can be evaluated.

When one is writing the objectives in a teaching and learning plan, Bloom's taxonomy is helpful because the objectives will be the framework for the instructional plan (Table 9–1).

PRINCIPLES OF LEARNING

Common learning principles have been identified. Using them when educating the client increases the likelihood that the client will *permanently learn*:

P *Perception* is necessary for learning to take place. It is the ability to mentally grasp and become aware of something by means of the senses. Learning is a multisensory process.

E *Emotional factors* affect learning. Although strong, negative feelings can hinder perception and learning, mild anxiety can contribute to seeking and retaining new knowledge.

TABLE 9–1 ▪ TAXONOMY OF EDUCATIONAL OBJECTIVES

Learning Domain	Action-Related Words
Cognitive Learning Domain	
Knowledge	
Have factual recall of materials	State, write, identify, select, define, describe
Comprehension	
Think more broadly	Describe, summarize main points, explain, give examples
Show in-depth understanding	
Application	
Use knowledge in a new situation	Discover, compute, demonstrate, prepare, change
Analysis	
Take materials and examine the pieces	Infer, relate, illustrate, select, outline
Synthesis	
Go beyond the present knowledge	Discuss relationships, compose, rearrange
Evaluation	
Use a system of judgment to critique ideas	Compare, conclude, explain, critique, appraise
Affective Learning Domain	
Receiving	
Develop awareness, consciousness	Listen, pay attention, ask, choose, locate
Responding	
Have willingness, satisfaction in response	Display an interest in, practice, conform, label
Valuing	
Have acceptance of a value, commitment	Assume responsibility for, complete, initiate, share
Organizing	
Use discussion, conceptualize a value	Adhere, modify, defend, explain, generalize, relate
Characterizing	
Live the belief, value	Discriminate, influence, listen, solve, revise, verify
Psychomotor Learning Domain	
Perception	
Receive sensory stimulation	Observe a skill, identify equipment, separate, choose
Set	
Have motivation	Begin, display, move, react, show
Guided response	
Use imitation, trial and error	Imitate a performance, assemble, build, manipulate, calibrate, construct, display
Mechanism	
Use a learned response	Same as for guided response
Complex overt response	
Use an automatic response	Same as for guided response
Adaptation	
Use an altering response	Adapt, alter, change, rearrange, revise
Origination	
Innovate with the response	Arrange, combine, compose, create, design

Adapted from Krathwohl, D. R., Bloom, B. S., & Masia, B. B. (1964). *Taxonomy of education objectives: The classification of educational goals: Handbook 2. Affective domain.* New York: Longman; and Bloom, B. S. (Ed.). (1987). *Taxonomy of educational objectives: Book 1. Cognitive domain.* New York: Longman.

R *Readiness* to learn means that the client has the cognitive ability and acknowledges the need to learn.

M *Motivation* is essential because the client must want to be successful in learning the information.

A *Active participation* of the learner improves interest and retention.

N *New learning* is based on past experiences. These provide not only a knowledge base but also an "emotional base," depending on the success or failure of past learning.

E *Environmental factors* affect learning. Privacy, physical comfort, good lighting, and fresh air add to a climate conducive to learning.

N *Negotiating* with the client about what the client needs and is willing to work for increases the success of learning.

T *Trial and error* is a learning process. Practice reinforces learning, whereas being able to "make a mistake" in a safe environment decreases fear and helps the learner find a correct solution.

L *Linking* learning style with past experiences, culture, class, and gender contributes to the success of learning.

Y *Your self-esteem* is increased when learning occurs.

L *Locating* educational and community-based resources helps the client to adapt and succeed in learning new materials and skills.

E *Emphasizing* the practical application of learning maintains interest and contributes to retention of knowledge.

A *Attitudes* or prejudices may distort a person's ability to learn.

R *Reinforcement* and feedback strengthen learning when given as soon as possible in a positive way.

N *Networking* with others who have similar learning needs encourages and supports the learner. Researchers found that the average performance of a small group is superior to that of an individual performing alone.

Each of these principles influences behavior, but two are outstanding in their impact on learning—readiness and motivation. *Readiness* of the learner is a vital factor. Unless the learner is cognitively, physically, and emotionally ready, learning cannot take place. The nurse has to be sure the client has the developmental and intellectual abilities to learn. The motivated learner is the successful learner. *Motivation* depends on many factors: the usefulness of what is to be learned, interest in the subject matter, and the self-confidence to be able to master the material. An enthusiastic nurse who is tuned in to the needs of the learner can add to the client's desire to learn, and as the learner participates in the process, motivation and desire to succeed are strengthened.

Clients learn more readily when they can apply what is learned to a practical situation. For example, being able to progress from crutch walking to using a cane gives the client fewer restrictions and more mobility. This and other external motivators, such as being able to return to work, encourage adult learners to engage in learning.

Internal motivation factors are even stronger drives toward learning. This motivation is self-directing in that the clients take responsibility for their own care. These clients receive a sense of accomplishment from learning and do not rely on constant guidance and reinforcement. Learning that results from internal motivation is long-lasting and enhances the self-esteem of the learner.

LEARNING STYLES

Each person has preferred ways to receive and communicate information. This is known as a *learning style* and is influenced by a variety of factors such as personality, intellect, physical state, personal goals, and learning environment. Models of learning styles help the educator investigate how an individual processes information in the learning situation. The learner is asked how he or she prefers to gather, interpret, organize, and think about information. For example, some clients look at problems from a global perspective, within a holistic view. Others look at problems singularly, being more interested in facts and details.

Learning styles can be identified by sophisticated inventories, by informal checklists, or even by asking key, directed questions. To discover the client's preferred learning style, ask simple questions such as "Do you find written materials helpful?" or "Would you rather listen to a tape about this or discuss it in a group?" If teaching strategies are planned around the client's preferred style, learning is more enjoyable and effective. It is helpful for the nurse and client team to be aware of learning styles and the team members' strengths and weaknesses as learners and teachers. It forces the teacher to look at a variety of teaching activities and adapt strategies to meet a broader range of the client's learning needs.

A classic model by Kolb (1984) identified four phases of learning. The first is *concrete experience* (feeling), in which the person engages in an activity in order to try to learn and master it. The second, the *reflective observation* (watching) phase, develops as the learner observes experience from a variety of perspectives. *Abstract conceptualization* (thinking) is the third phase, in which the learner develops theories and explanations from observations and experiences. The final phase, *active experimentation* (doing), is actually testing hypotheses and solving problems.

Phase 1: Concrete experience, or feeling, clients learn best when they

■ Are involved with other people who are looking at the problem as a team
■ Have the freedom to be actively involved in "the project"
■ Are challenged to solve a complex problem under time constraints and adverse conditions and with few resources
■ Are expected to "jump in" and "get started"
■ Are not restricted by precise, detailed instructions
■ Go ahead and try something without practicing
■ Are in a leadership role or are the "center of attention"

Phase 2: Reflective observation, or watching, clients learn best when they

■ Assume a passive role such as reading or listening to explanations of why and how to do things
■ Have time to "think about it" before taking any action
■ Can study and research every aspect of the problem
■ Have unlimited time for preparation
■ Have no outside pressures or deadlines to meet
■ Can finish a job completely before starting another
■ Can look back on what has been learned by this experience

Phase 3: Abstract conceptualization, or thinking, clients learn best when they

■ Feel free to investigate and ask questions in trying to find logical explanations

■ Consider a variety of ideas and concepts even though they don't seem relevant to the problem
■ Look at a problem as part of an overall model or theory
■ Approach a problem only after careful consideration about becoming involved
■ Rely on complex intellectual processes instead of emotions
■ Make decisions consistent with policies or principles
■ Are involved in structured activities that are complex and predictable

Phase 4: Active experimentation, or doing, clients learn best when they

■ Gain a reward as a result of the learning experience
■ See a clear connection between the subject matter and a solution to the problem
■ Can immediately use what has been learned
■ Are given instructions or techniques that are relevant to dealing with the problem
■ Have the opportunity to practice and then receive feedback from the teacher
■ Have clear purposes and can reach goals without obstacles
■ Can imitate someone else (a teacher, an expert) performing the task

Overall, clients are more satisfied and productive if they are working within a phase that is compatible with their preferred learning style. The nurse and client will find this information helpful when choosing teaching strategies that are compatible with the particular phase of learning.

TEACHING AND LEARNING PROCESS

Creating a teaching plan is a dynamic process for the nurse-client team that begins when the nurse and client first meet and continues with every meeting and communication. The nursing goal is to help the client learn within a teaching framework that is organized, well paced, and individualized to the needs, interests, and abilities of the client. Nurses have an advantage when working within the teaching and learning process because of its many similarities with the nursing process. In addition to establishing a partnership between the client and the nurse, the teaching process uses

■ *Assessment:* Collecting data to identify learning strengths and deficits
■ *Diagnosis:* Making an educational diagnosis

- *Planning:* Designing and preparing a teaching plan
- *Implementation:* Carrying out the teaching plan
- *Evaluation:* Checking the effectiveness of client learning

Like the nursing process, the teaching and learning process provides a framework for a rational, systematic approach to client care. This model is a continuous, accessible, and relevant collection of data about the learning needs of the client.

Assessment

Having access to health care records and talking with caregivers helps the nurse gain important information even before meeting the client. Sources of data in addition to the client include the support system, nurses, physicians, physical therapists, other professional health workers, caregivers, and health records. There is no need to spend time and energy investigating and repeating documentation of information that is already available within the client's record (e.g., health history). Instead, the nurse can now analyze the data for what is relevant and use the time with the client to validate areas of uncertainty and investigate concerns that have not been addressed.

In assessing data and on interviewing the client, the nurse needs to answer the following questions:

- Who is the client as a person? Where is the client from?
- Where does the client live, work, socialize?
- Who are included in the client's support system?
- What is the client's role in the family? Does it change if the client is sick?
- What does the client know about his or her current health status?
- Does the client know the diagnosis?
- How do the client and support system look on people with disabilities?
- What does the sick role mean to the client? Is it related to any religious beliefs; for example, is illness seen as the will of God?
- Will the client and the nurse be able to communicate effectively?
- Does the client speak and read English? If not, is someone (other than a family member) available to translate?
- How has the client cared for himself or herself in the past?

- What challenges or crises has the client faced in the past? How did the client cope?
- What challenge is the client now facing?
- Does the client want to be involved in making decisions about health, lifestyle, and so forth?
- What does the client think he or she needs to learn?
- What are the client's expectations?

In addition to developing a relationship with the client and gathering facts, the assessment phase of the teaching and learning process includes active and careful observation for nonverbal clues. This is the starting point for getting to know the client as a person and identifying actual and potential learning needs. The assessment phase leads to a learning diagnosis that will be the focus of the teaching plan.

An important component of this phase is assessing if the client has been compliant with treatment regimens in the past. Noncompliance is a major health issue in that it negatively affects the client's health status and the nurse-client relationship and is a drain on the financial resources of the health care system. This complex problem was studied by Lorig (1996), who explored how to help people with compliance (Fig. 9–1). Note that the levels in the chart offer actions, or choices of actions, that might be taken in response to a description of the problem.

Diagnosis and Planning

A teaching plan includes what the client sees as being important in gaining and retaining health. When the client's priorities are included in the plan, there is a greater chance for more participation and success in learning. Goals, objectives, content, and teaching strategies are tailored to the needs and interests of the client. A formal written plan is necessary to organize the teaching; to share with other members of the health team; for the client to refer to; and to use when evaluation takes place.

In developing a teaching plan focusing on areas of client needs, interests, and health state, the nurse needs to answer the following questions:

- What does the client want to know about his or her health status?
- Are the primary concerns of the client consistent with nursing observations and assessments?

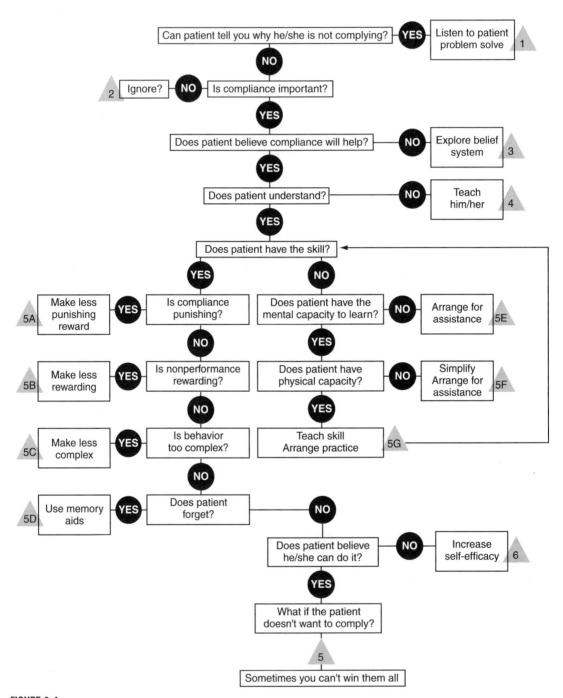

FIGURE 9–1

Improving patient compliance. (Redrawn from K. Lorig & Associates. [1996]. *Patient education: A practical approach* [2nd ed., p. 185]. Thousand Oaks, CA: Sase.)

- Do any cultural or religious beliefs conflict with these observations and assessments?
- What is the client's learning ability and level of reading ability?
- Does the client want to learn the content?
- Is the client physically and emotionally ready to participate in learning?
- Who will do the teaching?
- What teaching methods will be used?
- Where will the teaching take place?
- Will the time scheduled be convenient for the client and the teacher? Will the client need to be reminded of appointments?
- Who else needs to be taught? Are they capable and interested in learning?
- Who is the decision maker in the family? Does this person have to be included in health decisions?
- Does the client value the promotion and maintenance of health at this time?
- Can the behaviors to be learned be carried out in the client's daily environment? Are there resources there?

It is during this planning phase that the nurse and the client work together in formulating objectives—an important component of the teaching plan. They can be used as a guide to select and prioritize the learning content. Whether they are used as main objectives, addressing broad concepts, or are practical as subobjectives in which specific behaviors are "spelled out," they take into account what type of learning the client needs. As demonstrated in Bloom's (1987) classification system, both objectives and the choice of teaching methods should match the type of learning—cognitive, affective, or psychomotor. The methods should be congruent with the client's preferred learning style. Objectives should specify observable learner behavior; the conditions under which the behavior will be demonstrated and evaluated should be included.

Once the initial assessment has been completed and goals and objectives developed, the selection of content and teaching methods and a written formal plan follow. In addition to readiness and motivation of the client, time and resource allotment have great influence on the success of the planning stage. The nurse can refer to standardized teaching plans. They are readily available and can be helpful when used as a template with the client's individual needs, concerns, and abilities woven through the plan.

The choice of content is an important element in teaching. As the client has more input in deciding what content should be included in the session, his or her motivation and interest increase. The teaching should also be kept flexible to meet changing learning needs. Planning a teaching session should not be done in isolation. The teaching plan is more inclusive when other members of the client's health care team contribute information. Other nurses and members from various disciplines who have been and will be involved in the client's care should actively participate in all phases of the teaching plan. They also need to feel free to have access to and add documentation to the formal plan, as it is an important part of the client's permanent record.

Identifying learning goals and objectives directs the teacher as to what should be taught. The learning domain implied by the behavioral objectives determines what teaching methods might be used.

In selecting teaching approaches, the nurse needs to answer the following questions:

- What is the client's preferred method of learning?
- What teaching methods does the nurse enjoy using?
- What type of learning are the nurse and the client trying to achieve?
- How many teachers and students are involved in the sessions?
- How many sessions are needed?
- How much time should be allotted for each session?
- What instructional resources are available?
- Is there a need for and availability of assistive devices?
- Will there be time for practice and review?

Teaching Methods

Combining strategies in a teaching session keeps the learner's interest and promotes learning. It adds variety and challenges the teacher to judge what method or methods should be selected and the rationale for their use. Some of the following methods can be used.

Discussion

The technique of one-to-one discussion consists of the nurse's presenting information to the client. It can be very effective when done in a comfortable, informal fashion, at a level that can be understood by the learner. The client is actively engaged in the discussion, and it is tailored to the client's individual needs and interests.

Group discussion is a more efficient and economical way to teach several clients who have similar learning needs. In addition to presenting factual material, this method encourages the sharing of experiences and feelings.

The nurse acts as facilitator in presenting information and encouraging all members to explore, react to, and relate the information to their own lives. Group members have the opportunity to learn from each other, not just from the teacher. Discussion is a rich source of learning and appeals to the cognitive and affective domains.

Role Playing

Role playing is a technique in which clients act out a scene by taking on roles. The clients may play themselves or other people in the scene. The nurse-leader defines the problem and determines goals and the actual situation and roles to be played. Clear instructions are given to the players, and time is allotted for feedback and evaluation.

Role playing is effective when clients need to practice new behaviors or look at possible consequences of an unfamiliar situation. It is a safe environment to examine different attitudes and values and practice carrying out fresh ideas and decisions. Role playing helps clients explore the feelings and roles of others. Afterward, on reflection, clients are asked to identify feelings, concerns, and reactions to others in the scene. They then examine what seemed comfortable and uncomfortable and what alternative behaviors might have been more effective.

This technique helps clients understand themselves and others and prepare for upcoming real situations. When working with a group, those not participating should be observing for nonverbal behavior and how the players are responding to each other. Observers are expected to contribute to the discussion afterward by sharing interpretations, feelings, and ideas. Role playing is an effective teaching tool that stimulates creativity and problem solving. Presented in this formal way, with adequate time for in-depth discussion after the presentation, role playing is time-consuming in preparing, acting out, and evaluating.

Role playing is especially effective if an experienced teacher uses it spontaneously to address concerns about or strong reactions to what is being discussed. It is effective for the client who may be facing uncomfortable situations such as being aware of people star-

ing or when much effort and time are needed to gain access to public transportation. It has also helped family members understand and be more comfortable with their own feelings when accompanying clients in these situations. This is a method commonly used with the support system, coworkers, or classmates of people with chronic illness or those with disabilities. Role playing is a technique for teaching in the affective domain.

Demonstration and Coaching

The most common teaching strategy is demonstration and coaching, which helps the client perform a skill. Traditionally, it progresses through the following stages. The nurse demonstrates the procedure while explaining why it is done, how it is done, and when it is done. It is helpful if the nurse then slowly repeats the procedure while the client coaches the nurse on what is to be done next. The client is free to ask questions, handle the equipment, and practice parts of the procedure under the nurse's guidance and coaching. After several sessions, or as many as are required, the client performs the complete procedure while explaining what is being done and why. It is helpful when the client demonstrates the entire procedure using the same equipment and under similar conditions as when he or she will be performing the procedure independently. Coaching the client on how to recover from an error or make adjustments for unforeseen problems combines the cognitive to the overall psychomotor domain for this technique.

Teaching Aids and Instructional Technology

Books, pamphlets, outlines, instructional sheets, and printed cards can be helpful when used as preparation before a teaching session, to refer to during a session, or for review and reinforcement afterward. Pictures and diagrams also supplement learning and stimulate interest in a topic. They are available from state or federal agencies, special-interest groups, nonprofit organizations, professional groups, and communications programs within large computer networks, for example, the Internet (Table 9–2).

It is the nurse's responsibility to see that the materials chosen are accurate, complete, geared toward the client's learning needs, and presented on an appropriate educational level for the client. The materials should include terminology that will be understood and geared toward the client's reading ability.

TABLE 9–2 ■ INTERNET RESOURCES

A comprehensive Internet resource for consumer health information can be accessed easily. There are numerous world wide web (www) sites that will provide links to other sources of information. Following are examples:

http://www.health-infosys-dir.com/PtEd.html	Healthcare Information System Directory
http://www.acb.org	American Council of the Blind
http://www.medicinenet.com	Consumer Health Education
http://www.helix.com/	Health Education Learning and Information Exchange
http://www.reutershealth.com/	Health Information Services
http://www.healthtouch.com	Healthtouch
http://www.medmatrix.org/index.asp	Medical Matrix
http://www.medscape.com/	Medscape
http://www.cc.emory.edu/WHSCL/MedWeb.html	Med Web: Databases
http://www.shef.ac.uk/~nhcon/	Nursing and Health Care Resources on the Net
http://www.patient-education.com	The Patient Education Institute
http://text.nlm.nih.gov/medlineplus	Health Information
http://report.kff.org	Kaiser Family Foundation
http://www.noah.cuny.edu	New York Online Access to Health

Many people read at a low level and may not understand written or visual materials or videotapes. A client's appearance, verbal ability, or level of education does not always give an accurate estimate of literacy. The nurse should initiate teaching with simple materials if the client appears to have a low literacy level. The complexity of materials can be increased if the client progresses.

If English is not the client's primary language, the client may prefer reading materials in the native language. It may not be possible to find printed materials in languages that are not common in the area. In that case, nurses have been successful in networking with faculty sponsors of college- or graduate-level language clubs to have students translate as a community project. Another group that responded enthusiastically was a neighborhood social club whose retired members were very willing to translate health-related materials for people who speak their language. To ensure accuracy, translation of information occurs in two stages: translation from English to the client's language and then "back translation" to English by another person. This approach is recommended for translation of verbal communication as well. In the effort to maintain this objectivity, it is best if family members are not asked to act as translators.

Used to reinforce and supplement personal interaction between the nurse and the client, audiovisual aids add interest and stimulation to the teaching session. Videotapes, slides, flipcharts, films, transparencies, filmstrips, and computer technologies offer combinations of sound, sight, and touch. Having content presented in a visual fashion is helpful for many learners. Audiotapes and interactive computer programs add the dimension of hearing. Newer programs include an interactive element as the client touches the computer screen in response to a request. These sophisticated programs then respond to the client's input, give feedback, and either review present content in a different way or advance the client to the next level.

If audiovisual equipment is brought to a client's home, it should be portable, adaptable, and in working order. The nurse should be comfortable with its use, having practiced with the same equipment ahead of time and knowing how to contact technical assistance if necessary.

Clients must get the help they need to succeed in learning, and the nurse must give thought to how they might benefit from the use of technology. Nurses need to be familiar with the use of video magnifiers, close-captioned videos, and the newest computer and interactive programs. Many of these devices are geared specifically for people with disabilities. This may be a new concept for the client, yet many are already familiar with computer programs and devices that enhance learning. Some clients have adjusted equipment or made their own apparatus to help themselves.

It is common for computers and interactive multimedia to be used in accommodating students with different needs. Younger clients are often quite comfortable with these assisted-learning programs because many have had prior experience with computers. The nurse should become familiar with existing software instructional programs. Most computer-assisted instruction, modular learning, and self-paced educational programs are efficient and even incorporate evaluation as part of their content.

Advances in communication technology have been very exciting. Fiber-optic equipment, fax machines, and personal computer communication programs enable people thousands of miles away to communicate with each other in a matter of seconds. Many colleges are involved in distant learning programs in which students communicate from remote sites via video or teleconferencing. There are techniques using simultaneous live television or telephone presentations for a number of participants at different sites through intricate satellite or microwave systems. These options are already available at some large health care centers and will become more available in the near future.

An example of a computer-based program being used at the University of Wisconsin is the Comprehensive Health Enhancement Support System. Clients who are in need of information take the computer into their home for a period of 3 months, during which time they are taught to use it in finding information about current treatments and other areas of concern. They are able to read relevant bulletin boards, sign up for e-mail lists, or enter "chat rooms" and have dialogue with others who share the same condition: users have access to databases and health professionals for expert advice. It has been very successful, and clients have remarked that it has been a great support to interact with other clients and it has helped them make important decisions about their care (Films for the Humanities and Science, 1994).

Age Consideration

The age of the client affects learning because different age groups require different approaches to teaching. When dealing with children, it is important to consider the developmental stage, and the level of understanding to determine teaching strategies.

Preschoolers learn primarily from their parents but are responsive to other teachers and role models. It is usually reassuring for children to have parents present during teaching sessions with the nurse. This also helps parents reinforce the learning with their children. Three- to 5-year-old children ask many questions. These should be answered immediately in simple, clear language they can understand. Answering honestly increases trust, which is vital to children this age.

Play is an effective way for preschoolers to learn. For example, the nurse can demonstrate bandaging a favorite stuffed animal or use an age-appropriate coloring book. Many children of this age like to handle materials and supplies, and some like to practice procedures. As the nurse and child are involved in these activities, the nurse can be talking with the child about what to expect during the procedures. This is helpful in dealing with their fears. The preschooler is usually energetic but restless: teaching should be limited to 10-minute sessions.

School-aged children are generally eager to learn. They are beginning to develop logical reasoning and understand *cause-and-effect* relationships that help them problem-solve. Therefore, the child should be included in planning and setting goals. The nurse should answer all questions immediately and truthfully. A trusting relationship helps the child feel comfortable enough to express concerns.

Interacting with peers is important during school years, with parents taking a less dominant role. Six- to 12-year-old children enjoy arts and crafts activities and take pleasure in "winning"—they respond positively to teaching aids such as charts and colorful stickers. Pictures, diagrams, and printed materials regarding health conditions have been effective with this age group. The nurse should understand that a child's reading level may regress with sickness or hospitalization.

Most school-aged children are accustomed to a classroom atmosphere. Even if they are not in a typical school environment, they understand the scheduling of work and play. Teaching should be scheduled around other interests and activities that are important to them and are part of their daily routine: sessions should be no longer than 30 minutes in length.

Adolescent children's task is to establish their own identity separate from that of the immediate family: many prefer to learn without their parents present. Adolescents learn best when they see immediate benefits to themselves. They are becoming more adept at logical-reasoning and abstract-thinking skills. A problem-solving approach to learning has been successful with this age group and encourages them to take more responsibility for their own health.

Being accepted by peers is an important aspect of the adolescent child's development. This group often has difficulty following health regimens that make them feel different from others their age. Teenaged clients are usually responsive to group teaching because they feel understood and accepted by a peer group facing similar challenges. Emotional support and role modeling are important for the adolescent client.

Adolescents should be included in all stages of the teaching and learning process because they benefit by feeling more independent. Effective learning takes place when there is a trusting relationship between the nurse and the teenaged client. Acknowledging the client's value system and maintaining confidentiality enhances this relationship.

Printed materials have been helpful with adolescent learners, and these can be referred to and reviewed between sessions. The maximal length of a session for this age group should be from 45 to 50 minutes: they are accustomed to periods of this length in school.

Adults are the most numerous and fastest-growing population of health care consumers. Malcolm Knowles (1984) developed a concept of andragogy geared to the characteristics and needs of adult learners. It was based on assumptions that distinguished it from models based on the needs of young learners. One assumption was that adults need to know *why* they need to learn. They become motivated to learn when they perceive that it will help them deal with tasks and problems they confront in their daily life situations. Relatively healthy elderly adults can learn new materials and procedures if they see it as helping them remain well and independent. Knowles observed a strengthening of adult learners' self-esteem as they made the transition from dependent to self-directing learners. He viewed adult learners as being more heterogeneous in terms of background, learning styles, needs, interests, and goals than are a group of young learners.

Within the population of adult learners, the *elderly* population outnumbers the rest. Although general intelligence does not change with aging, learning and problem-solving abilities do decline.

When teaching elderly clients, the nurse needs to know that

- They have valuable past experiences on which to build and relate new materials.
- It is effective to incorporate daily habits into the teaching plan.
- They learn well when the pace is slow, with limited material presented at a single session.
- Large print in primary colors should be used for visual aids.

- Teaching sessions should be timed according to the client's stamina and level of interest. This usually does not exceed 20 minutes.
- Allowing time for the client to process new information is helpful—the ability to learn remains intact, but the time needed for processing increases.
- Multiple teaching sessions and frequent summaries enhance the material being taught.

In addition, when working with older clients, the nurse may have to make adjustments to account for diminished hearing, impaired vision, and other physical limitations or disabilities.

To facilitate expression and comprehension, the nurse needs to know that

- Acknowledging all communication efforts is important.
- The client needs adequate time to respond.
- "Filling in words" in anticipation of what the nurse thinks the client is trying to say is not helpful.
- Decreasing background noise and visual distractions is helpful.
- Speaking on eye-to-eye level, slowly and clearly and in a low voice enhances understanding.
- Using short sentences and not exaggerating articulation aids comprehension.

Implementation

The teaching plan is implemented more effectively when the teacher has full knowledge of the content being covered. Occasionally, questions that the nurse cannot answer at the time arise. The nurse should take this as an opportunity to model for the client how more information and answers can be found. This adds to the baseline of open communication, trust, and respect between the client and the nurse. After clients had been involved in formal teaching plans, several mentioned the benefit of seeing the nurse unable to answer a question. Observing the nurse in the process of finding a solution is helpful to clients. Knowing how to find information is a key factor in learning. There are numerous resources for people with disabilities (Table 9–3).

Scheduling the time of the session is important. Ideally, it should coincide with the time of day the client feels at his or her peak for learning, and it must also be convenient for the nurse. Good lighting, privacy, and

TABLE 9–3 ■ SOURCES FOR CLIENT EDUCATION MATERIALS

Administration on Developmental Disabilities
U.S. Department of Health and Human Services
200 Independence Avenue SW
Washington, DC 20201-0001
(202) 245-2980

American Association of Retired Persons
601 E Street NW
Washington, DC 20049
(202) 434-2277

American Cancer Society
90 Park Avenue
New York, NY 10016
(212) 599-3600

American Civil Liberties Union
132 W 43rd Street
New York, NY 10036-6599
(212) 944-9800

American Coalition of Citizens with Disabilities (ACCD)
1200 15th Street NW, Suite 201
Washington, DC 20005
(202) 785-4265

American Diabetes Association
1600 Duke Street
Alexandria, VA 22314-3447
(800) ADA-DISC
(703) 549-1500

American Juvenile Arthritis Organization
1314 Spring Street
Atlanta, GA 30309
(404) 872-7110

American Paralysis Association
PO Box 187
Short Hills, NY 07078
(800) 225-0292

Arthritis Foundation
1314 Spring Street NW
Atlanta, GA 30309
(800) 283-7800

Arthritis Rehabilitation Center
1234 19th Street NW
Washington, DC 20036
(202) 223-5320

Association of Rehabilitation Nurses
5700 Old Orchard Road, 1st Floor
Skokie, IL 60077-1057
(708) 966-3433

Better Hearing Institute
PO Box 1840
Washington, DC 20013
(800) 424-8576

Clearinghouse on Disability Information
    Office of Special Education and Rehabilitation Services
Room 3132, Switzer Building
330 C Street SE
Washington, DC 20202
(202) 732-1723
(800) 346-2742

Disability Rights Center
1346 Connecticut Avenue NW, Suite 1124
Washington, DC 20036
(202) 223-3304

Federation for Children with Special Needs
95 Berkeley Street, Suite 104
Boston, MA 02116
(617) 482-2915

Higher Education and Adult Training for People with
    Handicaps Resource Center
1 Dupont Circle
Washington, DC 20036-1193
(800) 544-3284

Information for Individuals with Disabilities
Fort Point Place
27–43 Wormwood Street
Boston, MA 02210
(617) 727-5540

Learning Disabilities Association of America
4156 Library Road
Pittsburgh, PA 15234
(412) 341-1515

Mainstream, Inc.
1030 15th Street NW, Suite 1010
Washington, DC 10005
(202) 898-1400

National Amputation Foundation
12–45 105th Street
Whitestone, NY 11357
(718) 767-0596

National Association for Home Care
519 C Street NE
Washington, DC 20002
(202) 547-7424

National Association for Visually Handicapped
22 West 21st Street
New York, NY 10010
(212) 889-3134

National Center for Youth with Disabilities
University of Minnesota
Box 721
420 Delaware Street SE
Minneapolis, MN 55455
(800) 333-6293

National Clearinghouse on Postsecondary Education for
    Individuals with Disabilities
HEATH Resource Center
One Dupont Circle NW
Washington, DC 20036
(800) 544-3284

National Council on Disability
899 Independence Avenue SW
Washington, DC 20591
(202) 267-3846

TABLE 9–3 ■ SOURCES FOR CLIENT EDUCATION MATERIALS *Continued*

National Council on the Handicapped
330 C Street SW, Room 3123
Washington, DC 20202
(202) 732-1276

National Head Injury Foundation
333 Turnpike Road
Southboro, MA 01772
(800) 444-6443

National Information Center for Handicapped Children and
   Youth (NICHCY)
National Information Center for Children and Youths with
   Handicaps
PO Box 1492
Washington, DC 20013
(703) 893-6061

National Injury Information Clearinghouse (USCPSC)
5401 Westbard Avenue, Room 625
Bethesda, MD 20207
(301) 492-6424

National Institute on Deafness and Other Communication
   Disorders Clearinghouse (NIDCD)
PO Box 37777
Washington, DC 20013-7777
(301) 565-4020

National Institute for Occupational Safety and Health
   (NIOSH)
NIOSH/CDC
1600 Clifton Road MS D36
Atlanta, GA 30333
(404) 639-3061

National Library Service for the Blind and Physically
   Handicapped (NLSBPH)
Library of Congress
1291 Taylor Street NW
Washington, DC 20542
(202) 707-5100

National Organization on Disability (NOD)
910 16th Street NW, Suite 600
Washington, DC 20006
(800) 248-ABLE

National Rehabilitation Information Center (NARIC)
8455 Colesville Road, Suite 935
Silver Spring, MD 20910
(800) 346-2742

National Spinal Cord Injury Association
600 W Cummings Park, Suite 2000
Woburn, MA 01801
(800) 962-9629

National Worksite Health Promotion Resource Center
777 North Capitol Street NE
Washington, DC 20002
(202) 408-9320

Office of Vocational and Adult Education
U.S. Department of Education
Policy Analysis Staff
Room 4525, Switzer Bldg.
330 C Street SE
Washington, DC 20202-0001
(202) 732-2251

Paralyzed Veterans of America
4350 West Highway, Suite 900
Washington, DC 20014
(202) 245-7246

Society for the Advancement of Travel for the Handicapped
327 Fifth Avenue, Suite 610
New York, NY 10016

The System-Accessible Design and Product Information
   System from Information
Development Corporation
360 St. Albin Court
Winston-Salem, NC 27104

Veterans Affairs Medical Center
Continuing Education Center (14B-JA)
St. Louis, MO 63125
(314) 894-6534

---

freedom from distractions and annoying noise levels all add to the comfort of the learning environment. If it is in the client's home, the first session might take longer than expected because of having to arrange the room in a way that is comfortable for learning. Attending to the client's comfort acknowledges the client as the focal point of the session. It is a good idea to rely on the client's choices because the client is aware of personal preferences and how he or she can be most productive as a learner.

When the teaching plan is implemented, the client needs to be ready emotionally—not too anxious, restless, or depressed. Being free from pain and physically comfortable is especially important. The environment and personal comfort are key elements to consider when the teaching session is taking place outside the familiar surroundings of the client's home or residence. The nurse can attend to the immediate environment. Ensuring that the client can travel to and gain access to the site where the teaching is taking place must be done well in advance. It helps the client remain more independent.

To teach sessions that are dynamic and productive, the nurse needs to answer the following questions:

- Is there flexibility to change direction, pace, or content as needs may change?
- Is the climate conducive to learning, taking into consideration cultural norms?
- Does the client feel free to question and challenge the teacher (an authority figure)?
- Are members of the support system included in all phases of the plan?
- Are the teaching aids that are being used helpful?
- Are the terms and vocabulary being used understood by the learner?
- Has time been allotted for clarification and review?

Evaluation

Evaluation takes place throughout the teaching and learning interaction, and modifications may be needed in the teaching plan during any of the four phases of the process. Evaluation is an ongoing process in which the client, nurse, and support system determine what has been learned. Evaluation is a measure to see if the client has been successful in mastering the learning objectives.

The predetermined objectives guide and direct the plan and help in the evaluation phase. Psychomotor learning is relatively easy to evaluate. The nurse observing the client carrying out a procedure is an example. Asking the client questions is a direct way to evaluate cognitive learning. It is more difficult to judge if attitudes or values have changed when attempting to see if affective learning has taken place. At times, this can be determined when talking with the client. Carefully listening to a client's responses can suggest a change in values or attitudes. The nurse might then observe changes in the client's behavior that are consistent with a new value; for example, a client who, in appraising his health, has decided to stop smoking to reduce susceptibility to further lung disease.

There are a variety of techniques to use for outcome assessment. Rating scales, checklists, questionnaire surveys, and written tests are among many instruments that measure if learning has occurred. Most are not time-consuming. One disadvantage is that clients may not be comfortable as they may feel they are being "tested."

When evaluation is ongoing, oral questioning is a reasonable method for the nurse to use. It promotes thinking about the subject under discussion. The nurse can check comprehension, test knowledge, and identify weak areas that will be readdressed. Because this takes place as a discussion, the client is usually not even aware that an evaluation is taking place.

Evaluation techniques are not limited to *if* and *what* the client has learned but also determine if the learning experiences were organized effectively and look at the efficiency of the guidance of learning. They encourage the nurse to evaluate the teaching and to be accountable for the nurse's role in the entire teaching and learning process.

When engaged in the evaluation phase, the nurse needs to answer the following questions:

- What does evaluation mean to the client?
- Does evaluation have cultural ramifications; for example, is failing a test considered an insult to the teacher?
- Are the client's behavioral outcomes consistent with the outcome criteria?
- What goals were not reached? Can the nurse-client team determine why?
- Did the content relate to and build on the client's previous knowledge and experience?
- Was the content logically organized?
- What kind of response or responses did the learner have throughout the phases of the process?
- Is it necessary to modify or repeat parts of the plan?
- If it appears that the client has not learned, is it possible that client actually learned content of the teaching plan but has chosen not to comply?

CASE STUDY AND TEACHING PLAN

The teaching plan, developed by the nurse, client, and support system, is the framework for organizing client teaching. The nurse has access to a variety of standardized teaching plans but is responsible to assess the individualized needs of the client.

This must be documented because it communicates to others what has taken place. It is part of the client's permanent record and can be referred to if further planning is necessary. Documentation provides evidence of a client's progress in achieving learning outcomes. It records what has been accomplished and demonstrates the cost benefit of having the client and support system take on more responsibility for self-care.

Following is a case study and customized plan. As data are collected in each phase of the teaching process, the plan becomes more thorough and personalized for the client. As learning preferences are identified, various teaching methods are introduced.

■ CASE STUDY 9–1

Carlo, 63 years old, was born in Italy and has been in the United States for 3 years. He came with his wife to be near his only family, a daughter with two adolescent sons. He and his wife live in a basement apartment in the daughter's home. Carlo and his wife do not speak English well and prefer to communicate in Italian.

Because their daughter works, they have taken on the responsibility of tending to household affairs: shopping, cooking, and caring for the grandchildren. Because they are not able to pay rent, Carlo and his wife feel obligated to help in these ways.

Their social life consists of being with the family and walking to the neighborhood church every morning for daily Mass. Afterward, they walk to the diner for a cup of espresso and pastries. In the afternoon, Carlo enjoys watching baseball games on television. His grandsons keep him updated, reading him the sports pages of the daily newspaper when they come home from school. This is the highlight of his day.

Five years ago, Carlo was diagnosed with rheumatoid arthritis when he experienced generalized joint pain with stiffness and some limitation of movement of both lower extremities. Pain was relieved by simple analgesics. He has not had to take medication and has been free from pain for the past year. The physician in Italy suggested a low-calorie diet because Carlo is 45 pounds overweight. Since coming to the United States, he has gained an additional 10 pounds because he has been cooking fried, high-fat food. His grandsons prefer this, because "it tastes like McDonald's."

Last week, Carlo fell on a patch of ice. He was hospitalized with a severe hip injury, but no fracture. He was recovering well from the injury but experienced a flare-up of rheumatoid arthritis. Carlo will have permanent limitation of movement in his lower extremities, and it has been suggested that his daughter find placement in an interim rehabilitation facility until her father regains his strength. Carlo has also been diagnosed with mild hypertension, which will be treated with a low-fat, low-sodium diet.

Carlo insists on returning home because he can't afford the hospitalization. He will be discharged in 2 days. His mobility is limited (he has practiced with a walker—taking only four steps on a flat surface before becoming fatigued). The physical therapist is scheduled for one home visit.

Carlo will be taking nonsteroidal anti-inflammatory agents for pain. His hospital record indicates a potential for injury because of pain and limited strength and movement of joints of the lower extremities. There is also a lack of knowledge in that Carlo is unfamiliar with the new diet and to date has used his walker only once, with supervision. His primary concern is that he wants to remain independent and does not want to "be a burden" to his family.

TEACHING PLAN

You are the nurse who will be visiting Carlo at home. The initial home visit is an opportunity to develop a positive relationship with Carlo while assessing his abilities, support system, environment, learning needs, and preferences.

Carlo and his wife are able to communicate slowly but effectively in "broken" English. Neither is able to read the English language. After the meeting with Carlo, his wife, and daughter, all agree that the main concern for the client and support system is to learn about Carlo's limitations in physical mobility related to rheumatoid arthritis and hip injury in order to allow him to return to maximal daily functions at home while maintaining an appropriate diet and being physically, spiritually, and emotionally comfortable.

Carlo learned some adaptive techniques 15 years ago after he fractured his right femur and both arms in an automobile accident. He remembers being actively involved with his therapy and getting started as soon as possible so he wouldn't need too much assistance from his wife. He is concerned that he is so much older now and hopes that he can get treatment very soon and be successful with therapy this time as well.

Carlo seems to be compatible with Kolb's (1984) *concrete experience* phase of learning. Learners partial to this stage do well when they have few restrictions and are able to take an active part and not focus on details or possible problems. The nurse will use a coaching approach incorporating diagrams and drawings in the teaching plan because Carlo has been successful with this method.

Table 9–4 shows the framework of a teaching plan that will be developed for this client. It will be updated and evaluated as members of the health care team contribute to Carlo's

TABLE 9–4 ■ TEACHING PLAN

Client Outcomes	Nursing Interventions	Learner Activities	Evaluation Method
1. C & SS will understand need for increased mobility and participate in progressive mobilization in seeking maximum level of functional ability.	Provide explanation for need to progress from active ROM exercises to functional activities to strengthen and restore function while preventing deterioration (demonstration/coaching, practice, videotaping). Plan sessions when client is not involved with baseball game on TV.	C & SS verbalize need for increased mobility and stamina to reach potential level of functioning.	Observe C performing ROM exercises and proper use of walker, with use of observational checklist of activities for C & SS. Review and discuss videotape session.
a) C will practice and safely demonstrate use of walker, increasing distance by 10–15 ft. each week, while increasing stamina.	Consult with PT as C learns proper use of walker by practicing with supervision and videotaping session. Provide for progressive mobilization.	C Practices and does return demonstration of ROM activities and use of walker (repetition, feedback, discussion of videotape practice). C & SS verbalize importance of and benefits of exercise and discuss adjusting routine and environs so C may increase activities in safe surroundings.	C adheres to exercise routine and ambulates with walker without injury. C & SS discuss ways to minimize safety hazards at home while making appropriate modifications to accommodate C's former lifestyle patterns as much as possible.
b) C will perform exercises to promote strength and mobility of lower extremities while including periods of rest.	Collaborate with PT in setting up exercise program. Team (nurse, PT, C, & SS) assesses C's mobility while monitoring level of fatigue. Demonstrate for C & SS How to sit in straight back chair that is high enough for his feet to remain flat on floor. How to wear properly fitting and supporting shoes to keep feet in alignment. How to use raised seat for toilet. How to safely transfer from seated to standing position. How to use handrails when preparing to bathe in tub or shower stall.	C is able to sit with feet supported; able to transfer without difficulty.	C's feet are in proper alignment.
c) C & SS will develop plan to adjust daily routine and environs to abilities and safety concerns.	Discuss with C & SS safety to establish access to and ability to maneuver within house.	C & SS verbalize understanding of barrier-free concept to remain safe while meeting mobilization needs. C prefers learning sessions of 20 min.	C makes suggestions as to changing placement of furniture, removal of throw rugs, etc., to prevent accidents. C remains safe in home environment. C does not tire after 20-min session.

TABLE 9–4 ■ TEACHING PLAN *Continued*

Client Outcomes	Nursing Interventions	Learner Activities	Evaluation Method
2. By 2nd visit, C & SS will understand basic process of rheumatoid arthritis and its connection with pain, alteration of abilities, and treatment plan.	Ask if C & SS have questions or concerns since last visit. After evaluating what C & SS already know, discuss rheumatoid arthritis as chronic, systemic, inflammatory disorder with exacerbation and remissions. Discuss fact that effective treatment exists and includes adherence to meds, diet, and balanced program of exercise and rest (discussion with C & SS, written materials with Italian translation, pictures, and diagrams of joint structure and arthritic changes if appropriate).	C & SS verbalize information accurately, discuss concerns, and ask appropriate questions. C & SS read materials, appear to understand content, and ask questions about treatment regimen. Grandsons are able to access, on computer, information, diagrams, etc. (presented in Italian), regarding C's condition.	Oral report. Direct observation during conversation and casual question and answer period with C & SS. C & SS verbalize concerns and appear less anxious. C appears to be interested and understands information.
3. By 3rd visit, C will understand pain reduction connection with rest and safe use of pain meds, including indications, effects, and side effects.	Ask if C & SS have questions or concerns since last visit. Provide verbal and written instructions and ask SS to interpret so C understands that NSAIAs should relieve mild to moderate pain in joints of his legs. It's best to take NSAIAs on empty stomach but they can be taken with milk or food to decrease GI symptoms. NSAIAs are to be taken as directed to maintain therapeutic blood level and promote effectiveness. Therapeutic effect may take up to 1 mo. Alcoholic beverages should be avoided. Periodic blood tests may be ordered to monitor for blood or liver changes. Blurred vision, ringing in ears, change in urine pattern, fever, blood in urine are side effects to be reported. NSAIAs do not cause addiction.	C & SS verbalize indication, effects, and side effects of NSAIAs. C understands medication regimen and takes as prescribed.	C & SS report that medication is effective in reducing pain. C appears relaxed and able to participate in exercise and mobility regimen and is able to sleep through night. Observations are validated by daughter's verbal report that her father and mother understand communication.

Table continued on following page

TABLE 9–4 ■ TEACHING PLAN *Continued*

Client Outcomes	Nursing Interventions	Learner Activities	Evaluation Method
a) C will incorporate relaxation skills and divisional activities for pain control.	Talk with C & SS about benefit of warm baths and application of warm compresses to affected areas to reduce pain, or application of cold compresses to swollen joints. Encourage use of stress reduction techniques, such as listening to music (maybe Italian), or methods he used that helped in the past.	C takes warm baths and practices making hot/cold packs and demonstrates their application. C reflects on techniques that have aided relaxation and verbalizes need to decrease activity if fatigued or in pain.	C reports he takes warm bath or finds relief in hot/cold pack applications. Measured by C's verbal understanding and willingness to investigate various methods.
4. By last visit, C will understand dietary restrictions and need for weight loss while participating in planning new dietary regimen.	Ask if C & SS have questions or concerns since last visit. Refer C & SS to dietitian for diet teaching prior to discharge. Check that C & SS receive information on "heart healthy" methods of buying, preparing, and cooking foods low in salt, fat, and calories, yet appealing to Italian cuisine. Discuss benefits of weight loss: control of hypertension and rheumatoid arthritis symptoms. Discuss and explain relationship of diet and obesity to hypertension and effects of excess weight on inflamed joints and mobility.	C verbalizes benefits of weight loss and connection to hypertension and joint inflammation. C & SS identify and prepare low-fat, low-calorie meals. C keeps food diary in identifying eating patterns. C helps with food planning and preparation, as before, using low-fat cheeses and oil and broiling instead of frying. C & SS understand how new eating habits benefit entire family.	Observe C & SS choosing and preparing foods of their choice that fit into new dietary and calorie regimen. Observe food preparation methods to reduce calories and fat content (e.g., boiling, broiling, omitting saturated fats and oils). Note amount of weight loss or gain.
5. By last visit, C will appreciate value of obtaining emotional, spiritual, and social support and how these reduce anxiety.	Check if there are questions or concerns since last visit. Give phone number where they can reach nurse when they have such concerns.	C & SS participate in discussion and seek support groups from community. C is willing to become involved with and accept help from outside family support system.	Observe C's interest and participation in support network in community.

TABLE 9–4 ■ TEACHING PLAN *Continued*

Client Outcomes	Nursing Interventions	Learner Activities	Evaluation Method
a) C will have sense of belonging and add to his present support system.	Expand C's support system to include community resources. Offer printed materials about various programs Investigate Italian social clubs, church and peer groups in neighborhood. (facilitate by phone calls, written referrals, etc.). Have grandsons get involved with doing chores C can no longer do. Teach C & SS process of accessing support in community, e.g., have Italian-speaking priest visit C at home, arrange senior van to transport C and wife to Mass.	C & wife gradually return to former daily routine as much as possible within new adaptations. C & SS contact others in church/social community. C teaches grandsons how to help out by taking on some responsibility for care of house and garden.	Direct observation and verbal reports. Expansion of C's support system to include resources in community. C appears interested in sharing some of his past activities with grandsons and in teaching them how to perform some household chores.

C, client; GI, gastrointestinal; NSAIA, nonsteroidal anti-inflammatory agent; PT, physical therapist; ROM, range of motion; SS, support system.

care. The client, family, and others in his support system will also contribute to this plan, because they are crucial to Carlo's success in understanding and adjusting to his altered abilities. ■

SUMMARY

For more than 100 years, nurses have incorporated teaching into their role. Client education is recognized today as a major responsibility of the professional nurse. It is seen as an integral component of care as nurses focus on accountability and the right of clients to be involved in their own care. Client education is especially challenging in a health care system that includes clients who are very ill and clients with altered abilities who are reentering a community with more limited professional, financial, and physical resources than in the past.

In developing a teaching plan, there is need to avoid making radical changes in the client's lifestyle. The nurse-client team should acknowledge the client's talents, abilities, and choices while incorporating daily habits into the plan. This plan is built on the client's belief system, based on the client's history, tradition, and culture. It is for this reason—the personal and cultural foundation—that each client needs an individual, personalized teaching plan.

The nurse's goal is to give the client and support system the best and most accurate information available to help the client attain and maintain wellness while remaining as independent as possible. In this way the client is encouraged to be his or her own advocate and to assume more responsibility for personal health care.

REFERENCES

Bloom, B. S. (Ed.). (1987). *Taxonomy of educational objectives—Book 1: Cognitive domain*. New York: Longman.

Films for the Humanities and Sciences. (1994). *Patient education and technology: Health on-line* [Film No. FFH 5113]. (Available from Films for the Humanities, Inc., Box 2053, Princeton, NJ 08543-2-53)

Knowles, M. (1984). *The adult learner—A neglected species* (3rd ed.). Houston: Gulf.

Kolb, D. (1984). *Experimental learning*. Englewood Cliffs, NJ: Prentice-Hall.

Krathwohl, D. R., Bloom, B. S., & Masia, B. B. (1964). *Taxonomy of educational objectives—The classification of educational goals—Handbook 2: Affective domain*. New York: Longman.

Lorig, K. (1996). *Patient education—A practical approach* (2nd ed.). Thousand Oaks, CA: Sage.

BIBLIOGRAPHY

O'Toole, M. (Ed.). (1997). *Miller-Keane encyclopedia & dictionary of medicine, nursing, & allied health* (6th ed.). Philadelphia: W. B. Saunders.

Redman, B. K. (1993). *The process of patient education* (7th ed.). St. Louis: C. V. Mosby.

Reilly, D. E., & Oerman, M. H. (1990). *Behavioral objectives: Evaluation in nursing* (3rd ed.). New York: National League for Nursing.

Simons-Mortan, B. G. , Greene, W. H., & Gottlieb, N. H. (1995). *Introduction to health education and health promotion* (2nd ed.). Prospect Heights, IL: Waveland Press.

Smith, C. E. (Ed.). (1987). *Patient education—Nurses in partnership with other health professionals*. Philadelphia: W. B. Saunders.

Smith, C. M., & Maurer, F. A. (1995). *Community health nursing—Theory and practice*. Philadelphia: W. B. Saunders.

PART II

Clinical Management

Concepts of Rehabilitation Nursing
Related to Patient and Family Care
in Chronic and Disabling Conditions

CHAPTER 10

Functional Assessment

Pat Quigley

Functional assessment gained a fundamental distinction among health care professionals during the 1990s, the decade of health care reorganization. Health care professionals have gained greater appreciation for assessing the individual's ability to function as independently as possible within the community. Health care teams incorporate functional status evaluations as an integral component of patient care assessment and treatment. As members of a nursing specialty, rehabilitation nurses have included the concept of functional evaluation as part of the rehabilitation nursing process (Kelly-Hayes, 1996).

Understanding the complexities of functional limitations of impaired individuals requires definition, clarity, classification, and measurement. In addition, scientific methods of measurement are needed in order to make generalizable interpretations regarding the type and amount of physical and social assistance required by providers to assist with community reintegration of disabled individuals and populations.

Even though functional evaluation is recognized among health care professionals, functional evaluations, practices, and outcomes vary among and within professions. Today, a consensus among rehabilitation disciplines does not exist for universal methods of functional evaluation measures.

Within this chapter, historical perspectives, definitions, and a conceptual model of functional assessment are discussed, including implications for rehabilitation nurses. Implications for rehabilitation practice for community reintegration of specialty populations, such as persons living with spinal cord injury and head injury, conclude this chapter.

HISTORICAL PERSPECTIVES

Functional assessment in rehabilitation has been a topic of concern in the United States for over half a century. In the early years following World Wars I and II, the concepts

of rehabilitation were very narrow and pathology oriented. Historical views of functional assessment were also limited in scope and failed to encompass environmental functioning and adaptation. The early work in functional assessment emphasized the physical disabilities associated with trauma and disease secondary to war. During the 1930s, health care professionals were concerned with addressing behaviors of individuals with physical as well as mental impairments. As a result of continued inquiry, functional assessment began to address the needs of those who acquired mental impairments, expanding to a holistic approach to rehabilitation.

The holistic philosophy broadened assessments to include appraisal of the client's physical, mental, social, and vocational needs. Assessment of functional status, central to all aspects of assessment, measures dynamic characteristics of functional abilities (Halpern & Fuhrer, 1984). Registered nurses understand the importance of obtaining and documenting specific information about a symptom, as well as the client's perception of the presenting problems and their impact on the client's ability to perform activities of daily living (ADLs). Through initial and ongoing assessment, nurses diagnose actual and potential health care problems and prioritize the need for nursing care (American Nurses Association, 1995). Nurses determine the clients' ability to meet their personal and physical needs while assessing their responses to clinical interventions and progress toward goals. However, nursing assessment has only recently expanded to include functional abilities related to ADLs, which requires training in functional evaluation (Kelly-Hayes, 1996).

The history of rehabilitation is significantly influenced by events in the early part of the 20th century. Frey (1984) conducted a historical analysis of functional assessment that was partially supported by a grant to the University Center for International Rehabilitation from the National Institute of Handicapped

TABLE 10–1 ■ FUNCTIONAL ASSESSMENT: HISTORICAL PERSPECTIVES

Rehabilitation Theme	Years	Rehabilitation Characteristics	Functional Assessment Characteristics
Cash value for disability	1920s–1940s	Financial reimbursement for physical loss of function	Loss of physical function Residual physical function
Rehabilitation rather than compensation	1940s–1960s	Adaptation to physical loss Utilization of residual capacities for maximal potential	Performance in activities of daily living Behavior patterns to function with loss Psychosocial integration
Rehabilitation accountability	1960s–1980s	Outcome achievements due to rehabilitation Focus on diagnostic groups	Skill-related performance per diagnostic group Functional outcomes per diagnoses Community reintegration

From Frey, W. (1984). Functional assessment in the 80's. In A. S. Halpern & M. J. Fuhrer (Eds.), *Functional assessment in rehabilitation.* Baltimore: Paul H. Brookes.

Research, Department of Education, Washington, DC. Frey presents a cumulative and holistic progression of functional assessment and rehabilitation in three periods (starting with the 1920s), categorized in Table 10–1.

1. Cash reimbursement for loss of physical function (1920s–1940s)
2. Expansion of services and effectiveness of services (1940s–1960s)
3. Focus on accountability of services within and among all human service networks (1960s–1980s)

Cash Value for Disability

During the first part of the 1900s, rehabilitation researchers were interested in quantifying the incidence of functional limitation in general populations. This information was obtained through health surveys seeking reports of activity restrictions due to physical impairments. After the passing of the first workers' compensation legislation in the United States in 1908, rehabilitation researchers made a sustained commitment to measuring residual functioning after chronic disease or injury. This legislation, the Federal Employees Compensation Act, entitled people to medical benefits and financial reimbursement for temporary or permanent physical inability to work.

By the 1920s, many states had invoked this law into statutory state regulations. Impaired persons were reimbursed for the physical loss of function. Assessments were performed to measure residual functions and loss of function. Assessments were done to link a loss of function to cash compensation. However, disagreement existed on how to measure a loss of function in a broader perspective other than the measure of anatomical loss. De-

termining the measure of loss in relation to job performance and cash value was primarily the physician's responsibility and was highly subjective. In 1931, Kessler developed a set of standards to measure functional abilities using physical units of degrees, pounds, range of motion, and muscle strength (Frey, 1984; Kessler, 1931). Standard tests and measures began to be developed. Other systems of measurement were developed during this time to measure physical impairment and related areas. However, in 1958, a committee of the American Medical Association (AMA) began to develop rating guides for physical impairment, distinguishing between evaluation of impairment and evaluation of disability (Halpern & Fuhrer, 1984). The AMA sought to distinguish between medical and nonmedical characteristics of rehabilitation, again reinforcing the shift of functional assessment to measure physical loss and impairment.

Rehabilitation Rather Than Compensation

As rehabilitation gained emphasis, the focus of rehabilitation expanded beyond reimbursement for the loss of a limb and subsequent loss of function. During this period, disability continued to be associated with trauma and traumatic losses. As a result of medical and surgical advances, death rates dropped and the population of impaired persons dramatically increased. Advances in antibiotic therapies extended the average life span. Therefore, the population requiring long-term care due to chronic disease, advanced age, and functional impairments increased. Rehabilitation professionals began to teach people how to use and adapt their residual capacities to their maximal potential. The philosophy of rehabilitation shifted from physical loss to holistic adaptation.

Legislation was passed during this period to further direct the progress and purpose of functional assessment. The Vocational Rehabilitation Act was adopted in 1943, and amended in 1954 and 1973, to ensure that all disabled people were entitled to vocational evaluations and adaptation or independent-living services.

Veterans' training programs extended rehabilitation services to both physically and mentally impaired people. Rehabilitation teams developed into multidisciplinary teams. Teams began to share responsibility for rehabilitation services with physicians. The team concept changed as new professionals emerged: physical therapists, occupational therapists, psychologists, and social workers. Technology advanced so that individuals were treated in hospitals and clinics rather than at home.

Functional assessments during this period focused on daily activities of everyday life, referring to behavior patterns related to individual performance. In 1945, Deaver & Brown grouped these daily activities as ADLs (Deaver & Brown, 1945; Halpern & Fuhrer, 1984). ADL scales proliferated without rigorous criteria for instrumentation. Rehabilitation programs grew in abundance. As programs developed, so did eligibility requirements for rehabilitation. In 1956, Social Security amendments were passed to require medical certification of disability for treatment in certain rehabilitation programs.

Rehabilitation Accountability

The 1960s witnessed a shift in rehabilitation programs, which were required to increase accountability for program development and outcomes measurement. An extensive proliferation of rehabilitation programs occurred. A wide range of policies, mandates, and programs affecting the lives of people with disabilities were established. In 1966, the Commission on Accreditation of Rehabilitation Facilities was established, emphasizing program accountability directly related to client preferences, goals, and outcome achievement. The Commission on Accreditation of Rehabilitation Facilities required valid and reliable functional assessment and outcome measures for program evaluation (Commission on Accreditation of Rehabilitation Facilities, 1998). Therefore, by the early 1980s, more than 100

federal agencies serving the disabled were established in a wide range of settings in which functional assessments were performed. Rehabilitation philosophies again expanded to embrace chronically ill and elderly people.

Throughout the years, rehabilitation professionals continued to struggle with a conceptual definition of functional assessment. Functional limitation became synonymous with disability. The AMA initiated efforts to further differentiate impairment from disability, in an effort to define medical and nonmedical issues related to workers' compensation. In 1958, the AMA defined *impairment* as a medical condition requiring a physician's management. *Disability* was defined as an administrative issue linking impairment with nonmedical or psychosocial factors. As defined, disability was no longer within the medical treatment domain. Thus, functional assessment instruments became skill-related and behavioral in nature. Functional and behavioral assessments proliferated.

With this proliferation, other problems were created. Because of the diversity of measurement instruments, rehabilitation professionals had difficulty communicating. They disagreed on rehabilitation goals and outcomes. Rehabilitation researchers lacked comparability in research efforts. Consistent aggregate data of rehabilitation populations were not available. Thus, a holistic perspective, proliferation of assessment instruments, and expansion of rehabilitation professionals contributed to a state of disorganization in the field of rehabilitation. Yet rehabilitation as a specialty gained recognition in the United States. In 1974, rehabilitation nurses organized a new nursing specialty organization, the Association of Rehabilitation Nurses (ARN) (Hoeman, 1996). Nursing theorists began to include rehabilitation as a concept in nursing curricula and practices.

Through the 1980s, health care organizations began to reengineer and reorganize. Conceptual clarity became a priority for rehabilitation professionals who had responsibility for demonstrating patient outcomes and the effectiveness of rehabilitation inpatient programs. Fundamental distinctions were necessary to understand factors affecting the disabled individual. As diagnosis-related groups were forced on the health care industry and rejected by rehabilitation professionals for function-related groups, rehabilitation professionals were again faced with a variety of definitions, divergent sources of data, and inconsistent methodology for identifying impairments and measuring outcomes. As a result, rehabilitation professionals from multiple specialty organizations, including ARN, made a commitment to definitional and contextual clarity, a systematic classification system, and test/measurement rigor.

DEFINITION: FUNCTIONAL ASSESSMENT

"*Functional assessment* is measurement of purposeful behavior in interaction with the environment, which is interpreted according to the assessment's intended uses" (Halpern & Fuhrer, 1984, p. 3). The absence of a definition of functional assessment before this time minimized the complexity of the field of rehabilitation. Yet, defining the term could endanger the field by constraining or confining its boundaries. However, having a definition enables rehabilitation professionals to focus attention on important characteristics within the previous definition: "measurement, purposeful behavior, environment, interaction, interpretation, and intended uses" (Halpern & Fuhrer, 1984, p. 3).

Measurement refers to both the method and the level of detail that are incorporated into processes of gathering assessment information and data. *Purposeful* refers to behavior that is goal-directed. *Behavior* is the object of performance for which the assessment is being conducted. *Environment* refers to the place where behavior is being observed and measured. *Interaction* refers to the dynamic relationship between the two concepts, behavior and environment, where the relationship is ever-changing. *Interpretation* requires that the clinician determine the meaning of data with respect to intended use, interpreting findings accurately and consistently based on the purpose and measurement system of the instrument. *Intended use* of the assessment instrument specifies the purpose of assessment instrument; for example, some assessment instruments have been designed to measure the client outcome, whereas others have been designed to classify the severity of disability.

The seven concepts within the definition of functional assessment are valuable criteria for the rehabilitation nurse when selecting an instrument or accurately interpreting findings.

FUNCTIONAL ASSESSMENT AND REHABILITATION NURSING

As the focus of functional assessment crystallized within the 1980s through to the 1990s, rehabilitation nursing emerged as a specialty area. In 1974, rehabilitation nurses from throughout the country joined together as the ARN to nationally address the rehabilitation nursing process, including functional evaluations. Rehabilitation nurses incorporated functional assessment into the domain and scope of nursing assessment, as evidenced in the first Standards of Rehabilitation Nursing Practice adopted by the American Nurses Association in 1977 (American Nurses Association, 1977). Rehabilitation nurses also contributed to the development of functional assessment instruments, measuring functional status based on valid and reliable measures, for example the Level of Rehabilitation Scales (LORS) and the Barthel Index (BI).

With the distinction as well as inclusion of rehabilitation nursing as a specialty among rehabilitation professionals, ARN became a pioneer in joining other specialty organizations to endorse requirements for conceptual clarity, uniformity in definitions and language, and measurement reliability and rigor for functional assessment measures. However, rehabilitation nurses, like all nurses, were increasingly familiar with the acuteness of patients' conditions and classification systems that also required the rigorous reliability and accurate interpretation necessary to determine appropriate staffing allocations.

Rehabilitation nurses shared in the professional and social accountability for quality outcomes as costs for health care rapidly increased. Yet, measurements of functional performance/outcome and client classification systems need to merge in order to determine rehabilitation nursing staffing needs. By assessing functional status and client levels of acuteness, nursing resources were matched to client care needs. In 1962, Bonney and Rothberg developed an instrument for nurses to determine nursing resources for clients that included functional status/dependence in ADLs (Ditmar, 1984). Many client classifications systems have been developed since then, recognizing an increased need for nursing resources on rehabilitation units based on client levels of independence.

Determining staffing needs based on the client's severity of disability requires that nurses accurately measure both functional performance and the acuteness of the client's condition. Barriers to this accurate measurement are not new. Barriers include problems with reliability in conducting ratings, the selection of classifications systems appropriate for rehabilitation, and acceptance of the importance of these measures as a determinant of resource allocation. In addition to determining staffing needs, functional assessment defines the need for rehabilitation nursing interventions. Rehabilitation nursing interventions can be prioritized based on the client's medical, nursing, and rehabilitation needs. Therefore, rehabilitation nurses are better equipped to integrate all aspects of care by the use of a functional assessment instrument, regardless of the methodology for measuring degrees of acuteness. A functional assessment instrument that is internationally accepted enables rehabilitation nurses to use language based on conceptual frameworks and definitions and consistent measures of functional status. Ultimately, standardized measures for rehabilitation nursing may be determined, followed by indicators' prediction of client outcomes and quality of care.

INTERNATIONAL ENDORSEMENT

Conceptual Clarity

The struggle for conceptual clarity of functional assessment continued for over half a century in this country, even longer in other countries. To that end, the World Health Organization adopted the Disablement Model (1980), providing definition clarity for three concepts that were internationally accepted: impairment, disability, and handicap. Even though this conceptual model has been endorsed now for 2 decades, continued confusion regarding these concepts exists throughout the health care system and community. One can travel communities and find parking spaces labeled as "handicapped parking" or "disabled parking." For purposes of this chapter, the concepts of the Disablement Model are defined in an effort to ensure conceptual clarity.

Disablement Model

The World Health Organization's Disablement Model defining three concepts as the conceptual framework (impairment, disability, and handicap) (Frey, 1984) offers rehabilitation clinicians a systematic, integrated method to comprehensively assess the needs of rehabilitation clients (Table 10–2). An *impairment* is any loss of normal function or structure that produces change in structure or function. The loss may be due to psychological, physiological, or anatomical conditions that result in the structural or functional loss, which may be permanent or temporary. Impairment occurs at the organ level instead of the cellular level associated with disease. Examples of impairment include hearing loss, amputation, neurogenic bladder, or hemiplegia.

Disability occurs when the impairment results in deficits related to ADLs, necessitating assistance. The assistance may include human assistance from another individual, structural assistance such as adaptive equipment and assistive devices, or prolonged time requirements. In other words, disability is any restriction or lack of ability to perform an activity within normal ranges. Disability focuses on the person's inabilities to perform essential ADLs, focusing on the "person" level of assessment. Examples include deficits in bathing, feeding, dressing, showering, and ambulating.

Handicap conceptually characterizes the disharmony that disability creates in the individual's personal and social community. Handicap represents socialization of the disa-

TABLE 10–2 ■ WORLD HEALTH ORGANIZATION DISABLEMENT MODEL: CLASSIFICATION OF IMPAIRMENTS, DISABILITIES, AND HANDICAP

Disease	Impairment	Disability	Handicap
Intrinsic abnormality or disease that occurs at cellular level	Loss or abnormality of psychological, physiological, or anatomical structure or function at organ level	Restriction or lack of ability to perform activity in normal manner	Disadvantage due to impairment or disability that limits or prevents fulfillment within personal and social roles
Examples:	Examples:	Examples:	Examples:
Peripheral vascular disease	Loss of limb	Decreased mobility	Loss of self-esteem
Spinal cord injury	Para-, or quadriplegia	Neurogenic bladder and bowel	Caregiver requirements
Stroke	Hemiplegia	Decreased activities of daily living	Social isolation
	Sensory/perceptual loss		

From World Health Organization. (1980). International classification of impairments, disabilities, and handicaps: A manual of classification relating to the consequences of disease. Geneva: World Health Organization.

bled individual within that person's valued cultural, social, economic, and religious environments. Handicap arises from problems with coping, adaptation, and transition. Examples of handicap include altered social integration, depression, economic dependency, and social isolation.

As one reviews the interrelationship, clearly an individual may be physically disabled but have a minimal handicap, for example, the paraplegic individual who adapts to living with spinal cord injury, enjoys a healthy relationship, and achieves economic security. Conversely, an individual could have minimal disability but severe handicap issues, for example, an individual with chronic low back pain who can independently walk, bathe, dress, and drive but is unable to maintain relationships or employment. Both exemplify needs for rehabilitation.

FUNCTIONAL ASSESSMENT INSTRUMENTS

Physical problems are easier to assess and better understood than psychosocial problems. Clients with neurological diseases and trauma have observable characteristics that are easily assessed as physical impairments. However, psychological and cognitive capabilities influence physiological or physical functioning and also must be assessed. With this understanding, the members of the American Congress of Rehabilitation Medicine and the American Academy of Physical Medicine and Rehabilitation suggested integrating psychosocial and medical rehabilitation models. Together with the efforts of multiple rehabilitation specialty organizations, including the ARN, these groups produced the Uniform Data System Functional Independence Measure (FIM) to offer a systematic framework and universal language to describe functional disabilities.

The goal of functional assessment instruments is to reliably measure an individual's capacity to perform ADLs systematically. Instruments have been designed to measure functional ability. The instruments presented in this chapter have been selected from the many available to describe three types of functional assessment scales: categorical assessment scales, ADL scales, and global functional assessment scales (Granger & Gresham, 1984). The categorical instruments address the unique functional profiles of clients with a particular disease or condition or profiles that

are limited to a single functional parameter. The ADL scales are most frequently used and focus on maximal independence in self-care and mobility. The global instruments provide an overall profile of the individual's functional ability.

All scales have been designed to objectively describe the individual's functional status at a given point in time. The scales can be used to sequentially measure changes in functional status over time, documenting outcomes of rehabilitation interventions. The functional assessment instruments also benefit the team process when used to improve practice for continuity of care. For example, functional assessment tools can enhance communication, referrals, and discharge planning among team members, patients, and family members. Linking objective measures of functions to jointly developed outcome goals can be extremely reinforcing to clients, families, and health care providers. When the functional assessments are displayed graphically, the individual and family members can view progress and functional areas of improvement. Lastly, a sound, valid, and reliable instrument offers data that can be used for research purposes.

The following functional assessment instruments are presented and critiqued for use by rehabilitation nurses. Two fundamental distinctions are evident in the conceptual models of functional assessment: the rehabilitation model (capability) and the psychosocial model (behavior). For example, the capacity to do an activity (capability) can be very different from the actual performance or what the individual actually does (behavior). This distinction is difficult for rehabilitation clinicians to measure and rate. The measures are distinct and cannot be substituted for one another. The differences between what someone can do versus what someone does do is a measure of behavior. Behavior is also influenced by environments. Environments can support rehabilitation performance negatively or positively. Therefore, environments also must by controlled for or captured within the context of functional performance.

Categorical Assessment Instruments

The categorical instruments address unique functional profiles of clients with a particular disease or condition or are limited to a single functional parameter. The categorical instruments to be presented include motor assessment scales that measure strength and isometric strength, and the Glasgow Coma Scale.

Motor Assessment Scales

Measurement of the motor system is usually performed by a clinician manually testing motor or muscle strength. Two standardized approaches to manual muscle testing have been used in the practice setting for a number of years. These include the Daniels and Worthingham techniques of manual examination of muscle testing and Kendall's method to measure muscle strength using percentages (O'Sullivan & Schmitz, 1988) Both methods assess muscle strength using resistance and gravity; Daniels and Worthingham's method is presented in detail.

The muscle testing method of measure is qualitative rather than quantitative. The clinician subjectively evaluates motor performance for strength, power, and endurance. More objective measures are made for range of motion. Over the last 70 years, several rating scales have been developed to assess muscle weakness in the clinical setting (Agre, 1984). Numerical values were used to simplify notation in the clinical chart, rather than to quantify muscle function.

Muscle Strength. Clinically, muscle strength is evaluated using a 6-point qualitative scale ranging from 0, no strength, to N, normal strength. The measures are as follows:

Absent	0	No strength, paralysis, no contraction felt
Trace	T	Muscle can be felt to tighten but has no visible movement
Poor	P	Produces movement with gravity eliminated, but cannot function against gravity
Fair	F	Can move or hold against gravity
Good	G	Can move or hold against moderate resistance and gravity
Normal	N	Can move or hold against maximal resistance and gravity

Pluses and minuses are used to designate further gradations in measurements.

The limitation with the manual muscle rating scale is that muscle strength is determined subjectively, relying on the judgment and experience of the clinician. Clinically, "normal" strength has not been subjected to scientific norms of validity and reliability.

Isometric Muscle Strength. Isometric measures of strength provided clinicians with more objective data of maximal muscle and muscle group strength in right and left upper and lower extremities. These data have been of value in client assessment and in the evaluation of progress. However, other important information may be missed if only maximal isometric force is measured. Strength can be defined simply as the maximal instantaneous force that a muscle or group of muscles can exert. However, the ability to perform most ADLs includes measures of both power and endurance. The ability to work at a certain rate is power. The ability to sustain the performance of an activity is endurance. New methodologies and instrumentation are being developed to quantify muscle strength, power, and endurance in disabled individuals. Accurate assessment of functional performance is of value in determining a client's progress in therapy more effectively and may ultimately result in the development of a better therapeutic program.

Glasgow Coma Scale

As the third categorical assessment scale, the Glasgow Coma Scale exemplifies an instrument designed to measure a specific aspect of function: the level of consciousness. Head injuries are classified as mild, moderate, or severe based on the Glasgow Coma Scale.

The client is scored for eye opening, motor responses, and verbal responses to voice commands or pain. Each of the three sections is scored separately on scales ranging from 4 to 6 points. The total score ranges from 4 to 15; the higher the score, the more responsive the client. The Glasgow Coma Scale is used for head injury as well as poststroke periods and has good face and predictive validity, as well as good interobserver reliability, and requires less than 2 minutes to administer (Agency for Health Care Policy and Research, 1995).

Activity of Daily Living Assessment Scales

The ADL assessment scales to be presented include the Barthel Index, Katz Index of Activities of Daily Living, and Kenny Self-Care Evaluation.

Barthel Index

The BI was developed by F. Mahoney and D. Barthel in 1965. Mahoney, a psychiatrist, and

Barthel, a physical therapist, wanted to develop a quick, valid, and reliable measurement of ADLs that could also monitor and quantify functional progress over time. The BI has been used in rehabilitation and rehabilitation research for over 30 years. The BI is easy to use, has excellent interrater reliability, and has been used in a variety of settings (Kidd et al., 1995; Shinar, Gross, & Bronstein, 1987; Wade & Collin, 1988). The BI indicates an individual's ability to perform 10 areas of functional activity:

1. Feeding
2. Wheelchair transfer
3. Grooming
4. Toilet transfer
5. Bathing
6. Level walking
7. Stairs
8. Dressing
9. Bladder control
10. Bowel control

Each of the 10 items is positively scored using a 3-point scale: independent (can do by myself), assistance needed (can do with help of someone else), and dependent (cannot do at all). The score ranges from zero to 100 and is scored positively; the higher the score, the more independent the individual. A BI of 100 points indicates an individual who is independent in ADLs, is continent, is able to walk a block (150 feet), and can ascend and descend a flight of stairs. The BI measures motor performance for ADLs. The BI does not measure cognitive processes or communication skills.

The BI has extensive use in research and has historically been the functional assessment instrument with predictive properties. If the BI score is equal to or less than 60, the client is predicted to need nursing home placement as community support is too great.

The BI has also been tested to determine the most predictive factors when predicting longitudinal community living resulting in a B4 subset. The B4 subset includes bladder and bowel control, eating, and grooming functions as the most predictive factors of the BI for individuals to be living in the community (Granger, Hamilton, Gresham, and Kramer, 1989). As a result of its advanced psychometric properties, rehabilitation professionals have utilized the BI for admission screening, formal assessment, monitoring, and maintenance.

Katz Index of Activities of Daily Living

The Katz Index of ADLs was developed by Katz and his coworkers in 1963 to classify self-care independence in heterogeneous diagnostic groups of primarily elderly clients (Katz, Ford, Moskowitz, Jackson, and Jaffe, 1963). The Katz Index of ADLs is unique in its purpose to capture recovered functional ability based on developmental theory that recovery is sequential. In other words, functional activity is lost and recovered according to a specific functional development sequence (Labi & Gresham, 1984).

The Katz Index of ADLs measures six areas of ADLs:

1. Bathing
2. Dressing
3. Toileting
4. Transfers
5. Continence
6. Feeding

Each ADL area is rated as dependent or independent based on the individual's ability to perform the tasks for each of the six ADLs. Overall functional status is assigned a grade of A to G. In other words, if the client is independent in all six areas of ADLs, the client receives an A rating. If the client is dependent in all six areas of ADLs, the client is assigned a G rating. The ordinal ranking A to G is based on descending levels of independence.

The strengths of the Katz Index of ADLs are that this instrument was carefully developed and tested for reliability based on a very large sample size of 1001 clients. The sensitivity for measuring the severity of disability is lost by the use of the grade designation, rather than assigned scores for the definition of functional performance.

Kenny Self-Care Evaluation

The Kenny Self-Care Evaluation was developed by Schoening, Anderegg, Bergstrom, and Iversen in 1965 to measure self-care and mobility in both individuals and groups (Schoening & Iversen, 1968). As another formalized functional assessment instrument, the Kenny Self-Care Evaluation focuses on ADLs. This ADL rehabilitation instrument measures the individual's ability to perform ADLs in six functional areas:

1. Bed mobility
2. Transfers
3. Locomotion

4. Dressing
5. Personal hygiene
6. Feeding activities

Each item is scored using a 5-point scale, with scores ranging from zero to 4. Each item is rated and weighted equally and positively, so that the higher the score, the more independent the individual. A score of zero is dependent, and 24 is independent. The Kenny Self-Care Evaluation was found to be more sensitive in measuring ADL functional status than the Katz Index. In addition, this instrument was originally designed to document and measure client outcomes as a result of the medical rehabilitation process (Granger & Gresham, 1984). Other unique factors of the Kenny Self-Care Evaluation are its use to quantitate the rehabilitation nursing workload, its method of simplifying ADL documentation, and its provision of valid efficacy outcome scores. Lastly, the authors emphasized the importance of summing scores as an index for monitoring changes in a specific area of ADL function.

Global Functional Assessment Scales

PULSES Profile

The PULSES Profile is credited with being the first formalized functional assessment instrument developed for use in medical rehabilitation settings; it was developed by Moskowitz and McCann in 1957 (Granger & Gresham, 1984). The PULSES Profile offered a more structured approach to functional assessment during the shift from compensation to rehabilitation to accountability. The PULSES Profile was designed to measure the client's ability to independently perform activities using all four extremities. The PULSES Profile also rates the presence of disease and the client's ability to correctly perceive and adequately interact with customary roles.

PULSES Profile addresses six items:

1. P — Physical conditioning
2. U — Upper limb functions
3. L — Lower limb functions
4. S — Sensory components
5. E — Excretory functions
6. S — Situation factors

The PULSES Profile is scored negatively; the lower the score, the more independent the individual. Each item is scored on a 4-point scale, 1 being independent and 4 being dependent or most impaired. The scores are summed so that a score of 6, the minimal score, indicates a client without systemic disease who is independent in activities requiring all extremities and can accurately perceive and interact with the environment. The client is also continent and able to perform customary roles.

Within the scale, levels 1 and 2 reflect an individual who is able to function without the assistance of another individual. Levels 3 and 4 reflect an individual who requires assistance from another individual.

The PULSES score of 12 correlates to the BI score of 60 in respect to differentiating less severe from more severe disability (Granger, Albrecht, & Hamilton, 1979).

Level of Rehabilitation Scale

Carey and Posavac adapted the Level of Rehabilitation Scale (LORS) from the Functional Life Scale to evaluate physical medicine and rehabilitation programs. The LORS assesses function in five categories: cognition, ADLs, activities in the home, outside activities, and social interactions. However, the four dimensions of performance (self-initiation, frequency, speed, and overall efficiency) were not retained. The staff at Lutheran General Hospital thought that the Functional Life Scale was too detailed and required too much time to complete the rating. Therefore, the staff recommended changes to the rating system.

During an interview with a person who has in-depth knowledge about the client, each LORS activity is rated on a 5-point scale (zero to 4). The scoring system was developed to specify behaviors for each of the five levels. The behaviors are scored as follows:

0—The client cannot or will not do the activity
1—The client requires physical assistance to do the activity
2—The client can perform the activity but standby assistance seems desirable
3—The client can perform the activity if special equipment or preparation is available
4—The client performs normally

Interviews of client performance are completed on admission, discharge, 6-week follow-up, and 4.5-month follow-up. Each subscale is scored, and the subscale scores are compared at each predetermined interval for trends in client performance and improvement.

Extensive psychometric testing has been conducted on validity and reliability properties of the LORS. Interrater reliability of scale scores was 0.96 or greater (Carey & Posavac, 1978). The interview is completed within 10 to 15 minutes and considered to be feasible for completion in the clinical setting. Use of the LORS has expanded beyond patient care assessment and evaluation to program evaluation, serving accreditation needs of rehabilitation units. In addition, the LORS provides an accumulation of improvement norms of stroke clients as a result of rehabilitation programs and after discharge. The LORS asserts the importance of follow-up evaluations as the real evidence of successful rehabilitation. The limitation of the LORS is that the scoring is conducted by interview, rather than observed performance over time, across settings, and with multiple people.

Uniform Data System for Medical Rehabilitation Functional Independence Measure

The UDSMRFIM is a minimum data set to measure the impact of physical or motor and psychosocial or cognitive disabilities on functional status (Fig. 10–1) (Uniform Data System, 1993).

The FIM is a measure of functional disability and status, based on ordinal measurement of 18 functional items using a 7-point Likert-like scale, 1 being dependent, unsafe to perform, or not performed, and 7 being independent, safe, and timely. The FIM results in subscale scores for self-care, continence, mobility, locomotion, communication, and social cognition. The first four subscales assess motor function, whereas the last two assess cognition and behavior. A total score is also obtained, indicating the overall severity of the disability or the burden of care.

Rehabilitation clinicians must successfully complete a credentialing test to measure the client using the FIM instrument. The range of scores is 18 (totally disabled/dependent) to 126 (totally independent). The FIM has good content validity and reliability properties and excellent test-retest results. The FIM is discipline-free in administration. In other words, functional items are not rated by an assigned discipline. The FIM has been used widely in rehabilitation research and in evaluating clinical functional outcomes. The motor subscale of the FIM has been correlated with the BI. The FIM is considered a global assessment scale of functional status because the FIM measures motor and cognitive functional items.

An individual's performance is rated based on the burden of care, observing performance over time, across settings, and among rehabilitation clinicians. Follow-up functional assessment is conducted 80 to 120 days after discharge from a rehabilitation program, generally by telephone interview, obtaining verbal reports of functional status rather than observed performance.

An integral part of the neurological assessment is functional status, the client's ability to perform not only neurological tests but also functional ADLs, safely and consistently across settings. In 1984, the ARN endorsed this universal method to measure, communicate, and compare disabilities and rehabilitation goals, thereby providing rehabilitation nurses and other rehabilitation professionals with a framework to examine functional disabilities.

Functional Assessment Measurement

Based on the diagnostic groups, neurological abnormality is a primary admitting diagnosis into rehabilitation. There was a need to systematically measure more complex cognitive functions, thus supplementing the FIM measurements. The Functional Assessment Measure (FAM), designed by Hall (1992), measures higher-level cognitive skills and provides an overview of functional assessment scales in brain injury. The FAM items include swallowing, car transfers, community access, reading, writing, speech intelligibility, emotional status, adjustment to limitations, employability, orientation, attention, and safety judgment. The FAM items are rated using the same 7-point rating scale as the FIM.

Use of the FIM and the FAM helps the nurse apply physical and psychological assessment findings to the client's ability or inability to perform daily living tasks. The severity of disability must also be accurately defined in order to direct, plan, implement, and evaluate the level of care and social and economic resources needed to optimize the client's independence and quality of life.

Patient Evaluation Conference System

The Patient Evaluation Conference System (PECS) was developed by Harvey and Jelli-

FIM™ instrument

L E V E L S	7 Complete Independence (Timely, Safely) 6 Modified Independence (Device)	**NO HELPER**
	Modified Dependence 5 Supervision (Subject = 100%+) 4 Minimal Assist (Subject = 75%+) 3 Moderate Assist (Subject = 50%+) **Complete Dependence** 2 Maximal Assist (Subject =25%+) 1 Total Assist (Subject = less than 25%)	**HELPER**

	ADMISSION	DISCHARGE	FOLLOW-UP
Self-Care A. Eating B Grooming C. Bathing D. Dressing - Upper Body E. Dressing - Lower Body F. Toileting			
Sphincter Control G. Bladder Management H. Bowel Management			
Transfers I. Bed, Chair, Wheelchair J. Toilet K. Tub, Shower			
Locomotion L. Walk/Wheelchair M. Stairs	W Walk C Wheelchair B Both	W Walk C Wheelchair B Both	W Walk C Wheelchair B Both
Motor Subtotal Score			
Communication N. Comprehension O. Expression	A Auditory V Visual B Both V Vocal N Nonvocal B Both	A Auditory V Visual B Both V Vocal N Nonvocal B Both	A Auditory V Visual B Both V Vocal N Nonvocal B Both
Social Cognition P. Social Interaction Q. Problem Solving R. Memory			
Cognitive Subtotal Score			
TOTAL FIM Score			

NOTE: Leave no blanks. Enter 1 if patient not testable due to risk

FIGURE 10–1
Guide for the Uniform Data Set for Medical Rehabilitation (including the FIM™ instrument), Version 5.1. Buffalo, NY 14214: State University of New York at Buffalo, 1997.)

nek in 1981 and is one of the most complex global functional assessment instruments in the field, measuring and graphically plotting profiles of patient progress (Harvey & Jellinek, 1983). The PECS contains 15 major categories and a total of 79 items to rate. The 15 categories are

1. Rehabilitation medicine
2. Rehabilitation nursing
3. Physical mobility
4. ADLs
5. Communication
6. Medications
7. Nutrition
8. Assistive devices
9. Psychology
10. Neuropsychology
11. Social issues
12. Vocational educational activity
13. Recreation
14. Pain
15. Pulmonary rehabilitation

Each item is scored on a scale of 1 to 7, 1 being dependent and 7, independent. Like the FIM, this scale measures degrees of independence (5 through 7) and measures degrees of dependence (1 through 4). The system is used throughout the client's rehabilitation program, setting functional goals and monitoring progress by changes in scores.

The items within the PECS are assigned to specific disciplines; for example, rehabilitation medicine is assigned to physicians for rating, and rehabilitation nursing to nurses. The PECS can be computerized as the documentation framework for the team. However, reliability becomes a problem due to the number of functional items for assessment using a 7-point scale.

IMPLICATIONS FOR SPECIAL POPULATIONS AND COMMUNITY REINTEGRATION

With the development of valid and reliable instruments to measure function, appropriate levels and settings for client treatment are now being determined based on functional levels. These decisions became evident when functional assessment measures were utilized to predict outcomes and community placement. Yet, when one is considering the needs of special populations (such as those persons living with head injury, spinal cord injury, or stroke) and community reintegration, functional status measures must be accompanied by psychosocial assessments. Rehabilitation nurses play an important role in discharge

planning, recommending assistance for care to clients and caregivers; suggesting environments that best meet the needs of both clients and caregivers; guiding both in understanding that differences exist in levels of nursing and rehabilitative care in institutions; and advising clients and caregivers in placement decisions.

Rehabilitation nurses are also aware of the shift in health care resources, limiting options for care, the duration of treatment, and the skill mix of institutional or community caregivers. This is all the more reason for rehabilitation nurses to accurately measure outcome indicators for quality and rehabilitation services.

SUMMARY

The contribution of rehabilitation nurses to determining the client's functional status must be stressed. There is no other discipline that assesses function across as many settings, with as many individuals, and at as many times of day as nursing. In addition, nurses cross functional boundaries. The history of nursing scopes of practice precedes that of physical therapists' and occupational therapists'. Functional assessment instruments are tools that measure the level of independence, severity of disability, functional ability, and outcome of a client. Many valid and reliable functional assessment instruments are available, depending on the client population, setting, and purpose of measurement.

Determining the functional status, progress, and outcome of clients has assumed a valuable place in outcome research, program evaluation, and clinical care management. A person's ability to perform functional activities is a significant determinant of the individual's ability to live independently within a community. The amount of nursing care needed to support the individual is an indicator of special economic and/or social assistance.

Assessment refers to a dynamic process of determining quantitative and qualitative needs of clients. Three kinds of assessment data are needed to organize and plan human service systems as advocated by the World Health Organization:

1. The nature of contacts made with the system
2. How the system responds to these contacts
3. The outcome of the contacts with the system

Many future challenges face all professionals involved in outcome data. One of the biggest challenges is to balance the usefulness of the data with the feasibility of the data. Many rehabilitation centers combine functional status outcome data with resource cost data for marketing services. If the cost is high and the outcomes are poor, programs will not be providers of choice. If the cost is high and outcomes are positive, providers will be used. Customers will pay the price for quality outcomes. Our responsibility is to ensure the reliability of data and the accuracy of data from which decisions are made. Additionally, data must be comparable among providers or health plans, hence the development of report cards.

Report cards are one strategy to differentiate among providers on the basis of performance (American Nurses Association, 1995a). Comparative information can also be provided in relation to cost and quality among competing providers. Report cards enable providers to conduct self-assessments and develop self-improvement strategies. Additionally, report cards can differentiate among individuals and organizations competing for the same resources (Wakefield, Hendryx, Uden-Holman, Couch, and Helms, 1996). In health care, both providers and consumers of care use report cards to identify the best practices and to serve as performance benchmarks.

In rehabilitation, program evaluation data can be reported in report cards. Relevant data may include the time after onset to rehabilitation admission (the number of days from the onset of disability to the day of admission to rehabilitation); functional gains (discharge functional status scores minus admission functional status scores); the length of stay efficiency (functional status gains divided by the number of days admitted to rehabilitation); and client safety (the number of falls resulting in injury divided by the number of falls). Caution is needed when developing and using report cards due to inherent limitations in valid and reliable measures, variations in performance measures, and data collection methods.

REFERENCES

Agency for Health Care Policy and Research. (1995). *Post stroke rehabilitation: Clinical practice guideline 16.* Washington, DC: U.S. Department of Health and Human Services, Public Health Service.

Agre, J. (1984). Quantification of muscle function. In A. Halpern & M. Fuhrer (Eds.), *Functional assessment in rehabilitation* (p. 117). Baltimore: Paul H. Brookes.

American Nurses Association, Division on Medical-Surgical Nursing Practice and the Association of Rehabilitation Nurses. (1977). *Standards of Rehabilitation Nursing Practice.* Kansas City, MO: Author.

American Nurses Association. (1995). *Standards of practice.* Kansas City, MO: Author.

American Nurses Association. (1995a). *Nursing report card for acute care.* Washington, DC: Author.

Bonney, V., & Rothberg, J. (1962). *Nursing diagnosis and therapy: An instrument for evaluation and measurement.* New York: National League for Nursing.

Carey, R., & Posavac, E. (1978). Program evaluation of a physical medicine and rehabilitation unit: A new approach. *Archives of Physical Medicine and Rehabilitation, 59,* 330.

Commission on Accreditation of Rehabilitation Facilities (1998). Medical Rehabilitation Standards Manual. Tucson, AZ: Author.

Deaver, G., & Brown, M. E. (1945). Physical demands of daily life. New York: The Institute for the Crippled and Disabled.

Ditmar, S. (1984). Functional assessment in rehabilitation nursing. In C. Granger & G. Gresham (Eds.), *Functional Assessment in Rehabilitation Medicine* (p. 194). Baltimore: Williams & Wilkins.

Frey, W. (1984). Functional assessment in the 80's. In A. S. Halpern & M. J. Fuhrer (Eds.), *Functional assessment in rehabilitation* (p. 11). Baltimore: Paul H. Brookes.

Granger, C., Albrecht, G., & Hamilton, B. (1979). Outcome in comprehensive medical rehabilitation: Measurement of PULSES profile and Barthel Index. *Archives of Physical Medicine and Rehabilitation, 57,* 103.

Granger, C., & Gresham, G. (Eds.), (1984). *Functional assessment in rehabilitation medicine* (p. 194). Baltimore: Williams & Wilkins.

Granger, C., Hamilton, B., Gresham, G., & Kramer, A. (1989). The stroke outcome study: Part 2. Relative merits of the total Barthel Index score and a four-item subscore in predicting patient outcomes. *Archives of Physical Medicine and Rehabilitation, 70,* 100.

Hall, K. M. (1992). Overview of functional assessment sacles in brain injury rehabilitation. *NeuroRehabilitation, 2*(4), 1992.

Halpern, A., & Fuhrer, M. (1984). *Functional assessment in rehabilitation.* Baltimore: Paul H. Brookes.

Harvey, R., & Jellinek, H. (1983). Patient profiles: utilization in functional performance assessment: *Archives of Physical Medicine and Rehabilitation, 64*(6), 268.

Harvey, R., & Jellinek, H. (1981). Functional Performance Assessment: A Program Approach. *Archives of Physical Medicine and Rehabilitation, 62*(9), 456.

Hoeman, S. (1996). *Rehabilitation nursing. Process and application* (2nd ed.). St. Louis, C. V. Mosby.

Katz, S., Ford, A., Moskowitz, R., Jackson, B., & Jaffe, M. (1963). Studies of illness in the aged. The Index of ADL: A standardized measure of biological and psychosocial function. *Journal of the American Medical Association, 94,* 185.

Kelly-Hayes, M. (1996). Functional evaluation. In S. Hoeman (Ed.), *Rehabilitation nursing. Process and application* (2nd ed.). St. Louis, C. V. Mosby.

Kessler, H. H. (1931). Accidental injuries. Philadelphia: Lea & Febiger.

Kidd, D., Stewart, G., Baldry, J., Johnson, J., Rossiter, D., Petruckevitch, A., & Thompson, A. (1995). The functional independence measure: A comparative validity and reliability study. *Disability & Rehabilitation, 17,* 10.

Labi, M., & Gresham, G. (1984). Some research applications in functional assessment instruments used in rehabilitation medicine. In C. Granger & G. Gresham

(Eds.), *Functional assessment in rehabilitation medicine.* Baltimore: Williams & Wilkins.

O'Sullivan, S., & Schmitz, T. (1988). *Physical rehabilitation: assessment and treatment* (3rd ed) (p. 113). Philadelphia: F. A. Davis.

Schoening, H. A., & Iversen, I. A. (1968). Numerical scoring of self-care status: A study of the Kenny self-care evaluation. *Archives of Physical Medicine and Rehabilitation, 46,* 221.

Shinar, D., Gross, C., & Bronstein, K. (1987). Reliability of activities of daily living scale and its use in telephone interviews. *Archives of Physical Medicine and Rehabilitation, 68,* 723.

Uniform Data System (1993). Guide for the Uniform Data Set for Medical Rehabilitation. Version 4.0 (1993). Buffalo, NY: State University of New York at Buffalo.

Wade, D., & Collin, C. (1988). The Barthel ADL Index: A standard measure of physical disability. *International Disability Studies, 10(2),* 64.

Wakefield, D., Hendryx, M., Uden-Holman, T., Couch, R., Helms, C. (1996). Comparing providers' performance: Problems in making the "report card" analogy fit. *Journal for Healthcare Quality, 18(6),* 4.

World Health Organization. (1980). International classification of impairments, disabilities, and handicaps: A manual of classification relating to the consequences of disease. Geneva: World Health Organization.

BIBLIOGRAPHY

Behner, K., Fogg, F., Fournier, L., Frankenbach, J., & Robertson, S. (1990). Nursing resource management: Analyzing the relationship between costs and quality in staffing decisions. *Health Care Management Review, 15,* 63.

Granger, C., & Clark, G. (1994). Functional status and outcomes of stroke rehabilitation. *Topics in Geriatric Rehabilitation, 9,* 72.

Granger, C., Hamilton, B., Linacre, J., Heinemann, A., & Wright, B. (1993). Performance profiles of the functional independence measure. *American Journal of Physical Medicine and Rehabilitation, 72,* 84.

Stineman, M., Escarce, J., Goin, J., Hamilton, B., Granger, C., & Williams, S. (1994). A case-mix classification for medical rehabilitation. *Medical Care, 32,* 366.

Stineman, M., & Williams, S. (1990). Predicting inpatient rehabilitation length of stay. *Archives of Physical Medicine and Rehabilitation, 71,* 881.

CHAPTER 11

Elimination

Karen Mandzak Fried, Guy W. Fried, and Catharine Farnan

Most people take for granted the ability to eliminate. Elimination is an intimate experience that is not often discussed in an in-depth manner. It is only when problems with bowel or bladder elimination become blatant that people are forced to confront elimination problems, often with embarrassment.

Rehabilitation nurses are frequently the first health care providers to detect and assess the extent of an individual's incontinence. It is the nurse who deals with the disabled individual across a variety of settings, including the acute hospital, rehabilitation facility, long-term care facility, and home environment. Often, it is the nurse who is in the position to assimilate the psychological, social, and cultural ramifications associated with problems of incontinence while assisting in the development of appropriate treatment strategies.

URINARY ELIMINATION

Urinary incontinence is a significant health care problem in the United States. It has been conservatively estimated that 13 million people suffer from urinary incontinence at a cost of $15 billion per year (Fantl, Newman, & Collins, 1996). This is a conservative estimate because many more people affected with urinary incontinence do not seek appropriate health care intervention for a variety of cultural and social reasons.

In Western culture, cleanliness and continence are assumed. Problems with incontinence are often hidden from view as they restrict lifestyles and impose a significant loss of self-esteem. Dougherty (1991) reported that incontinence can affect most aspects of daily life including clothing selection, decisions about food and fluid intake, occupational choices, leisure activities and travel, and sexual activities and intimacy.

Research within elderly populations (Ouslander, Morishita, Blaustein, Orzeck, & Sayre, 1987) has shown that incontinence affects the

"burden of care" on family members. Urinary incontinence is also a significant predictor of early nursing home placement, as family members share the pain, frustration, and limitations that incontinence often brings. According to an Agency for Health Care Policy and Research Clinical Practice Guideline (Urinary Incontinence Guideline Panel, 1992), "Incontinence imposes a significant psychological impact on individuals, their families and caregivers resulting in a loss of self-esteem, and a decrease in the ability to maintain an independent lifestyle."

At-Risk Populations

Many populations are at risk for urinary incontinence, the largest being the elderly. It has been estimated that urinary incontinence is a significant clinical problem that affects 15 to 35% of elderly people living in the community, 33% of elderly people in acute care settings, and at least 50% of institutionalized elderly persons (Fantyl et al., 1996). Although normal aging may predispose an elderly person to incontinence, it is not the cause of incontinence. It is now generally recognized that incontinence is a sign and that in most cases incontinence can be effectively managed.

Social and cultural variables may also influence the effective management of urinary incontinence. Chancellor & Blaivis, 1995) have identified the following variables as important in bladder management decisions: age; the desire to remain catheter-free; the desire to avoid surgery; economic resources; the ability to be educated; the cooperation and reliability of the family; hand function; mental status; motivation; the sexual activity status; and the rehabilitation prognosis.

Cultural variables cannot be underestimated with regard to patients' responses to management programs. Native Americans and Mexican Americans have strict codes for both sexes concerning privacy and modesty with bowel and bladder issues. Incontinence can be damaging to the self-esteem of men from African-American, Mexican-American, and Mediterranean cultures, and this may limit their seeking assistance (Hoeman, 1989). In the United States, the incidence of disability among African Americans is nearly twice that among whites, and "cultural mistrust" based on cultural differences may develop. When treating elimination problems, the rehabilitation nurse must be cognizant of the issues of intense intimacy in this area.

Other clinical populations most at risk for incontinence include patients with disabilities such as strokes, brain tumors, brain trauma, Parkinson's disease, multiple sclerosis, dementia, and spinal cord injury.

Micturition Process

Because the bladder slowly fills with urine, it maintains a low intravesical pressure. Continence is maintained as long as the pressure within the bladder is lower than the urethral pressure. As bladder volume increases, sensory receptors in the bladder wall are stimulated to transmit the sensation to the sacral reflex center (S2–S4). Sensory messages are then sent from the sacral reflex center in the spinal cord to the cerebral cortex through the posterior columns and the spinothalamic tract. Inhibitory centers in the frontal lobe prevent voiding from occurring until it is desirable. For micturition to be initiated, motor messages are sent back down through the corticoregulatory tract to the sacral reflex center. The messages then travel through the parasympathetic and somatic fibers to cause detrusor contraction, external sphincter relaxation, and bladder emptying (Chancellor & Blaivis, 1995).

Types of Dysfunction

There have been many classifications of urinary incontinence; however, two that are useful for the rehabilitation nurse are the symptom classification system identified by the Agency for Health Care Policy and Research (Urinary Incontinence Guideline Panel, 1992) and the neurological classification identified by Lapides and Diokno (1976) (Table 11–1). These classifications reflect the majority of patients with urinary incontinence seen by rehabilitation nurses.

Symptom Classification System

Stress Incontinence. Stress incontinence is the involuntary leakage of urine during activ-

TABLE 11–1 ■ TYPES OF URINARY DYSFUNCTION

Symptom Classification	Neurological Classification
Stress incontinence	Uninhibited neurogenic
Urge incontinence	Reflex neurogenic
Overflow incontinence	Autonomous neurogenic
Mixed incontinence	Sensory paralytic
Functional incontinence	Motor paralytic

Data from Urinary Incontinence Guideline Panel (1992). *Urinary incontinence in adults: Clinical practice guideline* (AHCPR Publications No. 92-0038). Rockville, MD: Agency for Health Care Policy and Research, Public Health Service, U.S. Department of Health and Human Services; and Lapides, J. (1976). *Fundamentals of urology.* Philadelphia: W. B. Saunders.

ities that increase intraabdominal pressure, such as coughing, sneezing, or laughing. This urinary leakage is not associated with an overdistended bladder or detrusor contraction. Stress incontinence is most often seen in women with urethral hypermobility when the intraabdominal pressure is raised. It may also be seen, on occasion, in men after prostatectomy.

Urge Incontinence. Urge incontinence is the involuntary leakage of urine preceded by a strong desire to void. Involuntary detrusor contractions or detrusor instability is almost always associated with urge incontinence. This detrusor instability can occur in "normal" individuals. In patients with neurological disorders such as stroke, spinal cord injury, or multiple sclerosis, the detrusor instability is known as *detrusor hyperreflexia*. In some patients with spinal cord injury and multiple sclerosis, detrusor hyperreflexia is evident and detrusor-sphincter dyssynergia also occurs, resulting in urinary retention, vesicoureteral reflux, and renal damage. In elderly persons, urge incontinence is often caused by detrusor hyperreflexia along with impaired bladder contractility. These patients have urgency related to the hyperreflexia, yet they must strain to empty their bladder and may do so incompletely.

Overflow Incontinence. Overflow incontinence is the involuntary loss of urine associated with bladder overdistention. This type of incontinence can be present as urge incontinence, stress incontinence, or constant urinary leakage. This type of incontinence is often due to the lack of detrusor contractility. In males, overflow incontinence may be coupled with outlet obstruction secondary to prostate enlargement. Overflow incontinence may be concurrent with detrusor-sphincter dyssynergia, which may occur in patients with spinal cord injury or multiple sclerosis.

Mixed Incontinence. In mixed incontinence, patients have both urge and stress incontinence symptoms. This type of incontinence is common in older women, and usually one symptom is more predominant than the other.

Functional Incontinence. Functional incontinence is the result of factors not directly related to the genitourinary tract, such as physical and cognitive impairments. In elderly patients, this type of incontinence can improve through behavioral and environmental changes such as timed toileting schedules, fluid restrictions, and mobility improvements.

Neurological Classification

Neurogenic bladders are classified by the urodynamic measurement of bladder function in combination with a functional description of the associated neurological lesion. There are five types of neurogenic bladder: uninhibited, reflex, autonomous, sensory paralytic, and motor paralytic.

Uninhibited Neurogenic Bladder. Uninhibited neurogenic bladder results from damage sustained in the corticoregulatory pathways in the brain that control voiding (Fig. 11–1). In this type of bladder dysfunction, there are strong uninhibited detrusor contractions with reduced bladder capacity and frequency, resulting in bladder emptying before its normal capacity is reached. The bladder usually empties with no residual volume, however, and reflexes are intact. Patients with this type of bladder can achieve continence by incorporating fluid restriction with a timed voiding program.

Reflex Neurogenic Bladder (Upper Motor Neuron, Spastic). A reflex neurogenic bladder results from damage in both the sensory and the motor tracts between the pontine micturition center of the brainstem and the sacral reflex center (Fig. 11–2). This dysfunction leads to involuntary and incomplete emptying owing to the lack of coordination, sensation, and cerebral control over voiding. Because the reflex arc is intact, voiding often occurs quickly and frequently at lower blad-

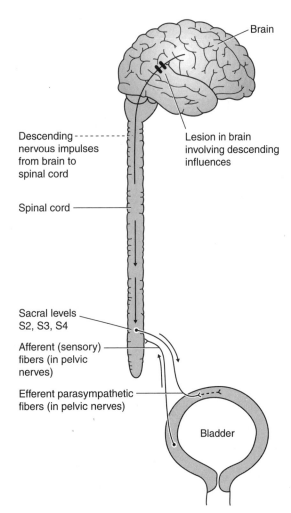

FIGURE 11–1
Uninhibited neurogenic bladder. (Redrawn from Pires, M., & Lockhart, P. [1992]. *Nursing management of neurogenic incontinence* [pp. 11–12, 14]. Skokie, IL: Rehabilitation Nursing Foundation.)

der capacities, often with high residual volumes. Also, with this type of neurogenic bladder, the detrusor often hypertrophies, causing vesicoureteral reflux and hydronephrosis, and the urethral sphincter often contracts, leading to detrusor-sphincter dyssynergia.

Autonomous Neurogenic Bladder (Lower Motor Neuron, Flaccid). Autonomous neurogenic bladder results from damage in the sacral region in the sacral micturition center at S2–S4 (Fig. 11–3). In this dysfunction, reflexes are absent or diminished, as are the detrusor contractions. Both sensory control and motor control are lost. This leads to massive bladder overdistention. The urethral sphincter is unable to hold the volume, and

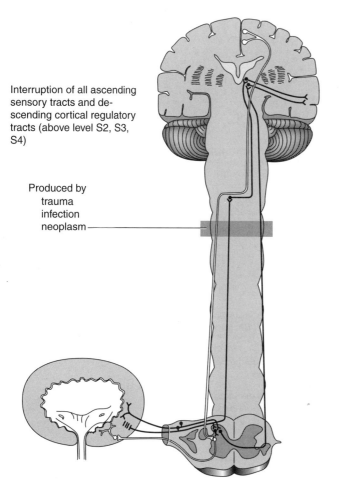

Interruption of all ascending sensory tracts and descending cortical regulatory tracts (above level S2, S3, S4)

Produced by
    trauma
    infection
    neoplasm

FIGURE 11–2
Reflex neurogenic bladder. (Redrawn from Lapides, J., & Diokno, A. C. [1976]. Urine transport, storage, and micturition. In J. Lapides [Ed.], *Fundamentals of urology* [p. 218]. Philadelphia: W. B. Saunders.)

overflow leakage or dribbling often occurs, with large residual volumes of urine remaining in the bladder.

Sensory Paralytic Bladder. Sensory paralytic bladder results from damage to the sensory half (dorsal roots) of the sacral reflex center. There is no sensation of bladder fullness; however, the patient can void voluntarily if the bladder has not become overdistended. Large residual volumes occur because of decreased tone and sensation of the bladder wall. The presence of reflexes is variable.

Motor Paralytic Bladder. Motor paralytic bladder results from damage to the motor half (ventral roots) of the sacral reflex center. Sensation is normal; however, the voluntary initiation and control of voiding are difficult because of the loss of motor functioning. In this dysfunction, the patient experiences the sensation of fullness and pain with increasing difficulty initiating voiding. Large residual

volumes occur because of the gradual stretching of the detrusor muscle.

Clinical Implications

Patients who have sustained cerebral damage from a stroke, brain tumor, or trauma frequently have an initial period of bladder areflexia, followed by bladder hyperreflexia with urinary frequency and incontinence. In these populations, however, voiding and complete emptying may be attained after careful assessment and bladder retraining.

In patients who have Parkinson's disease, there is often a 70% prevalence of bladder problems, with most having urinary frequency, urgency, and incontinence. Patients with Parkinson's disease may display symptoms similar to those of patients who have sustained a stroke, with hyperreflexia, poorly sustained contractions, and incomplete emptying. However, in Parkinson's, the patient's failure to empty is also a result of the bradykinesia that is experienced.

Patients with multiple sclerosis and spinal cord injury are very likely to experience urinary manifestations depending on the extent and completeness of the lesion. Ninety percent of patients with multiple sclerosis develop hyperreflexia and hypercontractility due to incomplete lesions. In spinal cord injuries, after the period of initial shock, the detrusor reflex usually returns, and this leads to reflex or overflow incontinence and to incomplete emptying due to the secondary effect of detrusor-sphincter dyssynergia. Patients who have sustained lesions in the conus/cauda areas of the spinal cord from trauma, tumor, or multiple sclerosis usually exhibit an areflexic, noncontractile, insensate bladder with severe overflow incontinence and decreased pelvic floor innervation. Many of these disease entities are associated with decreased mobility. As the patient has increased urgency, coupled with decreased mobility, urinary incontinence is more likely to occur.

Bladder Management Strategies

According to an Agency for Health Care Policy and Research Clinical Practice Guideline (Fantyl et al., 1996, p. 31): "The first choice should be the least invasive treatment with the fewest potential implications that is appropriate for the patient." There are three major approaches to treatment, which include behavioral, pharmacological, and surgical intervention, either alone or in combination.

In order to begin treatment, however, a thorough basic evaluation and assessment should occur. A basic evaluation consists of a history, a physical examination, and a urinalysis. The basic evaluation enables health care providers to confirm the presence of urinary incontinence as well as identify factors that may be contributing to the incontinence (Table 11–2). In addition, it serves as a guide to the appropriate bladder management program. It is also of the utmost importance that the rehabilitation nurse keep cultural and so-

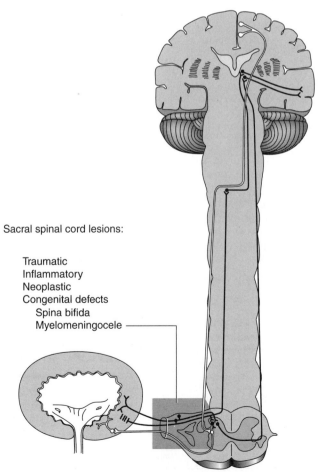

Sacral spinal cord lesions:

Traumatic
Inflammatory
Neoplastic
Congenital defects
　Spina bifida
　Myelomeningocele

FIGURE 11–3
Autonomous neurogenic bladder. (Redrawn from Lapides, J., & Diokno, A. C. [1976]. Urine transport, storage, and micturition. In J. Lapides [Ed.], *Fundamentals of urology* [p. 218]. Philadelphia: W. B. Saunders.)

TABLE 11–2 ■ FACTORS INFLUENCING THERAPY OPTIONS FOR THE MANAGEMENT OF INCONTINENCE

Age	Interest, reliability, cooperation
Desire to remain catheter-free	Hand function
	Mental state
Desire to avoid surgery	Prognosis of underlying
Economic resources	disease
Education of patient	Sexual activity
Cultural beliefs	Rehabilitation prognosis

cioeconomic considerations in mind when treating patients with incontinence, in order to maximize successful outcomes.

Behavioral Techniques

Behavioral techniques are low-risk interventions that decrease the frequency of urinary incontinence in most individuals when provided by knowledgeable heath care professionals (Fantyl et al., 1996). Behavioral techniques (Table 11–3) include educating the patient and providing positive reinforcement for effort and progress. These techniques usually require involvement of both the patient and the caregiver. When provided by caregivers, certain techniques can sometimes improve incontinence in cognitively impaired individuals. These strategies have no side effects and do not limit future treatment options. Often, the use of behavioral techniques alone can achieve continence; however, they may be combined with other modalities. Behavioral approaches often work best in patients with urge and stress incontinence and uninhibited neurogenic bladder. Patients with overflow incontinence are usually not candidates for behavioral interventions.

Toileting assistance includes scheduled toileting (or timed voiding), habit training, and prompted voiding. Scheduled toileting is provided by caregivers for patients who cannot

TABLE 11–3 ■ BEHAVIORAL TECHNIQUES FOR URINARY INCONTINENCE

Toileting assistance
    Routine scheduled toileting
    Habit training
    Prompted voiding
Bladder training
Pelvic muscle exercises
    With biofeedback
    With vaginal weight training

toilet independently. In this process, toileting occurs at regular intervals (usually every 2 to 4 hours), around the clock, in order to keep the patient dry. Studies have demonstrated improvements in continence in both males and females using this approach (Burgio, Stutzman, & Engel, 1989; Godec, 1994).

Habit training is toileting scheduled to match a patient's natural voiding pattern. In this process, after the natural voiding pattern is assessed, patients are toileted more and less frequently according to their own natural voiding pattern.

Prompted voiding consists of the three major elements of monitoring, prompting, and praising. The patient is monitored on a regular basis (usually every 3 hours) and asked if wet or dry. The patient is then prompted to use the toilet. Then the patient is praised for maintaining continence and attempting to void. Prompted voiding requires a patient who has enough cognitive ability to learn to recognize the need to void.

Bladder training is often used to manage bladder stability and urge incontinence. A bladder training/retraining program requires the patient to void according to a time schedule while resisting the urge in between. This type of program usually consists of three components: education, scheduled voiding, and reinforcement. The patient is taught to consciously delay voiding, beginning with a 2- to 3-hour interval, which is gradually increased using the relaxation techniques. Research by Fantl, Wyman, McClish, & Bump (1990) has demonstrated that bladder training can achieve both a reduction in incontinent episodes and complete continence.

Biofeedback techniques are used to enhance sphincter function by using computer readouts to illustrate the initiation and continuation of a contraction. Biofeedback is usually performed one or two times per week, usually incorporating pelvic muscle exercises.

Pelvic muscle exercises, also known as *Kegel exercises*, can also be used with vaginal weight training. These exercises are used to strengthen periurethral and paravaginal muscles that contribute to the closing force of the urethra. Pelvic muscle exercises are effective when used for both stress and urge incontinence in women and may be effective in reducing incontinence after prostatic surgery in men. Behavioral techniques combined with biofeedback have also been found effective with disabled patients who can voluntarily void and voluntarily contract their pelvic muscles (Fried, Goetz, Potts-Nulty, Cioschi, & Staas, 1995).

Pharmacological Management

Various drugs are used for the management of incontinence. Popular medications used in incontinence include anticholinergic agents, tricyclic antidepressants, α-adrenergic antagonists and agents, and estrogen. Table 11–4 identifies these drugs and the considerations involved in using them.

BOWEL ELIMINATION

Types of Dysfunction

Bowel function is not an openly discussed topic unless it is problematic. Fecal incontinence, although usually not life-threatening, has devastating financial and social consequences. Previous reports have estimated that in the United States, $8 billion per year was spent on fecal incontinence alone (Cardenas, Mayo, & King, 1996).

Problems with bowel incontinence range from 0.3% to approximately 6% in the general population, and from 10 to 50% among hospitalized or institutionalized elderly persons (Cardenas et al., 1996). As mentioned pre-

viously, both bowel and bladder incontinence are significant reasons for caregivers to place their loved ones in nursing homes.

The classification of bowel dysfunction is divided into nonneurogenic and neurogenic categories. Nonneurogenic bowel dysfunction includes diarrhea and constipation. Neurogenic bowel dysfunction includes uninhibited, reflex, and autonomous neurogenic bowel.

Nonneurogenic Bowel Dysfunction

Diarrhea. Diarrhea results from the rapid movement of waste through the bowel without sufficient time to absorb fluids, a normal function. The colon is responsible for absorbing water and electrolytes from solid waste in order to maintain normal cell homeostasis. Diarrhea can be very dangerous in infants, children, elderly persons, and debilitated persons, causing dehydration, electrolyte imbalance, renal failure, dysrhythmias, and even death.

Most diarrhea is caused by infection; however, lactose intolerance, food allergies, drugs, and even stress may cause diarrhea. Irritable bowel syndrome, which is characterized by diarrhea, abdominal pain, and gas, alternating with constipation, is caused by an ex-

TABLE 11–4 ■ PHARMACOLOGICAL MANAGEMENT OF INCONTINENCE

Medication	Action	Considerations
Anticholinergic Agents		
Oxbutynin chloride (Ditropan) Dicyclomine hydrochloride (Bentyl) Propantheline bromide (Pro-Banthine) Tolterodine (Detrol)	Blocks detrusor contractions	Avoid in patients with glaucoma; dry skin, blurred vision, mental status changes, nausea, constipation, tachycardia, possible urinary retention
Cholinergic Agonists		
Bethanechol (Urecholine)	Causes bladder contraction	Diarrhea, urinary urgency, asthmatic attacks
Tricyclic Agents		
Imiprimine (Tofranil)		Produces many adverse side effects
α-Adrenergic Agonists		
Phenylpropanolamine hydrochloride (Ornade)	Causes contraction and/or resistance of bladder neck	Nausea, xerostomia, itching, insomnia, rash, agitation, respiratory difficulty; use with caution
Adrenergic Antagonists		
Phenoxybenzamine (Dibenzyline) Terazosin (Hytrin) Doxazosin (Cardura) Tamsulosin (Flomax)	Inhibits smooth muscle activity at bladder neck	Hypotension
Estrogen	Restores urethral submucosa	

treme emotional response to stress. Diarrhea is also a mechanism for the body to eliminate infections. In bacterial or viral infections, the bowel becomes irritated and large amounts of fluid are secreted to wash the infection away. In most healthy adults, however, diarrhea is a symptom that something has disrupted the gastrointestinal tract, and it is not life-threatening.

Constipation.   Constipation is defined as bowel movements that are difficult to pass and infrequent for that particular person. Most people move their bowels between three times a day and three times a week; therefore, people are often considered constipated when they defecate one to two times a week.

Constipation is usually caused by irregular bowel habits (by suppressing the defecation reflex), immobility, diet, certain diseases, and emotional factors. Over time, failure to respond to the defecation reflexes results in constipation. Mobility is crucial for the normal propulsive movement of waste products through the digestive system. A patient who is immobile for any reason is at high risk for constipation. Dietary changes or a lack of adequate fiber in the diet is known to increase the transit time in the colon, and this results in constipation. Patients who are using narcotic pain medicines, such as codeine, or who have thyroid disease are also at risk.

Neurogenic Bowel Dysfunctions

The autonomic nervous system is responsible for the involuntary process of defecation, whereas the somatic nervous system is responsible for voluntary control. A neurogenic bowel results when there is damage to the brain or spinal cord and bowel function continues without voluntary cerebral control.

Uninhibited Neurogenic Bowel.   Uninhibited neurogenic bowel is caused by damage to the upper motor neurons in the brain as a result of stroke, multiple sclerosis, brain tumor, or trauma. Sensory impulses travel through the sacral reflex center to the brain; however, the brain is unable to interpret and suppress the urge to defecate. Elimination occurs involuntarily when the sacral reflex arc is activated (Fig. 11–4).

Reflex Neurogenic Bowel.   Reflex neurogenic bowel (or upper motor neuron bowel) occurs with damage to the upper motor neuron and sensory tracts in the spinal cord

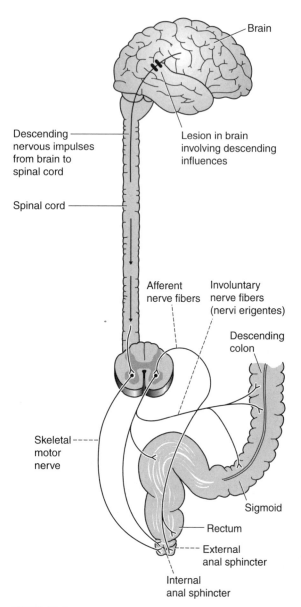

FIGURE 11–4
Uninhibited neurogenic bowel. (Redrawn from Pires, M., & Lockhart, P. [1992]. *Nursing management of neurogenic incontinence* [pp. 11–12, 14]. Skokie, IL: Rehabilitation Nursing Foundation.)

above the sacral reflex center. In this type of neurogenic bowel, sensation is often absent whereas the reflex arcs are intact. There is also partial or complete loss of voluntary sphincter activity. Defecation occurs as a mass reflex contraction stimulated by the rectal mucosa. This type of neurogenic bowel is most often seen in patients with quadriplegia, multiple sclerosis, vascular disease, or syringomyelia.

TABLE 11–5 ■ COMPONENTS OF A BOWEL PROGRAM

Clean bowel	Privacy
Timing	Positioning
Diet and fluid intake	Medications
Exercise	Digital stimulation

Autonomous Neurogenic Bowel. Autonomous or lower neuron neurogenic bowel occurs with damage at the sacral reflex center. In this type of neurogenic bowel, sensation as well as reflex activity is absent. No reflex emptying occurs, and both the internal and the external sphincters lack tone. This often leads to distention, oozing, and fecal incontinence.

Bowel Management Strategies

The overall goal of an effective bowel management program is regular evacuation of soft, formed stool, without incontinence or other complications. In order to achieve this goal, certain components must be evaluated and incorporated into the overall bowel program (Table 11–5).

A "clean" bowel is a requirement to begin any program. Medications or enemas may be used to eliminate any impaction before the initiation of any program. The timing of the program is also important. The bowel program must be scheduled at a time that incorporates the patient's preinjury schedule as well as future lifestyle. A morning bowel program may no longer be practical depending on the length of the patient's morning routine. It is important to note that the best time for a bowel program is one that is consistent and takes advantage of the gastrocolic reflex. In addition, the proper position, sitting, allows gravity to assist with the defecation process. From a dietary perspective, the two most important elements for enhancing soft, bulky stools are adequate fiber and water.

Although these interventions may be enough to correct some bowel problems, such as diarrhea and constipation, other interventions may be required. Medications such as suppositories, stool softeners, and mild bulk-forming laxatives (Table 11–6) may be necessary to initiate the bowel program, with the ultimate goal being to reduce or eliminate as much medication as possible. Digital stimulation performed by inserting a gloved, lubricated finger into the rectum and rotating until the sphincter relaxes also assists with reflex peristaltic activity and evacuation.

The most important variable to consider is privacy. In most cultures, privacy regarding the most intimate experiences of elimination and sexual activity is a necessity. Adequate privacy is often difficult to achieve in most health care institutions, and this affects the patient's, caregiver's, and visitor's comfort level with bowel and bladder programs. It is important to note that treatment refusals may occur for these reasons alone. Even a significant portion of the nondisabled population have difficulty in public restroom facilities.

It is of the utmost importance that the rehabilitation nurse educate both the patient and the caregivers adequately about elimination

TABLE 11–6 ■ MEDICATIONS FOR BOWEL MANAGEMENT

Medication	Action
Suppositories	
Glycerin	Draws fluid from bowel, distends bowel causing reflex peristalsis
Sodium bicarbonate/potassium bitartrate (Ceo-Two)	Activated in water before insertion
	Releases carbon dioxide, which distends bowel causing reflex peristalsis
Bisacodyl (Dulcolax)	Stimulates nerve endings in colon on contact, causing reflex peristalsis
Minienemas	
Ducosate (Therevac)	Already in liquid form; works quicker in stimulating evacuation
Fleet's bisacodyl	
Oral Stimulants	
Prune juice	Causes local irritation of mucosa leading to increased motility
Senna (Senokot)	
Bisacodyl tabs (Dulcolax)	
Oral Stool Softeners	
Ducosate (Surfax Colace)	Allows water to enter feces and soften stool

strategies that have been implemented. Retraining is truly a reeducation of both the body and the mind. In order for successful outcomes to occur, the rehabilitation nurse must perform the activities initially, while moving toward constant education/reeducation, so that the disabled individual and the caregivers can do or direct another to complete the task. This reeducation must occur while being attuned to the patient's cultural background and health beliefs in order for successful outcomes to occur.

REFERENCES

Burgio, K. L., Stutzman, R. E., & Engel, B. T. (1989). Behavioral training for post-prostatectomy urinary incontinence. *Journal of Urology, 141*, 303–306.

Cardenas, D. D., Mayo, M. E., & King, J. C. (1996). Urinary tract and bowel management in the rehabilitation setting. In R. L. Brad (Ed.), *Physical medicine and rehabilitation* (pp. 555–579). Philadelphia: W. B. Saunders.

Chancellor, M. B., & Blaivis, J. G. (1995). Practical Neurourology genitourinary complications in neurologic disease. Boston: Butterworth-Heinemann.

Dougherty, D. B. (1991). *Urinary and fecal incontinence nursing management.* St. Louis: Mosby–Year Book.

Fantl, J. A., Newman, D. K., Colling, J., et al. (1996). *Urinary incontinence in adults: Acute and chronic management, clinical practice guideline No. 2* (1996 update, AHCPR Publication No. 96-0682). Rockville, MD: U.S. Department of Health and Human Services, Public Health Service, Agency for Health Care Policy and Research.

Fantl, J. A., Wyman, J. F., McClish, D. K., & Bump, R. C. (1990). Urinary incontinence in community dwelling women: Clinical, urodynamic and severity characteristics. *American Journal of Obstetrics and Gynecology, 162*, 946–951.

Fried, G. W., Goetz, G., Potts-Nulty, S., Cioschi, H., & Staas, W. E. (1995). A behavioral approach to the treatment of urinary incontinence in a disabled population. *Archives of Physical Medicine and Rehabilitation, 76*, 1120–1124.

Godec, C. J. (1994). Timed voiding: A useful tool in the treatment of urinary incontinence. *Urology, 23*, 97–100.

Hoeman, S. P. (1989). Cultural assessment in rehabilitation nursing practice. *Nursing Clinics of North America, 24.*

Lapides, J., & Diokno, A. C. (1976). Urine transport, storage and micturition. In J. Lapides (Ed.), *Fundamentals of urology.* Philadelphia: W. B. Saunders.

Ouslander, J. G., Morishita, L., Blaustein, J., Orzeck, S., & Sayre, J. (1987). Clinical, functional and psychosocial characteristics of an incontinent nursing home population. *Journal of Gerontology, 42*, 631–637.

Urinary Incontinence Guideline Panel. (1992). *Urinary incontinence in adults; Clinical practice guideline* (AHCPR Publication No. 92-0038). Rockville, MD: U.S. Department of Health and Human Services, Agency for Health Care Policy and Research, Public Health Service.

BIBLIOGRAPHY

Ditmar, S. *(1989). Rehabilitation nursing process and application.* St. Louis: C. V. Mosby.

Dougherty, D. (1996). A physiologic approach to bowel training. *Journal of Wound Ostomy and Continence Nursing, 23*, 46–55.

Hoeman, S. P. (1996). Rehabilitation nursing process and application (2nd ed.). St. Louis: C. V. Mosby.

Opitz, J. L., Thorsteinsson, G., Schutt, A. H., Barrett, D. M., & Olson, P. K. (1988). Neurogenic bladder and bowel. In J. A. DeLisa (Ed.), *Rehabilitation medicine, principles and practice.* Philadelphia: J. B. Lippincott.

CHAPTER 12

Immobility

Karen Mandzak Fried and Guy W. Fried

Immobility is one of the most common yet most preventable causes of disability. The ability to successfully move around in one's environment is critical to the successful performance of activities of daily living, work, and leisure. Both chronically ill patients with functional and neurological impairments and the elderly are at the greatest risk for the hazards of immobility. Rehabilitation nurses usually care for these types of patients and play a key role in mobilizing them and preventing secondary disabilities.

The complications and symptoms that result from the restricted use of body systems have more recently come to be known as the "disuse syndrome" or "de-conditioning." According to Halar and Bell (1998), *de-conditioning* is defined as the reduced functional capacity of all body systems; it may be considered a separate disease entity from the original process that led to a curtailment of normal activity. Often, the complications of immobility can be more detrimental than the original injury or disease process. These complications can be devastating, even in an able-bodied population, and they often occur in a relatively short time.

HISTORICAL PERSPECTIVE

For many centuries, it was believed that exercise promoted health and that immobility led to physical decline.

This framework set the stage for generations of physicians to advocate exercise to prevent illness. Unfortunately, for a short time in the late 18th century, there was a philosophical shift from the benefits of exercise to the prescription of bed rest. However, that shift was often based on an exaggeration of information and a misapplication of research.

Today, current research and information obtained from the federal aerospace program have emphasized the importance of exercise and the avoidance of immobility because of its severe multisystem consequences. As dis-

covered in this and other research, these severe consequences can occur even in healthy people. For example, Taylor, Henschel, Brozek, & Keys (1949) found that 3 weeks of bed rest in healthy men caused de-conditioning, noted as increased heart rates in response to moderate work. It took 3 weeks for these men's bodies to counteract the effects of immobility and return to the prior state of conditioning. The adage "If you don't use it, you lose it" is true.

For these reasons, it is important for rehabilitation nurses to understand the consequences of even brief periods of immobility, in order to apply the appropriate interventions to limit its sequelae and return patients to their maximum level of functioning. It is the rehabilitation nurse, in conjunction with physical and occupational therapists, who mobilizes the patient and maximizes strength and endurance to counteract the global effects of immobility.

EFFECTS OF IMMOBILITY ON BODY SYSTEMS

Despite the overall discouragement of bed rest, there are times when bed rest or immobility is impossible to avoid. This occurs when normal demands exceed the body's ability to respond after illnesses such as myocardial infarction, pulmonary disease, and orthopedic trauma. It must be noted that when a person is immobilized, complications occur quickly. Immobility affects virtually every system of the body—musculoskeletal, integumentary, cardiovascular, metabolic-endocrine, respiratory, gastrointestinal, genitourinary, and neurological. The following discussions describe the effects of immobility and disuse on specific body systems (Table 12–1).

Musculoskeletal System

The musculoskeletal system enables the patient to perform two basic but completely

TABLE 12–1 ■ EFFECTS OF IMMOBILITY ON BODY SYSTEMS

System	Effect	Therapeutic Interventions
Musculoskeletal	Atrophy/weakness Contracture Osteoporosis	Encourage normal activity Proper positioning Muscle stretch and contraction to maintain strength Position joints in neutral position Range of motion Stretching with splinting/casting Weight bearing
Integumentary	Pressure sores	Adequate nutrition/hydration Frequent turning Weight shifting Use of pressure-relieving devices
Metabolic and endocrine	Negative nitrogen balance Calcium loss Glucose intolerance	Maintain adequate diet Exercise Maximal activity
Cardiovascular	Deconditioning Orthostatic hypotension Redistribution of body fluids Thromboembolus	Maintenance of sitting/standing positions Active/passive range of motion Isometric exercises Early mobilization Use of abdominal binder, elastic stockings, bandage wraps Medications to maintain blood pressure
Respiratory	Mucus plugging Atelectasis Pneumonia Pulmonary embolus	Encourage cough and deep breathing Aggressive pulmonary care Assistive coughing, coffolator
Gastrointestinal and genitourinary	Constipation Urinary retention/stasis Urinary stones, urinary tract infection	Small frequent feedings Fiber-rich diet, adequate fluids Bowel/bladder program
Neurological	Sensory deprivation Disorientation Anxiety/depression Impaired balance and coordination	Maintain sleep/wake cycle Frequent reorientation Frequent position changes

necessary functions, (1) mobilization of the body and (2) the performance of activities of daily living. The human body was made to function in an active, moving state. Movement and activity create a physiological balance in many body systems. Muscles are meant to flex and stretch, putting joints through their complete range of motion. When a person is immobile, the musculoskeletal changes that may occur are (1) atrophy and weakness, (2) contractures, (3) heterotopic ossification, and (4) osteoporosis.

Muscle Atrophy and Weakness

Research has demonstrated that even in completely healthy individuals, muscles will lose 1 to 3% of their strength per day. This means that a person who is immobilized for as little as 3 weeks could potentially lose half of his or her muscle strength (Halar & Bell, 1998). Muscle atrophy also contributes to impairment of metabolic and cardiovascular activity,

which subsequently affects endurance. Muscle atrophy and impaired range of motion are minimized by encouraging normal activities. Positioning is important in the development of atrophy, because stretching appears to delay atrophy. In addition, muscle strength can be maintained if daily muscle contractions are performed with self-care activities. It should be noted that the recovery of muscle strength may take two to three times as long as the original period of immobility.

Contractures

A contracture occurs as a result of a lack of joint mobilization throughout the full, allowable range. Spasticity, paralysis, or muscle strength imbalance hastens the development of contractures. Contractures can be classified into three groups on the basis of anatomical changes: (1) arthrogenic, (2) soft tissue, and (3) myogenic. It has been ascertained that the position in which a joint is immobilized also affects the severity of the underlying contracture by reducing muscle fibers. For these reasons, the joint should be immobilized in a neutral position to try to keep opposing muscles at equal length and tension. Also, it is commonly believed that contractures can be prevented by movement through the range of motion at least twice a day.

Arthrogenic contractures usually result from damage to the cartilage, synovium, or joint capsule itself. This type of a contracture usually occurs with arthritis but may also result from trauma or infection. Essentially, the pain of the cartilage damage from degenerative joint disease or the synovial inflammation from rheumatoid arthritis, trauma, or infection leads to a reduction in range of motion and, therefore, a contracture. Found most frequently in the shoulders, hips, spine, and knees, arthrogenic contractures affect all directions of joint movement.

Soft tissue contractures are often caused by burns. In this type of contracture, the damage occurs in the periarticular, subcutaneous, and cutaneous tissues and restricts range of motion in the same way arthrogenic contractures do. The difference is that range of motion is limited in one direction in a soft tissue contracture.

Myogenic contractures are due to the shortening of the muscle tissue itself as a result of replacement of muscle fibers with collagen. This replacement occurs with inflammation, degeneration, trauma, or neurological abnormalities. The limb is held in a flexed position. Prolonged malpositioning of the joint from neurological changes that cause flaccid or spastic paralysis also leads to myogenic contractures.

Heterotopic Ossification

Heterotopic ossification creates a contracture by a similar process; however, there is a deposition of bone instead of collagen in the muscle fibers. The exact cause of heterotopic ossification is not known, but it is believed that changes in metabolism may initiate the process. Heterotopic ossification is not caused by immobility itself but is found in patients who have experienced trauma.

Osteoporosis

Bone density is affected by mobility because activity stresses the bone and maintains the equilibrium between bone formation and bone reabsorption. Disuse that occurs with immobilization can lead to an almost 1% loss of vertebral mineral content per week. Children and young adults are especially at risk for hypercalcemia as a result of this bone loss.

Prevention

Rehabilitation professionals must be ever-vigilant about the prevention, treatment, and management of contractures, atrophy, weakness, and osteoporosis. The basic principles of treatment for musculoskeletal system changes are

- Stretching through active and passive range of motion
- Proper positioning
- Exercising or mobilizing to restore function

Stretching through active and passive range of motion is the best possible treatment for the musculoskeletal changes that occur as a result of immobilization.

For severe contractures, sustained stretching combined with heat (via ultrasound) maximizes the effects of stretching. Serial casting and dynamic splinting provide sustained stretching over a longer period (hours to days). *Serial casting* is the application of a well-padded cast on a joint immediately after a stretch. Initially, the cast is usually replaced in 2 or 3 days, after the skin is examined for areas of redness or breakdown. Subsequent serial casts may then be applied for up to 5 days. This method is most effective for the treatment of foot, knee, and elbow contractures.

Dynamic splinting is the application of a splint that allows for greater movement but provides dynamic tension to stretch the joint. This type of treatment is most effective in the upper extremities because it allows for function while providing stretch. In addition, continuous passive motion (CPM), provided through a CPM device, has become the standard in orthopedic postoperative care for the maintenance of joint mobility and prevention of contractures.

Proper positioning is another important treatment for an immobilized or paralyzed patient. A bed with a firm mattress, side rails, and a trapeze facilitates turning and mobility. Pillows are needed for support for side-lying and three-quarter-prone positions in bed. At all times while in bed the patient should wear foot guards or a similar type of foot positioner that attempts to relieve heel pressure while preventing plantar flexion.

The best method to minimize the musculoskeletal effects of immobility is to maximize the patient's time out of bed and encourage as much function as possible. Ambulation, wheelchair activities, physical therapy, occupational therapy, recreation therapy, and leisure activities encourage patients to be out of bed and strengthen and use their bodies to their maximal ability.

Integumentary System

A person who is immobilized is at high risk for the formation of pressure sores, which are a primary cause of disability and can lead to morbidity and mortality. It is a well-known fact that lying or sitting in bed creates pressure points greater than the capillary blood pressure, which is 30 mm Hg. As bony areas such as the occiput, ischium, sacrum, trochanters, and heels apply pressure over the skin, the capillary pressure is occluded. Necrosis owing to the lack of blood flow occurs quickly, and if it is combined with other variables, such as friction or shearing forces, incontinence, age, paralysis, edema, obesity, and infection, the damage can be rapid. If the patient is immobilized and does not move frequently, the skin is not adequately nourished.

The best method of treatment for pressure sores is prevention. Preventive measures include (1) frequent changes in position by turning and weight shifting, (2) proper nutrition, and (3) proper use of bed mattresses and wheelchair cushions.

Cardiovascular System

The changes that occur in the cardiovascular system as a result of disuse include cardiovascular de-conditioning, fluid balance changes, thromboembolism, and orthostatic hypotension. Cardiac efficiency is reduced by 25% after only 3 weeks of immobility and bed rest. In the supine position, the heart must work harder to pump the blood throughout the body because of increased venous return. There is also a concurrent decline in stroke volume and circulating fluid volume.

It has been discovered that a person does not have to be immobile to suffer the consequences of cardiovascular de-conditioning. Literature in the field of cardiac rehabilitation indicates that inactivity or a sedentary lifestyle is an independent risk factor for coronary heart disease.

During periods of immobility, the circulating blood plasma volume decreases, leading to increased viscosity and a potential for thrombus formation. Stasis in the lower extremities also occurs from the lack of movement of the muscles in the limbs. According to Virchow's triad, the first two of three variables for clot formation occur in immobility; these three variables are stasis, blood coagulability, and injury. Rehabilitative nurses can assess and observe for swelling and venous changes by measuring the calves and thighs of paralyzed patients. Other interventions, such as getting patients out of bed and assisting those who can ambulate, help decrease the risk.

Orthostatic hypotension is another common cardiovascular consequence of immobility. The cardiovascular system fails to adequately adapt blood pressure when the patient moves from a supine to an upright position. The physiological sympathetic response that counteracts hypotension in normal individuals no longer functions after a period of immobility. Reasons for the failure of this response are unknown, but it may be due to a diminished orthostatic neurovascular reflex. To prevent this complication patients should be placed in a sitting or standing position as soon as possible. Range of motion and early, progressive mobilization help prevent orthostatic hypotension. Also, the use of an abdominal binder, elastic stockings, and elastic bandage wraps (Ace bandage) is often required for quadriplegic and paraplegic patients.

Metabolic and Endocrine Systems

Periods of immobility also cause a negative nitrogen balance as a result of reduced muscular activity and breakdown of protein. Calcium loss is also related to inactivity, and a negative calcium balance can be difficult to counteract. Other minerals necessary for metabolic balance, such as sodium, sulfur, phosphorus, and potassium, are also reduced. Many hormones in the endocrine system, such as insulin, parathyroid hormones, androgens, and hydrocortisone, are affected by prolonged bed rest. Glucose intolerance is primarily due to changes in the peripheral muscle's sensitivity to circulating insulin. It is important for immobilized patients to have an adequate diet and as much exercise as possible, as soon as possible.

Respiratory System

When a person is immobilized, a decrease in diaphragmatic movement and chest excursion leads to a reduction in lung volumes due to mechanical resistance. Weaker chest and diaphragmatic muscles may limit the strength of expansion. Respiration often becomes shallow, resulting in an increase in respiratory rate. A decrease in the expansion of the muscles of respiration combined with a poor cough subsequently leads to a buildup of secretions in the lower lobes of the lungs, predisposing patients to mucus plugging, atelectasis, and pneumonia. This buildup of secretions may be further exacerbated by limited oral intake and dehydration.

Rehabilitation nurses enhance respiratory efforts through aggressive pulmonary toileting. The interventions include chest percussion, clapping, drainage, and assistive coughing techniques. Frequent changes of positions, deep slow breathing, and incentive spirometry also help maintain adequate respiratory function in a paralyzed patient.

Gastrointestinal and Genitourinary Systems

Immobility leads to constipation as a result of reduced peristalsis, dehydration, and a diminished appetite. In the supine position, there is a decrease in intraabdominal pressure, caused by abdominal muscle weakness and a lack of gravity. This makes it difficult to initiate voiding or a bowel movement. In order to prevent constipation, an appropriate bowel program should be initiated, consisting of (1) a fiber-rich diet, (2) stool softeners, (3) suppositories, and (4) scheduling of toileting.

The act of voiding the bladder in the supine position is frequently incomplete, leading to larger postvoid residuals and stasis. Urine stasis combined with an increase in calcium excretion leads to calculus formation and urinary tract infections. A bladder program may be required, depending on the patient's diagnosis and mobilization abilities.

Neurological System

The effects of bed rest and disuse on the neurological system are primarily sensory deprivation and time disorientation. These effects may lead to depression, anxiety, withdrawal, sleep disturbances, and emotional lability. The combination of bed rest, medications, and sleep deprivation have often led to the phenomenon known as "ICU psychosis." Coordination and balance may also be affected due to the physiological deterioration caused by immobility.

THERAPEUTIC INTERVENTIONS TO COUNTERACT THE EFFECTS OF IMMOBILITY

When a patient is immobilized, the rehabilitation nurse has the responsibility to maintain the patient's potential for possible remobilization and prevention of secondary disabilities.

Physical variables that must be taken into account for the remobilization process to occur are

- Range of motion
- Strength
- Balance
- Endurance
- Tone
- Proprioception

Range of motion, as mentioned before, is the full range of movement that a joint can normally perform. In *active* range of motion, the patient moves all of the joints through their full range at a minimum of twice a day. *Passive* range of motion is performed by the caregiver because the patient is unable to carry out the activity. The person performing passive range of motion places one hand above the joint to support it while using the other hand to move the joint through the range. In both active and passive range of motion, all joints are moved at least five times each. Range-of-motion exercises should be performed smoothly and gently and should not be forced past resistance.

Strength is the ability of the muscle to produce a physical force that is necessary to maintain function. Strength incorporates the normal state of balanced tension in the muscle, which is known as *tone*. *Balance*, the ability to sit and stand erect, occurs because of the integration of muscle strength and tone. *Endurance* is the ability to maintain the effort required for an activity. These variables combine to enhance smooth mobility activities, and they must be assessed and analyzed in order for any mobilization activity to occur.

Exercise is provided through repeated muscle contractions and endurance activities. Two types of active muscle contractions that can be used to provide exercise are isotonic contractions and isometric contractions. *Isotonic* contractions occur when a muscle and a joint are moved. In *isometric* or muscle-setting contractions, the muscle is tightened without apparent movement of the limb or joint. It has been revealed that electrical stimulation to muscles can cause isometric contractions that maintain or strengthen muscles in paralyzed patients. Rehabilitation nurses incorporate these and other therapeutic interventions in order to progressively mobilize their patients and maximize their function.

Culturally Competent Care. It should be noted that cultural variables may have an effect on a patient's response to mobilization activities. Health beliefs regarding the value of bed rest for healing may interfere with active mobilization. Indeed, the family's response to a life-threatening injury may be based on fear of causing another life-threatening event, and they may discourage attempts at mobilization. In most cultures, there is an automatic expectation of and response to sick people, and sick role behaviors and responses may be difficult to change. Also, the perceptions of the nurse as the caregiver, "doing for" patients rather than encouraging patients to do things for themselves, is a bias that is evident in most cultures. Rehabilitation nurses must continue to educate patients and families about their role on the interdisciplinary health care team as co-managers of care. Rehabilitation nurses must also be able to explain the concept of progressive mobilization and the prevention of secondary disabilities in terminology that expresses the maximizing of health as the ultimate outcome.

Activities in Bed

As mentioned previously, the proper therapeutic position in bed with correct support is necessary to prevent both contractures and pressure sores. The neutral position also keeps the limb in the best state for future exercise and activity to occur. Turning and repositioning should be based on an individual assessment of the patient. Although most patients can tolerate being turned every 2 hours, some may require it more frequently, and others may require less frequent turning.

Beds with the appropriate pressure-relieving mattresses are a requirement, as are pillows and foot positioning devices. If the patient is not paralyzed or unconscious, therapeutic positioning and bed mobility activities are the first step in progressive mobilization.

Bed mobility is the most basic stage of active mobilization. It consists of (1) turning from side to side, (2) redistributing pressure, (3) moving up, down, and sideways in bed, (4) bridging (being able to lift the hips/buttocks up off the bed), and (5) sitting up in bed. The patient may perform bed mobility activities independently or by using the side rails and a trapeze.

Activities Out of Bed

The second stage of mobility for patients to accomplish is transfers. A *transfer* is the activity used to move between the bed and a wheelchair, toilet, shower-commode chair, or car. Transfers can range from being completely dependent and requiring a caregiver or mechanical device, to being partially dependent, to being completely independent. In order for patients to be able to transfer safely, they must be able to adjust to sitting up in bed and then to dangling the legs on the side of the bed with assistance. Once the patient is transferred, mobilization activities can occur through either wheelchair or ambulation activities.

Wheelchair mobilization occurs with the patient either moving a wheelchair manually or moving a battery-operated power chair by controlling it with a joystick, sip-and-puff mechanism, or voice activation. All rehabilitation professionals should work together to maximize the patient's mobility both in therapy and on the unit by encouraging the patient to mobilize in the wheelchair as independently as possible.

For a patient to ambulate, therapy must work on preambulation activities, such as improvements in strength and sitting tolerance, and balance activities. Rehabilitation nurses must continue to emphasize with patients and families that mobilization is a slow and progressive process that is built upon the achievement of individual goals. Ambulation activities require adequate strength, balance, and coordination. Patients are assessed for appropriate assistive devices to enhance ambulation. Crutches, regular or wide-based canes, and walkers may be used either alone or in conjunction with bracing in order to achieve adequate stabilization for ambulation. Bracing is usually long-leg or short-leg and is made from a combination of metal and plastic. Prostheses, both temporary and permanent, are used for ambulation training of amputees. It is important to note that ambulation with assistive devices and bracing requires significantly more energy than unassisted ambulation by healthy persons and may not be the most efficient or functional technique for some patients.

Rehabilitation nurses realize the fact that no one can go through a traumatic injury or a prolonged period of bed rest and then get up and walk immediately. Patients and families, on the other hand, often express the goal of "walking" upon admission to the rehabilitation unit. It is only through consistent education and repetition that patients and families understand that bed mobility and "dangling" must occur before sitting or standing can even be tolerated. Consistent support and praise for each small achievement as one step closer to the ultimate goal will minimize the frustration experienced by patients and families during the long and difficult process of rehabilitation. This is where the interdisciplinary team and the art and science of rehabilitation nursing synthesize to bring the patient's physical, psychological, and emotional functioning to the highest level possible.

REFERENCES

Halar, E. M., & Bell, K. R. (1998). Immobility— physiological and functional changes and effects of inactivity on body functions. In J. A. DeLisa (Ed.), *Rehabilitation medicine principles and practice* (2nd ed., pp. 1015–1034). Philadelphia: Lippincott-Raven.

Taylor, H. L., Henschel, A., Brozek, J., & Keys, A. (1949). Effects of bed rest on cardiovascular function and work performance. *Journal of Applied Physiology, 2,* 223–239.

BIBLIOGRAPHY

Borgman-Gainer, M. F. (1996). Independent function: Movement and mobility. In S. P. Hocman (Ed.), *Reha-bilitation nursing process and application* (2nd ed., pp. 225–269). St. Louis: Mosby–Year Book.

Buschbacher, R. M. (1996). Deconditioning, conditioning and the benefits of exercise. In R. L. Braddom (Ed.), *Physical medicine and rehabilitation* (pp. 687–708). Philadelphia: W. B. Saunders.

Dean, E. (1993). Bed rest and sensory disturbances. *Neuroreport, 17,* 6–9.

Downs, F. S. (1974). Bed rest and sensory disturbances. *American Journal of Nursing, 74,* 434–438.

Glick, O. J. (1992). Interventions related to activity and movement. *Nursing Clinics of North America, 27,* 541–568.

Halar, E. M., & Bell, K. R. (1990). Rehabilitation's relationship to inactivity. In F. T. Kottke & J. F. Lehman (Eds.), *Krusen's handbook of physical medicine and rehabilitation* (pp. 1113–1133). Philadelphia: W. B. Saunders.

Hangartner, T. N. (1995). Osteoporosis due to disuse. *Physical Medicine and Rehabilitation Clinics of North America, 6,* 579–594.

Hoenig, H. M., & Rubenstein, L. Z. (1991). Hospital associated deconditioning and dysfunction. *Journal of the American Geriatrics Society, 39,* 220–222.

McCourt, A. E. (1993). *The specialty practice of rehabilitation nursing: A core curriculum* (pp. 108–121). Skokie, IL: Rehabilitation Nursing Foundation.

Monicken, D. (1991). Immobility and functional mobility in the elderly. In W. C. Chenitz, J. T. Stone, & S. A. Salisbury (Eds.), *Clinical gerontological nursing* (pp. 233–245). Philadelphia: W. B. Saunders.

Olsen, E. V., Johnson, B. J., & Thompson, L. F. (1990). The hazards of immobility. *American Journal of Nursing, 90,* 43–44.

Steinburg, F. U. (1980). *The immobilized patient: Functional pathology and management.* New York: Plenum Press.

Taylor, H. L. (1968). The effects of rest in bed and exercise of cardiovascular function. *Circulation, 38,* 1016–1017.

Umhaver, M. K. (1989). Movement. In S. Dittmar (Ed.), *Rehabilitation nursing process and application* (pp. 360–406). St. Louis: C. V. Mosby.

Vorhies, D., & Riley, B. E. (1993). Deconditioning changes in organ system physiology induced by inactivity and reversed by activity. *Clinics of Geriatric Medicine, 9,* 745–763.

CHAPTER 13

Sexuality

Helen Carmine

The topics of sexuality, sexual functioning, and sexual adjustment are critical issues in the lives of individuals and families who have experienced either a disability or a chronic illness resulting in disability. Over the past 20 years, sexuality, sexual behavior, and expanding attitudes and beliefs about people as sexual beings have been a major focus of society. Through excessive media attention and changing cultural values and mores, sexuality and sexual activity have become a common topic in the daily lives of many people. Since the late 1960s, health care professionals, including psychologists, social workers, physicians, physical and occupational therapists, and nurses, have received in their practices or curricula at least an introduction to sexuality and sexual behavior and their relevance to clinical practice.

The range of sexual issues for clients with physical and cognitive disabilities is broad and must be addressed by rehabilitation nurses and rehabilitation professionals. Now more than ever, rehabilitation nurses may be confronted with the challenge of addressing the individuals' issues and concerns. Because rehabilitation nurses' roles are expansive and exist throughout the range of health care, they have multiple opportunities to identify, explore, and support the patient, client, and significant others' needs in the area of sexual health and function. Across the continuum of care, from acute, trauma, and rehabilitation settings through lifetime community and follow-up care, the issues of sexual concern and the "how to's" of sexual functioning will be raised by individuals and their significant others. If we continue to provide a comprehensive and holistic approach to physical and psychosocial needs, the sexual needs of our patients will not go unaddressed. A holistic definition for sexual health was established in the 1970s and continues to provide a framework for health care professionals.

The World Health Organization (WHO) has defined sexual health as "an integration of somatic, emotional, intellectual, and social aspects of sexual being, in ways that are positive, enriching, and that enhance personality, communication and love" (World Health Organization, 1975).

In addition to this basic definition, health care professionals should provide the foundation for sexual health by supporting and facilitating the three basic tenets included in the WHO definition. Individuals are

1. To enjoy sexual and reproductive behavior in accordance with personal and social ethics
2. To have freedom from fear, shame, guilt, and false information—which impair a sexual relationship and inhibit sexual response
3. To be free of organic disease and disabilities that present barriers to sexual and reproductive functions

This definition supports the need to provide factual, timely, and appropriate information and to prevent complications that result from ignorance, lack of knowledge, and the inability to return to a healthy, restored sexual life.

As systems of care move patient groups into a disease management approach, patients and health care professionals *should* have more opportunities to discuss sexual needs as they are identified and experienced throughout the course of the disability or the life span of the individual. Although the opportunities for addressing sexual needs have broadened, individual and professional accountabilities for addressing these vital needs continue to be blurred in most settings. As patients move quickly to the next component of the continuum of care, many of their informational needs, fears, and concerns may go unaddressed.

It is *vital* that each care setting or system define the accountabilities of each health care professional as they relate to sexual education and counseling. Identifying needs and responding to the individual's issues and concerns in a timely manner through education, counseling, or referral to the proper setting or counselor remain paramount in appropriately managing this most basic human need.

Traditional sources of sexual information vary among individuals with disabilities and chronic illnesses. Unfortunately, despite much of our attention to the area of sexual health, it still is not uncommon for the issues and needs related to sexual health to go unaddressed and unexplored for such clients. A study completed by Tepper (1992) exemplifies the need for health care professionals to pay more attention to this basic need. This study involved a sample of Veterans Administration Hospital patients who were treated in their spinal cord systems of care. Of the 112 respondents, only 45% received sexual education or counseling. Another 76% reported that sufficient services, such as counseling, support, and education, were not made available to address their sexual needs. Those who had received sexual counseling wanted more counseling and education *after* being discharged, but the health care professionals they encountered did not offer it or were unable to respond to their issues.

The study by Tepper (1992) also highlighted the gender variations that occur with sexual counseling after the onset of disability. The odds of *not* receiving sexual education or counseling were about two times greater for females than for males in this research sample. An unpublished focus group study also has reinforced the need for sensitivity and attention to gender differences and marital status of patients with disability (Kraft-Fine, McGillin, Potts-Nulty, Lennon, & Cioschi, 1996). Female focus group participants, all of whom had spinal cord injuries, identified that although some issues were addressed by their health care providers, many were not, and often they were told that the answers to their questions were not scientifically explored. Many did not know what to ask or how to ask questions regarding sexual function or how to make sure their sexual health and function needs were met. In addition, many female patients were provided with incorrect or incomplete information about sexual health topics such as contraception, pregnancy, and delivery, and some experienced a bias about providing information based on their marital status; that is, not having an active partner was equated with not having sexual concerns.

Some interesting patterns can be observed in the field of sexuality research and disability. The early research into the sexual function and sexual needs of individuals with disabilities was most often conducted in men rather than women. Some compelling reasons for the dearth of literature on female sexual response and disability may be related to the epidemiological nature of traumatic injuries, the ease of studying physiological response in males, and, perhaps, the bias and the interest of the researchers. According to Sipski, Alexander, and Rosen (1995), female sexual physiology after disability has most recently begun to be assessed in a scientific and laboratory environment. These investigators have determined that although we know very little about the sexuality of women with spinal cord injury, even less information is available regarding the physiology associated with their sexual responses. A historical review of literature on sexual response in females with spinal cord injuries reflects the need for more scientific research, because much of what is known is based on questionnaire responses in which sexual response, intensity of response, and frequency of activity and resulting orgasms were self-reported.

Many clinicians are not well prepared or comfortable in addressing the sexual concerns of the individuals that they treat. Many continue to compartmentalize patient needs because of limited knowledge, their own fears or personal conflicts, or limited time and so fail to fully address their patients' sexual issues or concerns. A defined professional or programmatic approach may help to guide us through this process. For health care professionals working within a team environment, specific roles and responsibilities for identifying and addressing sexual health care needs may provide the structure, support, and desired outcome: increased patient knowledge and integration of information into life situations. In 1976, Anon developed a framework, the PLISSIT (*p*ermission, *l*imited *i*nformation, *s*pecific *s*uggestions, *i*ntensive *t*herapy) model, that continues to be applied to sexuality counseling and provides helpful guidelines. By addressing the level of intervention and the comfort of the health care professional, this model enables the right intervention to be provided at the right time for the patient and significant other. The model (1) enables the health care professional to provide a level of support, education, and counseling that is appropriate and (2) facilitates the integration of a team approach as consultants and experienced sex counselors and therapists are used for more in-depth management of sexual care needs (Table 13–1).

Other organized approaches have been established in a variety of settings to address the sexual needs of individuals with chronic illness and disability. In many organized systems of care and special disease management programs, education about alterations in sexual function is provided through individual and group teaching sessions. These sessions are augmented by individual and group educational sessions on topics such as sexuality, developing and maintaining relationships, social skills enhancement, and integration into community and social activities. These interventions reflect the broad continuum of sexuality and sexual function and the need for integration of rehabilitation skills into daily life skills so that the individual can regain and restore confidence in feeling and performance of his or her sexual life as well.

Another framework for addressing sexuality needs of individuals with disability is the Sexual Health Service approach that has been used in British Columbia over the past 20 years (Szaz, 1992). This service uses a sexual health care framework that addresses patient or client needs throughout the course of the disability and comprises a variety of levels of intervention. Perhaps the most interesting concept in this approach is the focus on sexual health as a lifelong requirement for which different issues and needs surface at different times. According to Szaz (1992), a group of individuals in the center are trained as sexual health care clinicians, and their roles incorporate visits and interventions ranging from admission through follow-up and postdischarge care to long-term care or care that is provided many years after onset of disability. This framework addresses the natural course of sexuality and sexual function throughout the life span but within the context of the disability. For example, 5 years after discharge from the rehabilitation setting, unmarried individuals may have entered significant relationships and others may have encountered divorce or widowhood. Given the changes that occur in relationships and individuals, this framework encourages the individual or couple to explore new issues or concerns as they arise through contact with the sexual health clinician. Referrals to specialists such as urologists and gynecologists, to further explore fertility, contraceptive, or sexual performance interventions, may also be recommended at future visits. These visits offer the opportunity to explore the patient's or couple's concerns about sexual response, sexual activity

capabilities, sexual interest and desire, fertility status, hygiene interventions related to bowel and bladder activity, and identification of additional goals.

Szaz (1992) further described two factors that seem to help the patients focus on realistic sex-related goals: (1) the presence of an active, varied, and satisfying sexual relationship before the injury and (2) the presence of an interested and adventurous partner (Zedjik, 1992). Although these recommendations are specific to individuals with spinal cord injury (SCI), they can be applied to other disabilities as well.

Nosek, Rintolk, and Young (1996) have offered an orientation for addressing the sexual needs of individuals with early-onset disabilities. In their study, the needs of individuals with congenital or early-onset physical disability, adolescence-onset disability, and late-onset disability were explored in relation to sexuality issues and concerns, including sexuality information, relationship development and maintenance, societal and environmental barriers and abuse, and health and sexual functioning. These investigators determined that sexual development and concerns in the early-onset disability group focused on needs and issues related to social and environmental challenges, lack of sexual knowledge, parental values and influences, peer relationships, and the ability and opportunity to develop sexual relationships. Concerns of individuals with adolescence-onset disability seem to be related to social adaptation, family issues, self-image, environmental factors including social opportunities, and the actual severity of the disability. Individuals with adult-onset or late-onset physical disability reported changes in sexual function and sexual patterns, interest, self-esteem, and intimacy.

Glass, Mustian, and Carter (1986) commented that "illness and disability remove the patient from accustomed personal, social and sexual interactions, changing the entire life pattern. Feelings of self-worth and attractiveness are threatened at a time when need for intimacy and belonging is greatest, causing a sense of loneliness and isolation." Nosek et al. (1996) pointed out that surveys show that people with physical disabilities may be lacking sexually related knowledge and skills but are unable to acquire needed information or training. In addition, these investigators indicated, individuals with disabilities would like to discuss their sexual problems with health care professionals. A study completed by Cole (1975) found that

TABLE 13–1 ■ PLISSIT MODEL FOR SEXUALITY EDUCATION: APPLICATION TO REHABILITATION PROFESSIONALS

Level of Intervention	Rehabilitation Nursing	Other Rehabilitation Professionals (Examples)
Permission	Rehabilitation nurses provide the patient with the opportunity to identify sexual health needs in the assessment. Identifying sexual health, including nonthreatening questions about menstruation, birth control, pregnancies, and sexual practices and concerns will open the door for discussion at a later time. In addition, a factual data-collecting approach as well as the openness to listen to premorbid and postmorbid sexual history will encourage further discussion. Rehabilitation nurses also have numerous opportunities in which questions or concerns are raised during special care activities, e.g., bladder and bowel routines, dressing activities.	Physical and occupational therapists can address functional issues during their assessment sessions as well. The ability to perform dressing activities, grooming, bathing and other activities of daily living as well as bed mobility, standing, and ambulation activities can be integrated into discussion regarding sexual health and function. Evaluation of the ability to integrate these functions into community and social skills related to dating or couple activity can be part of the baseline assessment. Give the client permission and comfort to explore the application of new routines to his/her sexual life throughout therapy education.
Limited information	The rehabilitation nurse provides limited information in the areas of sexual changes related to the disability or the chronic illness. Information regarding physiological changes and its impact on sexual performance and sexual health should be provided prior to discharge or at the time of the intervention (outpatient or home visit, etc.). Clients should be given literature on the sexual response cycle and how the illness or disability may influence the response.	Therapists and other rehabilitation professionals have the opportunity to provide limited information in the areas of incorporating activities of daily living and mobility methods into routine sexual activity. Patients will want to know that there is a way to incorporate the goals of therapy into other areas of life, including sexual life. A review of basic information for reinforcement or carryover will ensure that the patient has a basic understanding of sexual alteration and function related to activity. Often, the patient shares newly acquired information during therapy or individual or group counseling sessions and begins to request additional information or specific suggestions.
Specific suggestions	Rehabilitation nurses may provide specific suggestions about the management of bowel and bladder function to prevent accidents and to increase the comfort of partners. In addition, specific information regarding the use of safe sexual practices, including appropriate birth control interventions, may be discussed, as well as measures to prevent sexually transmitted diseases.	Therapists may provide specific suggestions about the use of certain positions, mobility aids, assistive devices, and certain techniques to optimize sexual activity. For example, safety techniques on incorporating wheelchair activities into sexual activity may be provided through diagrams and incorporation into therapy skills development. Other information regarding proper positioning to enhance function and avoid problems may also be reviewed.
Intensive therapy	Only nurses who are certified in sexual counseling and therapy should provide intensive therapy to individuals and couples. Nurses may become certified through a process identified by the American Association of Sex Educators, Counselors and Therapists.	Certified Sexual Therapists may provide intensive sexual therapy. Many of these therapists work in conjunction with rehabilitation psychologists and social workers to provide intensive therapy to couples while having a foundation of knowledge based on sexual alterations resulting from the disability.

Modified from Aron, J. S. (1976). The PLISSIT model: A proposed conceptual schema for behavioral treatment of sexual problems. *Journal of Sex Education Therapy, 2,* 1–15.

70% of subjects reported that no attention was given to their sexual adjustment issues during rehabilitation, yet 70% believed an active sex life important to their personal happiness, and 75% wanted explicit sexual information and counseling.

Ducharme, Gill, Beiner-Bergeman, and Fertitta (1993) proposed that health care professionals provide a comprehensive sex education curriculum for adolescents ˙ with disabilities; however, the curriculum's content is also applicable and relevant to adults with disabilities. A program following the curriculum recommended by Ducharme et al. (1993) might address the following topics:

- Basic anatomy and physiology
- Social skills training
- Assertiveness
- Sexual and personal values clarification
- Self-esteem
- Making choices for sexual lifestyle
- Birth control
- Genetic counseling
- Identifying and communicating feelings and sexual needs
- Managing sexual feelings
- Other topics, such as self-pleasuring/masturbation and safe sex practices

The assessment of and identification of patients' sexual needs as well as recommendation of interventions are vital in helping patients, clients, and their partners reestablish and restore a healthy and fulfilling sexual life.

Nosek et al. (1996) identified at least five major concerns of individuals with disabilities, particularly females, related to sexual function and sexuality: (1) the ability to satisfy a partner, (2) the need to feel sexually attractive, (3) the need to be perceived as sexually attractive, and (4) physical issues that influence sexual function and activity, including bowel and bladder management. These researchers also found that individuals with disabilities want more information and teaching about the "how-to" of coping with sexual function changes, helping a partner cope with limitations, and ways to achieve and give satisfaction. This information should be available throughout the individuals' lifetime as their needs and relationships change.

NURSING DIAGNOSIS: ALTERED SEXUALITY PATTERNS AND RELATED NURSING DIAGNOSIS

In addition to understanding the nurse's role in providing sexual health education and in-

terventions, the rehabilitation nurse must have a basic understanding of the impact of altered sexual function on the lives of the individuals for whom they provide care. As defined by NANDA, the nursing diagnosis Altered Sexuality Patterns is the state in which physical conditions or sexual behaviors cause an individual to express concern regarding his or her own sexuality. The major defining characteristics of altered sexuality patterns are difficulties, limitations, or changes in sexual behaviors or activities. Individuals experiencing alterations in sexuality patterns may also have related knowledge deficits concerning sexual changes and responses related to the disability.

For example, a sexually active adolescent male who sustains a complete T12 paraplegia may not understand that the loss of erectile function is due to his spinal cord injury. Losing sexual function while developing a sexual and personal identity compounds the physical losses and adjustments that this individual confronts. A C5-quadriplegic female who has not experienced a menstrual period since her injury 3 months before may believe that unprotected intercourse during a therapeutic home visit will not result in pregnancy. The spouse of the traumatically brain-injured individual may be fully unprepared for and unaware of the reasons for the sexually explicit, uninhibited behaviors that the injured person is displaying in the hospital or other social settings.

Rehabilitation nurses should anticipate corresponding factors that further influence the ability to reestablish sexual patterns. General related factors that contribute to alterations in sexual patterns include alterations in body structure and function. Examples are (1) the loss of or change in the sexual response cycle, (2) the impact of loss of intimate body functions, such as bowel or bladder control, on sexual spontaneity, and (3) the loss of a limb and its effect on body image, sexual function, and positioning. Another factor affecting sexual patterns is the availability of a significant other for a sexual relationship. Many disabled individuals report that the presence or absence of a partner raises or lowers the importance of sexual needs within their daily life. In a focus group of disabled women, the absence of a partner seemed to prevent the disabled female from being considered by health care providers as a sexually interested individual (Kraft-Fine et al., 1996).

Other examples of the influence and presence of a significant other on sexual patterns is observed in the elderly population, in which, if a spouse or significant other is absent, the sexual needs and concerns of the individual are assumed to be nonexistent or may go unaddressed by health care professionals. The concept that the elderly lose interest in sex is a myth that continues to distort societal attitudes, norms, and values, depriving the elderly of physical contact and having their sexual needs met. In addition, the loss of a partner may have an impact on sexual interest, importance, and sexual confidence. The failure of health care professionals to give attention to those issues may further enhance the feelings of isolation and diminished self-esteem that elders experience.

Other factors that further contribute to alterations in sexual patterns are mobility deficits, altered elimination patterns, pain, behavior and/or cognitive abnormalities, impaired verbal communication, and activity intolerance, including fatigue, muscle weakness, and pain or increased muscle tone/spasticity with movement.

Ineffective individual coping and the strain of assuming the caregiver role also contribute significantly to sexual pattern alterations in individuals who have experienced a disability or chronic illness. For the married or live-in partner, the role transition from sexual partner to caregiver may interrupt intimacy and reinforce a parent-child relationship, further affecting sexual roles and activity within the relationship. The rehabilitation nurse must assess for alterations in a variety of related areas.

ASSESSMENT OF SEXUALITY AND ALTERATIONS IN SEXUAL PATTERN

Sexuality and sexual function are typically addressed in the data assessment completed by nurses during the history and physical examination. Questions should include physiological "history" issues, such as preexisting medical conditions that might influence sexual performance, menstrual history, onset of sexual activity, history of sexually transmitted diseases, the use of safe sex practices, problems with sexual function or achieving sexual pleasure, birth control measures and use of condoms, medication regimens, use of over-the-counter products or natural vitamins or minerals, fertility issues, and number of pregnancies and births.

More in-depth discussion regarding sexual performance, sexual preferences and orientation, frequency of activity, and perceived or actual changes in sexual response and activity should also be explored. As a therapeutic relationship is developed, the nurse may obtain information about barriers to sexual pleasure and performance, including fears; physical limitations such as pain, mobility restrictions, plegia or paresis, and spasticity or flaccidity; positioning issues related to endurance, balance, or other motor issues; and sensory impairments. Many of these issues are assessed directly and in a less "threatening" manner by many members of the rehabilitation team as they proceed through their evaluation processes. Coordination of findings, either through an integrated documentation tool or through reporting at team conferences, could facilitate addressing those issues that are of immediate concern to the patient.

Some settings have specific sexual health clinicians who may meet with the patient and partner to explore, discuss, and relate the findings of the history, physical examination, and evaluation process and translate these findings into a plan for managing the patient's and partner's sexual concerns. Specific cultural and ethnic needs may need to be identified to best meet the patient's needs and comfort level when addressing sexual concerns. For some patients, having age-related or gender-related issues with a specific nurse or therapist may interfere with the patient's comfort with and ability to address sexual concerns. It is imperative that the nurse, physician, and members of the treatment team recognize and respect cultural differences and preferences of patients. Providing permission to discuss and explore issues with the physician, nurse, and any treatment team member with whom the patient is comfortable and who is prepared to inform and counsel provides an optimal outcome for the patient and partner. It is also crucial to reinforce with the patient that refusal to answer any questions or to discuss sexual issues will be respected by the nurse and the treatment team. Identifying key individuals who are accountable to the patient and the team for reporting and responding to sexual issues and concerns is paramount to meeting these issues, which may easily go unaddressed if each team member believes that "someone else" on the team has responded to these concerns.

With either an integrated history-taking session or a separate sexual counseling or history-taking session, the needs and issues of the patient will be determined. From this session, further counseling and follow-up interventions may be provided by the nurse or other members of the treatment team, depending on individual skill and knowledge and the patient's comfort.

The physical examination, completed primarily by the physician, nurse, physical therapist, occupational therapist, and speech therapist, provides a wealth of information that addresses the physical components of sexual activity and performance. The physical examination components, including breast and genitalia examination, offers an opportunity for the examiner and patient to discuss questions relevant to sexual concerns. The physician or nurse may introduce questions related to the history or may explore the patient's comfort with self-examination and discussion of other sexually related issues that may arise. For example, the patient's ability to perform bowel and bladder management and other hygiene activities will alert the team to issues relevant to sexual performance. The patient's ability to transfer, use bed mobility techniques, and perform dressing activities, and the assessment of other functional areas, will help the team and the patient identify issues that might contribute to sexual performance.

Additional components, including neurosensory examination, contribute to the sexual history and physical examination. Sensorimotor testing for pin, pain, and temperature in saddle sensation testing of sacral dermatomes (S2–S4) will help to determine extent of genital sensation, identify intact spinal centers, and identify whether the patient may experience orgasms. According to Yarkony and Chen (1995), the spinal centers related to erection are in the sympathetic preganglionic fibers from T11 to L2 and the parasympathetic fibers from S2 through S4. The parasympathetic and sympathetic systems work synergistically to produce erections. Reflex erections are mediated via the sacral parasympathetics with sensory input from the pudendal nerve, with T10 being the critical level for gonadal sensation. Sensation is transmitted through the afferent roots of these nerves, entering the spinal cord at the T10 level; if pain is elicited through testicle squeezing, reflexogenic and psychogenic erections are possible. When the pathways to the supraspinal centers are intact, psychogenic stimuli (tactile or visual stimuli, sexual thoughts) may inhibit or facilitate an erectile response. The presence of the bulbocavernosus reflex, which is elicited through compression of the penis or the clitoris during performance of a rectal will determine whether the sacral reflex arc is intact. If rectal tightening is obtained, then reflex activity in the sacral area is preserved and reflex erections will occur. The sensory component of the sacral reflex arc is elicited through the application of a pinprick to the anus; if the arc is intact, the pinprick will result in contraction of the anus. This sign is another positive indicator that reflex activity and erectile function are preserved.

Most often, these findings are sufficient to determine the extent of genital sexual response. Erections are a vascular phenomenon. On occasion, additional testing is completed, such as pharmacological injection of the penis with vasodilators. This test determines the integrity of the vascular system of the penis; if erection does not occur, vascular compromise is suspected. Penile biotheisometry and dorsal somatosensory-evoked potential testing will provide additional information regarding the intactness of sensory and dorsal nerves. If dorsal nerve endings are compromised, as seen in diabetes, alcoholism, and vascular insufficiencies, erectile dysfunction could result (Horn & Zasler, 1990). Other laboratory and diagnostic testing may be indicated, such as hormonal assays (helpful in determining low testosterone levels), vascular assessments, nocturnal penile tumescence with sleep electroencephalogram, and routine blood chemistry.

Finally, the ability to ejaculate and sperm quality, motility, and number may be compromised in the neurologically impaired male. Compromise of these areas is detected through sperm assays.

Inspection of the skin of the genitalia will alert the clinician and the patient to the presence of lesions, infection, discharges, mucosal dryness, irritation, and trauma and reveal the integrity of perineal, ischial, and sacral skin. Integration of questions regarding sexual practices and history of sexually transmitted diseases into the performance of the physical examination may help the patient feel more comfortable with the examination. Inquiring about safe sex practices and the use of condoms or other barrier methods may help the patient become comfortable with the clinicians. In this way, factual and informative integration of sexual health with information may be accomplished through the physical examination.

SEXUAL RESPONSE CYCLE: NORMAL PHYSIOLOGY AND RESPONSE

Nurses and other clinicians who provide information, education, and counseling to patients about sexual concerns and issues must have a basic understanding of the sexual response cy-

TABLE 13–2 ■ THE SEXUAL RESPONSE CYCLE IN MALES AND FEMALES

Phase	Control Centers	Male Response	Female Response
Excitement	Brainstem for arousal and alertness, thalamus, hippocampus, amygdala, frontal cortex, tactile centers, testosterone	Psychogenic (imagination) or reflexogenic (touch) arousal; nipples and penis erect, scrotal tightening and rising, testicular swelling and rising, ↑ heart rate (HR), BP, respiration	Psychogenic (imagination) or reflexogenic (touch) arousal; nipple, clitoral erection, skin flushing, breast swelling, vaginal lubrication, vaginal, labial swelling, cervix elevates, ↑ heart rate, BP, respiration
Plateau	High level of arousal in cortical and subcortical centers as listed above, sympathetic and parasympathetic responses	Increased testicular size and anterior rotation against perineum, vascular engorgement of penile shaft and glans, darkening and enlargement of glans, Cowper's secretion, increased muscle contraction	Continuation of vaginal expansion, clitoral and nipple erection, swelling, spreading of flushing to abdomen, breasts, and chest wall, increased muscle contraction
Orgasm	Triggered by neural reflex once stimulus threshold obtained; sympathetic control	Rhythmic contractions of penis, pelvic muscles, prostate; ejaculation of sperm, prostatic, vas deferens secretions; internal bladder sphincter closure; ↑ HR, BP, respiration	Rhythmic contraction of uterus, anal sphincter, outer third of vagina; peripheral muscle contraction, multiple orgasms possible; clitoral retraction; ↑ HR, BP, respiration
Relaxation/resolution	Reversal of vasocongestion; refractory period; sympathetic input decreased	Ejaculation will not occur again; erection may be maintained or lost; scrotal sac returns to size; muscle relaxation; nipple engorgement reduced	Uterus, vagina, and clitoris return to normal size and location; successive orgasms can occur; nipple engorgement reduced; muscle relaxation

Adapted from Masters, W. H., Johnson, V. E., and Kolodny, R. C. (1986). *Masters and Johnson On sex and the human body.* Boston: Little, Brown.

cle and the influence of major body systems on this cycle. Table 13–2 identifies the major components of the sexual response cycle and describes the changes that occur throughout these phases. Masters and Johnson (1966) identified the major stages of sexual response: (1) excitement, (2) plateau, (3) orgasm, and (4) resolution. The stages are part of a cycle or a process that individuals experience both physically and psychologically. Alterations in any stage of the sexual response cycle can occur with disability, chronic disease or illness, and other life-altering events.

Table 13–3 provides a framework for assessing the extent of sexual problems related to sexual performance.

ALTERATIONS IN SEXUAL ACTIVITY PATTERNS IN COMMON DISABILITIES

Stroke and Altered Sexual Activity Patterns

The individual who has experienced a cerebrovascular attack may experience a range of functional and cognitive impairments relative to the location, extent, and severity of the stroke. Although physiological mechanisms of arousal are thought to be preserved after a stroke, subjective aspects of arousal may be impaired by medications and other comorbid conditions such as diabetes. In addition, sensory deficits following a stroke may make arousal more difficult. Depending on the extent of cerebral damage, males may experience partial or absence of erection, retarded and/or retrograde ejaculation, and inability to maintain erection (Garlinghouse, 1987). Females may experience decreased vaginal lubrication, anorgasmia, pain, and altered sensation on the affected side, including the genital area. Other deficits are disinhibition or hypersexuality, decreased libido, lack of or poor erection, absence of ejaculation, poor vaginal lubrication, orgasmic difficulty, poor satisfaction or lack of enjoyment of sexual activity, and altered mobility from the plegia or paresis (Garlinghouse, 1987; Monga & Ostermann, 1995).

Some of the challenges that face the individual and sexual partner after a stroke are

TABLE 13–3 ■ ASSESSING THE EXTENT OF SEXUAL PROBLEMS RELATED TO SEXUAL PERFORMANCE

Nursing Diagnosis	Description
1. Sexual dysfunction, altered sexuality pattern.	Lack of or compromised ability to respond to those activities or behaviors associated with stimulation of the erogenous zones. Sexual dysfunction describes perceived problems in achieving sexual satisfaction and includes clients with limitations on sexual expression imposed by disease or therapy.
2. Body image disturbance, personal identity disturbance, self-esteem disturbance.	Lowered self-concept caused by impaired motor or sensory function, pain, fatigue, disfigurement, loss of control, loss of independence, social isolation, or depression. Body image disturbance is closely related to self-esteem disturbance and describes negative feelings or perceptions about characteristics, functions, or limits of the body or body parts.
3. Social isolation.	Lack of or limited ability for social interaction because of impaired motor or sensory function or self-imposed isolation. May result from voluntary or therapeutic isolation. Related factors include physical disability; cognitive impairment; emotional handicap, including but not limited to depression, anxiety; fear of embarrassment; rejection, environmental hazard, incontinence; body image changes; sensory losses; loss of employment; loss of transportation; insufficient community resources; dissonance.
4. Knowledge deficits.	Lack of knowledge regarding alternative ways to achieve sexual functioning; lack of knowledge regarding birth control; alternatives to usual sexual activities. Related factors include onset of disability; low readiness for reception of information, amotivation; cognitive impairments; psychomotor changes; uncompensated memory loss; inability to use materials or information due to language or cultural barriers.

From Eneco, S. (1995). *Rehabilitation nursing: Process and applications.* Chicago: C. V. Mosby.

- Acknowledging and adjusting to altered libido and, possibly, frequency (increased or decreased)
- Personality changes and, possibly, depression
- Decreased excitement
- Impaired pleasure response due to fear, pain, or psychological issues
- Altered mobility and physical performance due to paralysis
- Altered communication processes from aphasias and visual alterations, which may interfere with verbal and nonverbal cuing during sexual activity

Personality changes resulting from hemispheric damage contribute to the complexity of poststroke sexual adjustment for the individual and partner. For example, the patient with a stroke affecting the left hemisphere may be cautious, hesitant, and labile, whereas the patient with a stroke in the right hemisphere may be impulsive and uninhibited. Role change, self-esteem, body image alterations, grief, and depression as well as fear of a second stroke further influence the dynamics of the individual as a sexual person and

the dynamics of any relationship (Ducharme et al., 1993).

It is critical that accurate information be provided to the stroke survivor and partner. Probably the most significant concern related to sexual function is the fear that sexual excitement and activity will bring on another stroke. Research in stabilized ischemic stroke indicates that recurrence or progression of a cerebrovascular accident as a result of sexual activity is unlikely (Agency for Health Policy and Research, 1995). Health care professionals must reassure the individual and partner that sexual activity is not contraindicated after a stroke.

Individuals who have experienced motor changes resulting in problems of coordination or balance as well as weakness or spasm may benefit from incorporating positioning techniques that will support the hemiplegic side with pillows. Use of the pillows leaves the unaffected side available for touching and caressing. The side-lying position allows freedom of movement for both partners while increasing comfort and support for the paralyzed side. Supine positioning with the affected extremities supported may also be helpful for the hemiparetic patient if shoulder pain is present. Although sensory dysfunction may be present in the hemiplegic patient, sexual stimulation and sensory arousal may still occur through the visual stimulus of watching one's partner touching the entire body. Both partners need to recognize and adjust for the effects of motor, sensory, and attention deficits and for easy fatigue during sexual activity. Planning for intimacy may help increase the likelihood of a positive and pleasuring experience for both partners.

A few successful strategies are communicating needs for touching as well as expressing needs in an unhurried manner. Allowing adequate time for positioning and pleasuring might also help to avoid fatigue and stress for the couple (McCormick, 1986; Sjorgen & Fugl-Meyer, 1981).

As discussed earlier, erectile dysfunction may occur as a result of the stroke, comorbid conditions (e.g., vascular disease, diabetes), and some medications used to control hypertension or depression, including antidepressants, hypnotics, and thiazides. History taking at poststroke visits should address both medication compliance and any side effects that may result in an alteration in function,

including sexual function (U.S. Department of Health and Human Services, 1996).

For individuals experiencing erectile dysfunction, a few invasive and noninvasive options exist. The use of a vacuum erection device, such as the Erec Aid Hand Pump System or the Erec Aid–Plus Battery Operated System, help to produce and maintain an erection. Through the vacuum-like suction, the penis is able to become erect, and a rigid ring is placed at the base of the penis to help sustain the erection for approximately 30 minutes. The device must be prescribed by a physician, and counseling must be provided as to the use of the device, because damage to the penile shaft, tissue, infection or irritation to the urinary tract could result from improper use. Occasionally, ejaculation and pain or numbness may also result from use of such devices. Education of the user and partner is essential in preventing complications and maintaining awareness of early signs of infection or tissue trauma (Fig. 13–1).

Another more widely used intervention that helps to sustain erections is the use of penile pharmacological injections of vasodilator agents, such as papaverine, phentolamine, and alprostadil (prostaglandin E$_1$). The injec-

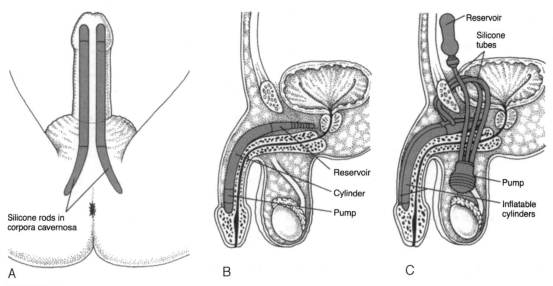

FIGURE 13–1

Penile prostheses. *A*, Semirigid prosthesis consists of rods inserted into the corpora cavernosa via a perineal or dorsal penile incision. The penis remains in a constant state of semierection. *B*, Self-contained penile prosthesis consists of a pump, a cylinder, and a reservoir, all in a single unit. The client squeezes the pump just below the head of the penis to fill the cylinder and achieve erection. *C*, Inflatable penile prosthesis consists of two hollow silicone cylinders, an abdominal reservoir, and a scrotal pump. The client squeezes the pump to fill the cylinders and achieve erection. (From Ignatavicius, D. D., Workman, M. L., and Mishler, M. A. [1999]. *Medical-surgical nursing across the health care continuum* [3rd ed.]. Philadelphia: W. B. Saunders).

tion, which is inserted directly into the penile shaft (corpus cavernosum), affects erection through vasodilation. Occasionally, subcutaneous bleeding from improper injection technique can occur. Priapism, a sustained erection lasting longer than 4 hours, which could result in penile tissue damage, ischemia, and necrosis, may also occur. Individuals should be instructed about (1) the potential adverse effects of this intervention, (2) when and how to seek emergency medical treatment, and (3) the importance of adhering exactly to the prescribed medication regimen for injection (Girdley, Bruskewitz, & Feyzi, 1988).

Another alternative for the treatment of erectile dysfunction is the use of surgical penile implants. Semirigid and inflatable implants (see Fig. 13–1) are available and provide an alternative to the injection and vacuum suction options. Surgical implants for erectile function have been widely accepted since the 1970s. Individuals and partners may find this a more acceptable and "natural" alternative, in that they are not externally applied and are easily incorporated into sexual activity (Golgi, 1979). Other noninvasive interventions for erectile dysfunction include oral medication agents such as L-dopa and yohimbine. Yohimbine hydrochloride, a natural α-adrenergic blocking agent, depresses the inhibitory fibers that prevent erections and may increase libido. Controlled clinical trials demonstrated that this agent has only limited efficacy whether it is used as monotherapy or in combination with methyltestosterone and vitamins or a caffeine-containing stimulant. The use of testosterone injections to increase libido and erectile function in individuals whose erectile dysfunction may be secondary to low serum testosterone levels has also been a treatment option (Horn & Zasler, 1990).

In 1996, sildenafil (Viagra), a phosphodiesterase inhibitor that was originally developed to treat angina pectoris, was found to be a very effective agent for the treatment of impotence. Sildenafil inhibits type V cyclic guanosine monophosphate (cGMP), which is the predominant phosphodiesterase enzyme. Inhibition of the phosphodiesterase enzymes causes the smooth muscle cells of the corpus cavernosum to relax, increasing the blood flow into the cavernosal spaces. This greater blood flow leads to higher intercavernosal pressure, a major factor in producing an erection (Boolell, Gepi-Attee, & Gingell, 1996). The adverse effects of sildenafil include headache, flushing, dyspnea, and muscle aches. Sildenafil potentiates the hypotensive effects of nitrates, so its administration to patients who are currently using organic nitrates in any form is contraindicated. Deaths have been reported in individuals who are using nitrates and sildenafil (Anonymous, 1996).

For females who have experienced a stroke, sexuality and sexual functioning issues are minimally addressed and underreported. Issues such as loss of interest, lack of initiation, lack of active or passive role playing, lack of communication of sexual needs, provision of adequate and supportive positioning, and facilitation of sexual pleasure, including the ability to achieve sexual satisfaction and pleasure, continue to be minimally addressed in the literature. Concerns regarding vaginal lubrication and diminished genital sensation are reported. The use of topical agents for vaginal lubrication, such as water-soluble lubricants or estrogen creams, may help minimize the discomfort of sexual activity. Exploring the genital areas and other erogenous zones for areas that have preserved sensation will help the patient and partner to restore touching and pleasuring through exploration as part of their sexual routine.

For stroke survivors of both sexes, instruction about and reinforcement of safe sex practices might not be reinforced or reviewed because of the health care practitioner's age bias or belief that exposure to sexually transmitted diseases is limited in these patients. The practitioner should be aware of this bias.

Brain Injury and Altered Sexual Activity Patterns

Alterations in sexual activity patterns in the brain-injured patient usually mirror the extent of cognitive, emotional, and psychosocial issues experienced by the individual. According to Zasler and Horn (1990), traumatic brain injury can result in sexual problems due to both cognitive and genital dysfunction. Genital dysfunction may result in erectile dysfunction, ejaculatory problems, orgasmic dysfunction, problems with vaginal lubrication, and vaginismus. Nongenital problems that may adversely affect sexual intimacy include sensorimotor deficits, linguistic-pragmatic deficits, perceptual deficits, limited joint range of motion, neurogenic bowel or bladder dysfunction, dysphagia with or without problems controlling secretions, motor dyspraxias, posttraumatic behavioral deficits, and alterations in self-image and self-esteem (Horn & Zasler, 1990).

Major cortical and subcortical centers that

are affected during brain assault influence the extent of alterations in sexual performance. At the cortical level, both frontal and temporal areas are involved in sexual behavior; most often, these areas are directly affected by brain trauma. Damage to the frontal areas may result in disinhibition of or loss of initiative or interest in sexual activity. Temporal lobe injuries may result in behavioral alterations, including reduced sexual drive. Although once considered common, hypersexuality in the brain-injured adult is rare and is usually associated with damage to the amygdala. Increased sexual activity as a result of the disinhibition of behavior is common in patients with frontal lobe injuries. Subcortical centers such as the hypothalamus may occasionally be affected by head injury, resulting in altered sexual behavior as a result of changes in control and production of hormones.

Other alterations from brain injury include emotional lability and cognitive alterations resulting in alterations in problem-solving, planning, and sequencing of activities. As patients begin to recover through the phases of rehabilitation, a variety of issues related to sexual function, behavior, and relationships are observed.

During the acute stage of recovery, self-stimulation, including genital fondling, oral stimulation, and masturbation, may be observed by the nurse and the treatment team. Patients should be provided with privacy for these behaviors but also should be given socially appropriate feedback about them. For example, patients may need behavioral reinforcement and cuing regarding the social inappropriateness of performing these behaviors in public settings.

Health care practitioners must treat sexually explicit behavior and communications in a behaviorally controlled manner, providing feedback to the individual while also helping the partner or caregivers understand the nature of and stimulus for these behaviors. Basic reeducation in socially appropriate skills related to social-sexual behaviors is essential in the reintegration of the brain-injured client into the community. The treatment teams in acute and postacute care settings must work together to establish appropriate behavior patterns.

Often, persistent sexual dysfunction may lead to relationship dissatisfaction and separation. The partner of the patient in whom sexual apathy has occurred may experience frustration and dissatisfaction with the relationship. Counseling in this situation can address how to manage or restore sexual interest in a safe, simplified, nonthreatening manner.

For patients who are disinhibited, behavioral management and intervention become the focus of the team, the partner, and the family. Cognitive retraining for impulse control, desensitization of the patient for public or social situations, and preteaching of the patient to avoid behaviorally inappropriate behaviors in social situations may help reduce disinhibition within social contexts. Redirection, providing alternative motor activities for distraction, changing the environment and stimuli, and using positive reinforcement for socially appropriate behaviors reinforce the desired behavior.

Significant role changes occur after a brain injury. Most often, the patient is impaired in thought processing and memory, changes that may significantly influence current or future relationships. Sexual and individual identity is confused and disrupted. According to Greco (1995), sexual function is a high-level social skill that requires planning, preparation, and anticipation. Each of these areas is affected in traumatic brain injury and will alter the individual's ability to perceive and anticipate the needs of a partner. Intimacy and sexual expression may be significantly affected. Confusion regarding sexual behavior, orientation, and relationships is common. Significant impact on self-esteem and self-image should be anticipated.

Partners and family members may also exhibit difficulties with managing these cognitive and behavioral changes. Often, partners and sometimes parents of the head-injured individual may be affected by the injury because it affects their relationship, roles, and role functions. Parents who assume the responsibility of caregiver for the adult child may experience anger, frustration, and guilt in their relationship. Partners of the injured individual may be unable to manage the caregiver role and the conflict associated with being a sexual partner. Attention to verbal and nonverbal or indirectly expressed concerns regarding sexual behavior and sexual needs must be addressed by the team. Providing an ongoing assessment of behavior and related concerns helps the brain-injured individual, partner, and family members develop consistent interventions and determine the success of those interventions.

Patients who have experienced traumatic brain injury, their partners, and their family members will benefit from basic sex education as well as instruction about alterations in function as a result of the injury, fertility and contraceptive issues, and social-sexual behavioral interventions. Areas that may be discussed in individual and group sessions include

- Adjustment to the injury
- Impact of the injury on the individual, partner, couple, and family system
- Social and sexual values and norms
- Relationship issues
- Family and role adjustment

Incorporation of role playing as well as the relearning of socially appropriate expectations, interactional skills, basic social activities, and the consequences of behavior will help the brain-injured individual relearn and reintegrate with more opportunity for social success and safety.

Contraception management remains a crucial concern for clients with brain injury and their partners. Executive function impairments affect the ability to organize, plan, reason, and judge situations. Providing for proper planning, cuing, and incorporating birth control methods into routines is essential. In addition to concerns about contraception, the individual must have a simple, practical plan for avoiding unsafe sex practices. Reinforcement of the use of condoms and other barrier methods with sexual activity is probably the simplest "take home" message that should become an automatic behavior to minimize risk of contact.

Prelearning about safe sex practices and awareness of the influence of other medication regimens on birth control measures are crucial. Medications such as antileptics and antibiotics may interfere with the effectiveness of oral contraceptives. The patient or caregiver must be aware of potential problems related to possibly unprotected sexual activity in these situations and may need to take an active and intervening role in ensuring safe sex practices and contraceptive interventions. For the brain-injured client, choices regarding birth control, including oral, barrier, and surgical methods, must be reviewed and explored and consultation provided so that the best choice can be made by the individual. Guardian intervention in this area remains challenging and presents ethical dilemmas in preserving the right of the individual while providing for client sexual safety.

Spinal Cord Injury and Alterations in Sexual Activity Patterns

The typical profile of a person who sustains a spinal cord injury (SCI) is young, male (82%), usually between the ages of 16 and 45 years (79.6%), single (53.5%), and either employed or a student at the time of injury. The remaining 18 to 20% of spinal cord injuries are sustained by females.

These trends, which have been reported over a 20-year period by the Model System's National Spinal Cord Injury Database, define a pattern of incidence and attention to male sexual function with this disability. According to Stover, DeLisa, and Whiteneck (1996), this attention is primarily due to the higher ratio of males to females with SCI. It may also be due to the external nature of men's genitalia (and perhaps the ease of studying the effect of SCI) and the previous societal bias that women's sexual functioning is limited to procreation. As described earlier in this chapter, the sexual needs and concerns of the male with SCI have been investigated thoroughly over the past 20 years. Much is known about the anticipated changes and interventions for alterations in erection, ejaculation, fertility, and other areas of sexual function. Most data and information regarding females and alterations in sexual function, until recently, have been anecdotal or identified through surveys and self-reporting. Sipski, Alexander, and Rosen (1995) have attempted to provide more clinical data on women with SCI and sexual function and life after injury.

After an SCI, men experience alterations in erection, ejaculation, fertility, sexuality, role, and sexual behavior. According to Szas (1992), the neurological site of the mental or sensory aspect of orgasmic experience is unknown. However, the physical events associated with orgasm, including ejaculation, vaginal lubrication, and vaginal response, seem to be located in the T12 to L2 and S2 to S4 segments of the spinal cord. Ejaculatory function is controlled through T12 to L2 spinal cord segments, which influence sperm motility, contraction of the seminal vesicles, injection of semen into the prostate, prostatic fluid secretion, and closure of the internal sphincter of the bladder neck. At the same time, the S2 to S4 segments send signals to relax the external sphincter of the bladder and to initiate contraction of the urethra, causing forward ejaculation of the seminal fluid. In females, the T12 to L2 and S2 to S4 segments provide for innervation of the vaginal walls, resulting in their swelling, lubrication, and widening.

As defined by Szas (1992), the neurological sites mediating the orgasmic sensations are unknown; however, the spinothalamic tracts are the main signal conductors between the genitalia and the thalamus region of the brain. The extent and type of motor and sensory cord damage as well as the level of injury determine the extent of alterations to the normal sexual response cycle in the male or female with SCI. In complete injuries, the brain becomes disconnected from the spinal cord segments below the level of injury, and a disconnect in ascending and descending neural responses occurs. In incomplete injuries, motor or sensory preservation at and below the level of the spinal cord injury influences the extent of sexual function and the alterations experienced.

It is important to note, however, that incomplete injuries may not always result in more preservation of sexual function. According to Szas (1992), the degree of preserved sexual function depends on the extent of damage to specific pathways and cellular structures. Incomplete injuries to the spinal cord may result in an interference with reflex arc function but may also receive additional inhibitory control from preserved cortical pathways that may further influence or impair sexual response.

Physiological changes in males with SCI are as follows. Individuals who have an intact sacral reflex arc will have preserved erectile function. These injuries are typically classified as upper motor neuron injuries. In upper motor neuron injuries, the sacral reflex arc (S2–S4) is intact, and stimulation to these nerve roots through tactile, pressure, pain, or other sensory input results in an erection. Sensory input to the S2 to S4 nerve roots through touching, oral stimulation, pressure, or certain positioning helps sustain erections. Comarr (1970), an earlier researcher of SCI dysfunction, noted that 93% of males with upper motor neuron injuries had reflex erections, and only 4% of these individuals were able to have ejaculations. Comarr also determined that males with upper motor neuron complete injuries were unable to have psychogenic (or psychologically induced or controlled) erections. Males with incomplete SCI, in which motor and sensory function are preserved, may have a greater chance of achieving psychogenic and reflexogenic erections; the rate of ejaculatory ability also increases from 4 to 32%.

Spinal cord injuries that result in complete lower motor neuron damage—that is, damage directly to the sacral reflex arc (S2–S4)—result in alterations of erectile and ejaculatory functions. In this type of injury, the touch-stimulation based erection is not achievable; however, a psychogenic erection resulting in penile swelling, a mild erection, and seminal fluid leakage may occur. Men who have experienced incomplete lower motor neuron injuries have a greater likelihood of experiencing combined reflex and psychogenic erections (90%) and are more likely to experience ejaculation (70%).

Sperm motility, production, and concentration are decreased after a SCI. Recurrent urinary tract infections and retrograde ejaculations into the bladder significantly alter fertility. Over the past 20 years, techniques to improve ejaculatory function and sperm retrieval have been explored and enhanced (Brindley, 1981). Electroejaculation is used to harvest sperm through transrectal electrical stimulation of the hypogastric plexus, with an anoscopy performed before and after stimulation to assess for mucosal damage. This electrical stimulation procedure results in sperm emission. Bladder catheterization is also completed at the end of the procedure to harvest sperm that have traveled retrograde. The sperm are then harvested, and follow-up in vitro fertilization, embryo transfer, and artificial insemination trials have resulted in successful pregnancies. Individuals with injuries above T6, who are susceptible to autonomic dysreflexia, may be treated prophylactically during the procedure to avoid a hyperreflexic episode due to the electrical stimulation. Another technique that is successful in sperm retrieval is electrovibration to the tip of the penis, which may result in ejaculation and can be performed independently by the client and his partner. This technique is effective in men with injuries above T10 and may produce seminal emissions. This technique may also stimulate autonomic hyperreflexia and should only be used under the direction of a physician and by individuals who are aware of interventions to minimize or avoid hyperreflexia. More work needs to be done on fertility and the man with SCI and his partner. Despite the techniques and an increased attentiveness to the urological and sexual health of men with SCI, only a small number of successful births have resulted from these fertility interventions to date (Stover et al., 1995).

Interventions for achieving and maintaining erections were described in the discussion of stroke. Since 1970, penile implants have been used for erectile dysfunction in men with SCI. Concerns about the occurrence of urinary tract and soft tissue infections with the use of such implants were identified in this population. Today, other methods, including the corpus cavernosum injection and vacuum suction, have been widely applied. Model System SCI data show that 22 of 72 men reported complications with the injections, whereas of 19 men who used penile implants, 15 reported mechanical failure, 9 reported infections, and others reported late erosion of the implant through the urethra. Of the 19 patients who reported penile implant use, many had second surgical implantations. However, 14 of the 19 patients reported satisfaction with their implants. Vacuum constriction devices (suction) have been successfully used since 1986. Complications reported for this intervention in the man with SCI include skin irritation, edema, sweating, and penile erythema.

The newest intervention for achieving and maintaining erections is the surface application of nitroglycerin, which causes vasodilation of the corpus cavernosum. The introduction of a male transurethral suppository (MUSE) has provided men with erectile dysfunction with another alternative for the treatment of impotence. Because (1) the long-term risks of repeated corpus cavernosum injections remain a concern and (2) many experience aversion to penile self-injection, this alternative noninvasive treatment option may prove to be safer and as effective. The transurethral applicator is inserted 3 cm into the urethra, a button on the end of the applicator is pressed, and the medication, alprostadil, is deposited against the urethral mucosa (Hellstron, Gesundheit, et al., 1996). Local absorption relaxes smooth muscle, resulting in rapid arterial inflow and penile rigidity. The erectile process is initiated within 5 to 10 minutes of application. Use of no more than two systems (applications) of the suppository is recommended within a 24-hour period. Reported side effects of this use of alprostadil include mild to moderate transient urogenital pain, hypotension, and dizziness. Sustained erection was rarely reported by the study trial's participants.

When priapism occurs in a man with SCI, pseudoephedrine promotes resolution. Use of a transurethral suppository is contraindicated in clients with anuria, a long-term indwelling catheter, prior penile surgery, sickle-cell disease, unstable angina, recent myocardial in-

farction, poorly controlled diabetes, and congestive heart failure.

Sildenafil, the oral medication for erectile dysfunction described earlier in the discussion of stroke, has also been reported to have provided significant improvement in erectile response in 83% of trial subjects with SCI. However, men with SCI who use this agent should be assessed for its potentiated hypotensive effect.

Women with SCI experience alterations in their ability to experience orgasms and may have altered genital response to sexual stimulation, both tactile and psychogenic. Sexual response in females is influenced at the T11 to L1 and S2 to S4 spinal segments. Vaginal changes, including swelling of the vagina, expansion of the inner third of the vagina, clitoral erection, and vaginal lubrication, occur as a result of sensory or tactile stimulation of the genitalia or psychic stimulation. After a spinal cord injury, alterations in these areas as well as in orgasmic response have been reported. Through stimulation of areas that are sensorily and motorly intact, sexual pleasure may be achieved. If an injury is incomplete, physiological orgasms may be achieved in women with SCI. Sipski et al. (1995) reported that 50% of women with SCI can achieve orgasm. Charlifue, Gerhart, Menter, et al. (1992), in their study of sexual issues of women with SCI, noted that either genital or genital and breast stimulation was frequently used in achieving orgasms, although the orgasms reported were less intense and took longer to achieve. Both of these studies identified variability in quadriplegic and paraplegic females in achieving orgasms; however, perceived orgasms were not related to the level of injuries. Subjects in these studies also reported the ability to achieve multiple orgasms after injury.

Leyson studied the physiological response of 10 women with SCI to sexual stimulation. This work represents one of the few studies actually measuring physiological response, consisting of vaginal and rectal contractions, blood pressure, heart rate, respirations, and other responses. Sipski et al. (1995) also emphasized the need to study lubrication responses using psychophysiological techniques, including vaginal photoplethysmography, to determine the extent of reflex or psychologically mediated lubrication.

Another sexual alteration experienced by women with SCI is amenorrhea for at least 3 to 5 months after onset of the injury. Studies indicate that dysmenorrhea remains present after injury and that dysreflexia (autonomic hyperreflexia) is also common during menstruation. Some women with SCI also experience the challenge of managing feminine hygiene with compromised upper extremity and hand function and mobility challenges. A focus group of women with SCI identified that tampons were the preferred method for feminine hygiene and rated instructing attendants to help with insertion and changes of tampons as an important task in activities of daily living, in order to avoid the risk of toxic shock syndrome from infrequent tampon changing. Sipski et al. (1995) reported that many women with SCI have requested hysterectomy as a functional convenience to allow for greater independence and to avoid having to manage these problems. Clearly, this choice may seem a drastic intervention and should be evaluated carefully, with consideration given to all issues related to future family planning needs.

Women with SCI continue to be fertile after injury. Therefore, they must use birth control measures. Table 13–4 identifies common birth control measures and their implications and considerations for women with SCI. More research is needed in the area of oral contracep-

TABLE 13–4 ■ CONTRACEPTIVE INTERVENTIONS FOR WOMEN WITH DISABILITIES

Method	Lowest Expected Failure Rate	Intervention/Evaluation for Women with Disabilities
Spermicidal jellies, creams, and foams	3%	Requires ability to grasp inserter with universal cuff or other assistive device; or partner participation with insertion.
Diaphragm	6%	Requires ability to flex diaphragm for insertion, abduct extremities, and be able to check for placement. May require additional evaluation if female has had chronic UTI. Partner may assist with insertion. May need to empty bladder prior to insertion to avoid bladder emptying if female has neurogenic bladder.
Cervical cap	6%	Should be used with all sexual activity to avoid risk of STD and HIV. Partner will need to assist females with limited hand function, if activity is incorporated into sexual foreplay.
Condom	2%	Male partner will need to assist with holding condom with penile withdrawing post coitus.
Combination pills	0.1%	May be contraindicated in disabilities causing significant mobility/motor impairment due to incidence of deep vein thrombophlebitis secondary to decreased venous return, increased risk for undetected lower extremity trauma. Studies exploring risk. Female may choose to take OC with knowledge of risk and will need to sign consent regarding understanding of increased risk.
Progestin-only pills	0.5%	
Depo-Provera	0.4%	
Progestin	0.04%	
Intrauterine device	0.8% 2.0%	Many state that this method is contraindicated due to risk for infection since S&S of infection may go undetected (PID, UTI). Many disabled females, however, choose this method as the most convenient, least risky, and more predictable form of contraception. Decreases feelings of dependency on others and partners. May need to sign release with knowledge of risks and side effects noted.
Tubal ligation	0.2%	Should be considered permanent. May be suggested in females with traumatic brain injury and other significant cognitive impairments wherever contraceptive steps may be confused or may be not followed due to memory impairments. Controversial/ethical issue regarding competency/self-determination in long-term management of TBI; MR.

From Burtosa, H., Zellura, M., Pierro, L., & Rothacker, C. (1993). Women with spinal cord injuries require sensitive reproductive care. *Maternal Child Nursing Journal, 8,* 254–257.

HIV, human immunodeficiency virus; MR, mental retardation; OC, oral contraceptives; PID, pelvic inflammatory disease; S&S, signs and symptoms; STD, sexually transmitted disease; TBI, traumatic brain injury; UTI, urinary tract infection.

tive measures because oral methods have been linked to higher incidence of deep vein thrombophlebitis in noninjured women with a history of cigarette smoking. Because of their limited mobility, venous stasis, and possible prior history of deep vein thrombophlebitis, women with SCI must avoid oral contraceptives; these agents must be prescribed very cautiously, with close monitoring of the client, who should be informed of the increased risk for thrombophlebitis and its sequelae.

Intrauterine devices (IUDs) have also been identified as potential problems for women with SCI. The use of these devices may lead to pelvic infections or pelvic inflammatory disease, whose signs and symptoms may go undetected in the insensate woman with SCI whose urinary system is compromised. Reviewing safe sexual practices remains critical in educating all patients about sexual function. Tables 13–5 and 13–6 describe how to address sexual activity concerns related to sexually transmitted diseases and adherence to safe sex practices with partners.

Because only 20% of all SCIs occur in females, research in the areas of pregnancy and childbearing is also limited. Challenges related to managing pregnancy and SCI include

- Preventing or minimizing chronic urinary tract infections
- Monitoring, maintaining, or modifying bowel and bladder programs to promote adequate and planned emptying as the pregnancy progresses so that optimal health and functional ability are maintained
- Avoiding pressure ulcers due to increased weight and difficulty with transfer activities
- Preventing respiratory complications due to increased diaphragmatic pressure and diminished respiratory capacity

Anemia and altered nutritional status may also occur and further influence overall health and skin integrity, increasing the woman's susceptibility to pressure ulcers. Other structural and hormonal changes may occur, including a higher risk for deep vein thrombophlebitis due to increased venous stasis and the potential for greater bone loss in a woman with preexisting osteoporosis.

Mobility and activities of daily living of the pregnant woman with SCI also need to be reevaluated for the greater need for assistive devices or mobility aids. Reevaluation might indicate a change to a power chair from a manual chair to aid mobility, speed, and ease; changes in wheelchair size throughout the

TABLE 13–5 ■ COUNSELING CHECKLIST FOR SEXUALLY TRANSMITTED DISEASES

____ Help the client to relax and express concerns or fears.
____ Reassure client that he or she has assumed responsibility for personal well-being and is better off knowing diagnosis and receiving treatment than going undiagnosed.
____ Without imparting guilt, help client understand how his or her specific sexual behavior relates to the sexually transmitted disease (STD) or other STDs.
____ Help client understand the specific disease, its transmission, and its clinical picture.
____ Help client understand how the disease is treated and what is involved with the treatment protocol.
____ Explain any medication, dosage, administration routine, side effects, and rationale for adherence to routine.
____ Assist client with partner notification strategies–role playing, rehearsing, or script writing may be indicated.
____ Provide written information to client on diagnosis, treatment, follow-up, partner notification, and supportive services.
____ Discuss contraceptives in terms of STDs. Discuss contraceptive strategies to reduce future exposure to and risk of STDs.
____ Remind the client to avoid intercourse until cured.

From Alexander, L. (1992). Sexually transmitted diseases: Perspectives on this growing epidemic. *The Nurse Practitioner: The American Journal of Primary Healthcare, 17,* 10. Copyright 1992 by Springhouse Corporation; reprinted with permission of the publisher.

pregnancy to accommodate the increase in body proportions; and a greater need for assistive devices such as reachers.

Perinatal care provided by an obstetrician experienced in high-risk pregnancies, in concert with rehabilitation team members, will result in a pregnancy and postpartum plan that will meet the medical, functional, and parenting needs of the mother with SCI. Early labor is not uncommon in the woman with SCI because of the incidence of urinary tract infections and other factors. Undetected labor or labor that is perceived as increased spasticity is also common. Autonomic dysreflexia in women with injuries above T6 may also be experienced throughout pregnancy and labor; it should not be confused with preeclampsia and must be treated carefully and in a timely manner. Labor is reported to be shorter, with a higher incidence of cesarean deliveries.

Support after delivery and throughout the first few parenting years for the woman with SCI and her partner is critical. Helping to monitor changes in function and supporting the role and functions of the parenting partner in managing the infant's needs optimize the experience and environment so that child care can be most easily provided. As the child grows, ongoing support from a functional and social perspective can and should be provided through periodic functional and environmental evaluations by therapists, rehabilitation nurses, and physiatrists.

The management of bowel and bladder function remains a critical issue for men and women after a SCI as they plan their sexual lives. Bladder management prior to sexual activity might consist of (1) emptying the

TABLE 13–6 ■ SEXUALLY TRANSMITTED DISEASES—BEHAVIORAL COUNSELING MESSAGES WITH SPECIFIC SEXUALLY TRANSMITTED DISEASES (STDs)*

Disease	Behavioral Counseling Message
Chlamydia	Condom use; refer partner(s) for evaluation.
Cytomegalovirus	Condom use; refer symptomatic partner(s) for evaluation.
Human papillomavirus	Weekly or biweekly treatment until lesions resolve; early treatment to reduce sequelae; examine partner(s) for warts; abstain from sex or use condoms during treatment; women should have annual Papanicolaou smear.
Gonorrhea	Avoid sex until patient and partners are cured; return for evaluation 2 to 3 days after treatment; take medications as prescribed; ensure examination of partner(s) as soon as possible; return early if symptoms persist or recur.
Hepatitis B	Condom use; refer partner(s) for evaluation.
Herpes	Keep lesion area clean and dry; abstain from sexual contact in areas of lesion while symptomatic; realize undetermined risk for transmission during asymptomatic intervals; use condoms for further protection during asymptomatic periods; women should have annual Papanicolaou smear.
Syphilis	Return for follow-up serologies 3, 6, 12, and 24 months after treatment; refer sexual partner(s) for evaluation and treatment; avoid sexual activity until patient and partner(s) are cured; use condoms to prevent future infections.

*For all STDs, voluntary, confidential HIV-antibody testing, coupled with pretest and posttest counseling, and evaluation should be routinely offered when the results may contribute either to the clinical management of the person or to the prevention of further disease transmission.

From Alexander, L. (1992). Sexually transmitted diseases: Perspectives on this growing epidemic. *The Nurse Practitioner: The American Journal of Primary Healthcare, 17*, 10. Copyright 1992 by Springhouse Corporation; reprinted by permission of the publisher.

bladder through intermittent catheterization or the Credé method, or (2) taping the Foley catheter to the abdomen or thigh of a woman or covering the catheter with a condom for a man. Male external urine-collecting devices may be removed before and reapplied after sexual activity. Bladder augmentation procedures and artificial bladder sphincters also provide mechanisms for bladder emptying without a Foley catheter and may free the woman with SCI from catheter use, improving self-esteem and feelings of sexual attractiveness.

Avoiding bowel accidents and incontinent episodes remains a primary concern for clients with SCI. Maintaining and adhering to a bowel routine that is consistent and provides for routine evacuation through either digital stimulation or the use of liquid or solid suppositories may help to reduce the fear of bowel elimination during sexual activity. Instructing the client to plan ahead and to inform his or her partner about the possibility of an accident may help decrease performance anxiety. Many clients with SCI use their attendants for these preparations to help minimize the effects of caregiving on the partner. This intervention, when possible, helps to preserve the sexual roles of the couple and does not detract from the sexual intimacy or the relationship.

With all of the focus on function—ejaculatory, erectile, or orgasmic—and fertility, it is critical to remember the sexual-social issues of the client with an SCI. Sexuality is greatly affected in the adolescent or adult with such an injury. Role changes, role adaptation, self-image, self-esteem, sexual desire, and feelings of sexual attractiveness influence the sexual lives of people after the onset of their injuries. Sexual desire is lessened after an SCI, and the change may be related to any of these issues as well as to the availability of a partner and the comfort with social skills and opportunities that may result in sexual activities and relationships. After the onset of any disability, reduced self-esteem and diminished personal social and sexual interactions may result in decreased sexual interest, satisfaction, and activity patterns. Partner satisfaction and intimacy in a relationship will be directly affected.

When these elements are combined with only limited information provided by health care providers, clients with SCI may retreat from and alter their sexual lives. People who experience any disability need to be given the opportunity to understand, explore, and rediscover their self-esteem and sexual selves.

MULTIPLE SCLEROSIS: ALTERATIONS IN SEXUAL FUNCTION AND SEXUALITY

Many of the issues previously identified for clients with spinal cord injury and brain injury may also apply to the individual experiencing multiple sclerosis (MS). A progressive disease with multiple clinical presentations and, for many, an unpredictable course, MS may have from minimal to extensive influence on sexual function and sexuality. It may cause lesions throughout the central nervous system, altering the transmission of neural impulses and possibly leading to an altered sexual response cycle, diminished sensation, and paresthesias. Cortical lesions may affect the ability, interest, and desire to initiate and have a sustained interest in sexual activity or, depending on the location of the lesion, may result in disinhibition of sexual activity. The sequelae of MS may cause secondary complications that may also influence function or desire.

Valleroy and Kraft (1984) identified the common complaints of MS patients through the University of Washington MS Project, in which 656 individuals responded to questions about issues and concerns in relation to sexual function. Female respondents identified their most common sexual symptoms or function issues since onset of the disease to be weakness; fatigue; anxiety; decreased sensation, libido, or orgasm; anorgasmia; difficulty with arousal; and frequent urinary tract infections. Male respondents identified the following issues: difficulty achieving and maintaining erection, decreased sensation, decreased libido, difficulty with ejaculation or orgasm, frequent urinary tract infections, and spontaneous morning or night erections. The most common symptoms of MS, including problems with balance, mobility, motor weakness, spasticity, emotional lability, memory, and speech and communication problems, were also reported as contributing factors to alterations in the respondents' sexual responses. As with any chronic illness or disability, alterations in self-esteem and body image may have a direct effect on an individual's interest in and performance of sexual activities.

The most commonly reported problem in men with MS is erectile dysfunction, which is reported to occur in more than half of men with the disease (Grana). Erectile function, which is primarily mediated through reflexogenic (via autonomic sacral parasympathetics), may be affected by lesions in the thoracolumbar segments of the spinal cord. Psychogenic erections may be influenced by supraspinal lesions but also by decreased libido, depression, and other psychosocial factors.

Pregnancy and its impact on the course of MS has also been studied. Women with MS tend to avoid pregnancy and suggested that this avoidance may be related to the level of individual disability. Most studies are limited, however, in that they do not include a large enough sample of a range of women with MS from the least disabled to the most disabled. These studies supported previous studies concluding that no association could be demonstrated between the number of pregnancies and the worsening of MS in relation to pregnancy. Epidemiological studies have suggested a greater frequency of exacerbations of the disease in the first 3 to 6 months after delivery.

Thompson, Nelson, Burks, and Franklin (1986) also studied the course of MS throughout pregnancy and post partum in 178 women. They found no effect of pregnancy on subsequent or overall MS disability. They also studied the immunological role of pregnancy and MS and demonstrated that the immunosuppressant effect of estrogen on T-helper cells and the loss of that effect with the precipitous drop in estrogen levels in the postpartum period may be important, with women having more exacerbations after delivery, but that the ultimate course of the disease is not affected by pregnancies.

The Summer 1998 issue of *Inside MS*, a consumer periodical about MS, quoted the Multiple Sclerosis Society's Chief Medical Officer, Dr. Stanley van den Noort, regarding MS and pregnancy (*Inside MS*, Summer 1998). He concluded from his experience of treating MS for more than 40 years that symptoms and attacks decrease during pregnancy and may increase the first 6 months after birth without any long-term effect on the course of the disease. He recommended that all MS treatment be stopped during pregnancy, including use of interferon beta-1a (Avonex), interferon beta-1b (Betaseron), and glatiramer acetate (Copaxone), which might otherwise increase the risk of miscarriage. The postpartum use of these drugs and their effect on nursing have not been studied. Therefore, Dr. van den Noort suggested that mothers may either create a nursing schedule around drug administration (holding off nursing for 12 hours after administration) or delay resuming treatment with these MS drugs while lactating. He suggested that intravenous corticosteroids may be used safely during pregnancy. Dr. van den Noort suggests that the major consideration for women with MS who are considering pregnancy and parenthood may be the degree of disability from a mobility, cognitive and the extent of the physical disability on parenting.

As with the dearth of information on females and sexual response and sexual alterations after disability, there is very little information on the impact of menopause on women with MS and other disabilities. The issue of *Inside MS* just described has also been helpful in identifying individual women's responses to menopausal changes (*Inside MS*, Summer 1998). More research and focus are needed on the effect of hormone replacement therapy, its values, and its limitations in this population and other mobility-impaired women. Preexisting risk factors such as obesity, smoking history, heart disease, previous clotting abnormalities, and osteoporosis may influence the individual's ability to use hormone replacement therapy.

MUSCULOSKELETAL DIAGNOSES AND SEXUAL ALTERATIONS

One of the most common reasons for admission to a comprehensive, subacute, or outpatient rehabilitation program is the management of functional and related problems associated with musculoskeletal disorders. According to Lim (1995), musculoskeletal conditions constitute the largest single category of diseases that result in impairment of self-care, ambulation, or ability to carry on the usual activities of daily living. Osteoarthritis, rheumatoid arthritis, and ankylosing spondylitis may result in pain, physical limitations, fatigue, genital lesions, depression, anxiety, decreased self-esteem, role changes, altered mobility, and altered ability to perform activities of daily living. Decreased desire and satisfaction and a concomitant reduction in sexual activity are common scenarios in these conditions. In addition, some of the medications that are taken to control the disease symptoms, such as steroids, may reduce libido and alter self-image through secondary physical complications (hirsutism, truncal obesity, buffalo hump).

Interventions that will aid in the management of sexual issues in this group of individuals are directed at alleviating symptoms such as pain and fatigue. Instructing clients to take pain medications prior to sexual activity, use heat or cold to decrease pain, and integrate massage and other forms of deep touching may help to decrease muscle spasms and stiffness and promote mobility during activity. Warm-up exercises with the application of heat may help prior to activity so that the individual can achieve decreased tone and increased flexibility.

Special positioning techniques should be experimented with to minimize painful sexual experiences. The use of bolsters, pillows, and other cushions may help with leg positioning or back support. Any position that reduces pain on the affected areas (extremities, hips), such as rear entry, lateral positioning, or the unaffected partner on top, may be helpful. According to Malek and Brower (1984), muscle relaxation techniques and mental imagery are also helpful for promoting comfort. Typically, individuals find these sexual problems decreased or eliminated by surgical replacement of joints.

After hip replacement, certain positioning restrictions are indicated. The surgeon may instruct the patient to avoid exaggerated abduction, external and internal rotation, and flexion. Typically, the patient is instructed to avoid these positions for 6 to 12 weeks after surgery to avoid displacement of the prosthesis. Sexual positions to be avoided after a total hip arthroplasty or replacement include posterior entry and side-lying positions because of the need for hip flexion greater than 90 degrees, and adduction or abduction. The optimal postoperative position is supine to reduce the risk of prosthesis displacement. Individual surgeon restrictions should be reinforced with each patient, because the specific limitations on and period for limitation of types of sexual activity may vary (Lim, 1995).

AMPUTATION AND SEXUAL ALTERATIONS

According to Lim (1995), sexuality in amputees is a neglected subject, possibly because of the older age of the majority of amputees and the reluctance of health professionals to address these issues.

Unlike individuals with other disabling conditions, many individuals who experience a traumatic or nontraumatic amputation may not have sufficient information on how to manage the resulting challenges. Significant alterations in body image, self-esteem, mobility, ability to perform activities of daily living, depression, phantom sensation, and phantom pain may further affect the individual's sexuality and sexual activity.

Health care providers may focus entirely on the restoration of function and limb replacement and may overlook the need to address these complex issues, which may influence overall patient outcomes and success in managing life after amputation. Positioning and foreplay may be influenced by pain and alterations in mobility and balance. Loss of a dominant upper limb may decrease sexual foreplay. Finding alternatives to positioning and avoiding stimuli that trigger a pain response are advised (Conine & Evans, 1982).

Alterations in erection and ejaculation may also occur in men with vascular disorders who experience an amputation. Transurethral suppositories of alprostadil, as already described for men with SCI, may enhance erection if significant vascular compromise has not occurred. Other erectile interventions, including vacuum pumps, may produce variable responses depending on the individual and the extent of vascular compromise.

Body image, self-esteem, and role alterations may influence sexual self-image and sexual activity after an amputation. Through individual, group, and peer counseling, the amputee can experience a restored sense of self after mourning the lost extremity. Acceptance of the individual with an amputation, as well as helping the individual to accept the loss, will assist with coping and restoring interest in sexual relationships.

AIDS AND SEXUAL ACTIVITY

Emphasizing safe sexual practices when providing sexual information and counseling is critical. Acquired immunodeficiency syndrome (AIDS) continues to occur in epidemic proportions in the United States and other countries because of the failure to practice safe sex. AIDS has become the sixth leading cause of death for women between 25 and 44 years of age, because of both the absence of safe sex practices and the belief that "it couldn't happen" this time or with this person.

The principles of safe sex are the same for everyone and should include the following:

- Abstinence
- Talking about safe sex before doing it
- Using barriers (condoms, dental dams, plastic wrap, latex gloves or finger cots between all organs, orifices, body fluids, and sexual aids/devices)

Clinicians must obtain a careful past medical and sexual history to assess a client's or patient's risk for human immunodeficiency virus (HIV), including as much detail as possible about past and present sexual practices, substance abuse, and transfusions. Over the past 15 years, extensive research has resulted in various algorithms that support early intervention and perhaps a preventive approach for the individual who is HIV seropositive. Early diagnosis and treatment through HIV specialty programs provide a comprehensive approach to the medical and psychosocial interventions needed by individuals, their partners, and their support systems. It is critical that individuals who believe that they may have HIV seek early counseling and medical management. Also, talking to partners or potential partners about HIV status is essential.

Upon evaluation, an inclusive sexual history will help to highlight individual practices, partner and relationship issues, and sexual and other potentially high-risk practices that will require support and intervention.

Lynch and Ferri (1997) have written an outstanding article facilitating health care professionals' awareness of the sexual health care concerns of bisexual individuals, lesbian women, and gay men. Reading it will help any health care provider understand and avoid the common pitfalls in the care of individuals with same-sex partners.

Other sexually transmitted diseases also appear to be increasing in incidence, and some, such as *Chlamydia* infection, are reaching epidemic status. The sexually transmitted diseases commonly treated in a sexually active individual include *Chlamydia* infection, cytomegalovirus, human papillomavirus, gonorrhea, hepatitis B, herpes, and syphilis. Alexander (1992) provides a helpful approach for the clinician counseling the individual for specific treatment and preventing transmission of the sexually transmitted disease among partners (see Table 13–5). Specific treatment interventions for each disease is beyond the scope of this chapter; however, the following recommendations can easily be integrated into rehabilitation nursing practice:

- Taking an inclusive, nonjudgmental history
- Identifying sexual practices and partners
- Strictly reinforcing the need for the patient or client to fully complete the therapeutic regimen, even if asymptomatic
- Alerting all sexual contacts within the previous 60 days so they can be treated to prevent further transmission
- Reinforcing safe sexual practices

It is critical to review with the infected individuals and their partners the importance of barrier methods, including condoms and diaphragms, and the use of these methods with spermicides that contain nonoxynol 9. Routine screening after unprotected sex or for individuals who engage in high-risk practices allows for early intervention and reduces transmission of these mostly silent infections. Incorporating early intervention, prevention, and screening into rehabilitation settings will help control the incidence of sexually transmitted diseases. Assuming that individuals with disabilities are not at risk for such disorders reinforces sexual stereotypes and ignorance and prevents the delivery of optimal health care.

REFERENCES

Alexander, L. (1992). Sexually transmitted diseases: Perspectives on this growing epidemic. *The Nurse Practitioner, 17,* 10.

Aron, J. S. (1976). The PLISSIT model: A proposed conceptual schema for behavioral treatment of sexual problems. *Journal of Sex Education Therapy, 2,* 1–15.

Boolell, M., Gepi-Attee, S., & Gingell, J. C. (1996). Sidenafil, a novel effective oral therapy for male erection dysfunction. *British Journal of Urology, 76,* 257–261.

Brindley, B. S. (1984). The fertility of men with spinal cord injury. *Paraplegia, 22,* 337.

Charlifue, S. W., Gerhart, K. A., Menter, R. R., Whiteneck, G. C., & Scottmanley, M. (1992). Sexual issues of women with spinal cord injuries. *Paraplegia, 30,* 192–199.

Cole, T. (1975). Sexuality and physical disabilities. *Archives of Sexual Behavior, 4,* 389.

Comarr, A. E. (1970). Sexual function among patients with spinal cord injury. *Urologia Internationalis, 25,* 134–168.

Conine, T. A., & Evans, J. H. (1982). Sexual reactivation of chronically ill and disabled adults. *Journal of Allied Health, 11,* 261–270.

Ducharme, S., Gill, K. M., Beiner-Bergeman S., & Fertitta, L. (1993). Sexual functioning: Medical and psychological aspects. In J. A. DeLisa (Ed.), *Rehabilitation medicine: Principles and practice* (2nd ed., pp. 763–782). Philadelphia: J. B. Lippincott.

FDC Reports. The pink sheet. May 3, 1996 a; 58, T&G12–13.

Garlinghouse, N. M. (1987). Sexuality of male cerebral vascular accident victims. *Sex and Diseases, 8*(2), 67–72.

Glass, J. C., Mustian, R. D., and Carter, L. R. (1986). Knowledge and attitudes of health care providers toward sexuality in the institutionalized elderly. *Educational Gerontology, 12,* 465.

Girdley, F. M., Bruskewitz, R. C., Feyzi, J., Grauersen, P., & Gasser, T. (1988). Intracavernosus self-injection for impotence: A long-term therapeutic option? Experiences in 78 patients. *Journal of Urology, 140,* 972–974.

Golgi, H. (1979). Experience with penile prostheses in spinal cord injury patients. *Journal of Urology, 121,* 288–289.

Grana, E.(1995). Sexuality issues in multiple sclerosis. *Physical Medicine and Rehabilitation: State of the Art Reviews, 9*(2), 377.

Greco, S. (1995). Sexuality education and counseling. *Rehabilitation Nursing: Process and Applications.* (2nd ed., pp. 594–623). Chicago: C. V. Mosby.

Hellstron, B., Gesundheit, N., Kaiser, F., Lue, T., Padma-Nathan, Peterson, C., Yam, P., Todd, L., Varady, J., & Place, V. (1996). A double blind, placebo-controlled evaluation of the erectile response to transurethral alprostadil. *Urology, 48*(6), 851–856.

Horn, L., & Zasler, N. D. (1990). Neuroanatomy and neurophysiology of sexual function. *Journal of Head Trauma Rehabilitation, 5*(2), 1–13.

Kirkeby, H. J., Poulsen, E. U., Petersen, T., & Dorup, J. (1988). Erectile dysfunction in multiple sclerosis. *Neurology, 38,* 1366–1371.

Kraft-Fine, C., McGillin, L., Potts-Nulty, S., Lennon, D., & Cioschi, H. (1995–1996). *Not just surviving...Women living a full life with a spinal cord injury* [Videotape] (Model Project 3MP 116). American Association of Spinal Cord Injury Nurses. Jackson Heights, NY.

Lim, P. (1995). Sexuality in patients with musculoskeletal diseases. *Physical Medicine and Rehabilitation: State of the Art Reviews, 9*(2), 401–415.

Lynch, M., & Ferri, R. (1997). Health needs of lesbian women and gay men. *Clinician Reviews, 7*(1), 85–89.

Malek, C. J., & Brower S. S. A. (1984). Rheumatoid arthritis: How does it influence sexuality? *Rehabilitation Nursing, 9,* 26–28.

Masters, W. H., Johnson, V. E., & Kolodny, R. C. (1986). *Masters and Johnson's On sex and the human body.* Boston: Little, Brown.

McCormick, R. (1986). Coital positioning for stroke affected couples. *Rehabilitation Nursing, 11*(2), 17–19.

Nosek, M, Rintolk, D., & Young, M. (1996). Sexual functioning among women with physical disabilities. *Archives of Physical Medicine and Rehabilitation, 77,* 106–113.

Sipski, M., Alexander, C., & Rosen, K. (1995). Orgasms in women with SCI. *Archives of Physical Medicine and Rehabilitation, 76*(12), 1097–1102.

Sjorgen, K., & Fugl-Meyer, A. R. (1981). Sexual problems in hemiplegia. *Int Rehabil Med, 3*(11), 28–31.

Stover, S., DeLisa, J., & Whiteneck, G. (1995). *Spinal cord injury: Clinical outcomes from the model systems.* Baltimore: Aspen Publications.

Szaz, G. (1992). Sexual health care in the management of SCI. In C. M. Zedjlick (Ed.), (2nd ed., pp. 175–201). Boston: Jones and Bartlett.

Tepper, M. (1992). Sexual education in SCI rehabilitation: Current trends and recommendations. *Sexuality and Disability, 10*(1), 15–31.

Thompson, D. S., Nelson, L. M., Burks, J. S., & Franklin, G. M. (1986). The effects of pregnancy in multiple sclerosis: A retrospective study. *Neurology, 36,* 1097–1099.

U. S. Department of Health and Human Services. (1996). *Post stroke rehabilitation: Guidelines for clinical practice.* Vol 7, Number 12, December 1995. Public Health Service Agency for Health Care Policy and Research, Rockville, MD, pp. 607–623.

Valleroy, M. L., & Kraft, G. H. (1984). Sexual dysfunction in multiple sclerosis. *Archives of Physical Medicine and Rehabilitation, 65,* 125–128.

World Health Organization. (1975). *Education and treatment in human sexuality: The training of health professionals* (WHO Testimonial Report Series No. 572 1975).

Younglan and Davis. Women's Health. ISBN#0-8385-1230-5.

Zasler, N. D. (1989). Managing erectile dysfunction with external devices. *Practical Diabetology, 8*(1).

Zasler, N. D., & Horn, C. G. (1990). Rehabilitation Management of Sexual Dysfunction. *Journal of Head Trauma and Rehabilitation.* 5(2), 14–24.

BIBLIOGRAPHY

American Red Cross. (1992). *Talking to your partner about AIDS.* American Red Cross.

Anon. (1996, May 17). *SCRIP World Pharmaceutical News,* p. 24.

Captain, C. (1995). The effects of communication skills training on interventions and psychosocial adjustment among couples living with SCI. *Rehabilitation Nursing Research, 4*(4), 111–118.

Coslett, H. B., & Heilman, K. M. (1986). Male sexual function: Impairment after right hemisphere stroke. *Archives of Neurology, 43*(10), 1036–1039.

Drench, M., & Losie, R. (1996). Sexuality and sexual capacities of elderly people. *Journal of Rehabilitation Nursing, 21*(3), 118–123.

Fahey, J., & Fitzpatrick, M. (1995). Pharmacological update: Emerging post coital contraceptive therapies. *Journal of the American Academy of Nurse Practitioners American Academy of Nurse Practitioners, 7*(10), 505.

Felenstein, D. (1995). Sexually transmitted disease. In K. E. Carlson (Ed.), *Primary care of women* (pp. 115–125). Philadelphia: Mosby.

Friend, R. (1987). Sexual identity and human diversity: Implications for nursing practice. *Holistic Nursing Practice, 1*(4), 21–41.

Griffith, E. R., & Trieschmann, R. B. (1983). Sexual dysfunction in the physically ill and disabled. In C. C. Naddsen & D. B. Marcotti (Eds.), *Treatment interventions in human sexuality* (pp. 241–277). New York: Pleener Press.

Hudson, L., & Green, S. (1995). Parenthood after SCI: The personal side. *Topics in Spinal Cord Injury Rehabilitation, 1*(2), 62–64.

Osbon Medical Systems. (1996). *Impotence is treatable.* Augusta: Osbon Medical.

Sachs, P. (1995). *Aging and sexuality.* Paper presented to Penn Council for Relationships. Philadelphia.

Santana, J. (1989). Sexuality and sexual function. *Rehabilitation Nursing: Process and Applications,* 407–427.

Sonya, P., & Fulgemiti, P. (1992). Sexual functioning of women with complete SCI: Nursing implications. *Sexuality and Disability, 10*(2), 103–117.

CHAPTER 14

Self-Care

Diana M. L. Newman

This chapter presents a discussion of Dorothea Orem's theory of self-care, theory of self-care deficit, and theory of nursing systems (Orem, 1995). The concepts of self-care are applied to activities of daily living (ADLs). Specific focus on rehabilitation nursing is included with attention to a multicultural perspective.

The importance of self-care to the discipline of nursing is attested to by the frequency with which it appears in the literature. The numerous publications underscore the value of using explicit nursing models and theories to guide nursing practice. Rehabilitation nurses are particularly interested in self-care, emphasizing the patient's becoming independent in self-care activities. Orem's self-care framework can be classified as a conceptual model of nursing because it is "a set of abstract and general concepts and propositions that integrate those concepts into a meaningful configuration" (Fawcett, 1995, p. 2). Professional nursing practice emphasizes nursing's unique contribution to health care. It is based on a scholarly and scientific foundation. Professional nurses must use and systematically evaluate nursing conceptual models to enhance developing nursing knowledge.

THEORY OF SELF-CARE

The theory of self-care is "the voluntary regulation of one's own human functioning and development that is necessary for individuals to maintain life, health, and well-being" (Orem, 1995, p. 95). Individuals intellectually process their experience and make decisions about self-care action based on their reflections. People's perception of their own health includes their views about their mental, biological, interpersonal, social, and human characteristics. This perception also includes their ability to grow when new situations require change.

Self-care is influenced by a person's self-concept, level of maturity, culture, and knowledge. Self-care requisites are insights about actions necessary to regulate an aspect of human functioning. Self-care requisites express the goals of self-care (Orem, 1995). Three types of self-care requisites have been identified: the universal self-care requisites, the developmental self-care requisites, and the health deviation self-care requisites.

Universal Self-Care Requisites

The universal self-care requisites comprise the basic needs that must be met to achieve or maintain optimal functioning, health, and well-being. They are common to all persons throughout each stage of the life cycle. The following, as described by Orem (1995), are typically considered to be universal self-care requisites:

1. The maintenance of a sufficient intake of air
2. The maintenance of a sufficient intake of water
3. The maintenance of a sufficient intake of food
4. The provision of care associated with elimination processes and excrements
5. The maintenance of a balance between activity and rest
6. The maintenance of a balance between solitude and social interaction
7. The prevention of hazards to human life, human functioning, and human well-being
8. The promotion of human functioning and development within social groups in accord with human potential, known human limitations, and the human desire to be normal, in accord with the characteristics of the individual

Developmental Self-Care Requisites

The developmental self-care requisites include the dimensions of growth and development; the psychic dimensions, including cognition and emotions; and the personal dimension, with the subdimensions of personality, character formation, and mental health. Developmental self-care requisites take into account associations among the dimensions and the dynamic process that occurs between people and their environment. The typical life-cycle stages with developmental stages are (Dennis, 1997)

1. Fetal, including birth
2. Neonatal
3. Infancy
4. Childhood and adolescence
5. Adulthood
6. Pregnancy in either adolescence or adulthood

There are three sets of developmental self-care requisites (Orem, 1995):

1. Provision of conditions that promote development
2. Engagement in self-development
3. Prevention of life situations that can adversely affect human development

Health Deviation Self-Care Requisites

The health deviation self-care requisites "exist for persons who are ill or injured, have specific forms of pathology including defects and disabilities and who are under medical diagnosis and treatment" (Orem, 1995, p. 200). Deviations in structure and function, in behavior, and in capacity to perform ADLs may require changes in self-care. These changes may mean that the self-care agent (the person who engages in a course of action or has the power to do so) needs a dependent care agent. A dependent care agent is a person who is responsible for meeting the therapeutic self-care demands of a person who is socially dependent on the agent or on a person who regulates the other person's self-care agency (Orem, 1995). The term *therapeutic self-care demand* specifies the total care measures necessary for optimal health and well-being in relation to a person's conditions and circumstances (Dennis, 1997; Orem, 1995). Six health deviation self-care requisites have been identified (Orem, 1995, pp. 201–202):

1. Seeking and securing appropriate medical assistance in the event of exposure to specific physical or biological events and states, or when there is evidence of genetic, physiological, or psychological conditions known to produce or be associated with human abnormality
2. Being aware of and attending to the effects and results of pathological conditions and states, including effects on development
3. Effectively carrying out medically prescribed diagnostic, therapeutic, and rehabilitative measures directed toward preventing specific types of pathological processes, to the pathological process itself, to the regulation of human integrated functioning, to the correction of deformities or abnormalities, or to compensation for disabilities
4. Being aware of and attending to or regulating the discomforting or deleterious effects of medical care measures performed or prescribed by the physician, including the effects on development
5. Modifying the self-concept (and self-image) in accepting the self as being in a particular state of health and in need of specific forms of health care
6. Learning to live with the effects of pathological conditions and states and the effects of medical diagnostic and treatment measures in a lifestyle that promotes continued personal development

Rehabilitation nurses who intend to use the theory of self-care to guide their practice should identify self-care requisites of their patients, choose ways in which the requisites can be met, and describe actions that can be taken to meet each self-care requisite. The effectiveness of self-care practice is determined by the therapeutic value it achieves. More specifically, self-care practices are therapeutic if they (1) support life processes, (2) maintain normal human structure and function, (3) support development in accord with human potential, (4) prevent injury and pathological states, (5) contribute to the regulation or control of the effects of injury and pathological processes, (6) contribute to the cure or regulation of pathological processes, and (7) promote general well-being (Orem, 1995).

Self-care needed by people is influenced by their basic conditioning factors and the health care services available to them. The basic conditioning factors affect therapeutic self-care demand. Ten basic conditioning factors have been identified: "(1) age; (2) gender; (3) developmental state; (4) health state; (5) sociocultural orientation; (6) health care system factors; for example, medical diagnostic and treatment modalities; (7) family system factors; (8) pattern of living including regular activities; (9) environmental factors; (10) resource availability and adequacy" (Orem, 1995, p. 203).

Self-Care Agency and Dependent Care Agency

The terms *self-care agency* and *dependent care agency* stand for specific powers of individuals to act to meet continuing requirements for care of self or care of other. The adequacy of self-care and dependent care is measured against therapeutic self-care demands. The therapeutic self-care demands include the maintenance of life processes, the prevention of personal harm or health deterioration, health maintenance, health promotion, and promotion of well-being under existing conditions. It is essential that the adequacy of self-care agency be determined so that nurses can assess self-care deficits, plan nursing actions, and design nursing systems. The adequacy of self-care agency can be determined by identifying self-care behavior, assessing the benefits of that behavior, and suggesting changes in self-care activity when new self-care requisites may be needed. Self-care agency is characterized by the operations of estimating or knowing self-care requisites and the means of meeting them. It also includes the transitional ability to make judgments and decisions about self-care and production, or the ability to act to meet self-care requisites. As components of self-care agency, human powers are necessary for the production of self-care operations, which are activities for the preparation and performance of self-care measures. The power components are (Orem, 1995, p. 221)

1. The ability to maintain attention and exercise requisite vigilance with respect to the self as self-care agent and internal and external conditions and factors significant for self-care
2. The controlled use of available physical energy that is sufficient for the initiation and continuation of self-care operations
3. The ability to control the position of the body and its parts in the execution of the movements required for the initiation and completion of self-care operations
4. The ability to reason within a self-care frame of reference
5. Motivation (i.e., goal orientations for self-care that are in accord with its characteristics and its meaning for life, health, and well-being)

6. The ability to make decisions about self-care and to put these decisions into operation
7. The ability to acquire technical knowledge about self-care from authoritative sources, to retain it, and to put it into operation
8. A repertoire of cognitive, perceptual, manipulative, communication, and interpersonal skills adapted to the performance of self-care operations
9. The ability to order discrete self-care actions or action systems into relationships with prior and subsequent actions toward the final achievement of regulatory goals of self-care
10. The ability to consistently perform self-care operations, integrating them with relevant aspects of personal, family, and community living

The foundations of self-care are evident in people's knowledge and reasoning capabilities. Furthermore, people's willingness to look at themselves as self-care agents and their acceptance of themselves as in need of particular self-care measures are key to self-care agency. In addition, their health habits and concern about health have an impact on the effectiveness of self-care.

Self-care activities have internal and external orientations. Externally oriented activities include knowledge seeking; assistance/resource seeking; expressive, interpersonal actions; and actions to control external factors. Internally oriented activities are those that use action sequences to control internal factors or to control one's thoughts, feelings, and awareness. Clearly, these external- and internal-oriented activities are purposeful and goal directed. Self-care can be said, therefore, to be deliberate action (Orem, 1995). Self-care agency is in continuous development. The phases of self-care such as knowledge, decision making, and production can be at different levels for a particular person at a specific time and circumstance. People can be conditioned by human and environmental factors in such a way that self-care is affected. Self-care agency can be undeveloped, developing, developed but not stabilized (in need of continued development or in process of continued development or in need of redevelopment or in process of redevelopment), developed and stabilized (in need of redevelopment, in process of redevelopment, or redeveloped and stabilized), and developed but declining (Orem, 1995).

Rehabilitation nurses need to assess self-care agency in the patients for whom they care. They need valid and reliable methods to describe self-care systems of individuals. Data obtained with these methods inform nurses about the therapeutic self-care demand of patients and how to help patients with their self-care operations. In adverse conditions, when self-care demands cannot be met, the nurse must assess the self-care limitations and the therapeutic self-care demand to determine the self-care deficit.

THEORY OF SELF-CARE DEFICIT

The self-care deficit theory of nursing describes the inability to care for the self or for dependents because of the state of health or the health care needs of the recipient of self-care. Deficit represents the relationship between the action required by the individual and the responses of that individual for self-care or dependent care. In this context, deficit is not a defect but rather a relationship (Orem, 1995). The theory of self-care deficit can be used to explain nursing practice as the reply to real and potential human responses to health deviations. Self-care deficits exist when competencies for self-care are limited and cannot meet the therapeutic self-care demand. Self-care deficits comprise the number of self-care deficits and the components of the therapeutic self-care demand. Self-care deficits exist when the therapeutic self-care demand exceeds the abilities of self-care agency (Dennis, 1997). Self-care deficits arise if the following are present (Orem, 1995, p. 240):

1. An absence of ongoing engagement in self-care or gross inadequacy of what is done to meet self-care requisites
2. Limited awareness or loss of awareness of self and environment, excluding that due to natural sleep
3. An inability to recall past experience in the control of conduct
4. Limitations in judgment and decision making about self-care associated with a lack of knowledge about and unfamiliarity with internal and external conditions
5. Events indicative of disordered or impaired functioning giving rise to new health deviation self-care requisites and necessitating adjustments in one or more or all of the universal self-care requisites
6. Needs of individuals to incorporate newly prescribed complex self-care measures into

their self-care systems, the performance of which requires specialized knowledge and skills to be acquired through training experiences

Self-care deficits can be complete, in which there is no ability to meet a therapeutic self-care demand, or partial, in which there is limited ability to meet therapeutic self-care demands (Orem, 1995). An example of an existing self-care deficit is the case of an individual with a new amputation who has to learn how to use a prosthesis. When the known future change in therapeutic self-care demand will require more than the current self-care agency, the self-care deficit is said to be projected (Dennis, 1997). An example of a projected self-care deficit is the case of an individual with a new amputation who has no knowledge of the lifestyle changes he or she will have to make in relation to the use of a prosthesis; teaching about changes in diet, activity, and hygiene may improve compliance with the treatment regimen.

Nursing Assessment of Self-Care Deficits

Nursing assessment that is focused on the universal, developmental, and health deviation self-care requisites can determine self-care deficits. After the needs for self-care are determined, the patient's capabilities and limitations for meeting the specific self-care requisites must be determined. The nursing assessment of self-care agency is based on the foundational abilities, power components, and self-care abilities associated with the estimative, transitional, and productive self-care operations (Dennis, 1997). Restrictions in knowing, in judging and decision making, and in meeting goals are self-care limitations. These self-care limitations are associated with the three self-care operations (estimative, transitional, and productive) (Table 14–1). The association between self-care limitations and self-care operations allows each association to be applied to any of the self-care requisites for a particular patient. Both self-care limitations and self-care operations may contribute to the self-care deficit; self-care limitations may have a major impact on self-care deficits (Dennis, 1997).

Self-care abilities may be lacking because they are not developed or because they are not operable at the present time. If self-care is lacking, therapeutic self-care demands are not met. When therapeutic self-care demands

TABLE 14–1 ■ LINKING TYPES OF SELF-CARE LIMITATIONS WITH SELF-CARE OPERATIONS

Types of Self-Care Limitations	Self-Care Operations
Knowing	Estimative
	Transitional
	Productive
Judging and decision making	Transitional
	Productive
Engaging in result-achieving actions	Estimative
	Productive

From Dennis, C. M. (1997). *Self-care deficit theory of nursing. Concepts and applications* (p. 74). St. Louis: Mosby–Year Book.

are not met, patients demonstrate a need for nursing. Because the ultimate goal of nursing is to ensure the achievement of therapeutic self-care demands, patients who have health-related self-care deficits are legitimate patients of nursing (Dennis, 1997; Orem, 1995).

Dependent Care

Dependent care actions, like self-care actions, are deliberate nursing interventions directed toward meeting self-care requisites. "Dependent care is the continuing health-related personal regulatory and developmental care provided by responsible adults for infants and children or persons with disabling conditions" (Orem, 1995, p. 9). The person performing the care over time is the dependent care agent. The dependent care agent is a responsible adult who cares for someone who is socially dependent. The person who is socially dependent is called the dependent care recipient (Dennis, 1997). Both the dependent care agent and the dependent care recipient may vary according to cultural and social group norms. The dependent care agent role and the dependent care recipient role are modified by the self-care requisites and therapeutic self-care demands of each role. The similarities between dependent care and self-care include the following (Dennis, 1997, pp. 76–77):

1. Action is deliberate with estimative, transitional, and productive operations.
2. Actions are logically ordered and sequentially performed.
3. Actions are intended to meet known self-care requisites of the person receiving care.

4. Actions are performed by persons having specialized abilities.
5. Actions are influenced by basic conditioning factors.
6. Care is learned in a sociocultural context, most often the family.
7. Care may or may not produce the desired outcome.
8. Care may or may not be therapeutic.
9. Dependent care is necessary to meet requisites for care in those acknowledged by society as legitimately dependent.
10. Dependent care has new or altered needs because of the presence of health deviations.

Dependent care is unlike self-care in the following ways (Dennis, 1997, p. 77):

1. Actions are performed for the benefit of another. Dependent care requires interactions between at least two persons.
2. Dependent care is intended to meet the self-care requisites of another.
3. Dependent care has as its goal self-care agency of the dependent care recipient. Continuing evaluation of dependent care agency is required. The exception is the dependent care recipient who is socially dependent for life.

Dependent Care Recipient

Dependent care recipients are persons who legitimately need assistance in meeting self-care requisites because of self-care deficits. Delivery of this assistance requires identification of who will be the care provider and who will be the care recipient. The therapeutic self-care demand is calculated specific to the self-care requisites of the dependent care recipient. The complexity of the relationship between the dependent care agent and the dependent care recipient lies in the manner in which the care is focused only on the self-care deficits of the recipient. Whenever possible, the dependent care agent and the dependent care recipient should cooperate in moving toward self-care in dependent care systems (Dennis, 1997).

Dependent Care Agency

Dependent care agency is similar to self-care agency in the following ways (Dennis, 1997, pp. 79–80):

1. The focus is on abilities for carrying out care actions.

2. Dependent care agency consists of foundational capabilities, power components, and abilities associated with estimative, transitional, and productive operations of deliberate action.
3. Dependent care agency is modified by basic conditioning factors.
4. Nursing assessment consists of the appraisal of the estimative, transitional, and productive operations of deliberate action.
5. Dependent care agency may be a combination of abilities and limitations. Dependent care limitations are analogous to self-care limitations in that they are constraints in the performance of action.
6. Abilities are learned and developed over time within the family system and the sociocultural, spiritual, and educational systems.

Dependent care agency is unlike self-care in the following ways:

1. Dependent care actions may be both similar to and different from those of self-care. For example, bathing oneself is similar to yet different from bathing another.
2. Dependent care agency results in dependent care.
3. Dependent care agency requires at least two persons. Cooperation and interaction are essential.

A dependent care deficit can exist if the therapeutic self-care demand of the dependent care recipient is greater than the self-care agency of the dependent care recipient and the dependent care agent. This relationship must take into account the efforts of the dependent care recipient toward self-care and the role of the dependent care agent to develop self-care agency in the dependent care recipient.

Theory of Nursing Systems

Nursing is a human service derived from nursing knowledge. The specialized knowledge of nursing enables nurses to respond to persons with needs for self-care. The human service provided by nursing is a helping service based on scientific nursing knowledge that guides practice. Nursing practice is a sequential series of actions that compensates for health limitations that restrict persons' own functioning and development and that of their dependents. Nursing systems as helping systems are produced from the deliberate, discrete actions of nurses and patients in nursing situations. Six helping methods have been identified: (1) doing for or acting for another, (2) guiding and directing another, (3) providing physical support, (4) providing psychological support, (5) providing an environment that supports development, and (6) teaching (Table 14–2) (Orem, 1995, p. 305).

Nursing Agency

The proficiencies that nurses have that are used for the benefit of society are collectively called nursing agency. Nursing agency is similar to self-care agency, but it is used to help others. Nursing agency is comparable to self-care agency in the following ways (Dennis, 1997):

1. Nursing agency is a combination of abilities, learned and developed over time, and limitations that affect the extent of nursing agency at any point in time.
2. Nursing agency is altered by the basic conditioning factors.
3. The appraisal of nursing agency involves the evaluation of deliberate action in the performance of estimative, transitional, and productive operations of nursing care.

Nursing agency differs from self-care agency in the following ways (Dennis, 1997):

1. Competencies of nursing agency include the social, interpersonal, and professional-technological dimensions of nursing practice.
2. Nursing agency involves at least two persons and involves nursing actions with social and interpersonal components; therefore, nursing agency is similar to dependent care agency.
3. The goal of nursing agency is nursing care that may or may not be similar to the goals of self-care agency.
4. The educational process for professional nursing is the basis for nursing agency, which provides a specific body of knowledge that is not required for self-care agency.

The power components of nursing agency include knowledge of the social, interpersonal, and professional-technological operations of nursing practice. These components empower nursing agency. The characteristics of nursing agency included in the social domain are awareness of the social and legal dimensions of nursing situations. Cultural and economic differences between groups significantly affect nursing agency. Social

TABLE 14–2 ■ NURSE'S AND PATIENT'S ROLES IN NURSING SITUATIONS AS SPECIFIED BY METHODS OF HELPING

Method of Helping	Nurse's Role	Patient's Role
Doing for or acting for another	A person who acts in place of and for the patient	Recipient of care to meet the therapeutic self-care demand and to compensate for self-care limitations Recipient of services relevant to environmental control and resources
Guiding and directing another	Provider of factual or technologic information relevant to regulation of self-care agency or the meeting of self-care requisites	Receiver, processor, and user of information as self-care agent or as regulator or self-care agency
Providing physical support	A partner cooperating in performing self-care actions to regulate the exercise of or value of self-care agency by patient	Performer of actions to meet self-care requisites or regulator of the exercise of or the value of self-care agency in cooperation with a nurse
Providing psychological support	An "understanding presence"; a listener, a person who can institute the use of other methods of helping if necessary	A person confronting, resolving, and solving difficult problems or living through difficult situations
Providing an environment that supports development	Supplier and regulator of essential environmental conditions and a significant other in a patient's environment	A person who is confronted with living and caring for himself or herself in a way and in an environment that supports and promotes personal development

Teaching	Teacher of
	  Knowledge describing and explaining self-care requisites and the therapeutic self-care demand
	  Methods and courses of action to meet self-care requisites
	  Methods of calculating the therapeutic self-care demand
	  Methods of overcoming or compensating for self-care action limitations
	  Methods of managing self-care
		Learner engaged in the development of knowledge and skills requisite for continuous and effective self-care

From Orem, D. E. (1995). *Nursing concepts of practice* (5th ed.). (p. 305). St. Louis: Mosby–Year Book.

skills, including communication and interpersonal relations, are areas for continued development in nursing. Professional behavior demands that nursing recognize the boundaries of its discipline while being able to establish working relationships with other professions.

Because nursing is primarily an interpersonal profession, competencies in this area are paramount throughout nursing situations, for the beginner through the advanced practitioner. Psychosocial expertise includes knowledge of factors that enhance and impede interpersonal functioning. Nurses need competency in communication skills with individuals and families throughout the life span. In addition, the nurse needs to be attuned to verbal and nonverbal communications that signify the vast range of human responses in nursing situations.

The professional-technological operations of nursing include the nursing process. In this context, the nursing process is composed of diagnostic, prescriptive, regulatory, treatment, and evaluative operations. These operations meet the therapeutic self-care demands of patients including the universal, developmental, and health deviation self-care requisites. They also develop, protect, and regulate the exercise of self-care agency. In order to accomplish these operations, nurses must be continually updating their education to deepen their knowledge. The nurse must also be comfortable with these operations in nursing situations that are emergent in nature or continuing over a long period of time (Orem, 1995).

Additional power components support the social, interpersonal, and professional-technological operations of nursing agency. These components are intellectual and practical skills pertaining to the three areas of nursing agency; enduring motives; a willingness to provide nursing; an ability to unify different action sequences toward result achievement; consistency in the performance of nursing operations; making adjustments according to conditions; and an ability to manage self as the essential professional operative in nursing practice situations (Orem, 1995, p. 248).

Nursing practice situations consist of three stages: the stage of initial contact, the stage of continuing contacts, and the stage of preparation for discharge. The stages vary in duration and in the sequence of operations performed by nurses. However, all nursing practice situations contain helping relationships. It is necessary to ask the following questions within the framework of these helping relationships to classify the nursing system: (1) Who can and should perform the actions through which components of patients' therapeutic self-care demands are met according to current prescriptions for them? (2) Who can and should regulate patients' exercise or development of their powers of self-care agency? The answers to these questions assist the nurse in developing the structure for a nursing system in which all the helping methods can be identified.

If the patient is totally unable to engage in self-care activities, the system is called wholly compensatory. In this instance, the nurse compensates for the patient's total inability to engage in self-care activities. If the patient can perform some but not all self-care activities, the system is called partly compensatory. If the patient can perform all self-care activities, the system is called supportive-educative (Orem, 1995, p. 306) (Table 14–3).

Wholly Compensatory System

Regardless of the degree of compensation necessary for patient care, nursing must make every effort to ensure that the universal, developmental, and health deviation self-care requisites are met. When the patient is unable to engage in self-care actions needing self-directed, controlled movement either by self-limitation or by medical prescription (a health deviation self-care requisite), the nursing system required is wholly compensatory. Three subtypes of nursing systems have been recognized for patients with these limitations.

The first subtype is suitable for patients who are unable to engage in any form of deliberate action and are unable to control their position and movement in space. These patients are unresponsive to stimuli or are responsive to internal and external stimuli through hearing and feeling. These patients are also unable to control the environment and convey information to others because of

TABLE 14–3 ■ BASIC NURSING SYSTEMS

Wholly Compensatory System

Nurse's action
   Accomplishes patient's therapeutic self-care
   Compensates for patient's inability to engage in self-care
   Supports and protects patient

Partly Compensatory System

Nurse's action
   Performs some self-care measures for patient
   Compensates for self-care limitations of patient
   Assists patient as required
Patient's action
   Performs some self-care measures
Nurse's and patient's actions
   Regulate self-care agency
Patient's action
   Accepts care and assistance from nurse

Supportive-Educative System

Patient's action
   Accomplishes self-care
Nurse's and patient's actions
   Regulate the exercise and development of self-care agency

From Orem, D. E. (1995). *Nursing concepts of practice* (5th ed.). (p. 307). St. Louis: Mosby–Year Book.

a loss of motor ability. Because these patients can only be moved by others, they must be protected and cared for. In the helping method of doing and acting for, they should be spoken to frequently in a conversational tone and handled frequently and gently, and their environment should be monitored to promote typical functioning. Patients in a coma typically are cared for in a nursing system of this subtype.

The second subtype of nursing system is suuitable for patients who are aware and who may be able to make observations, judgments, and decisions about self-care but who are unable to move. These patients may have varied degrees of awareness and ability to communicate with others. However, movement is not feasible because of abnormality; the results of injury; medical restriction; treatment; weakness; or debility. Although these patients may be involved in exercising self-care agency that does not involve movement, they may have to make adjustments and be willing to be cared for by others for an undetermined period of time. Nurses must consider development, psychological support, guidance, and teaching while doing and acting for the patient. Nursing agency must involve stimulation and the promotion of self-care agency for the patient whenever possible to counteract the effects of social isolation, loneliness, and dependency.

The last subtype of nursing system is suitable for patients who are conscious but unfocused. They have a short attention span and can make decisions about some of their ADLs only with constant guidance. They need protection and safety measures for themselves and others in their environment. Helping methods include promoting development; guiding and directing; supporting; and doing or acting for the other.

The social, interpersonal, and professional-technological dimensions of wholly compensatory nursing systems involve very compromised patients. Nursing agency provides a major portion of the universal, developmental, and self-care requisites. Family members must be included in the design of nursing systems. Care must be taken to advocate for patient and family rights and responsibilities.

Partly Compensatory Systems

Partly compensatory systems are characterized by flexibility in the sharing of responsibility between nurse and patient for the meeting of patient self-care requisites. This sharing of responsibility is contingent on the patient's restriction in movement, the knowledge and skills necessary, and the patient's psychological readiness to meet self-care requisites. These systems take into account all six helping methods. They are particularly appropriate when the patient is learning new health care measures.

Supportive-Educative Systems

Supportive-educative systems are focused on support, guidance, provision of a developmental environment, teaching, and consultation. The patient is able to meet his or her therapeutic self-care demand with assistance in the areas of decision making, behavior control, and acquiring knowledge and skills. The nurse who designs a supportive-educative nursing system should be able to exercise nursing agency in a flexible manner with particular attention to patient responses.

Designing nursing systems helps to define nursing responsibilities with legal, professional, and ethical backing. The end result of designing and implementing nursing systems is the monitoring of patients' self-care agency and the meeting of their self-care requisites. The three types of nursing systems could be used for nursing situations in health care agencies or communities. For example, the commonalities of patients in need of rehabilitation could specify necessary roles and assistive techniques. These specifications could be used in designing nursing systems for use in nursing administration, education, and research.

SELF-CARE AND ACTIVITIES OF DAILY LIVING

Self-care promotes effective nursing practice because it is a response to current trends in health care. Current cost-control measures, the unequal distribution of health care providers, a shift from acute to chronic health problems, and a gradual change with clients more in control of themselves undergird the movement toward self-care (Dodd, 1988). Self-care can empower the patient to gain control over his or her illness in the face of unknowns about the future. The fulfillment and identity reinforced by self-care practices enhance patient dignity and reduce excessive reliance on the medical care system (McLaughlin & Zeeberg, 1993).

Cultural Implications

Self-care practice must be culturally based to achieve its goals. Some non-Western cultures value care by others more than self-care. They may prefer relationships with their caregivers that emphasize interdependence, interconnectedness, understanding, being with, and being responsible for, rather than self-care. Nurses who care for patients who prefer these caregiving situations must adapt their practice to be culturally congruent with the preferences of the care recipient (Leininger, 1992). Culturally based health care can enhance client satisfaction, support recovery from illness in a timely fashion, and increase client responsiveness. Culturally specific and culturally congruent nursing care takes into account culture defined as "the lifeways of a particular group with its values, beliefs, norms, patterns, and practices that are learned, shared and transmitted intergenerationally" (Leininger, 1996, p. 73). Recognition of culturally specific care includes the differences and universals among peoples. The practice of nursing within a cultural perspective includes nurse-patient interactions that emphasize preservation and maintenance, accommodation and/or negotiation, and restructuring and repatterning. These interactions are based on the dimensions of the culture care concept, which include the following factors: technological; religious; philosophical; kinship and social; cultural values and lifeways; political and legal; economic; and educational (Leininger, 1996). Clearly, culture enriches the relationship between the nurse and the patient. It provides a wealth of information to enhance the design of nursing systems.

Activities of Daily Living

A review of the literature about self-care and ADLs suggests that patients in American, Asian, and European rehabilitative settings prefer independence in these activities (Anderson, 1991; Blair, 1995; Boake & High, 1996; Clark et al., 1995; Fidler, 1995; McLaughlin & Zeeberg, 1993; Morales-Mann & Jiang, 1993; Prescott, Soeken, & Griggs, 1995; Russell, 1996; Vogelpohl, Beck, Heacock, & Mercer, 1996; Yu, 1995). Although some nursing home residents may be independent in ADLs when they enter a nursing home, their self-care agency may decrease because of excessive helping by nurses. In some instances, nurses encourage dependency, because they feel more altruistic when they are doing total care. Patients who are independent may get less attention from the nurse than those who are dependent. Induced physical dependency can lead to a loss of control and a higher mortality rate.

To enhance self-care in ADLs, nurses should collaborate with patients in establishing mutual goal setting by prompting, shaping, and providing reinforcement. This encouragement will enable patients to perform more ADLs (Blair, 1995). Older patients who live independently may suffer a loss of self-worth and feel self-neglected, powerless, worthless, and like failures if their control over ADLs is lessened and their dependency increased. Nurses working with community-based elderly people can enhance self-care agency by suggesting greater physical activity and encouraging family members to facilitate the older person's independence (Yu, 1995). Persons who are demented and have diminished cognitive capacity still have reserves that can be activated by an individualized, supportive, caregiving approach (Vogelpohl et al., 1996). The Strategies to Promote Independence in Dressing method matches the caregiver's approach with the patient's cognitive and physical abilities and disabilities. This rehabilitative, reactivating method is an alternative for accomplishing routine self-care tasks. It mobilizes the latent cognitive and physical reserves and maximizes the utiliza-

tion of the person's functional capacity (Vogelpohl et al., 1996). An example of a behavioral intervention for a dressing activity is as follows (Vogelpohl, 1996, p. 40):

1. Establish a routine that provides both structure to decrease the person's stress and flexibility to accommodate for normal fluctuations in cognition.
2. Modify environmental conditions that contribute to dressing deficits.
3. Strengthen environmental conditions that support dressing independence.
4. Alter the interactions between the caregiver and the person.
5. Provide immediate reinforcers when the person successfully performs a dressing task.

The coping abilities of people affect their degree of disability. A person with a severe physical problem who has excellent coping skills may have a lesser degree of disability or impairment than a person who has a mild physical defect and very few coping skills (Clark et al., 1996). Hospitalized patients are discharged earlier than in the past, with the expectation that they will recover at home rather than in the hospital. This recovery is based on adequate home health care services, which should prevent rehospitalization of the patient. Patients who are discharged must have an adequate assessment of their self-care agency for ADLs. They must be given information about available community services and how to manage at home. Nurses with an acute care perspective may not be able to identify patient self-care agency for ADLs after discharge (Prescott et al., 1995). Self-care agency for ADLs and physical function should be determined at hospital discharge. Self-care deficits in these areas are predictors of nursing home placement (Prescott et al., 1995). The reader is encouraged to investigate specific empirical measures for self-care agency (Dodd, 1988; Gulick, 1988; Hagopian, 1988; Jones, 1988). Carefully collected data about patients' self-care agency capabilities and patterns of living including meeting universal self-care requisites can inform the nurse about patient self-care agency and ADLs. Table 14–4 presents a nursing history developed in two sections with different goals. Section 1 is identified as a nursing history with two parts designed to explicate the self-care situation of a patient. Part 1 identifies changes in a patient's therapeutic self-care demand; part 2 is concerned with the self-care agency of the patient. Section 2 of

TABLE 14–4 ■ NURSING HISTORY

SECTION 1

Goal: explication of the self-care situations of a patient
Part 1: Changes in the Therapeutic Self-Care Demand

A. In relation to your present condition (name the condition and elicit confirmation or adjustment from the patient) have you:

    A.1 Used new regulatory measures in your daily or periodic self-care, for example, restricting your activities, taking additional rest, eliminating certain foods, taking prescribed or unprescribed medications? If so, please name them.

        How did you come to use these measures?

        Did you know how to perform them or did you have to learn how?

        If you had to learn, how did you go about this?

        Are these measures still a part of your daily or continuing self-care? All_____ Some_____ None_____

        When did you discontinue the measures that are no longer a part of your self-care regimen?

        Why did you discontinue them? Give names of measures.

        Of all the measures named, which ones do you judge to have been or to be of value in your present situation?

    A.2 In relation to your present condition, have you made specific observations about your own functioning, for example, when you experience being tired, when your body temperature is elevated? If so, will you name what you have observed that you see as relevant to your needs for periodic or continuing self-care?

        Did you (do you) follow a systematic plan for making these observations? If so, describe it.

        Did you seek help in making observations? Did you seek help to learn the meaning of what you observed? If yes, from whom did you seek help?

    A.3 What, if any, parts of your routine of self-care have been changed by your present conditions and circumstances? Routine of self-care has been added to? Yes_____ No_____

        Usual routine care measures are unaffected_____; affected in this way_____;

        virtually eliminated: Yes_____ No_____

    A.4 In relation to your present condition, what do you suggest as in need of special attention by nurses as they develop with you a program of nursing care?

Part 2: Self-Care Agency Focus

A. After or during childhood, when did you come to bear or take on responsibility for your daily and periodic care to regulate your own functioning and development as related to your health and well-being?

    Partial responsibility at age of_____. Who bore or bears responsibility with you?

    Full responsibility at age of_____.

    What sources of help, if any, did you use when you did not know what to do or how to manage your own care?

    What sources of help do you presently use when you have self-care problems that you do not know how to handle?

B. Are there aspects of your self-care that you

    B.1 Attend to regularly? Yes_____ No_____

        If yes, what are they?

    B.2 Have questions about? Yes_____ No_____

        If yes, what are they?

    B.3 Tend to forget? Yes_____ No_____

        If yes, what are they?

    B.4 Ignore? Yes_____ No_____

        If yes, what are they?

        Why do you ignore them?

C. In your contacts with physicians, have you been able to talk to your physicians about self-care questions? Yes_____ No_____ If yes, give an example of a self-care matter that you described to or discussed with one or more physicians.

    What was the outcome in terms of your subsequent self-care?

    If no, will you tell why you have not or do not discuss your self-care questions with your physician?

D. In the past, have you had episodes of illness or disability when you were unable to provide your own daily self-care? Yes_____ No_____ If yes:

    D.1 Were you cared for? Yes_____ No_____

        If yes, by whom?

        What was your response to being cared for?

    D.2 What was the extent of your inability to provide care for yourself? Could you perform some measures of care? Yes_____ No_____

    D.3 With what conditions in yourself or your environment did you associate your inability to care for yourself?

E. How do you describe your past performance in providing self-care in order to regulate your own functioning? Consider completeness and effectiveness.

    E.1 On a day-to-day basis.

    E.2 When suffering illness or injury.

    E.3 In terms of performance over time.

Table continued on following page

TABLE 14–4 ■ NURSING HISTORY *Continued*

F. How would you describe yourself in relation to your present condition as being personally able to provide self-care that you consider essential for your health and well being? Able_____ Not able_____ If able, why?
   If unable, why not?
   F.1 Provided it is judged safe by your nurse(s), what parts of your routine daily self-care can you perform without placing yourself under stress?
   No part_____ These parts by name:_____
   F.2 What parts of your routine of daily self-care do you judge that you will have difficulty in performing?
   No part_____ Will have difficulty with_____
   Do you judge yourself able to cooperate with and give needed guidance to persons who will help you with the difficult parts of your care? Yes_____ No_____

G. What are your present interests and concerns about
   G.1 Meeting your known existent needs for day-to-day self-care?
   G.2 Recognizing and meeting emerging needs for self-care?
   G.3 Learning about and taking on a reasonable role in your own care according to your state of health?
   G.4 Becoming more knowledgeable about and skilled with respect to your own care
       a. In making observations relevant to your care?
       b. In making judgments and decisions about care?
       c. In performing and observing results of specific care measures?

SECTION 2

Goal: explication of the conditions and pattern of living of a patient including residence features, activity mix, environmental conditions, routine of self-care

A. Residence
   A.1 Do you live in a home with your family? Yes_____ No_____
   If yes, who lives in the home with you?
   A.2 If no, do you live alone? Yes_____ No_____
   If you do not live alone, with whom do you share your living space?
   A.3 Do you live in a house, apartment, room, or other? Write in.
   A.4 Is where you now live your permanent residence or a temporary residence?
   A.5 Are you responsible for the costs and day-to-day upkeep of your place of residence? Yes_____ No_____
   If no, who bears this responsibility?
   A.6 What activities are routinely part of your daily living within your residence?

	Yes	No
Food storage after purchasing	——	——
Meal preparation	——	——
Eating meals	——	——
Care and storage of clothing	——	——
Washing of clothing	——	——
Washing of linen (bed)	——	——
Care of bed(s) and bedding	——	——
Resting and sleeping	——	——
Hygienic care of self	——	——
Recreational activities and hobbies	——	——
If yes, name.		
Work	——	——
If yes, describe.		
Social engagements with		
One to two persons	——	——
More than two persons	——	——

   A.7 Do you feel pressed for space in the place where you live? Yes_____ No_____
   If others live with you, do they feel the same as you feel? Yes_____ No_____
   A.8 Do you have concerns about your place of residence that are relevant to your present condition and circumstances?
   Yes_____ No_____
   If yes, what are these concerns?

TABLE 14–4 ■ NURSING HISTORY *Continued*

B. Activity mix
   B.1 What is the nature of the actions in which you routinely engage each day?
      _____ Special education:_____
      _____ Extended education:_____
      Work outside the home:_____
      Household routines:_____
      Care of dependents: Children by age:_____
                          Adults by age and relationship:_____
      Community projects:_____
   B.2 Has your routine related to the above changed because of present conditions and circumstances? Yes_____ No_____
      If yes, in what way(s) has it changed?
   B.3 Have you experienced or are you experiencing particular problems or difficulties in accomplishing your usual routine of activities within or outside the home? Yes_____ No_____. If yes, would you tell about the problems that are of special concern to you?
C. Environment: What concerns, if any, do you have about environmental factors?
   C.1 Air quality? Yes_____ No_____. If yes, describe.
   C.2 Living area
      a. Cleanliness of living areas? Yes_____ No_____. If yes, describe.
      b. Freedom from vermin? Yes_____ No_____. If yes, describe.
      c. Other? Name and describe.
   C.3 Adequacy of water for

	Yes	No		Yes	No
Drinking quality?	—	—	Quantity?	—	—
Cooking quality?	—	—	Quantity?	—	—
Bathing quality?	—	—	Quantity?	—	—

      Other uses, describe:_____
   C.4 Adequacy of food supplies
      a. Quality? Yes___ No___.   Quantity? Yes___ No___
      b. Access to food supplies? Yes___ No___
   C.5 Freedom from hazardous conditions stemming from
      a. The numbers and relationships of individuals with whom you interact? Yes___ No___
      b. The health of persons with whom you associate? Yes_____ No_____
      c. The trustworthiness of these persons? Yes_____ No_____
D. Routine for self-care
   D.1 Do you routinely or periodically use care measures to facilitate your intake of air, your breathing? Yes___ No___
      If yes, what are they?
      When do you use them?
      In what ways do they help you?
      When did you start using them?
   D.2 How much water do you drink during the 24 hours of a day?
      How much water do you usually drink at one time?
      When during the 24 hours do you drink water?
      Has your consumption of water changed? Yes___ No___
      When?
      How?
   D.3 Eating patterns
      a. Think about what you consider an ordinary day and identify what and when you would eat.
      b. How does what you eat at other times differ from your described eating on an ordinary day?
      c. Has what you eat and when you eat changed? Yes___ No___
         When?
         How?
      d. Do you suffer from:
         Not having enough food? Yes___ No___
         Not having the right kind of food? Yes_____ No_____

Table continued on following page

TABLE 14–4 ■ NURSING HISTORY *Continued*

D.4 Elimination
  a. Do you have any concerns or problems about bowel or bladder functioning?
  b. If you use any special care measures related to the following, name the measures.
     Passing of urine:_____
     Bowel elimination:_____
     Hygienic care after urination or defecation:_____
  c. Describe the patterns of your bladder and bowel functioning in terms of frequency and time.
  d. Do you note the color and amount of urine you pass? Yes____ No____
     If the color and amount of urine changed from the usual color and amount, would you be observant of the change?
     Yes____ No____
     Have you observed such changes? Yes____ No____
     What are they?
D.5 Rested emotions
  a. What do you usually do to rest yourself when you experience a need for rest?
     Under what circumstances do you experience a need for rest?
     How frequent are these experiences?
     When you feel that you need to rest, are you usually able to do so? Yes____ No____.
  b. Do you have regular hours for sleeping? Yes____ No____
     If yes, what are they?
     How do you feel when you get up after your usual hours of sleep?
     Do you have a routine for preparing for sleep?
     If so, what is it?
     Do you know of conditions and circumstances under which it is difficult for you to have a restful sleep?
  c. How many hours of the day do you estimate that you are

     Walking_____ Doing mental work_____
     Standing_____ Doing physical work_____
     Sitting_____   Light____ Heavy____ Strenuous____
     Reclining_____
     Engaged in physically active recreational activities_____
     Engaged in the use and movement of your body or its parts for therapeutic purposes_____
  d. When not actively engaged in work requiring concentration, are you relaxed_____or tense_____?
  e. How frequently do you experience the following: Fear_____ Anger_____ Other emotions_____?
     What is the duration of these emotional experiences?
     How do you feel after such experiences?
  f. What is your judgment about the balance you maintain between high-energy-consuming activities and experiences and restorative, restful activities and experiences including sleep?
D.6 Social communication
  a. How much time during a usual day do you spend alone?
     During this time are you in proximity to other persons in the same general area?
     Or are you quite isolated from other persons? How do you feel about being alone?
  b. How many persons and of what ages and relations to you do you have contact with during a usual day?
     What is the length of your contacts?
     What kinds of communication occur?

From Orem, D. (1995). *Nursing concepts of practice* (5th ed.) (pp. 422–430). St. Louis: Mosby–Year Book.

the history illustrates the conditions and pattern of living of a patient including residence features, activities, environmental conditions, and the routine of self-care.

PROCESS OF NURSING

The process of nursing is a combination of social, interpersonal, and professional-technological elements. Nursing practice is composed of these elements happening concur-
rently in the context of a nursing situation. The social element includes a professionally educated nurse in a situation in which the "patient is open and willing to receive nursing care" (Dennis, 1997, p. 102). The interpersonal element implies cooperation between the nurse and the patient. This cooperation is mediated by the basic conditioning factors and the patient's family or significant others. The interpersonal relationship between the patient and the nurse is affected by communi-

cation, compassion, confidence, personality style, and empathy (Dennis, 1997). The professional-technological element is composed of the assistance that nurses provide with existing and projected self-care deficits and "accomplishing therapeutic self-care through regulating the exercise and development of self-care (or dependent care) agency" (Dennis, 1997, p. 104). The nursing process is the operational definition of the professional-technological element. Nursing process is constructed from "nurses' performance of diagnostic, prescriptive, and regulatory or treatment operations with associated control operations including evaluation" (Orem, 1995, p. 268). These operations take into account the interpersonal and contractual elements of nursing. They identify persons with self-care or dependent care deficits, "provide and regulate the kind and amount of nursing care needed to assist patients with achieving therapeutic self-care, and lead to formation of appropriate judgments about the effectiveness of the nursing care provided them" (Dennis, 1997, p. 104). The application of the nursing process in the context of a nursing situation typically is most effective in a sequential rather than a linear manner. Nursing process is based on the theories of self-care, self-care deficit, and nursing systems. Other sources of nursing knowledge are contributed from empirical, esthetic, ethical, and personal ways of knowing (Carper, 1978).

Nursing process is a common practice throughout the discipline of nursing. Yura and Walsh (1988) have established the four steps of the nursing process as (1) assessment and diagnosis, (2) planning, (3) implementation, and (4) evaluation. These familiar steps are often considered the generic nursing process (Dennis, 1997). Orem (1995) suggests the following steps in the nursing process, which are more consistent with the self-care deficit theory of nursing: "Step 1: Diagnosis and prescription; Step 2: Design and plan; Step 3: Regulate and control" (Dennis, 1997, p. 106) (Table 14–5). Table 14–6 compares the generic nursing process and the steps in nursing process in the self-care deficit theory of nursing.

Step 1: Diagnosis and Prescription

The first step of the nursing process involves data collection including interviewing, taking vital signs, physical assessment, and reviewing medical information. This information is assessed with consideration of the ba-

sic conditioning factors. It is collected to enhance nursing assessment of therapeutic self-care demand and self-care agency. It will be used as a basis for nursing diagnosis, the nursing judgments made at the end of step 1. The first step of the nursing process "(1) assesses self-care agency in light of the basic conditioning factors; (2) determines therapeutic self-care demand and analyzes self-care agency; (3) identifies self-care deficits expressed as nursing diagnosis statements" (Dennis, 1997, p. 107). The first step of the nursing process establishes the contractual and cooperative relationship between the nurse and the patient. The basic conditioning factors must be prioritized in the assessment of self-care agency. The most important basic conditioning factors are the patient's age, development, and health. The basic conditioning factors, along with the patient's perception of his or her health, contribute to the appraisal of self-care agency. In addition, the patient's understanding of his or her health has an impact on self-care agency (Dennis, 1997; Orem, 1995). The nursing assessment of the patient's self-care requisites is key in the calculation of the patient's therapeutic self-care demand. The compatibility of the nurse's assessment of patient self-care requisites and the patient's assessment of his or her self-care requisites must be determined. Patient self-care agency for specific self-care requisites must also be established.

The assessment of self-care agency includes the patient's ability for sensation (use of the five senses) and communication. Other abilities foundational to self-care agency are the attending, processing, and storing of information and the use of reason. Self-awareness and self-examination are also important. Careful attention must be paid to the person's capacities in the estimative, transitional, and productive operations in each of the self-care requisites. In the estimative self-care operation, the person's ability to know his or her self-care requisites and their meaning and value needs to be determined. In addition, the patient's understanding of the outcome of self-care in terms of what needs to be done (therapeutic self-care demand) in relation to what is currently being accomplished needs to be assessed (Dennis, 1997). The specific ability of the person to seek out information regarding current and future self-care requisites and the behaviors necessary to attain self-care agency is an important determination. The transitional self-care operation in-

TABLE 14–5 ■ STEPS IN OREM'S NURSING PROCESS

Step 1: Diagnosis and Prescription

Therapeutic Self-Care Demand				Self-Care (Dependent Care) Agency				Self-Care Deficits (Nursing Diagnosis Statements)
Particularized SCR	Related SCRs			Abilities	Limitations	Adequacy		
	U	D	HD			Yes	No	
Air	x			Breathes without difficulty; skin warm, dry, normal for client		x		
					Smokes cigars		x	Potential for respiratory problems related to smoking
Water	x			Fluid intake sufficient; no edema; skin turgor normal for age		x		
Food	x			2000-calorie ADA diet	Does not adhere to diet Weight: 225 lb. Height: 68 inches Blood sugar check bid usually between 90 and 130 mg/dL Decreased appetite Increased alcohol consumption	x	x x x	Potential for deterioration of physiological health status related to noncompliance, overweight, decreased appetite, and increased alcohol ingestion
Elimination	x			Voids without difficulty; last bowel movement [insert date]			x	
Activity/rest	x				Difficulty sleeping; never feels rested		x	Ineffective sleep patterns related to underlying depression; ineffective pain and movement control related to inappropriate pain medication schedule and physical therapy schedule
					Unable to garden related to joint pain and stiffness		x	
Solitude/social interaction	x			Nuclear and extended families provide support; socializes with Greek-American club; his children visit him daily to bring meals they have cooked		x		
Prevention of hazards	x				Lives alone; mobility is compromised		x	Potential for falls/injury related to living alone

Promotion of normalcy		X
Maintenance of developmental environment	Has good relationship with nuclear and extended families; enjoys social interaction with members of Greek-American club	X
Seeking of medical assistance when health status altered		X
Potential for increased health deterioration related to inadequate nutrition	Decreased appetite and increased alcohol consumption since wife died	X
Potential for diabetic complications, decreased mobility related to chronic health conditions	Bilateral hearing deficit; poor vision left eye; hypertension; rheumatoid arthritis; type 2 diabetes mellitus	X

Step 2: Design and Plan Selected Nursing Diagnosis (Conclusion of Step 1)	Type of Nursing System with Rationale and Expected Patient Outcome	Step 3: Regulate and Control*
1. Potential for respiratory problems related to smoking	1. *Supportive-educative:* Provide teaching materials to help patient stop smoking. Provide support from family and peers; perhaps a stop-smoking support group. *Partly compensatory:* Monitor patient's lungs and breathing patterns to identify any abnormalities. *Expected patient outcome:* Patient will stop smoking and not develop any smoking-related abnormalities. Patient will initiate this response with full understanding.	
2. Potential for deterioration of health status related to noncompliance with diet, overweight, and increased alcohol ingestion	2. *Supportive-educative:* Provide peer counseling with diet for increase in compliance. Teach about appropriate exercise for loss of weight that would not aggravate arthritis. Provide individual and/or group therapy to help patient deal with problems of loneliness and decrease alcohol intake.	
3. Ineffective sleep pattern related to underlying depression; ineffective pain and movement control related to inappropriate pain medication schedule and physical therapy schedule	3. *Partly compensatory:* Discuss with patient kinds of medications he is taking for sleep and pain relief. Also review physical therapy schedule. Encourage patient to discuss these concerns with physician and physical therapist. Provide information to physician and physical therapist to advocate for patient's health.	
4. Potential for falls and injury related to living alone	4. *Supportive-educative:* Provide patient with electronic devices to notify friends and family if he falls. Remove any unsafe areas from his environment. *Partly compensatory:* Monitor patient on daily basis to determine advisability of his living alone.	

* Regulate and control operations would be done to regulate the self-care (dependent care), which includes monitoring the plan of care and data needed for judgments about adequacy of the nursing system. SCR, self-care requisite; U, universal health care requisites; D, developmental health care requisites; HD, health deviation health care requisites; ADA, American Diabetes Association. Format for steps in nursing process from Dennis, C. M. (1997). *Self-care deficit theory of nursing* (pp. 122–123). St. Louis: Mosby-Year Book.

TABLE 14–6 ■ COMPARISON OF STEPS IN "GENERIC" NURSING PROCESS TO STEPS IN NURSING PROCESS IN SELF-CARE DEFICIT THEORY OF NURSING (SCDTN)

Generic Nursing Process	SCDTN Nursing Process
1. Assessment and diagnosis	
2. Planning	1. Diagnosis and prescription
3. Implementation	2. Design and plan
4. Evaluation	3. Regulate and control

From Dennis, C. M. (1997). *Self-care deficit theory of nursing. Concepts and applications* (p. 106). St. Louis: Mosby–Year Book.

volves the person's ability to ascribe value and meaning to particular self-care actions, to reflect on the consequences of specific actions, and to know the resources to enact self-care agency (Dennis, 1997). Also included in transitional operations are judging and decision making concerning effective, therapeutic self-care actions and the willingness to be an advocate for the person's self-care. The productive self-care operations include observing and evaluating outcomes. Self-care actions should be continued or changed based on the evaluation of outcomes. Psychomotor skills and resources required for the performance of these skills are part of this operation (Dennis, 1997).

The relationship between therapeutic self-care demand and self-care agency determines the self-care deficit or deficits. Self-care deficits are limitations in self-care agency that justify the need for nursing care. In addition to identifying self-care limitations, the nurse must determine why these limitations exist and what the underlying factors are. The future of patient self-care agency must be carefully estimated (Dennis, 1997). At the end of step 1, a nursing diagnosis is formulated.

Step 2: Design and Plan

By reviewing the therapeutic self-care demand and self-care actions necessary to fulfill self-care or dependent care, the nurse decides what type of nursing system to employ. This decision is also based on the nursing diagnosis, which includes all the self-care deficits. The achievement of therapeutic self-care includes a plan of care. The plan of care states the roles that are to be fulfilled and who will perform specific actions in a sequence to en-

act therapeutic self-care. The plan of care includes necessary equipment and resources and the type, amount, and duration of necessary nursing care (Dennis, 1997).

Step 3: Regulate and Control

In the first part of step 3, actions of the nursing process should achieve therapeutic self-care demand. These care actions performed by the nurse or patient are classified as nursing actions that regulate the plan of care. These nursing actions are production and management actions. The second part of step 3 concerns desired and expected patient outcomes. The plan of care must be evaluated for adequately meeting the therapeutic self-care demand and exercising, protecting, and developing self-care agency. Points to consider in this part of step 3 include the usefulness of nursing actions in meeting agreed-upon patient outcomes, the achievement of patient outcomes, the resolution of self-care deficits posed by the nursing diagnosis, and the accomplishment of the goal of nursing care. This deliberate action can produce effective care for patients and satisfaction for professional nurses.

The following case study illustrates the Orem nursing process as applied to an older adult with chronic health problems.

■ CASE STUDY 14–1

Anthony Stavros is a 75-year-old retired bus driver. He retired 10 years ago after working for public transportation for 25 years. Previous to that he had worked as a gardener and a construction worker. His wife died 5 years ago after a 2-year battle with chronic myelogenous leukemia. His current health problems include a bilateral hearing deficit, cloudy vision developing in his left eye, hypertension, rheumatoid arthritis, and type 2 diabetes mellitus. His medications include aspirin 1.3 g orally twice daily and atenolol 50 mg orally per day. He is allowed 650 mg of aspirin for pain, not to exceed four doses in 24 hours. He has a hearing aid for his left ear, but it works only erratically. He wears glasses at all times because he has hyperopia, myopia, and presbyopia. His blood glucose readings are high, but his diabetes is managed by diet alone. He is 5 feet 8 inches tall and weighs 225 pounds. Mr. Stavros emigrated from Greece to the United States in 1935 at the age of 13 years with his parents and two brothers and two sisters. The whole family became naturalized American citizens. He served in the U.S. Army in World War II and was wounded in the right knee. His father died in 1970 from a cerebrovascular accident; his mother died in 1977 from a heart attack. He is the eldest of his siblings. The siblings are George, aged 72 years; Helen, aged 68 years; Frederick, aged 64 years; and Lillian, aged 60 years. He does not know the health status of his siblings, except that his brother George has "the sugar diabetes." His family of origin all live within a 50-mile radius of each other and see each other on all the major holidays and significant family events such as weddings, funerals, and family reunions. His religion is Greek Orthodox and is important to him. He has seven children: Anthony Jr., aged 55 years; Claudia, aged 53 years; Helen, aged 51 years; Robert, aged 45 years; Joseph, aged 40 years; and twin daughters, Maria and Sophia, aged 39 years. He is closest to his eldest son, Anthony Jr., who lives 2 miles from his father. He is also close to his daughters Maria and Sophia, who live in the same town. He has 17 grandchildren.

His health problems include a limitation in mobility that prevents him from attending to his garden, which he loves. He enjoyed eating in the past, and his children alternate cooking meals for him and bringing them to his house. He has suffered a decrease in appetite during the past 2 weeks. He has lived alone since his wife died, and his children have been encouraging him to move in with one of them, but he is reluctant to give up the home he has built up over the last 50 years. His socialization includes membership in the local Greek-American Club, where he goes to play cards. He receives spiritual support from membership in the local Greek Orthodox church. He smokes one or two cigars every day. He drinks wine or beer with dinner and states that since his wife died his ingestion of alcohol has gradually increased. Mr. Stavros has been having difficulty sleeping over the past 6 months and usually sleeps only 3 to 4 hours per night. He naps in the afternoons but never feels really rested. He still has a driver's license and owns a 1990 car that is in good condition because his son Anthony Jr. provides the maintenance. His sources of financial security are a pension from the city where he was employed as a city worker, a

union pension, and social security. His health insurance is Medicare. This income is adequate since his house mortgage was paid off 15 years ago. His current household expenses include taxes, insurance, maintenance, and repairs. ■

REFERENCES

Anderson, J. M. (1991). Immigrant women speak of chronic illness: The social construction of the devalued self. *Journal of Advanced Nursing, 16,* 710–717.

Blair, C. E. (1995). Combining behavior management and mutual goal setting to reduce physical dependency in nursing home residents. *Nursing Research, 44,* 160–165.

Boake, C., & High, W. M. (1996). Functional outcome from traumatic brain injury. *American Journal of Physical Medicine and Rehabilitation, 75,* 105–113.

Carper, B. (1978). Fundamental patterns of knowing. *Advances in Nursing Science, 1,* 13–23.

Clark, F., Carlson, M., Zemke, R., Frank, G., Patterson, K., Ennevor, B. L., Rankin-Martinez, A., Hobson, L., Crandall, J., Mandel, D., & Lipson, L. (1995). Life domains and adaptive strategies of a group of low-income, well older adults. *The American Journal of Occupational Therapy, 50,* 99–108.

Dennis, C. M. (1997). *Self-care deficit theory of nursing. Concepts and applications.* St. Louis: Mosby–Year Book.

Dodd, M. J. (1988). Measuring self-care activities. In M. Frank-Stromberg (Ed.), *Instruments for clinical nursing research* (pp. 171–184). Norwalk, CT: Appleton & Lange.

Fawcett, J. (1995). *Analysis and evaluation of conceptual models of nursing* (3rd ed.). Philadelphia: F. A. Davis.

Fidler, G. S. (1995). Life-style performance: From profile to conceptual model. *The American Journal of Occupational Therapy, 50,* 139–147.

Gulick, E. E. (1988). The self-administered ADL scale for persons with multiple sclerosis. In C. F. Waltz & O. L. Strickland (Eds.), *Measurement of nursing outcomes: Vol. 1: Measuring client outcomes* (pp. 128–159). New York: Springer-Verlag.

Hagopian, G. (1988). The measurement of self-care strategies of patients in radiation therapy. In O. L. Strickland & C. F. Waltz (Eds.), *Measurement of nursing outcomes: Vol. 4: Measuring client self-care and coping skills* (pp. 45–57). New York: Springer-Verlag.

Jones, L. C. (1988). Measuring guarding: A self-care management process used by individuals with chronic illness. In O. L. Strickland & C. F. Waltz (Eds.), *Measurement of nursing outcomes: Vol. 4: Measuring client self-care and coping skills* (pp. 58–75). New York: Springer-Verlag.

Leininger, M. (1992). Self-care ideology and cultural incongruities: Some critical issues. *Journal of Transcultural Nursing, 4,* 2–4.

Leininger, M. (1996). Culture care theory, research, and practice. *Nursing Science Quarterly, 9,* 71–78.

McLaughlin, J., & Zeeberg, I. (1993). Self-care and multiple sclerosis: A view from two cultures. *Social Science and Medicine, 37,* 315–329.

Morales-Mann, E. T., & Jiang, S. L. (1993). Applicability of Orem's conceptual framework: A cross-cultural point of view. *Journal of Advanced Nursing, 18,* 737–741.

Orem, D. E. (1995). *Nursing concepts of practice* (5th ed.). St. Louis: Mosby–Year Book.

Prescott, P. A., Soeken, K. L., & Griggs, M. (1995). Identification and referral of hospitalized patients in need of home care. *Research in Nursing and Health, 18,* 85–95.

Russell, C. K. (1996). Elder care recipients care-seeking process. *Western Journal of Nursing Research, 18,* 43–62.

Vogelpohl, T. S., Beck, C. K., Heacock, P., & Mercer, S. O. (1996). I can do it! Dressing: Promoting independence through individualized strategies. *Journal of Gerontological Nursing, 22,* 39–42.

Yu, S. (1995). A study of functioning for independent living among the elderly in the community. *Public Health Nursing 12,* 31–40.

Yura, H., & Walsh, M. (1988). *The nursing process: Assessing, planning, implementing, and evaluating* (5th ed.). Norwalk, CT: Appleton & Lange.

CHAPTER 15

Family Dynamics

Judy Winterhalter

When a person suffers from a chronic illness or disability, the family is affected as well. The effects reverberate throughout the family system and create demands on both the client and the family (Gillies, 1987; Minuchin, 1974, 1985), which often must cope with unexpected hospitalizations, treatments, and uncertain outcomes and prepare for a life with a disability. Indeed, the hallmark of chronic illness or disability is that individuals and their families must cope with uncertain demands for the rest of their lives (Power, Dell Orto, & Gibbons, 1988; Woods, Haberman, & Packard, 1993; Woods, Yates, & Primomo, 1989). It is documented in the literature that this presents a formidable challenge to clients, families, and nurses (Caine, 1989; Kleeman, 1989; Winterhalter, 1992; Wright & Leahey, 1994). This chapter presents family theory, psychosocial assessment, and interventions to provide comprehensive rehabilitation nursing care to clients and their families.

FAMILY-CENTERED CARE

The client with a disability may be dependent on family caregivers during both the acute and the long-term phases of rehabilitation. Family-centered care is espoused by the nursing profession, and families are routinely included in the plan of care. However, both nurses and clients often describe dissatisfaction with care. Nurses report feeling inadequate or uncomfortable (or both) in their skills and knowledge to intervene with families. Empirical evidence indicates that family needs are not consistently addressed (Fawcett & Whall, 1990; Gilliss, 1993; Whall, 1993; Wright & Leahey, 1994).

In the current health care climate, meeting the needs of families is a challenge. With decreased lengths of stay, clients may progress more quickly through the acute care setting, often with more severe residual disabilities. Thus, nurses are caring for clients with higher levels of acuteness and may have little time,

energy, or knowledge to care for families. This is particularly problematic in relation to the role of the family in the rehabilitation of clients with a disability or chronic illness. Clinical research has documented the importance of the family in rehabilitation outcomes. For example, in studies involving family members with chronic renal disease, hypertension, and diabetes mellitus, a direct relationship has been found between treatment compliance and family functioning (Gilliss, 1989).

With family support, a client with a disability copes more effectively and achieves a better outcome. In response to shortened lengths of stay, families must be included early in the client's care. For this inclusion to be effective, family support and interventions need to be an integral aspect of nursing care. If the family is supported during rehabilitation, family members may be more effective in supporting the client and in adapting to the long-term consequences of the disability (Campbell & Patterson, 1995; Kleeman, 1989; Power, 1985).

FAMILY AS A SYSTEM

Certain concepts of general systems theory are relevant to understanding the family as a system. A *system* is composed of a set of objects with certain attributes and the relationships among those objects. A family can be viewed as a system of interrelated parts forming a whole. Systems theory views the family comprehensively in terms of the relationships, associations, and connections that occur in a dynamic interacting whole. It may be helpful to visualize the family as a mobile suspended in space. *Nonsummativity* refers to the notion that the whole is greater than the sum of its parts. In keeping with this notion, the family (like a mobile) as a combined effort produces a greater and different effect than the sum of individual efforts. This whole includes the family's uniqueness—its history and dynamics. *Wholeness* means that a change in one part of a system triggers a compensatory change in other systems and parts of the system. Much as touching one piece of a mobile causes all of its pieces to shift and move, a change in one member of a family in response to chronic illness or disability creates changes in other family members (Minuchin, 1985; Minuchin & Fishman, 1981).

Systems and families strive to maintain *homeostasis*—a dynamic equilibrium or balance among the many forces that operate within and upon it. All systems need to balance themselves within a range of functioning in which the work of the system can be accomplished. Family homeostasis depends on each member's knowing and carrying out his or her role and adhering to the values and communication patterns of the family. If a family depletes most of its energy to maintain this balance, little energy remains for growth of the family or its individual members (Minuchin, 1974, 1985; Minuchin & Fishman, 1981). Homeostasis may best be understood as a balance between change and stability, with the family needing to respond to constant change. Thus, change and stability coexist within the family (Wright & Leahey, 1994). In the mobile example, picture what happens when a breeze hits a "stationary" mobile and how it eventually settles into its usual "balance" again. If one piece is lost, the mobile needs to adjust and achieve a new balance.

It is also important to note that balance or homeostasis does not imply "normality." Families may attain and maintain a balance that is dysfunctional and acutely painful for an individual member. An example is a chronically ill child who functions as a "ping-pong ball" between two warring parents, or a family member who carries out a sick role prescribed by the family.

All systems are viewed along a continuum of being *open* to being *closed*—referring to the system's ability to adapt to changes in the environment. Openness allows flexibility, growth, and change. Thus, an open family responds to *feedback*, or information from the outside, in order to change and grow. Feedback may also come from inside the system and provide information on the family's functioning. This may include how behavior affects others and how actions are perceived.

Boundaries define who participates in the system, the extent of differentiation permitted, the amount of intensity of emotional investment, the amount and kinds of experiences available outside the system, and ways to evaluate experiences in terms of the family

system. In a family, boundaries may be too rigid and not allow growth and change or may be too diffuse—such as a child's becoming "parentified"—taking on adult, parental roles and functions when a parent becomes chronically ill or disabled. In the mobile, if two pieces become tangled together, the mobile will remain balanced if other pieces shift.

The *structure* of systems and families includes the *suprasystem*—or outside systems—such as school, church, and sports activities. The *subsystems* include subdivisions within the family such as the spousal, parental, and sibling subsystems and others that function according to boundaries, roles, and interests.

Subsystems are formed on a hierarchical basis, and boundaries should be clear. Subsystems are created by generations, gender, interest, or function. Each person in a family usually belongs to several subsystems (Minuchin, 1974, 1985). The *spousal subsystem* is a refuge that fosters learning and creativity within each spouse's psychological territory. Children should not perceive the boundary as diffuse or share spousal roles and functions. The *parental subsystem* achieves the child-rearing functions of guidance, nurturance, and control. Children should be socialized without loss of the emotional support between the spouses. There should be a differentiated use of authority, a balance of autonomy and guidance, which changes over time as children mature. The *sibling subsystem* provides opportunities to experiment with peer relationships and learn how to negotiate, cooperate, and compete. Older siblings bring new knowledge and skills from the "world" to younger siblings (Minuchin, 1974).

Power in a family is usually structured as a hierarchy in which adults wield power—usually in an authoritative way. As children grow, there is an increased diffusion of power and an increase in the democratic process. Power creates a safe environment for individuals to grow and develop and allows the family as a system to operate effectively (Minuchin, 1974, 1985). *Family roles* are established by families to accomplish family development tasks, according to family rules. Examples of family roles include breadwinner, peacekeeper, nurturer, and decision maker. *Role conflict* may occur if family members are unable or unwilling to perform assigned roles during chronic illness or disability; for example, a father who sustains a spinal cord injury may no longer be the breadwinner in the family. Family members fulfill various roles depending on the setting—thus, a woman may be a powerful executive at work but may be a "little girl" in the presence of her parents. Some family roles are assigned before birth.

Behavior, or patterns in a family system, is characterized as circular—meaning that each person's behavior is both a cause and an effect at the same time. In a family, each member engages in behavior that influences the other members. The process may be viewed as circular patterns of uninterrupted sequences of interchanges. Picture the pieces of a mobile bumping against each other. It is the cycle of interaction (for example, interaction between the caregiver and the chronically ill family member) that is the irreducible unit, and change must occur within this cycle (Minuchin, 1985). The range of behaviors within a family depends on the family's capacity to absorb and incorporate information from extrafamilial systems, for example, the health care team. During chronic illness or disability, the family's coping response depends on its ability to respond to the demands and make changes in order to accomplish necessary family tasks (Minuchin, 1985). However, during times of stress, families tend to hold onto previously used patterns of behavior, whether or not they are effective (Wright & Leahey, 1994).

FAMILY DEVELOPMENT TASKS

Each family develops its unique personality and methods of performing the tasks that society expects. Various family models describe these tasks. The family sociologist Evelyn Duvall (1977) listed the developmental tasks of American families (Table 15–1).

During chronic illness and disability, a family needs to change roles, rules, and functions in order to accomplish these developmental tasks. The entire family will experience life with a chronic illness or disability and must cope with the chronicity for their remaining life together. An additional and critical family role is added—that of family caregiver. The family's strength depends on its ability to mobilize alternative patterns in response to the demands of chronic illness or disability (Minuchin, 1974, 1985).

FAMILY LIFE CYCLE

Family systems evolve over time according to family life-cycle stages. Just as individuals in a family go through developing stages, so do

TABLE 15–1 ■ DUVALL'S FAMILY DEVELOPMENTAL TASKS

Physical maintenance (food, shelter, clothing, health care)

Resource allocation (material goods [family expenses, space], emotional goods [affection, respect, authority])

Division of labor (who does what)

Socialization of family members (mature patterns of expressing aggression, sexuality)

Reproduction, recruitment, and release of family members (birth, adoption, child rearing, including new members and establishing policies for including others, e.g., in-laws)

Maintenance of order (administrative sanctions to conform to family and social norms)

Placement of members in larger society (interaction with community, school, church)

Maintenance of motivation and morale (rewarding members for achievements, developing philosophies of life, family loyalties, rituals and celebrations, meeting personal and family crises)

families as a whole. Carter and McGoldrick (1988) identify family life-cycle stages as (1) single young adults leaving home; (2) the new couple—joining of families through marriage; (3) families with young children; (4) families with adolescent children; (5) middle-aged couples—launching children and moving on; and (6) older couples—families in later life. Mastery of each stage affects subsequent stages of adaptation and is affected by internal and external demands placed on the system. Periods of transition from one stage to another usually involve people's entering or leaving the system and necessitate changes in order to maintain homeostasis.

NORMATIVE FAMILY FUNCTIONING

Family function is the purpose that the family serves for individual members, the family as a whole, and other social systems. Family functions allow the family to do the work required of the family unit in contemporary life. The functions of the family influence, and are influenced by, the health status of individual family members and the family as a whole. Family health care requires the rehabilitation nurse to first assess the family's functioning in order to assess the effect of the family on health status, assess the impact of chronic illness or disability, and work with the family in the development and implementation of a care plan to improve the family's health (Table 15–2) (Ballard, 1996).

TABLE 15–2 ■ CHARACTERISTICS OF A FUNCTIONAL FAMILY

There is maintenance of a homeostatic balance and flexibility to adapt to change during transitional stages of family life and periods of stress.

Problems are viewed as partially a function of each person, rather than residing entirely in one family member.

Emotional contact is maintained across generations and between family members without blurring necessary levels of authority.

Overcloseness is avoided, and distance is not used to solve problems.

Each dyad or twosome is expected to resolve problems between them.

Bringing in a third person to settle disputes or to take sides is discouraged.

Differences among family members are encouraged to promote personal growth and creativity.

Children are expected to assume age-appropriate responsibilities and to enjoy age-appropriate privileges negotiated with their parents.

Preservation of a positive emotional climate is more highly valued than doing what "should" be done or what is "right."

Within each spouse there is a balance of affective expression, careful rational thought, relationship focus, and care taking, and each spouse can effectively function in his or her respective role (Minuchin, 1974; Walsh, 1993). The marital relationship is the basic foundational unit of the family, and it is the most critical factor in the quality of family functioning (Beavers, 1985).

IMPACT OF CHRONIC ILLNESS OR DISABILITY ON THE FAMILY

Crisis theory provides several concepts relevant to assessing and supporting families experiencing chronic illness or disability (Aguilera, 1994). In the acute phase of rehabilitation, family members are most in need of and amenable to intervention. Whether family members experience the event as a crisis is affected by three balancing factors that must be assessed: perception of the event, coping mechanisms, and social support.

The onset of the disability may affect *perception of the event*. An acute event such as an injury or trauma may present increased difficulties because the client and family cannot engage in anticipatory work as they might do during the insidious progression of a chronic illness (Lundin, 1984; Rando, 1983). The demands of the illness are the events or experiences that clients and families attribute to the illness that may burden the family in relation to personal, social, and economic resources. The client with a chronic illness or disability experiences the demands due to the direct effects of the disease such as loss of function and social isolation (Woods et al., 1993; Woods et al., 1989). Families experience demands in dealing with the extended family, suprasystems such as school and work, and pressure to change internal processes such as family roles and functions.

Since the demands are the perceptions of individuals, they may vary over time and may differ among family members. Indeed, family members appraise the chronic illness or disability differently depending on their age, gender, role in the family, and prior experience. Families must struggle to achieve a shared understanding (McCubbin & McCubbin, 1993). In the situation of chronic childhood illness, families have more effective coping and outcomes if they view the event as a challenge and an opportunity for growth and endow the illness with meaning (Holaday, 1989; Venters, 1986).

Chronic illness requires lasting alterations in how the family functions from day to day. The family reorganization that occurs during an acute illness when the family focuses on the ill member's care cannot continue over the long term. In progressive chronic illness such as some cancers or Alzheimer's disease, the family member declines over time—either rapidly or slowly. Caretaking demands increase over time, and the family caregivers may become burned out. In illnesses or disabilities with a more constant course (spinal cord injury or cerebrovascular accident), the family must adapt to the lessened but rather stable functioning of the family member. Family caregivers are affected by the constancy of the changed family. In relapsing or episodic illnesses (cancer or multiple sclerosis), the individual and family as a whole experience stable periods punctuated by exacerbations. This requires family flexibility in moving between a crisis mode and a daily functioning mode. Family members may be in a constant state of alertness for change (Rolland, 1988, 1994).

Thus, the response to chronic illness or disability in a family member may depend on the nature and course of the illness and its variability and on family members' perceived demands of the illness (Woods et al., 1993; Woods, et al., 1989). Wright and Leahey (1994) emphasize that the family's perception of the illness event has the most influence on their ability to cope.

Coping mechanisms and *social supports* need to be assessed. It is normal for family members to feel helpless, overwhelmed, and fearful. Families need to be supported in order for them to help support the client with a chronic illness or disability. This is particularly important since the family's ongoing physical, emotional, and social health may be the standard against which the client measures his or her rehabilitation progress (Wright & Leahey, 1994). According to McCubbin and McCubbin (1993), families are more likely to adapt successfully if

- They are less vulnerable because fewer other stressors or family changes are occurring at the time.
- They have patterns of functioning that are more adaptive (e.g., there is more emotional closeness among family members, and they are more flexible and able to change roles, boundaries, and rules when necessary).
- They define the situation positively and view it as something they can master and have some control over.
- They have good coping and communication skills.

FAMILY NEEDS THROUGHOUT THE REHABILITATION PROCESS

Family needs may differ according to the phase of the rehabilitation process: the acute, adjustment, or adaptation/long-term phase (McCubbin & McCubbin, 1993).

Acute Phase

The acute phase begins when the injury or trauma occurs or the chronic illness is diagnosed. The family and client are often faced with an unexpected hospitalization, the uncertainty of the outcome, and the need for the family to begin to make internal changes in response to the chronic illness or disability.

Family needs during the acute phase have been identified in the literature (Lynn-McHale & Smith, 1993; McCubbin & McCubbin, 1993; Rolland, 1994; Winterhalter, 1992; Wright & Leahey, 1994) as

- The need for information
- The need to manage emotional distress
- The need to maintain family functioning
- The need to utilize coping skills
- The need to manage uncertainty

Managing the uncertainty associated with a chronic illness or disability may be a critical task of adaptation (Mishel, 1988, 1990). According to Mishel, there are four forms of uncertainty in the illness experience: ambiguity concerning the state of the illness, complexity regarding care and treatment systems, a lack of information about the treatment and severity of the illness, and the unpredictability of the course of the disease and its prognosis. Managing chronic uncertainty can produce growth and change through a new worldview. The client and family should be encouraged to develop new methods for valued activities and to consider new alternatives in coping with the changing nature of the illness (Mishel, 1990; Mishel & Sorenson, 1991).

The client and family begin to realize they must prepare for a life with chronic illness or disability when they make the transition from the acute to the chronic state. If the family members are supported during the acute phase, they will be better prepared to plan and give care, participate in discharge planning, and make the transition through the health care system. During the acute phase, the family is most amenable to intervention. Family members are experiencing a period of tremendous stress and will probably "band together" to support each other and the client. Supporting families during the crisis of the acute phase is critical in optimizing client and family recovery (Campbell & Patterson, 1995; Rolland, 1994; Woods et al., 1993).

Adjustment Phase

This phase usually occurs during the period of hospitalization following the injury or diagnosis of chronic illness. At this point, the family must deal with two major issues. They are relieved that the client won't die, but they must confront the reality of long-term disability. This phase is a period of transition from an acute to a chronic illness status.

The family needs to make internal changes in order to effectively respond to the demands of the chronic illness or disability. The family must meet the needs of the well family members as well as those of the "ill" member. This usually involves adjusting to changes in roles and lifestyle. Indeed, it is critical for family members to learn new role behaviors. The client needs to learn new behaviors associated with the chronic illness or disability, while the family must learn new behaviors associated with the caregiving role. In general, families experiencing chronic illness or disability tend to experience role overload in family members and role constriction in the client (Leahey & Wright, 1985).

The family and client may need to manage issues of uncertainty of the prognosis or outcome and prepare for the client to be discharged to home or a rehabilitation facility. Families need skills and support to prepare to take the client home. This may present several challenges. The family may have 24-hour responsibility for care and need home modifications and special equipment. Although teaching, support, and anticipatory work are helpful, the family can never be totally prepared for the client's return home. Research evidence indicates that this phase usually lasts up to 1 year after diagnosis in the acute setting. If the family is the primary caregiver, this phase usually lasts 1 to 2 years (Clubb, 1991; Gaynor, 1990; Jacob, 1993; Sayles-Cross, 1993).

Adaptation Phase

The hallmark of chronic illness is the variability in disease response and the long-term nature of symptom management and psychological adaptation (Woods et al., 1993; Woods et al., 1989). The demands of chronic illness or disability are many. The family may have economic concerns related to the cost of care, lost wages, and insurance limits. Even if the family has adequate financial resources and insurance, family members often spend an incredible amount of time and energy engaged in the process of record keeping, claim filing, and "working the system" to advocate for appropriate care for the family member. Access to community services may be limited or unknown to the family. In general, research documents that many families do not receive needed services whether it be for case management, respite care, support groups, transportation, or home care (Hoeman, 1992).

FAMILY COPING

Families may cope by defending against the impact of the event or may actively deal with it through physical, cognitive, or affective coping skills. Effective strategies include cognitive reframing or positive reappraisal in which the person makes comparisons with someone in a similar situation, focuses on the positive, and expresses optimistic beliefs. Selective ignoring can provide temporary relief from the situation, whereas information seeking and problem solving attempt to deal directly with the impact of the chronic illness or disability (Mishel, 1990; Mishel & Sorenson, 1991; Wright & Leahey, 1994).

Rehabilitation clients and their families may use different coping strategies to deal with the demands of the illness. In one study of women with cancer and their spouses, the women were more inclined to do something about their situation (problem-focused and cognitive restructuring), whereas their husbands tended to hope that the problems would go away (threat minimization) (Zacharias, Gilg, & Foxall, 1994).

In the situation of chronic childhood illness, normalization is an effective strategy for family coping. The child is viewed as not different in any significant way. The family separates the illness or disability aspects from nonillness aspects of the child's life. The family recognizes the impact of the chronic illness or disability but emphasizes the normal. In this way, the disability is acknowledged but the significance of social stigma is diminished. The family depicts life as normal and substitutes actions when needed (Deatrick & Knafl, 1990; Holaday, 1989; Knafl & Deatrick, 1990).

FAMILY CAREGIVING

Family caregiving may be perceived as a burden or an act of love and caring, or both. One person usually assumes the major role of caregiver, and this is usually a married woman in the family. In fact, 85% of family caregivers are female (Jacob, 1993). The demands of caregiving may require physical, emotional, economic, and social sacrifices. The research literature has documented the burdens of caregiving related to depression, chronic fatigue, physical symptoms, lowered self-esteem and well-being, and social isolation (Collins, Stommel, Wang, & Given, 1994; Gaynor, 1990; Robinson, 1989; Sayles-Cross, 1993). Most families need respite care but rarely ask for assistance or complain (Robinson, 1989). Even 3 to 4 hours of respite care per week would provide a "safety net" to families who are caregiving.

Younger caregivers seem to suffer the most stress of caregiver burden (Gaynor, 1990). This may be due to the "sandwich" effect of caring for a family member while juggling the demands of children and a career. Long-term caregivers have higher perceived burden and more physical illnesses. A cycle of neglect may exist in these women as they age and endure the stress of prolonged caregiving. Caregiver stress seems to peak at 2 to 4 years—perhaps owing to the loss of home health services, decreased family support, and/or the onset of caregiver fatigue (Quint, Chesterman, Crain, Winkleby, & Boyce, 1990). These findings are supported in studies of technology-dependent children receiving nursing care at home (Fleming et al., 1994; Quint et al., 1990; Teague et al., 1993).

In a qualitative study of family caregivers of family members with varied chronic illnesses, family caregivers reported a feeling of isolation or aloneness. Feelings of isolation also included neglecting personal needs, being unable to have or maintain an outside job, and decreasing family or social contacts. However, these caregivers were unwilling to share care with others, even refusing respite care when their own health declined. Their universe included the caregiver–care recipient dyad. There was little "giving up" or "giving away" of other role responsibilities. These caregivers perceived their caregiving as a "solitary joining" to which they were totally committed in the face of uncertainty and challenges (Boland & Sims, 1996).

Respite care, support groups including Internet mailing lists, and hotlines would provide a mechanism for family caregivers to deal with fatigue, guilt, resentment, and social isolation (Bull, Maruyama, & Luo, 1995; Fink, 1995; Jacobs, 1993). In one study of families with a technology-dependent child receiving respite care at home, the extent of family use of services was directly related to a decreased perception of stress and lower sibling strain. The mothers who were primary caretakers expressed a decrease in both somatic symptoms and the number of hospitalizations while using increased rates of respite services (Sherman, 1995).

The family needs to be supported and educated during the chronic trajectory of remissions and exacerbations or the gradual physical decline of the family member. There is an increased need for support and education during the integration of treatment activities into activities of daily living, when there is a change in the pattern and intensity of symptoms, and when the family recognizes the progression of the chronic illness or disability or terminal phase (Fink, 1995; Jacob, 1993). In one study, 63% of caregivers reported that health professionals had not answered questions about managing the member's care (Bull et al., 1995).

When a child is chronically ill or disabled, the family has a central role in managing the child's care. The child's prognosis depends on the family's ability to exert continual efforts on its own behalf (Battle, 1975; Deatrick & Knafl, 1990; Sterling, 1990). The parents often experience "chronic sorrow" in that they do not have the hoped-for "normal" child and the chronic illness or disability will not ever go away. At developmental milestones, family life-cycle events, or changing physical states, the parents may experience a reemergence of acute grief (Clubb, 1991; Damrosch & Perry, 1989). Empirical evidence shows that there are critical times for families (Gilliss, 1989; Winterhalter, 1989):

- At the time of diagnosis
- When there is an increase in the child's or family members' needs
- When there is a change in the support structure
- When there is an increase in the severity or number of physical symptoms
- At the time of transferring self-care to the child—often occurring during adolescence

Strained family relationships may occur because of a variety of factors (Gallo, Breitmayer, Knafl, & Zoeller, 1992; Winterhalter, 1989; Wright & Leahey, 1994):

- Overprotectiveness of the child
- Coalitions between the primary caretaker and the child
- Scapegoating and blaming of the child or parent
- Overt or covert rejection of the child
- Worry or resentment over extended parenting/caregiving responsibilities
- Sibling competition for parental time and affection
- Sibling comparisons and discrepancies related to growth and development
- An overall increase in tension and conflict

Research evidence supports the concept that family activities and goals must be modified owing to less flexibility with leisure time, vacations, career changes, and the decision to have more children. The burden of increased tasks and time commitments related to the medical regimen takes its toll in economics, social isolation, fatigue, and personal goals and activities (Fleming et al., 1994; Gallo et al., 1992; Teague et al., 1993; Winterhalter, 1989; Winterhalter & Burke, 1996). Parents are often overwhelmed with advocating for their child in relation to competent home care, maintaining parental authority, and obtaining appropriate school experiences (Hazlett, 1989; Quint et al., 1990; Williams, Lorenzo, & Borja, 1993).

There is empirical evidence that mothers and fathers perceive different burdens and goals and use different coping mechanisms (Benson & McLaughlin, 1996; Winterhalter, 1989; Winterhalter & Burke, 1996). Sibling responses reported in the literature include both positive and negative aspects of living with a sibling with a chronic illness or disability (Gallo et al., 1992; Leonard, Brust, & Nelson, 1993; Winterhalter, 1989; Winterhalter & Burke, 1996).

However, there is evidence that parents caring for a chronically ill child in the home have less stress than parents who are not the primary caregivers (Leonard et al, 1993; Teague et al., 1993). Along with a decrease in caregiver stress, a significant decrease in sibling strain was noted in families in which respite care was used to provide for the chronically ill child. Although the relationship between caring for a chronically ill child in the home and intrafamily and marital stress has been widely documented, many families believe and report that they would not have changed their decision and claimed that their ability to provide care for their child was the best aspect of their situation (Teague et al., 1993).

However, research findings indicate that health care professionals may not be meeting the needs of families receiving care in the home. Although health care professionals and home care nurses were named most frequently as resources for the family, they were also perceived by families as the most significant barrier to care (Ray & Ritchie, 1993; Sharer & Dixon, 1989). Investigating the relationship between parents and health care workers providing care to the medically fragile child in the home, Patterson, Jernell, Leonard, and Titus (1994) stated that parents reported both positive and negative aspects associated with interactions with the nurses who were providing care to their child. On the whole, parents reported that they felt the nurses were competent, genuinely cared for the child, and were supportive of the family's needs, but they stated that often they experienced difficulties with scheduling, staff turnover, and cancellations. Parents also said they felt that their privacy was being invaded by having the nurses in the home and felt the nurses demonstrated a lack of respect toward other family members. The parents participating in the study completed by Sharer and Dixon (1989) stated that many of the home care nurses lacked empathy for the parents, made them feel inadequate as parents, or interfered with their parenting and the parent-child relationship.

FAMILY SOCIAL SUPPORT

Social support for the family is conceptualized as an interaction of reciprocity, emotional involvement, and advice or feedback (Kane, 1988). Reciprocity is achieved by sharing resources and asking for and receiving help. The emotional involvement factor includes traits such as caring, compassion, and warmth. The advice or feedback factor involves family members' sharing their perception of themselves and of the family as a whole with others and receiving appraisals on how others view the family. In this way, family social support enables the family to function with resourcefulness and flexibility. As previously discussed, this is a critical attribute when the family is attempting to cope with the internal and external demands brought on by chronic illness or disability.

Different sources of support—professionals, family, and friends—may best provide different types of support. For example, information sources might include professionals with specific expertise or nonprofessionals whose experiences have made them experts (family members farther along in the rehabilitation process). Professionals who are expert in the therapeutic use of self and in conducting family assessments and interventions may be an appropriate source of emotional support. This may be especially needed during the acute crisis phase of rehabilitation if family members are unable to give support to or receive it from each other or the client. Otherwise, emotional support may best be provided by extended family or friends. The best source of expressive or affective support is probably family, friends, and families coping with the same chronic illness or disability (Kane, 1988; Woods et al., 1993; Woods et al., 1989).

In one study of family resources and demands, social support was found to have a direct effect on family well-being. Also, the perception of having resources available and viewing life changes as challenges maintained a sense of well-being in the face of stressful situations. Family confidence in problem solving and the ability to work together were important factors in maintaining well-being (Fink, 1995).

FAMILY SUPPORT GROUPS

If the family is supported during the acute phase of rehabilitation, family members may be more effective in supporting the client and in adapting to the long-term consequences of the chronic illness or disability. In the author's experience, the use of a family support group assists families in resolving the crisis of the acute phase and facilitating a smoother transition through the health care system (Richmond, Metcalf, & Winterhalter, 1987; Winterhalter, 1992). Early involvement in a family support group may promote client and family adaptation through linkage to sources and types of support needed in the acute phase of rehabilitation.

The author helped to develop a family support group to help meet the needs of family members of neurosensory clients in a major tertiary care setting. Most of the attendees were parents and spouses of clients in the neurosensory intensive care unit, although the group was available to family members of all neurosensory clients. Most of the clients had sustained head and/or spinal cord trauma. Goals were developed on the basis of identified family needs and input from the interdisciplinary group. The group focused on supporting families in coping with an acutely ill family member and in preparing for the long-term needs of the client with chronic deficits. Although specific to this client group, the goals are germane to family members in the acute phase of the rehabilitation process. The goals of the family support group included (Winterhalter, 1992)

- Providing emotional support to families
- Facilitating anxiety reduction
- Facilitating the sharing of common concerns and stresses related to the illness or injury and its treatment
- Reinforcing effective coping skills and identifying maladaptive ones
- Facilitating a smooth transition through the health care system

Identifying nurse facilitators, practical logistics, and advertising are key organizational components for developing and maintaining a family support group. The reader is referred to the literature for details of organization and implementation (Winterhalter, 1992; Richmond et al., 1987). Common themes that emerged in family support groups and their interventions are outlined in Table 15–3.

The positive outcomes of attending family support groups are many. The sense of camaraderie with other families in similar circumstances is supportive. Family members are grateful for a safe place to verbalize their feelings and fears. Family members often report that group sessions provide the only vehicle for expressing their true feelings, especially if they are maintaining a "strong" position in the family and keeping everybody and everything "together." The family members may have temporarily lost the person most supportive emotionally to them—the client. When the entire family is suffering, family members may not be able to support each other and probably need extrafamilial support.

In a group setting, family members learn

TABLE 15–3 ■ COMMON THEMES IN FAMILY SUPPORT GROUPS AND RELATED INTERVENTIONS

Need to relive the incident leading to hospitalization, particularly when the admission is unexpected. The family member should be encouraged to relive the incident and express feelings related to it. However, one group member cannot monopolize group time.

Unpredictability of the client's prognosis. Facilitators should encourage ventilation of feelings and fears while teaching family members that chronic uncertainty is a normal aspect of chronic illness or disability. The family is supported during the "roller coaster" ups and downs during the acute phase.

Need for basic information. Facilitators should provide basic information related to the treatment of the client's illness or injury. However, specifics of individual needs and care should be discussed on a one-to-one basis outside the group. Basic information is often necessary to begin anxiety reduction and have family members responsive to emotional support.

Need to express anger. Facilitators should accept anger in a nonjudgmental manner as a normal part of the experience. If family members feel comfortable, they may express anger toward the client, the health care team, the illness or injury, and the losses. Limits may need to be set if family members become uncomfortable.

Need to grieve. Verbalizing their sense of loss and its effect may facilitate the work of mourning. Perceived and anticipated losses are often multiple and profound.

Difficulty in maintaining family functioning, such as changes in roles, task fulfillment, power, and communication. Facilitators should encourage family members to express the impact of the illness or injury, use social supports, and use effective coping skills. Family members need to accept that they cannot meet the needs of the "ill" member while maintaining the usual daily life for the family as a whole. Family members should be encouraged to meet their own needs and their need for respite from a bedside vigil.

Need to facilitate communication. Depending on the client's injury or illness, family members may need help in developing alternative communication techniques such as touch, reading, or audiotapes. Families may need support in order to communicate assertively with the health care team. Facilitators may need to initiate referrals on behalf of family members.

Need for early discharge planning. Family members need support during teaching for caregiving after discharge. Family members often feel overwhelmed and incompetent.

that their feelings and actions are normal to the situation and that their expression facilitates adaptation. Anxiety reduction occurs through the verbalization of affect, the use of adaptive coping skills, and the use of social support. The support group facilitator can help family members negotiate the health care system by the provision of information, the encouragement of assertive communication, and the provision of assistance with discharge planning. Most importantly, family members learn to accept that their needs are important, are shared by others, and must be met (Winterhalter, 1992).

FAMILY NURSING PROCESS: FAMILY ASSESSMENT

The rehabilitation nurse needs to assess the family as a system and determine whether the family was functional or dysfunctional before the chronic illness or disability occurred and to assess the current status of the family. Can the family accomplish needed tasks? Can the family get the work done? Can it meet the needs of the family as a whole and of each individual member? Does the family encourage growth and autonomy? In general, functional families are more open, flexible, and adaptable to changes in response to internal and external demands. Dysfunctional families are more closed and rigid. Assessment can occur by observing family interactions, by using a formal data collection process, and by using family assessment tools.

The rehabilitation nurse needs to assess family dynamics within the context of the family's culture and ethnicity. Family values, roles, power, communication patterns, and coping are shaped by the family's culture. Effective assessments and interventions must be based on the client/family cultural milieu (Antai-Ontong, 1995; Friedman & Ferguson-Marshalleck, 1996) (Table 15–4).

In summary, the family's strength depends on its ability to mobilize alternative patterns when stressed by internal or external changes such as chronic illness or disability. McMaster (1982) has identified areas of family function that contribute most significantly to healthy outcomes in times of crisis or change (Epstein, Baldwin, & Bishop, 1983):

- Problem solving that provides for basic human needs
- Communication that is clear, congruent, and direct
- Role allocation that family members can adhere to and that allows role sharing

- Affective involvement in which family members are sensitive to each other's needs
- Affective responsiveness in which emotions are expressed freely, validated, and accepted
- Behavior control in the form of flexible rules and feedback mechanisms

It is particularly important for the nurse to assess if there are family issues that would interfere with the rehabilitation process and to plan interventions to minimize their effects. For example, a family with ineffective communication patterns may be unable to dialogue effectively with staff and to be involved in care or discharge planning. In a disengaged family, family members may be unavailable or unwilling to participate in care and support the ill family member. In overinvolved families, there may be a bedside vigil and a lack of client participation in planning and self-care.

FAMILY NURSING DIAGNOSES

Although other alterations may occur in response to illness and caregiving demands, the following nursing diagnoses are particularly relevant to the family during chronic illness or disability (Ross, 1996):

- Altered family process
- Alteration in parenting
- Altered role performance
- Altered sexuality patterns
- Decision conflict
- Family coping: potential for growth
- Ineffective family coping: compromised
- Ineffective family coping: disabling
- Parental role conflict
- Potential altered parenting

FAMILY NURSING INTERVENTIONS

Interventions to Maintain the Family as the Unit of Care

The rehabilitation nurse may intervene to help maintain the family as the unit of care in the following ways:

- Intervention with the family as a whole throughout the rehabilitation process.
- Advocating for the family in relation to family adaptation with the health care delivery system.
- Keeping a focus on the present needs of the family.

TABLE 15–4 ■ A MODEL OF FAMILY ASSESSMENT

Family Structure

Family constellation
Generational history of family patterns
Participants of family subsystems
   Spousal
   Parental
   Sibling
   Other alliances
Boundaries across family subsystems
Degree of closeness among family members (enmeshment/
   disengagement)
Degree of autonomy among family members (autonomy/
   diffusion)

Family Function

Adequacy of role performance
   Formal roles and performance
   Informal roles and performance
   Degree of family agreement on assigned roles and
      performance
   Presence of role strain, conflict, or overload
   Changes in roles in response to the chronic illness or
      disability
Family rules
   Rules that foster maintenance and stability
   Rules that foster dysfunction
   Modification of rules in response to the chronic illness or
      disability
   Respect for differences
Family communication
   Communication patterns, verbal and nonverbal
   Provision of information to family members
   Channels of communication
   Quality of messages
   Responsiveness to feedback within and from outside the
      system
   Changes in response to chronic illness/disability
Family power
   Who speaks for the family
   Degree to which family members participate in family
      functions
   How interpersonal conflicts are handled
   Methods of conflict resolution
   Methods of decision making
   Methods of task allocation
   Changes in response to chronic illness/disability

Family subsystems
   Adequacy of functions
   Role of alliances in family stability
   Interaction of subsystems and family as a whole
Family development tasks
   Meeting of physical, emotional, and social needs of the
      family as a whole
   Meeting of physical, emotional, and social needs of
      individual family members
   Family resources to meet needs
   Conflicts between individual and family needs
   Degree to which family goals and values are adhered to by
      individual and family members
   Extent to which family will permit pursuit of individual goals
      and values
   Family coping styles and adherence by individual family
      members, congruence with individual coping styles
   Family social supports and utilization
   Changes in response to chronic illness/disability

Family Life Cycle

   Chronological stage of family
   Adaptation and/or problems with transitions
   Shifts in family process over time
   History of earlier stages

Family Demographics

   Economic resources
   Employment of family members
   Cultural and ethnic identification and practices
   Religious identification and practices
   Living arrangements
   Education of family members

Family Assessment Instruments

Family Systems Stressor-Strength Inventory (FS³I)
   (Mischke-Berkey & Hanson, 1991)
The Friedman Family Assessment Model (short form)
   (Friedman, 1992).
The Calgary Family Assessment Model
   (Wright & Leahey, 1994).
Family APGAR (Smilkstein, Ashworth, & Montano, 1982).
(McMaster) Family Assessment Device (FAD)
   (Epstein, Baldwin, & Bishop, 1983)
Family Functioning Index (Pless & Satterwhite, 1973)
F-COPES (Olson, Russell, & Sprenkle, 1980)
Feetham Family Functioning Survey (FFFS)
   (Roberts & Feetham, 1982).

- Incorporating knowledge of family history and dynamics as appropriate. For example, if there is a high level of emotional fusion in the family, family members may need to keep a "vigil" at the bedside. They may "burn out" faster and suffer caregiver fatigue, thereby requiring more respite care. If family members are disengaged from each other, the nurse should hold meetings with the entire family when planning care.
- Helping the family to achieve a realistic perception of the event and to frame the chronic illness or disability as a family challenge.
- Encouraging family members to ventilate affect related to the event.
- Providing hope-enhancing strategies.
- Assisting the family in balancing the needs of the client, the individual family members, and the family as a whole.

Interventions to Enhance Family Functions

Following are ways the nurse can intervene to help enhance family functions:

- Assisting the family in negotiating the reallocation of role performance in response to the demands of the chronic illness or disability
- Identifying family rules that interfere with the rehabilitation process
- Offering consistent information and education related to the client's condition
- Holding family care planning meetings
- Facilitating the family's open communication with family members and health care providers
- Teaching alternative communication techniques for the client as appropriate
- Teaching assertive communication techniques as appropriate
- Assisting the family with conflict resolution and decision making; if the family is disagreeing, holding family meetings and temporarily functioning as "peacemaker"
- If power is very centralized in one family member, meeting with that person first and early to supply information, assist with decision making, support reallocation of family tasks, and provide for caregiving and discharge
- Giving "permission" for family members to take care of their own needs
- Assisting the family in mobilizing social support, as needed, e.g., other professionals, extended family, families in similar circumstances, family support groups
- Teaching alternative coping mechanisms, as needed
- Providing additional support and resources if the family life cycle is at a period of transition, e.g., a birth, a child going to school or college
- Assisting the family in normalizing the client's life as much as possible
- Providing adequate discharge teaching, including written materials
- If the family is dysfunctional, interfering with the rehabilitation process, and/or highly anxious after 4 to 6 weeks, referring the family to a mental health professional for assessment and counseling
- Encouraging the use of supportive home care services, including respite care
- Coordinating services for the client and family along the care continuum

FAMILY OUTCOMES

Following are desired family outcomes:

- The maintenance of open, effective communication and problem-solving among family members, the client, and the health care team
- Mutual support given and received among family members
- Utilization of appropriate resources and supports
- The maintenance of family stability, hope, and optimistic views
- Effective family involvement in client care and planning
- The meeting of the ill family member's needs and the needs of the family as a whole through appropriate task allocation
- A family with a sense of mastery over events

REFERENCES

Aguilera, D. (1994). *Crisis intervention. Theory and methodology.* St. Louis: C. V. Mosby.

Antai-Otong, D. (1995). *Psychiatric nursing.* Philadelphia: W. B. Saunders.

Ballard, N. (1996). Family structure, function and process. In S. Hanson and S. Boyd (Eds.), *Family health care nursing* (pp. 57–78). Philadelphia: F. A. Davis.

Battle, C. U. (1975). Symposium on behavioral pediatrics. Chronic physical disease. Behavioral pediatrics. *Pediatric Clinics of North America, 22,* 525–531.

Beavers, W. (1985). *Successful marriage: A family systems approach to couple therapy.* New York: W. W. Norton.

Benson, E., & McLaughlin, S. (1996). *Family functioning and well-sibling self-concept of technology-dependent chil-*

dren receiving nursing care at home. Unpublished master's thesis, Gwynedd-Mercy College, Gwynedd Valley, PA.

Boland, D., & Sims, S. (1996). Family care giving at home as a solitary journey. *Image: The Journal of Nursing Scholarship, 28,* 55–58.

Bull, M., Maruyama, G., & Luo, D. (1995). Testing a model for posthospital transition of family caregivers for elderly persons. *Nursing Research, 44,* 132–138.

Caine, R. (1989). Families in crisis: Making the critical difference. *Focus on Critical Care, 16,* 184–189.

Campbell, T., & Patterson, J. (1995). The effectiveness of family interventions in the treatment of physical illness. *Journal of Marital and Family Therapy, 21,* 545–548.

Carter, B., & McGoldrick, M. (Eds.), (1988). *The changing family life cycle: A framework for family therapy.* New York: Gardner Press.

Clubb, R. (1991). Chronic sorrow: Adaptation patterns of parents with chronically ill children. *Pediatric Nursing, 17,* 461–466.

Collins, C., Stommel, M., Wang, S., & Given, C. (1994). Caregiving transitions: Changes in depression among family caregivers of relatives with dementia. *Nursing Research, 43,* 220–225.

Damrosch, S., & Perry, L. (1989). Self-reported adjustment, chronic sorrow, and coping of parents of children with Down syndrome. *Nursing Research, 38,* 25–29.

Deatrick, J., & Knafl, K. (1990). Management behaviors: Day-to-day adjustments to childhood chronic conditions. *Journal of Pediatric Nursing, 5*(1), 15–23.

Duvall, E. (1977). *Family development.* Philadelphia: J. B. Lippincott.

Epstein, N., Baldwin, L., & Bishop, D. (1983). The McMaster family assessment device. *Journal of Marital and Family Therapy, 9,* 171–180.

Fawcett, J., & Whall, A. (1990). Family theory development in nursing. In J. Bell, W. Watson, & L. Wright (Eds.), *The cutting edge of family nursing* (pp. 17–23). Calgary, Alberta, Canada: University of Calgary.

Fink, S. (1995). The influence of family resources and family demands on the strains and well-being of caregiving families. *Nursing Research, 44,* 139–145.

Fleming, J., Challela, M., Eland, J., Hornick, R., Johnson, P., Martinson, I., Nativio, D., Nobes, K., Riddle, I., Steele, N., Sudela, K., Thomas, R., Turner, Q., Wheeler, B., & Young, A. (1994). Impact on the family of children who are technology dependent and cared for in the home. *Pediatric Nursing, 20,* 379–388.

Friedman, M. (1992). *Family nursing: Theory & practice.* Norwalk, CT: Appleton & Lange.

Friedman, M., & Ferguson-Marshalleck, E. (1996). Sociocultural influences in family health. In S. Hanson & S. Boyd (Eds.), *Family health care nursing* (pp. 81–98). Philadelphia: F. A. Davis.

Gallo, A., Breitmayer, B., Knafl, K., & Zoeller, L. (1992). Well siblings of children with chronic illness: Parents' reports of their psychological adjustment. *Pediatric Nursing, 18,* 23–27.

Gaynor, S. (1990). The long haul: The effects of home care on caregivers. *Image: The Journal of Nursing Scholarship, 22,* 208–212.

Gillies, D. (1987). Family assessment and counseling by the rehabilitation nurse. *Rehabilitation Nursing, 12,* 65–69.

Gilliss, C. (1989). *Toward a science of family nursing.* Menlo Park, CA: Addison-Wesley.

Gilliss, C. (1993). Family nursing research, theory, and practice. In G. Wegner & R. Alexander (Eds.), *Readings in family nursing* (pp. 34–42). Philadelphia: J. B. Lippincott.

Hazlett, D. (1989). A study of pediatric home ventilator management: Medical, psychosocial, and financial aspects. *Journal of Pediatric Nursing, 4,* 284–294.

Hoeman, S. (1992). Community-based rehabilitation. *Holistic Nursing Practice, 6*(2), 32–41.

Holaday, B. (1989). The family with a chronically ill child. In C. Gilliss, B. Highley, B. Roberts, & I. Martinson (Eds.), *Toward a science of family nursing* (pp. 300–321). Menlo Park, CA: Addison-Wesley.

Jacob, S. (1993). Support for family caregivers in the community. In G. Wegner & R. Alexander (Eds.), *Readings in family nursing* (pp. 340–344). Philadelphia: J. B. Lippincott.

Kane, C. (1988). Family social support: Toward a conceptual model. *Advances in Nursing Science, 10,* 18–25.

Kleeman, K. (1989). Families in crisis due to multiple trauma. *Critical Care Nursing Clinics of North America, 1,* 23–31.

Knafl, K., & Deatrick, J. (1990). Family management style: Concept analysis and development. *Journal of Pediatric Nursing, 5,* 4–14.

Leahey, M., & Wright, L. (1985). Intervening with families with chronic illness. *Family Systems Medicine, 3,* 60–69.

Leonard, B., Brust, J., & Nelson, R. (1993). Parental distress: Caring for medically fragile children at home. *Journal of Pediatric Nursing, 8,* 22–30.

Lundin, T. (1984). Long-term outcome of bereavement. *British Journal of Psychiatry, 145,* 424–428.

Lynn-McHale, D., & Smith, A. (1993). Comprehensive assessment of families of the critically ill. In G. Wegner & R. Alexander (Eds.), *Readings in family nursing* (pp. 309–328). Philadelphia: J. B. Lippincott.

McCubbin, M., & McCubbin, H. (1993). Families coping with illness: The resiliency model of family stress, adjustment, and adaptation. In C. Danielson, B. Hamel-Bissell, & P. Winstead-Fry (Eds.), *Families, health, & illness: Perspectives on coping and intervention* (pp. 21–63). St. Louis: C. V. Mosby.

Minuchin, S. (1974). *Families and family therapy.* Cambridge: Harvard University Press.

Minuchin, S. (1985). Families and individual development: Provocations from the field of family therapy. *Child Development, 56,* 289–302.

Minuchin, S., & Fishman, C. (1981). *Family therapy techniques.* Cambridge: Harvard University Press.

Mischke-Berkey, K., & Hanson, S. (1991). *Pocket guide to family assessment and intervention.* St. Louis: Mosby–Year Book.

Mishel, M. (1988). Uncertainty in illness. *Image: The Journal of Nursing Scholarship, 20,* 225–232.

Mishel, M. (1990). Reconceptualization of the uncertainty in illness theory. *Image: The Journal of Nursing Scholarship, 22,* 256–261.

Mishel, M., & Sorenson, D. (1991). Coping with uncertainty in gynecological cancer: A test of the mediating function of mastery and coping. *Nursing Research, 40,* 167–171.

Olson, D., Russell, C., & Sprenkle, D. (1980). Circumplex model of marital and family systems: 2. Empirical studies and clinical intervention. In J. P. Vincent (Ed.), *Advances in family intervention, assessment, and theory* (pp. 88–97). Greenwich, CT: JAI Press.

Patterson, J., Jernell, J., Leonard, B., & Titus, J. (1994). Caring for medically fragile children at home: The parent-professional relationship. *Journal of Pediatric Nursing, 9,* 98–106.

Pless, I. B., & Satterwhite, B. (1973). A measure of family functioning and its application. *Social Science and Medicine, 7,* 613–621.

Power, P. (1985). Family coping behaviors in chronic illness: A rehabilitation perspective. *Rehabilitation Literature, 46*, 78–83.

Power, P., Dell Orto, A., & Gibbons, M. (1988). *Family interventions throughout chronic illness and disability.* New York: Springer-Verlag.

Quint, R., Chesterman, E., Crain, L., Winkleby, M., and Boyce, T. (1990). Home care for ventilator-dependent children. *American Journal of Diseases of Children, 144,* 1238–1241.

Rando, T. (1983). An investigation of grief and adaptation in parents whose children have died from cancer. *Journal of Pediatric Oncology, 8,* 3–20.

Ray, L., & Ritchie, J. (1993). Caring for chronically ill children at home: Factors that influence parents' coping. *Journal of Pediatric Nursing, 8,* 236–247.

Richmond, T., Metcalf, J., & Winterhalter, J. (1987). Support group for families of acute neurological patients. *The Journal of Neuroscience Nursing, 19,* 40–43.

Roberts, C., & Feetham, S. (1982). Assessing family functioning across three areas of relationships. *Nursing Research, 31,* 321–335.

Robinson, K. (1989). Predictors of depression among wife caregivers. *Nursing Research, 38*(6), 359–363.

Rolland, J. (1988). Family systems and chronic illness: A typological model. In F. Walsh & C. Anderson (Eds.), *Chronic disorders and the family* (pp. 143–168). New York: Haworth Press.

Rolland, J. (1994). *Families, illness, and disability: An integrative treatment model.* New York: Basic Books.

Ross, B. (1996). Nursing process and family health care. In S. Hanson & S. Boyd (Eds.), *Family health care nursing* (pp. 125–144). Philadelphia: F. A. Davis.

Sayles-Cross, S. (1993). Perceptions of familial caregivers of elder adults. *Image: The Journal of Nursing Scholarship, 25,* 88–92.

Sharer, K., & Dixon, D. (1989). Managing chronic illness: Parents with a ventilator-dependent child. *Journal of Pediatric Nursing, 4,* 236–247.

Sherman, B. (1995). Impact of home-based respite care on families of children with chronic illness. *Children's Health Care, 24,* 33–45.

Smilkstein, G., Ashworth, C., & Montano, D. (1982). Validity and reliability of the family APGAR as a test of family function. *Journal of Family Practice, 15,* 303–311.

Sterling, W. (1990). Resource needs of mothers managing chronically ill infants at home. *Neonatal Network, 9,* 55–58.

Teague, B., Fleming, J., Castle, A., Kiernan, B., Lobo, M., Riggs, S., & Wolfe, J. (1993). "High-tech" home care for children with chronic health conditions: A pilot study. *Journal of Pediatric Nursing, 8,* 226–232.

Venters, M. (1986). Family life and cardiovascular risk: Implications for the prevention of chronic disease. *Social Science and Medicine, 22,* 1067–1074.

Walsh, F. (1993). *Normal family processes.* New York: Guilford.

Whall, A. (1993). The family as the unit of care in nursing: A historical review. In G. Wegner & R. Alexander (Eds.), *Readings in family nursing* (pp. 34–42). Philadelphia: J. B. Lippincott.

Williams, P., Lorenzo, F., & Borja, M. (1993). Pediatric chronic illness: Effects on siblings and mothers. *Maternal-Child Nursing Journal, 21,* 111–121.

Winterhalter, J. (1989). *Family functioning and sibling self-concept of diabetic children: An exploratory study.* Unpublished D.N.Sc. dissertation, University of Pennsylvania, Philadelphia.

Winterhalter, J. (1992). Group support for families during the acute phase of rehabilitation. *Holistic Nursing Practice, 6*(2), 23–31.

Winterhalter, J., & Burke, S. (1996). Family functioning and well-sibling self-concept of technology-dependent children receiving nursing care at home [Abstract]. In *Fourth National Nursing Research Conference: Nursing care contributions to health outcomes* (p. 123). White Sulphur Springs, WV: Charleston Area Medical Center.

Woods, N., Haberman, M., & Packard, N. (1993). Demands of illness and individual, dyadic, and family adaptation in chronic illness. *Western Journal of Nursing Research, 15,* 10–30.

Woods, N., Yates, B., & Primomo, J. (1989). Supporting families during chronic illness. *Image: The Journal of Nursing Scholarship, 21,* 46–50.

Wright, L., & Leahey, M. (1994). *Nurses and families: A guide to family assessment and interventions.* Philadelphia: F. A. Davis.

Zacharis, D., Gilg, C., & Foxall, M. (1994). Quality of life and coping in patients with gynecologic cancer and their spouses. *Oncology Nursing Forum, 21,* 1699–1706.

CHAPTER 16

Psychosocial Issues for the Person with Chronic Illness or Disability

Judy Winterhalter

When a chronic illness is diagnosed or disability occurs, the affected person experiences a psychological reaction to the event. This reaction may be profound and may range from feeling numb to feeling devastated. The event may be perceived as a crisis or as a challenge. Coping techniques are equally varied. Nurses working with clients with a chronic illness or disability are challenged to support clients and their families through the process. The hallmarks of chronic illness are its duration; the variability of symptoms, disease progression, and individual responses; and the need for ongoing care by self and/or others. The progression of chronic illness may be viewed as a trajectory with peaks and valleys of exacerbations and remissions. In certain chronic illnesses or disabilities, there is a gradual decline or a progression that is unpredictable (Lubkin, 1986; Rolland, 1987). This chapter presents psychosocial issues within the context of the adjustment process following chronic illness or disability. Concepts such as denial, grieving, self-concept, uncertainty, and hope are discussed within a coping framework. The role of the rehabilitation nurse in psychosocial assessments, planning, intervention, and evaluation is outlined.

MODEL OF THE ADJUSTMENT PROCESS

Using a model of an adjustment process can facilitate understanding for the client and for the nurse. However, there are advantages and disadvantages in using a stage model as a theoretical base for psychosocial interventions in chronic illness and disability. One must be cautious not to apply the model indiscriminately, disregarding vast individual differences in response. Not all clients move through a set sequence, and the nurse may tend to underestimate the amount of time required to recover. As a "label," a stage theory may give the illusion of understanding and may relieve nurses of the responsibility for how their own behavior affects the client. Nevertheless, the advantages of using a stage theory outweigh the disadvantages.

A model of adjustment (Table 16–1) may be clinically useful in that it implies progress or other change. A stage model provides a sense of predictability and a framework for understanding common psychological reactions to chronic illness and disability. Prugh and Eckhardt (1980) developed a model of the adjustment process that has shown clinical utility in rehabilitation settings. This model comprises three stages:

- Impact
- Recoil
- Restitution

TABLE 16–1 ■ MODEL OF THE ADJUSTMENT PROCESS WITH PSYCHOLOGICAL CONCEPTS

Impact
Perception of the event
Coping skills
Reactions of others
Recoil
Coping framework
Denial
Grieving
Self-concept
Uncertainty
Hope
Restitution
Adaptation
Social support
Chronic illness management

Using a three-stage model allows individual differences to be maximized. Although most individuals with a chronic illness or disability progress through these stages, the duration in each stage varies widely among individuals: the actual progression of psychological adjustment is unpredictable and unique for each client.

First Stage—Impact

The impact stage begins when the illness is diagnosed or injury occurs. Examples include a person's being informed of a diagnosis of cancer, acquired immunodeficiency syndrome, or arthritis; suffering an acute myocardial infarction; sustaining a spinal cord injury in a motor vehicle accident; or being severely burned in a worksite fire. Psychological disequilibrium may occur. The person feels overwhelmed, fearful, helpless, and vulnerable and usually is preoccupied with questions such as "Will I live?" or "What will I be able to do?" According to crisis theory, there are three factors mediating whether someone is so stressed that he or she will be in crisis: perception of the event, coping mechanisms, and social support (Aguilera, 1994). These three concepts are discussed throughout the model of adjustment.

Perception of the Event

Each person's unique personality attributes, life experiences, and lifestyle affects the *meaning of events* in this stage. The meaning of the event goes beyond the actual illness or injury. The person often feels a threat to physical safety and self-concept including self-esteem and body image. People diagnosed with a chronic illness or disability attribute symbolism to the event. Thus, a woman with a myocardial infarction may perceive that her heart is the "core" of her identity, which is now damaged. A man with a spinal cord injury may perceive that his sexuality is irreparably damaged and he is no longer a "man." A diagnosis such as cancer or acquired immunodeficiency syndrome may be equated with a death sentence. The chronic illness or disability may be viewed as a punishment or "act of God." People may ask: "Who am I?" "Who will I become?" "Will my family still care about me?"

Children with a chronic illness or disability respond, in part, according to their developmental/cognitive level. Thus, a preoperational child may perceive a diagnosis of a disability as a punishment for thinking a "bad thought" or being a "bad child." Adolescents are preoccupied with their physical bodies, and any illness may pose a particular threat to their evolving identity.

Coping Skills

In this impact stage, the person attempts to use usual *coping skills* related to past life experiences in order to deal with the chronic illness or disability. This may be hindered by the actual illness or injury. For example, a person who usually reduces stress by engaging in physical activity such as jogging, cleaning, or shopping is hindered if the illness or injury prohibits such activity. As previously mentioned, the person's unique perception of the event affects the style of coping and response.

Reactions of Others

The person's perception of the event and his or her coping skills are also influenced by the *reactions of others* in the environment. According to Wright (1983), several psychosocial concepts have relevance for understanding reactions to a person with a chronic illness or disability. The research literature supports the concept that attitudes toward people with a disability are correlated with attitudes toward other minority groups and to people with underprivileged status. Thus, people with disabilities suffer hardships owing to restrictions imposed by a dominant majority and also by devaluative feelings about the self and the specific disability. Wright (1983) describes several concepts that affect the perception and lead to devaluation of a person with a disability.

The concept of *spread* refers to the power of a single characteristic to evoke inferences about the person. People make judgments partly based on their beliefs about the effects of the disability. For example, people might perceive a wheelchair-bound person as more empathic because of "how much she has suffered" or speak more loudly to someone who is blind. The disability is usually perceived as more severe than it actually is. Any disability is viewed as a tragedy from which there is no reprieve.

This concept is closely linked to *physique as prime mover,* in which traits are automatically attributed to the physical characteristics of the person. Thus, a person paralyzed from amyotrophic lateral sclerosis is a genius or overachiever "in response to his illness"—not due to his inherent intelligence and abilities. In this example, positive motives are seen as compensatory conditions attributed to the person rather than the environment.

Overprotection of a person with a disability may be a consequence of spread. Parents may underestimate a child's total capabilities owing to spread effects. Excessive spread of physique is seen in the attitude that people who have a disability stand apart from, rather than being a part of, the rest of the community. This is reinforced by the view that physical differences are the major force in every situation. Unfortunately, the spread effects also tend to foster the view that people with a disability are psychologically different kinds of people (Wright, 1983). In summary, the impact stage is a period of stress and vulnerability for the client with a chronic illness or disability. The reactions of significant others and the rehabilitation team influence the client's perception of the event and, in turn, the process of psychological adjustment.

Second Stage—Recoil

During the recoil stage, the person with a chronic illness or disability responds to the event. Time has elapsed since the illness was diagnosed or the injury occurred. Researchers and clinicians support the premise that the psychological response to physical disability or chronic illness is not necessarily distressing and may not necessarily end in maladjustment. Rather, the person's resources are many and varied, usually with a broad capacity to adapt. Most people respond to chronic illness or disability as they have to other life events and in relation to specific personality traits, not the situation or specific diagnosis (Pollock, Christian, & Sands, 1990; Wright, 1983). Again, most individuals respond not to the physical condition but to the unique personal meaning of it.

Coping Framework

By using a coping framework, people are able to deal with difficulties and begin to appreciate their abilities and identities as people with intrinsic value. Through education and training, individuals learn new skills and restructure their value system. The extent of the chronic illness or disability may be mitigated by treatments and environmental changes. One hopes that the individual will seek new solutions and find new satisfaction in living

with a chronic illness or disability, viewing it as one aspect of a rich and full life.

Moos (1984) has identified *seven coping skills* common to clients during illness and hospitalization:

- Denying or minimizing the seriousness of a crisis
- Seeking relevant information
- Requesting reassurance and emotional support
- Learning specific illness-related procedures
- Setting concrete, limited goals
- Rehearsing alternative outcomes
- Finding a general purpose or pattern of meaning in the course of events

Many of these coping skills are behaviors that the client can learn and practice. They can be used at various times and are not sequential or ordered. Coping with a chronic illness or disability is a process that takes place over time. Rehabilitation nurses need to support clients and help them to develop an effective coping style.

Caring effectively for clients with a chronic illness or disability necessitates that rehabilitation nurses and significant others support a coping framework. Wright (1983) and others caution that clinicians and family members may safeguard their own values by exaggerating the suffering of those considered less fortunate. The *requirement of mourning* may occur, in which the person with a chronic illness or disability is expected to suffer and be distressed in response to the others' projection of their perception. This may help caregivers to maintain a superior status. If there is a gap between the expected and the apparent reality, the affected person or the caregiver may experience *expectation discrepancy*. When expectations exceed observations, there is anguish and disappointment. For example, this would occur if a family member expected a client with a cerebrovascular accident to be responsive but the client remained aphasic or unresponsive. Surprise occurs when observations exceed expectations.

In summary, spread, physique as prime mover, the requirement of mourning, and expectation discrepancy are important concepts in understanding both a person's response to chronic illness or disability and the response of significant others and rehabilitation nurses.

Denial

Denial is often observed in clients after a diagnosis of chronic illness or disability and is particularly evident after a cerebrovascular accident, traumatic head injury, myocardial infarction, or spinal cord injury. Through denial, the person disavows the aspects of reality affected by the condition. Experts view denial as both a primitive defense that may be problematic and a method of healthy coping (Lazarus, 1983; Lazarus & Golden, 1981).

Lazarus and Golden (1981) view denial in two forms. It may be an emotionally focused method of coping, an internal and psychically oriented process, or a problem-focused coping method that is active and externally focused, such as participating in a rehabilitation program. These two forms are not mutually exclusive, and an individual may use both types of coping. Lazarus's (1983) topology includes

- Denial of the fact—"I do not have a spinal cord injury"
- Denial of implication—"I will walk again"
- Denial of affect—"I am not upset about what has happened to me"

The process of denial begins with the appraisal of the stress-inducing information, for example, being told of paralysis from a spinal cord injury or a diagnosis of multiple sclerosis. Thus, an awareness of the event is required. The greater the perceived threat, the more profound the initial level of denial. Denial can be either explicit (verbally expressing minimization of the event) or implicit (nonverbal/behavioral refusal to comply with the rehabilitation regimen). Particularly relevant to rehabilitation clients is the concept of *pathogenic denial* (Janis, 1983). This involves an ambiguous circumstance in which the probability of threat is high but is difficult to ascertain until there are further changes or developments. In this situation, the rehabilitation client may minimize the threat or engage in a process of suppression of upsetting thoughts and selective inattention to certain threatening aspects coupled with equally selective acceptance of more encouraging facts. Clients may also use denial/partializing by focusing on one aspect (often trivial) of their physical condition to find hopeful signs, thus creating a discrepancy between what they have been "told" ("You will never walk again") and what they know ("I can feel my toe, so I will walk again"). Thus, clients may exhibit complete denial ("Nothing has happened"), denial of a major disability ("I know this injury isn't serious"), minimization ("It doesn't matter if my leg is gone"), or denial of affect

("I'm not upset about my paralysis") (Lazarus & Golden, 1981; Wright, 1983).

Most clinicians agree that in the early stages of chronic illness and disability, denial is an adaptive response that prevents psychological disintegration and affords the individual time to marshal needed coping resources. It allows gradual acknowledgment of aspects of the event. This is especially helpful in relation to chronicity in that the problem won't heal or go away, and there may be incomplete awareness of the permanence of the condition.

There is empirical evidence that early denial plays a positive role in long-term adjustment but that its persistence inhibits the rehabilitation process (Lazarus, 1983; Lazarus & Folkman, 1984; Lazarus & Golden, 1981). It is important for the rehabilitation nurse to determine whether the denial facilitates or interferes with the acquisition of disability-appropriate behavior. Thus, verbal denial may be indulged as long as there is no behavioral denial inhibiting the rehabilitation process. The use of denial is variable, fluctuating, subject to uncertainty, challenging, and subject to dissolution in the face of facts and evidence. With the passage of time and the continuation of the chronic illness or disability, the use of denial becomes untenable. However, some degree of denial is probably necessary for the rehabilitation client to have hope.

Grieving

The rehabilitation client may begin to grieve after the initial shock has worn off. This grief involves being preoccupied with perceived losses, such as the inability to walk, a decline in self-esteem, or a loss of functioning in terms of activities of daily living. Feelings characteristic to the grief process include sadness, anxiety, anger, and feeling isolated, overwhelmed, and vulnerable. There is disagreement as to whether grief is universal in response to loss and whether it is a necessary precondition to adjustment.

Some people confine their sense of loss more narrowly to the loss itself and "deal with it and go on from there." Some people become more pervasively depressed. With intense mourning, the loss aspects dominate the person's emotional state. In the extreme case, the loss seems to pervade all aspects of the person's life. Then there is no differentiation between areas of the person that are and are not disability-connected (Wright, 1983). The person may also become numb and apathetic.

The person with a disability may experience losses in terms of physical, personal, and social functions that are thought to be impossible. The feelings of despair and suffering may be all-encompassing and overwhelming. For rehabilitation clients, the change from their former state may be so overpowering that the suffering seems boundless—both in extent and in time.

The *work of mourning* typically includes going through stages of grieving in order to facilitate acceptance of the loss. As described by Engel (1964), these stages include shock and disbelief, developing awareness, restitution, and resolution. Kubler-Ross (1969) delineates the stages of grieving as denial, anger, depression, bargaining, and acceptance. Although the grieving process is individualized, almost everyone who grieves demonstrates signs of denial, a period of reality awareness, and a gradual resolution of the mourning process.

During chronic illness and disability, there are factors that may prolong and/or inhibit the bereavement process. Rehabilitation clients often need to hold onto their preferred, preillness or preinjury state, thus keeping the past in the present and not "giving it up." Clients may also need a certain amount of time to begin to incorporate the new changes into their sense of self and body image. In comparing the present to the past state, the rehabilitation client often focuses on the changes and ignores the sameness. The things that stand out in this comparison are the ones that are different. Since the disability is the difference, the client's loss may be perceived as the main feature of the new state (Wright, 1983).

Rehabilitation clients are able to finish the work of mourning when they realize that there is meaning to life and that all is not lost because of the chronic illness or disability. At the moment of deepest despair—perhaps even contemplating suicide—rehabilitation clients may reclaim the value of life with a renewed feeling of strength and hope. When rehabilitation clients see others with different disabilities, their own assets may finally be acknowledged. In comparing disabilities, people usually feel "better off" than others. Through this process, people may become aware of their own assets and capabilities and that they and others can participate in their own way in the world (Wright, 1983).

The sheer necessity of meeting one's needs, and of living on a daily basis, may contribute to dealing with the here and now versus the past. Mastering activities of daily living early in the rehabilitation process is important in this regard. A rehabilitation client can maintain emotional despair for only so long. The person may finally become "satiated" with mourning, may feel "wrung dry." Then the dominance of loss subsides and the person rediscovers a wider world. This may permit a person to "snap out of" a feeling of grief or hopelessness (Wright, 1983).

The period of mourning is a healing process during which the "wound" is numbed and then gradually "closed," leaving the least scarring. The period of mourning cannot be rushed or minimized. It should be recognized as a period that can help people prepare themselves before meeting the challenges that lie ahead. Although the work of mourning must be completed in order to adjust to life with chronic illness or disability, it is not a state a person passes through smoothly and then leaves behind. It continues to be experienced intermittently after the deepest suffering has been mitigated (Horowitz, 1985; Lipowski, 1983; Wright, 1983).

It may be difficult to distinguish grieving from clinical depression after a diagnosis of chronic illness or disability. Although clinical depression is relatively rare in the rehabilitation population, the boundary between grieving and depression is not clear (Lipowski, 1983). Whether rehabilitation clients become depressed is dependent on personal and social resources, their appraisal of the impact of the chronic illness or disability, and their own coping responses.

The physical sequelae of a chronic illness or disability may overlap with symptoms of a major depression, for example, psychomotor retardation, anorexia, and sleep disturbance. Conservation withdrawal may be mistaken for clinical depression. As described by Weiner and Lovitt (1979), conservation withdrawal is a self-limited biological reaction pattern of withdrawal and inactivity that protects against overstimulation or excessive deprivation. The behavioral symptoms of low energy, apathy, and feelings of being overwhelmed and unable to exercise control resemble those of depression.

The concept of *learned helplessness* (Seligman, 1975) may also present similarly to depression, particularly in relation to the inability to exercise control. The reemergence of hope and some restoration of a degree of personal efficacy produce remission in the symptoms of learned helplessness. Thus, behavior seen as depression may represent the person's strenuous efforts to attain some level of adaptive coping. Determinants of depression include the rehabilitation client's premorbid level of emotional and cognitive development, premorbid tendencies for depression, attributions, socioeconomic status, and cultural values. Clinical depression is not an inevitable or necessary psychological response to chronic illness or disability (Lipowski, 1983; Weiner & Lovitt, 1979). If extended and untreated, it may be counterproductive to adjustment and compliance with rehabilitation. In addition, rehabilitation clients who continue to feel helpless and hopeless are at a high risk for suicide or other self-destructive behaviors.

Self-Concept

The *self-concept* is one's conscious awareness of the varieties of self-perceptions; one's characteristics, abilities, and values; and one's idea of self in relationship to others (Wylie, 1979). It is the totality of individual thoughts and feelings having reference to one's self. It is not necessarily the real self, but one's picture of self. Self-concept is a multidimensional superconstruct that includes body image, sexual identity, and self-esteem (Rosenberg, 1979). The self-concept is viewed as a characteristic of age and developmental level.

Theorists also emphasize the social nature of the development of the self with regard to family, school, peer group, and work in that people define and perceive themselves as others do. Thus, the self-concept develops through interactions with others. The constructivist view of self-concept emphasizes that people throughout their life span attempt to maintain or enhance their level of self-regard. The standard for self-evaluation and the current self-evaluation are functions of social interaction (Harter, 1983). The centrality of the self-concept in maintaining physical and psychosocial well-being has been widely recognized by nurses in practice. A person's beliefs, feelings, and expectations about the self play a fundamental role in shaping health outcomes (Stein, 1995). Thus, after a chronic illness is diagnosed or disability occurs, rehabilitation clients may alter their self-concept based on the meaning of the event and reactions from others.

Body image, a component of self-concept, involves the perceptions, attitudes, feelings, and personal reactions relative to one's own body. A person's perception of body image is dynamic and continually changes over time. However, the integration of body experiences develops slowly. Thus, after chronic illness or disability, a person's mental picture of the body changes slowly over time in relation to the physical condition (Drench, 1994; Price, 1993).

There is a direct relationship between one's body image and the overall concept of self and one's sense of worth as a human. Body image is influenced by one's outward appearance; internal and somatic sensations; the reactions of significant others; values; culture; and religion. It is important to note that one's body image may not be the same as the actual body structure or function (Drench, 1994; Price, 1993; Wright, 1983). Clothing, assistive devices such as wheelchairs, and the environment may become part of one's body image. All that we perceive, think, and believe takes place within the context of body experiences.

Body image is also profoundly affected by the psychological significance or symbolism assigned to various body parts and functions (Wright, 1983). The importance of a body part or function is partially explained by how close it is to the "core of the self." For example, the face seems to be a more intimate part of the person than the hands or legs. Gender identification is often a central personal characteristic that defines the person to self and others. After chronic illness or disability, the rehabilitation client needs to grieve for the loss of valued body parts or functions and the resultant change in overall image.

Self-esteem, another component of self-concept, is the general evaluation of the self as a worthy or an unworthy person. Four antecedents of self-esteem are (Coopersmith, 1981)

- The power to control one's behavior and influence others
- A sense of being loved, being respected, and belonging
- A sense of personal moral values
- A belief in one's competency in expected roles for self and by others

An injury or illness may be viewed as a punishment. In order to preserve self-esteem, the rehabilitation client may act "as if" the disability doesn't exist. Wright (1983) cautions that early in the process, rehabilitation clients may idolize normal standards and therefore devaluate themselves by supporting inferiority and guilt feelings. A single attribute, such as paralysis, is more likely to influence self-esteem if the affected body part is closely connected to the person's self core and if it has a high status value. Status value refers to the relevancy of an aspect of self for the appraisal of personal worth or self-esteem. If the essential *I* of the person is centrally associated with an intact body and if the status value is high for "body beautiful, body whole, and body well," (Wright, 1983, p. 232) the person's self-concept may be severely damaged. This may be so severe that the new body image is never integrated into the self-concept.

Uncertainty

Uncertainty has particular relevance for the rehabilitation client. Uncertainty is defined as the inability to determine the meaning of illness events. Managing the uncertainty associated with an illness or injury may be an essential task in adaptation (Mishel, 1988, 1990; Mishel & Sorenson, 1991). It is a cognitive state in which the person cannot adequately structure or categorize an event because of a lack of cues. The person either cannot place value on an event or is unable to accurately predict outcomes. However, the rehabilitation client needs to subjectively interpret the illness or disability, treatment, and hospitalization. If this cannot be done, uncertainty results.

In illness, uncertainty includes four forms: (1) ambiguity concerning the state of illness, (2) complexity concerning treatment and systems of care, (3) a lack of information regarding the diagnosis and seriousness of the illness, and (4) unpredictability of the course of the illness and prognosis. Uncertainty can be viewed as a danger or an opportunity. If the event is perceived as dangerous, the individual uses coping strategies to reduce the uncertainty. Uncertain events viewed as opportunity imply a positive outcome, and coping strategies to maintain uncertainty are used. In either case, if the coping strategies are effective, adaptation occurs.

Chronic illnesses, with their remissions and exacerbations, may present a pattern of symptom inconsistency that hampers a definition of the illness state and thus causes uncertainty. Uncertainty can be influenced by factors that provide structure, such as education, social support, and trust and confidence in health care providers. In situations in which the person is helpless to influence the outcome or in which the outcome has a negative, downward trajectory, the person may depend on uncertainty to maintain a sense of hope (Mishel, 1988; Mishel & Braden, 1988).

Mishel (1990) and Mishel and Sorenson (1991) report that uncertainty has been associated with a pessimistic outlook, depression, and increased anxiety in studies involving acute and chronic illness. However, evaluating uncertainty as an opportunity may be particularly helpful to clients facing a negative outcome or downward trajectory. Hope is then possible and may allow the client to wish or wait for new treatments and increase compliance with the current treatment. Indeed, chronic uncertainty can produce growth and change through a new worldview.

Rehabilitation nurses should encourage clients to develop new methods for valued activities and to consider new alternatives in coping with the changing nature of the illness. The phase of the rehabilitation process and the client's location (e.g., hospital or home) may have an effect on mediating factors for uncertainty. During hospitalization or doctor or clinic visits, evaluation of uncertainty may be blunted as the client is preoccupied with treatment issues. Evaluation of the implications of the uncertainty may be delayed until further along in treatment as the impact of the illness becomes evident in daily life. Coping activities may be suspended during active treatment when there is no well-developed sense of opportunity or danger (Mishel, 1990; Mishel & Sorenson, 1991; Wineman, 1990).

Hope

Hope is an emotion, an expectation, an illusion, and a disposition. It is a powerful, sustaining force that may motivate people by giving them the vitality to live and cope. Hope allows a person to view a crisis as an opportunity for growth. Hope can be the counterpoint to despair during chronic illness and disability (Miller, 1985, 1989; Miller & Powers, 1988). Wright (1983) emphasizes that the following aspects of hope are more helpful to use than dichotomizing *hope* versus *reality.*

1. *The content of hope:* Can it be supported?
2. *The time dimension:* For the immediate future, realistic tasks are important; for the longer term, new discoveries and treatment may be considered.
3. *Probabilities and possibilities:* These are probabilities based on realistic expectations for

the present and possibilities of hoped-for treatments.

4. *Hoper characteristics:* These involve the person's coping versus "waiting for miracles."

It is important to ground hope in reality, thus differentiating it from expectations. Four cognitive-affective tasks of coping include (Wright, 1983)

1. *Reality surveillance:* Coordinating hopes with reality in order to ensure the maintenance of hope

2. *Encouragement:* Motivating, sustaining, and comforting the person

3. *Worry:* The affective counterpart to cognitive uncertainty; it forces the person to re-examine reality

4. *Mourning:* The affective consequence of having to relinquish hope

In a recent study by Morse and Dobuneck (1995), the concept development of hope (Table 16–2) included various attributes (left column). One group used for confirming the conceptual components was spinal cord–injured clients. These clients' qualitative responses are included as examples in the right column.

The uncertainty arising from not knowing how much movement they would regain caused these spinal cord–injured clients to

TABLE 16–2 ■ CONCEPT DEVELOPMENT OF HOPE

Hope Attribute	Manifestation in Person with Spinal Cord Injury
Realistic initial assessment of predicament or threat	Immediate realization of ramifications of injury, e.g., permanent paralysis
Envisioning alternatives and setting goals	Working for small gains and life skills versus becoming completely dependent
Bracing for negative outcomes	Preparing for increasing probability that mobility will not improve
Realistic assessment of personal resources and of external conditions and resources	Recognizing dependence on others and constant need for assistance, planned modifications to home
Solicitation of mutually supportive relationships	Getting support from other spinal cord injury patients and often spouses or boyfriends or girlfriends
Continuous evaluation for signs that reinforce selected goals	Focusing on tiny physical gains
Determination to endure	The greater the determination, the greater the progress

Adapted from Morse, J., & Dubuneck, B. (1995). Delineating the concept of hope. *Image: The Journal of Nursing Scholarship, 27*(4), 277–285.

modify their hopes to meet reality. They realized the delicate balance between hope and reality. They braced for negative outcomes by celebrating each small gain in function and learned activity. They braced for reactions of others by rebuffing stares and comments from others. They were scared to reintegrate into the community because everyone else was "beautiful and in shape." These clients were able to realistically appraise supports and modifications needed in home settings. They "buddied" with other spinal cord–injured clients and learned from them.

Clients reported it took several months to realize what their limitations were. They carefully watched how other persons with similar injuries handled their disability, developed a sense of camaraderie, and worried together. They carefully aimed for small gains and endured, because they realized they had no choice. They modified their hoped-for goals as they came to realize the permanence of their limitations and downsized their goals, celebrating every small gain. Goals varied according to how much movement the client had. Attaining each goal required a tremendous amount of work. They had to relearn the simplest tasks. They realized the importance of physical and occupational therapy and their own efforts necessary to achieve their goals. Hope was manifested by working toward small incremental gains, each requiring extraordinary self-discipline and the determination to achieve small and important goals. Morse and Dobuneck (1995) labeled this as *incremental hope.*

The degree of threat to personal safety is the principal factor contributing to the intensity of hope and serves as a motivating force. It is important for rehabilitation nurses to discuss current planning for care based on reality without destroying hope for future improvements. The emphasis on the reality of the future should be based on the client's readiness to know it. Shocking a person into "reality" has doubtful value. A person needs time and experience with a chronic illness or disability to face it. Accepting the disability does not banish hope (Wright, 1983).

The empirical literature has documented the role of hope in successful adjustment to chronic illness and disability (Raleigh, 1992; Wineman, 1990; Wright, 1983). In one study, subjects most commonly reported sources for maintaining hope as family, friends, and religious beliefs. They were able to identify specific ways in which these sources supported their hope. The majority of the subjects reported positive attitudes about their illnesses (cancer and chronic illness), with transient periods of lowered hope associated with illness variables. They also could describe specific cognitive and behavioral strategies that helped to maintain their hope. These included getting busy doing something, praying or religious activity, thinking about other things, and talking to others. Other people were helpful to them by visiting, listening, talking, and providing physical help (Raleigh, 1992).

Third Stage—Restitution

In the restitution phase after chronic illness or disability, the rehabilitation client achieves an *adaptation* to the condition. Adaptation to chronic illness or disability may best be defined as a process of discarding both false hope and destructive hopelessness so that there is meaning and purpose to living that transcends the limitations imposed by the illness (Feldman, 1974). Problem solving, coping skills, and social support play a central role in this process of achieving a hopeful perspective.

Social support has been shown to be a significant factor in a person's adaptation to chronic illness or disability. Perceived support has been shown to be related to a wide variety of outcomes that include physical health, mental well-being, and successful social functioning. The receipt of instrumental social support, such as practical help, advice, and feedback, significantly contributed to positive well-being in persons with Parkinson's disease (MacCarthy & Brown, 1989), women with rheumatoid arthritis (Lambert, Lambert, Klipple, & Mewshaw, 1989), and women with diabetes mellitus (White, Richter, & Fry, 1992). Controlling for disease severity and duration did not change the results.

In a study of 50 functionally disabled, wheelchair-bound individuals, the perception of the availability of social support, not the use of social support, was significantly related to coping effectiveness through the mediating variables of problem-focused and emotion-focused coping (McNett, 1987). In a study of men and women with multiple sclerosis, the perceived supportiveness of social network interactions was directly related to their sense of purpose in life but not to depression. For the person with an unpredictable chronic illness who is feeling devalued by society, social support through being loved, cared for, and needed by important people in that person's life may play a central role in fostering a sense of meaningfulness. The feeling of be-

longing to a social network may confirm the individual's value as a person—redefining beliefs, reaffirming values, and renegotiating roles as the need arises relative to living with others with an unpredictable chronic illness (Wineman, 1990).

Individuals with chronic illness or disability are influenced not only by normative changes and life events but also by the stressors produced by the uncertainties of the illness course and the *changing demands required to manage the chronic illness throughout its course* (White et al., 1992). Research findings document that it probably takes at least 1 to 2 years after a diagnosis of chronic illness or disability to make the necessary psychological adjustments (Lubkin, 1986; Pollock et al., 1990; Rolland, 1987). Often the true meaning of the condition and resultant losses do not become clear until the client goes home for the first time.

As previously described, rehabilitation clients must make major changes in how they relate to the world. There is no clear evidence of an association between the type of chronic illness and disability and particular personality characteristics or between the physical disability itself and psychological adjustment (Pollock et al., 1990). When rehabilitation clients have accepted the disability and restructured their sense of self, they will view themselves as people first and as people with a disability second.

PSYCHOSOCIAL NURSING ASSESSMENT

Nurse's Self-Awareness

Assessment of the rehabilitation client begins with the nurse's self-awareness of personal values. The nurse's perceptions, values, and emotions regarding chronic illness or disability affect nursing care provided to the client and family. These subjective issues are self-assessed by answering the following questions:

1. What is my reaction to disability? Do I view it as a tragedy or as a challenge?
2. What value do I place on particular body parts and functions?
3. Do I believe that psychological adaptation to a chronic illness or disability is attainable?
4. How do I respond to ambiguous or uncertain conditions?
5. Do I believe problems are an inevitable part of the adjustment process?

6. Do I believe in maintaining hope for the client with a chronic illness or disability?

Honest answers by rehabilitation nurses determine their ability to therapeutically care for the psychosocial needs of rehabilitation clients.

Client Psychosocial Assessment

Need for Assessment

A comprehensive psychosocial assessment of both objective and subjective client data is critical for appropriate planning and intervention. If the rehabilitation client is unable to engage in the assessment process, the nurse obtains information from family and/or significant others.

Cultural Values

Understanding cultural values, beliefs, and traditions is critical in working with individuals and families because ethnicity determines norms and values associated with caretaking, problem solving, conflict resolution, and family functioning. Appreciating the uniqueness of culture and its intergenerational transmission enhances the effectiveness of nurses' caring for clients and families. Culture can provide a sense of belonging, comfort, and self-validation for individuals and family systems.

When assessing a client, the nurse needs to incorporate cultural values related to language; personal space and the use of touch; authority issues; trust; the gender of the nurse and the client; differences in time orientation; health care practices; traditional cultural practices; socioeconomic status; religious beliefs; and alternative medical practices (Antai-Otong, 1995).

Assessment

The assessment of the mediating factors discussed throughout this chapter can be accomplished by using the following questions.

Perception of the Chronic Illness or Disability
- Can you describe what has happened to you?
- What was happening in your life before this event occurred?
- Describe how you are feeling right now.
- What has bothered you the most about this illness?

- How has this event affected your life?
- Do you know anyone with this chronic illness or disability?
- How did the chronic illness or disability affect them?
- How do you see this event affecting your future?

Knowledge of the Chronic Illness or Disability
- What have you been told about your chronic illness or disability?
- What treatment will you be receiving?
- How long do you expect to be hospitalized?
- What do you expect your condition to be when you are discharged?
- What follow-up services will you receive?
- Are you satisfied with the information you have received?

Coping Mechanisms
- What do you usually do to feel better?
- What have you tried to do this time? Has it worked?
- How has your chronic illness or disability affected your usual way of handling stress?
- How would you describe how you are feeling right now?
- What is the most difficult event you've had to deal with in your life?
- What did you do then?
- Have you thought about killing yourself?
- In general, how do things usually turn out for you?

Situational Supports
- With whom do you live?
- To whom do you talk when you feel upset?
- Whom do you rely on most or expect will be most helpful for you now?
- Who else is available to help you?
- What social, community, or religious activities do you attend?

Family and Lifestyle Resources
- What is your occupation?
- What are your hobbies or leisure-time activities?
- Where do you live? House? Apartment?
- What is your family income?

SPECIFIC PSYCHOSOCIAL ASSESSMENTS, PLANNING, AND INTERVENTION

Coping Mechanisms

Assessment of Coping Mechanisms

The assessment of coping mechanisms was described previously.

Possible Assessment Instruments

Possible assessment instruments include the following:

Schedule of Recent Events (Holmes & Rahe, 1967)

Ways of Coping Checklist, Revised (Lazarus & Folkman, 1984)

Revised Ways of Coping Checklist (Vitaliano, 1987)

Jalowiec Coping Scale (Jalowiec, Murphy, & Powers, 1984)

Beck Anxiety Inventory (Beck, Epstein, Brown, & Steer, 1988)

Planning and Nursing Diagnoses

Planning and nursing diagnoses related to difficulties in coping with a threatening situation include (Gordon, 1993)

- Ineffective individual coping
- Defensive coping
- Altered thought process
- Altered family process
- Anxiety (moderate/severe/panic)

Nursing Interventions

Following are appropriate nursing interventions:

- Be knowledgeable about the usual responses to a given illness so that the client's behavior can be properly evaluated.
- Accept the client's feelings and behavior as the best response the client can have at the present time.
- Educate the client and the client's significant others about the reactions the client and others may have to the illness.
- Know what the client is likely to be struggling with (i.e., the developmental tasks at the client's age and stage of life).
- Allow the client the opportunity to try out new ways of being (e.g., talking about feelings with a nurse).
- Listen to clients solve problems out loud and provide feedback without giving direct advice.
- Give information (e.g., the relationship between anxiety and pain).
- Provide referrals to other resources (e.g., self-help groups, specialists, or other clients).
- Help the client to manage the hospital environment, thereby increasing the client's sense of control and competence.
- Develop written contracts with clients.

- Separate your own personal responses from those of the client.

Denial

Assessment of Denial

Ways to assess denial include the following:

- Assess the client in different situations at different times, with a variety of people.
- Assess the duration of denial.
- Assess whether denial is verbal or behavioral.
- Assess the degree of the client's control over the situation.
- Assess outcomes of denial—are they adaptive or maladaptive at this point?

Planning and Nursing Diagnoses

Planning and nursing diagnoses associated with the use of denial by rehabilitation clients may include (Gordon, 1993)

- Ineffective denial
- Impaired adjustment
- Defensive coping
- Ineffective management of the therapeutic regimen
- Noncompliance

Nursing Interventions

Following are appropriate nursing interventions (Wilson & Kneisl, 1996):

- Provide information regarding the client's condition and implications at optimal times, when requested.
- If the client does not request information, convey the promise of a therapeutic commitment. Be truthful but somewhat ambiguous so the client can interpret information in ways consistent with his or her needs.
- Before providing information, clarify what other professionals have told the client.
- Acknowledge and reflect but do not reinforce or counter disbelief and denial.
- Solicit information from the rehabilitation team concerning the client's adjustment.
- Permit some degree of hope. Recognize the multilevel characteristics of denial. Verbal denial may be an expression of hope and may not inhibit the rehabilitation process. Recognize that some degree of denial is probably necessary for hope.
- Be aware of the staff's need to confront or encourage denial to meet their own needs.
- Provide continuous emotional support.

Grieving and Depression

Assessment of Grief and Depression

To assess grief and depression, ask the following questions:

- Can you distinguish between grieving and depression?
- Does the client acknowledge a recent loss?
- Does the "depression" seem normal to the client? What is the history of the depression?
- Is there a loss of self-esteem?
- Is there a pervasive feeling of guilt?
- In which stage of the grieving process is the client?
- Does the client feel hopeless or helpless?
- Does the client meet the *Diagnostic & Statistical Manual of Mental Disorders* (4th ed.) criteria for a major depression (American Psychiatric Association, 1994)?
  - Depressed or sad mood
  - Loss of interest or motivation
  - Changes in appetite, concentration, and sleeping patterns
  - Social isolation
  - Feelings of hopelessness
  - Decreased libido and energy

Possible Assessment Instruments

Possible assessment instruments include

Beck Depression Inventory (Beck & Beamesderfer, 1974)
Multiscore Depression Inventory for Adolescents and Adults (Berndt, 1986)

Planning and Nursing Diagnoses

Planning and nursing diagnoses associated with grieving and depression include (Gordon, 1993)

- Anticipatory grieving
- Dysfunctional grieving
- Self-esteem disturbance
- Ineffective coping
- Spiritual distress
- Impaired social interaction
- Powerlessness
- High risk for self-directed violence

Nursing Interventions

Following are appropriate nursing interventions:

- Spend time talking with and listening to the client. Use silence and touch therapeutically.

- Validate the bereaved's experience.
- Allow the expression of sadness, despair, anger, and so forth.
- Reassure the client that grieving is a process that requires time.
- If clinical depression and/or suicidality is suspected, request a consultation from a mental health professional.

Self-Concept, Self-Esteem, and Body Image

Assessment of Self-Concept, Self-Esteem, and Body Image

To assess self-concept, self-esteem, and body image, ask the client the following questions:

- How do you see yourself?
- How has your illness or disability affected how you perceive yourself?
- When did this change occur?
- How do you think other people perceive you?
- How will any changes affect your lifestyle?
- How would you describe your body?
- How has your illness or disability affected your view of your body?
- Are you satisfied with your overall sense of yourself and your body?

Possible Assessment Instruments

Possible assessment instruments include

Beck Self-Concept Test (Beck, Steer, Epstein, & Brown, 1990).
Self-Observation Scales (Katzenmeyer & Stenner, 1979).
Rosenberg Self-Esteem Scale (Rosenberg, 1965).
Piers-Harris Children's Self-Concept Scale (Piers-Harris, 1983).

Planning and Nursing Diagnoses

Planning and nursing diagnoses associated with self-concept, self-esteem, and body image include (Gordon, 1993)

- Body image disturbance
- Self-esteem disturbance
- Personal identity disturbance

Nursing Interventions

Appropriate nursing interventions include the following:

- Encourage and support clients in mourning the loss of the "ideal" former self.

- Create opportunities for the client to discuss the disability, its meaning, and the problem of compensating for the loss.
- Help family and friends to overcome any negative attitudes toward the chronic illness or disability.
- Teach and encourage anticipatory guidance in relation to expected change or outcomes.
- Develop the client's ability for self-care.
- Offer appropriate praise and recognition for the client's accomplishments.
- Involve the client in planning and scheduling care activities.

Hope

Assessment of Hopelessness

To assess hopelessness,

- Observe the client's behavior. Is the client withdrawn, despondent, participating less in self-care?

Ask the client the following questions:

- Do you feel empty, drained?
- Do you feel irritable? tense? Do you have a lump in your throat?
- Do you feel vulnerable, helpless, or overwhelmed?
- Do you feel despair?

Possible Assessment Instruments

Possible assessment instruments include

- The Hopefulness Scale (Miller & Powers, 1988)

Planning and Nursing Diagnoses

Planning and nursing diagnoses associated with hopelessness include (Gordon, 1993)

- Hopelessness
- Powerlessness
- Spiritual distress

Nursing Interventions

Appropriate nursing interventions include the following:

- Emphasize sustaining relationships.
- Support family members to sustain the client.
- Radiate hope through faith and confidence in client abilities. Focus on the person, not the disability.

- Discuss the disability and explain options and alternatives.
- Expand the client's coping repertoire.
- Teach effective coping behaviors and relaxation techniques.
- Teach reality surveillance, in which the client reconstructs past events and assigns meaning to them, compares self to others with the same condition, plans for self-care activities, and makes realistic plans.
- Provide information on self-help groups.
- Help the client to devise and revise goals.
- Help the client renew his or her spiritual self

EVALUATION AND FOLLOW-UP

In general, rehabilitation clients have met the challenges of psychosocial adjustment to chronic illness or disability if they accomplish the following:

- Setting reasonable goals for self-care, vocation, and social roles
- Describing positive attitudes
- Demonstrating a sense of self and self-esteem
- Being an active participant in decision making
- Performing self-care activities within capabilities
- Seeking support and assistance as needed

After the client's discharge, the rehabilitation nurse should arrange for follow-up care in order to monitor the client's progress, to facilitate continuation of needed care, and to manage any concerns that were not present or evident before discharge. Comprehensive services through case management for the client and family will optimize the client's functioning.

REFERENCES

Aguilera, D. (1994). *Crisis intervention: Theory and methodology.* St. Louis: C. V. Mosby.

American Psychiatric Association (1994). *Diagnostic and statistical manual of mental disorders* (4th ed). Washington, DC: Author.

Antai-Otong, D. (1995). *Psychiatric nursing.* Philadelphia: W. B. Saunders.

Beck, A., & Beamesderfer, A. (1974). Assessment of depression: The Depression Inventory. *Psychological Measurements in Psychopharmacology, 7,* 151–169.

Beck, A., Epstein, N., Brown, G., & Steer, R. A. (1988). The Beck Anxiety Inventory. An inventory for measuring clinical anxiety: Psychometric properties. *Journal of Consulting and Clinical Psychology, 56,* 893–897.

Beck, A., Steer, R., Epstein, N., & Brown, G. (1990). The Beck Self-Concept Test. Psychological assessment. *Journal of Consulting and Clinical Psychology, 2,* 191–197.

Berndt, D. (1986). *Multiscore Depression Inventory.* Los Angeles: Western Psychological Services.

Coopersmith, S. (1981). *The antecedents of self-esteem.* Palo Alto, CA: Consulting Psychologists Press.

Drench, M. (1994). Changes in body image secondary to disease and injury. *Rehabilitation Nursing, 19,* 31–36.

Engel, G. (1964). Grief and grieving. *American Journal of Nursing, 64,* 93.

Feldman, D. (1974). Chronic disabling illness: A bibliography. *Journal of Chronic Disease, 27,* 16–24.

Gordon, M. (1993). *Manual of nursing diagnosis 1993–1994.* St. Louis: Mosby–Year Book, 1993.

Harter, S. (1983). Developmental perspectives on the self-system. In P. Mussen (Series Ed.) & E. Hetherington (Vol. Ed.), *Handbook of child psychology: Vol 4. Socialization, personality, and social development* (4th ed., pp. 275–385). New York: Wiley.

Holmes, T., & Rahe, R. (1967). The Social Readjustment Rating Scale. *Journal of Psychosomatic Research, 11,* 213–218.

Horowitz, M. (1985). Psychological responses to stress. *Psychiatric Annals, 15,* 161–167.

Jalowiec, A., Murphy, S., & Powers, M. (1984). Psychometric assessment of the Jalowiec Coping Scale. *Nursing Research, 33,* 157–161.

Janis, I. (1983). Preventing pathogenic denial by means of stress inoculation. In S. Breznitz (Ed.), *The denial of stress* (pp. 35–77). New York: International Universities Press.

Katzenmeyer, W., & Stenner, J. (1979). *Self-observation scales.* Durham, NC: NTS Research Corp.

Kubler-Ross, E. (1969). *On death and dying.* New York: Macmillan.

Lambert, V., Lambert, C., Klipple, G., & Mewshaw, E. (1989). Social support, hardiness and psychological well-being in women with arthritis. *Image: The Journal of Nursing Scholarship, 21,* 128–131.

Lazarus, R. (1983). The costs and benefits of denial. In S. Breznitz (Ed.), *The denial of stress* (pp. 35–77). New York: International Universities Press.

Lazarus, R., & Folkman, S. (1984). *Stress, appraisal, and coping.* New York: Springer Publishing.

Lazarus, R., & Golden, G. (1981). The function of denial in stress, coping, and aging. In J. McGaugh & S. Keisler (Eds.), *Aging: Biology and behavior* (pp. 286–307). New York: Academic Press.

Lipowski, S. (1983). Psychosocial reactions to physical illness. *Canadian Medical Association Journal, 128,* 1069–1072.

Lubkin, I. (1986). *Chronic illness: Impact and interventions.* Boston: Jones and Bartlett.

MacCarthy, B., & Brown, R. (1989). Psychosocial factors in Parkinson's disease. *British Journal of Clinical Psychology, 28,* 41–52.

McNett, S. (1987). Social support, threat, and coping responses and effectiveness in the functionally disabled. *Nursing Research, 36,* 98–103.

Miller, J. (1985). Inspiring hope. *American Journal of Nursing, 1,* 22–25.

Miller, J. (1989). Hope-inspiring strategies of the critically ill. *Applied Nursing Research, 2,* 23–29.

Miller, J., & Powers, M. (1988). Development of an instrument to measure hope. *Nursing Research, 37,* 6–10.

Mishel, M. (1988). Uncertainty in illness. *Image: The Journal of Nursing Scholarship, 20,* 228–232.

Mishel, M. (1990). Reconceptualization of the uncertainty in illness theory. *Image: The Journal of Nursing Scholarship, 22,* 256–262.

Mishel, M., & Braden , C. (1988). Finding meaning: Antecedents of uncertainty in illness. *Nursing Research, 37,* 98–103.

Mishel, M., & Sorenson, D. (1991). Coping with uncertainty in gynecological cancer: A test of the mediating function of mastery and coping. *Nursing Research, 40,* 167–171.

Moos, R. (Ed.), (1984). *Coping with physical illness* (Vol 2). New York: Plenum.

Morse, J., & Dobuneck, B. (1995). Delineating the concept of hope. *Image: The Journal of Nursing Scholarship, 27*(4), 277–285.

Piers, E., & Harris, D. (1983). *Piers-Harris Children's Self-Concept Scale.* Los Angeles: Western Psychological Services.

Pollock, S., Christian, B., & Sands, D. (1990). Responses to chronic illness: Analysis of psychological and physiological adaptation. *Nursing Research, 39,* 300–304.

Price, M. (1993). Exploration of body listening: Health and physical self-awareness in chronic illness. *Advances in Nursing Science, 15,* 37–52.

Prugh, D., & Eckhardt, L. (1980). Stages and phases in the response of children and adolescents to illness or injury. *Advances in Behavioral Pediatrics, 4,* 181–194.

Raleigh, E. (1992). Sources of hope in chronic illness. *Oncology Nursing Forum, 19,* 443–448.

Rolland, R. (1987). Chronic illness and the life cycle: A conceptual framework. *Family Process, 26,* 203–221.

Rosenberg, M. (1965). *Society and the adolescent self image.* Princeton, NJ: Princeton University Press.

Rosenberg, M. (1979). *Conceiving the self.* New York: Basic Books.

Seligman, M. (1975). *Helplessness.* San Francisco: W. H. Freeman.

Stein, K. (1995). Schema model of the self-concept. *Image: The Journal of Nursing Scholarship, 27,* 187–193.

Vitaliano, P. (1987). *Manual for revised ways of coping checklist (WCCL).* Seattle: Stress and Coping Project.

Weiner, M., & Lovitt, R. (1979). Conservation-withdrawal versus depression. *General Hospital Psychiatry, 1,* 347–349.

White, W., Richter, J., & Fry, C. (1992). Coping, social support, and adaptation to chronic illness. *Western Journal of Nursing Research, 14,* 211–224.

Wilson, H., & Kneisl, C. (1996). *Psychiatric nursing* (5th ed.). Redwood City, CA: Addison-Wesley.

Wineman, N. (1990). Adaptation to multiple sclerosis: The role of social support, functional disability, and perceived uncertainty. *Nursing Research, 39,* 294–299.

Wright, B. (1983). *Physical disability—A psychosocial approach.* New York: Harper & Row.

Wylie, A. (1979). *The self concept* (Vol 2). Lincoln: University of Nebraska Press.

CHAPTER **17**

Cognition

Janet M. Farahmand

Contact with clients who have altered cognition is occurring more frequently for rehabilitation nurses in all settings. This contact is increasing because of greater longevity and the technology available to sustain life after trauma, birth defects, and chronic illnesses. Because of changes in the financing of health care, the rehabilitation nurse must be able to (1) rapidly identify and assess clients with cognitive dysfunction, (2) plan interventions to facilitate clients' achievement of optimum potential for independence, and (3) provide for their smooth transition to selected community settings. The rehabilitation nurse must have a knowledge base consisting of scientific, developmental, psychosocial, and nursing principles that provide an understanding of the nature of cognition and the structures and functions of the brain and related sensory organs necessary for cognition to occur. The nurse with such understanding can

1. Assess the level of cognitive function
2. Identify nursing diagnoses relevant to the client with cognitive dysfunction
3. Choose appropriate nursing interventions in planning care
4. Implement the plan holistically
5. Evaluate the outcomes
6. Adjust the plan of care to achieve goals

The rehabilitation nurse often functions as a member of an interdisciplinary health care team, whose ultimate goal is to assist culturally diverse clients and their families to return to their communities. The World Health Organization (WHO) is promoting the use of community-based rehabilitation programs to improve the delivery of rehabilitation services to underserved populations, such as refugees, victims of open conflict, ghetto inhabitants, and nomads. Underserved populations are located in limited resource settings.

Decentralization of care to give more responsibility to local communities for meeting the needs of the disabled is encouraged.

WHO estimates that from 7 to 10% of the world's population are citizens with disability. With the known relationships between head injury and violence, inadequate nutrition, and substance abuse, the risk of brain injury is likely higher in many of these underserved populations, although there are no current statistics supporting this assumption. The Second World Injury Congress, held in Seville, Spain, in May 1997, estimated the incidence of brain injury (mild, moderate, and severe) to be 150 cases per 100,000 population (Melvin, Graham, Graham, & Olsen, 1997). Community-based rehabilitation programs rely heavily on the services of family members and trained rehabilitation workers, who learn through manuals and workshops. Because clients with cognitive dysfunction often need continuing care throughout their lives, case management is increasingly being employed to provide for comprehensive services as clients' needs change, especially in the more highly developed countries. Individuals with impaired cognition require multilevel assistance regardless of the setting.

COGNITION AND COGNITIVE PROCESSES

Cognition comprises all mental activity or states involved in knowing and the mind's functioning: perception, attention, memory, imagery, language functions, developmental processes, problem solving, and the area of artificial intelligence (which is outside the discipline of psychology) (Corsini, 1994).

A problem encountered in the rehabilitation of clients with cognitive dysfunction is that the process of thinking cannot be witnessed. What is seen is the product of cognition—behavior—which itself is usually inferred from the client's response to a problem. However, one needs to consider that cognition is a response to internal and external stimuli and, thus, that human emotions become a factor in bringing about changes that enable clients to achieve independent living. Cognitive processes are generally held to involve (1) gathering of information, (2) processing of information, (3) generating ideas and solutions, (4) carrying out responses, (5) storing and retrieving those responses, and (5) incorporating them into life activities (Table 17–1).

For cognition and its processes to be functional, the nervous system must be intact. Within the nervous system, the brain receives information (both internal and external information) from the body, processes the information, and determines the response of the body to the information. This response relies on cell and organ function, nerves, and the hormonal systems. In addition, the response is shaped by one's culture, genetic make-up, previous experiences, and emotional composition. Damage to the brain leading to altered functional outcomes with respect to cognition may occur not only from external causes (traumatic) but also from a large variety of neurological conditions (vascular, degenerative, neoplastic). It is best to examine the functional significance of each part of the brain of the organism to clarify the effects of damage to it.

STRUCTURES AND FUNCTIONS NEEDED FOR COGNITION TO OCCUR

For optimum cognition to occur, the central nervous system (brain and spinal cord), peripheral nervous system, and autonomic nervous system must be intact. Only the brain and the structure lying within it will be briefly discussed here.

The Brain and Associated Structures

The brain is the largest structural unit of the central nervous system, and its most prominent structure is the cerebral cortex, an outer shell of gray matter enclosing the other brain structures. Large bundles of white matter, which are nerves, connect the various parts of the brain with the spinal cord. Buried within these nerve tracts are a number of subcortical neurological structures—thalamus, hypothalamus, basal ganglia, and brainstem (Fig. 17–1).

Cerebrum (Cerebral Cortex)

The most important component of the nervous system in relation to cognition is the

TABLE 17–1 ■ COGNITIVE PROCESSES AND THEIR DEFINITIONS

Process	Definition
Orientation	The ability to know the self and the relationship of self to the environment. Evaluation of self to time, place, and person are conducted. Loss of orientation to time occurs, first, then to place, and finally, loss of orientation as to who one is as a person.
Alertness	The ability to be ready to respond to stimuli from the environment.
Attention span	Ability to listen, select important stimuli from those not important for a sustained period.
Concentration	Ability to make an effort to maintain focus on relevant stimuli for a sustained period.
Memory (short-term and long-term)	Complex processes of retaining, filing, and retrieving information when and where it is needed. Short-term memories are subject to displacement (usually last from 1 minute to 1 hour). Long-term memory is information stored in a conceptually meaningful mode for a lifetime, and is considered limitless.
Thinking	Requires memory, planning, organizing, use of abstraction, and ability to transfer knowledge from one situation to another. It is the highest order of intellectual functioning.
Problem-solving skills	Involves the ability to identify a problem, analyze it, compile a range of solutions or options, then choose one and put it into action.
Learning	Acquisition of knowledge, information skills, and attitudes measured by a change in behavior. It depends on memory.
Information processing	The ability to input information, organize it, sequence it, store it, and retrieve it to produce an overt response or goal-directed behavior.

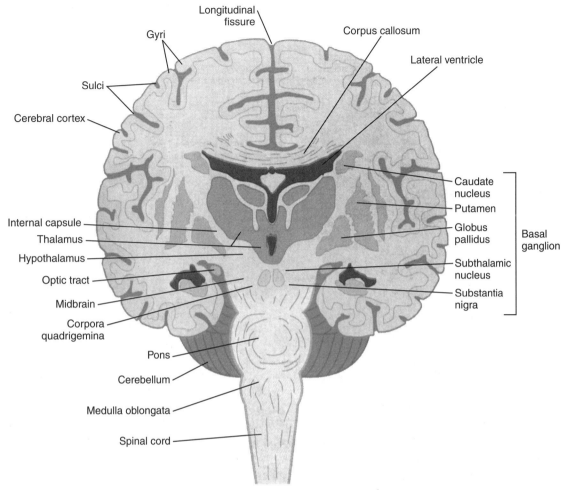

FIGURE 17–1
The structures of the brain (coronal section). (From Black, J. M., & Matassarin-Jacobs, E. [1997]. *Medical-surgical nursing: Clinical management for continuity of care* [5th ed., p. 691.] Philadelphia: W.B. Saunders.)

cerebral cortex. The cortex has two hemispheres, the right and the left, which are connected by a thick bundle of nerve tracts, the corpus callosum. Each cerebral hemisphere is divided by major sulci into five lobes (frontal, temporal, parietal, occipital, and central [insula]).

The lobes in each hemisphere of the cortex have three zones (Fig. 17–2):

- Primary sensory zones, which receive information from the sensory organs
- Primary motor zones, which activate specific muscular functions
- Association zones, both motor and sensory

Both the left cortex and the right cortex function to interpret sensory data, store memories, learn, and form concepts. The left cortex is better able to carry out sequential analysis in an orderly, logical assessment of parts, and thus to handle language, mathematics, abstraction, and reasoning. The right cortex is better able to process whole sensory experiences and thus to handle visual-spatial information and activities, such as listening to music, appreciating art, and dancing.

Frontal Lobes.   The frontal lobes have areas designated as prefrontal and frontal. The *prefrontal* areas control attention span and executive functions (motivation, plan, initiate, maintain, and terminate activities) and use feedback. Clients with prefrontal lobe damage are unable to initiate or maintain activities, have short attention span, look apathetic, and do not problem solve. In addition, the prefrontal areas inhibit the limbic and vegetative areas of the cerebrum.

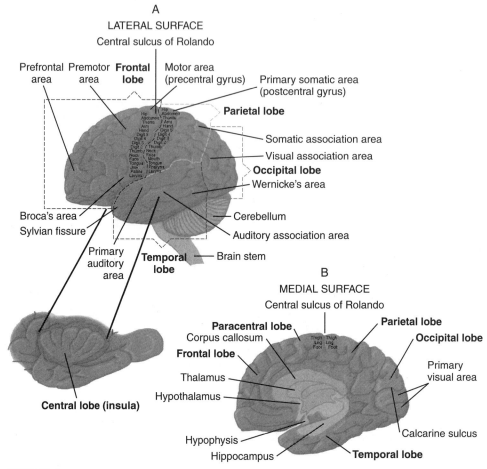

FIGURE 17–2
The lateral *(A)* and medial *(B)* surfaces of the cerebral cortex. (From Black, J. M., & Matassarin-Jacobs, E. [1997]. *Medical-surgical nursing: Clinical management for continuity of care* [5th ed., p. 692.] Philadelphia: W.B. Saunders.)

The *frontal* lobes in the precentral gyrus control voluntary motor activity. Damage to this area results in involuntary motor perseveration.

Temporal Lobes. The temporal lobes (see Fig. 17–2*A*) have a primary auditory receptive area and secondary auditory association areas (store spoken language memories), nonlanguage sound memories (music and other environmental sounds) that are stored in the right temporal auditory areas. The primary olfactory cortex, located in the dorsomedial portion of the anterior temporal lobe, provide an emotional context to the interpretation of smells.

Parietal Lobes. The parietal lobes are associated with tactile reception and association areas. The postcentral gyrus and the posterior portion of the paracentral lobule (see Fig. 17–2*A*) primarily receive tactile sensations. Association areas take up the rest of the parietal lobe. The right parietal association area handles spatial orientation and body awareness. The left parietal association area handles written language, reading, right-left orientation, and mathematics.

Occipital Lobes. The occipital lobes contain visual reception and association areas. Each of the two occipital lobes has a primary visual receptive area and an association area. Visual reception areas are located on each side of the calcarine sulcus (see Fig. 17–2*A*). The remaining areas of the occipital lobes are visual association areas, where visual memories are stored to enable recognition and understanding of the environment.

Limbic Lobe. The limbic lobe, located at the core of the cerebrum, mediates affect. Also, the limbic structures control the transfer of short-term (recent) memory into permanent memory stores. Permanent stores are held in the association areas of the parietal, occipital, and temporal lobes. Amnesia results if this transfer system is damaged.

Central Lobes (Insula).   The insula lies hidden in the lateral sulcus. It is a triangular area that forms the floor of the lateral cerebrum fossa. It is surrounded by the frontal, temporal, and parietal lobes.

Basal Ganglia

Lying deep inside the white matter of the cerebrum are areas of gray matter called basal ganglia or cerebral nuclei. The cerebral nuclei consist of the caudate nucleus, globus pallidum, and an associated structure, the internal capsule. The four structures collectively make up the *corpus striatum*, which appears striped because of the connections between its gray matter and white matter in the internal capsule (see Fig. 17–1). The cerebral nuclei are believed to contain multiple connections to various regions of the central nervous system and to initiate and fine-tune voluntary motor movement and responses.

Brainstem

Reticular Activating System.   Throughout the brainstem, special cells that make up the reticular formation tissue are responsible for controlling awareness or alertness. The reticular activating system has abundant connections with the brain, the rest of the brainstem, and the cerebellum because many sensory fibers branch and end in the reticular formation tissue.

The brainstem (diencephalon, medulla oblongata, pons, and midbrain) holds most of the structures below the cerebral cortex (see Fig. 17–1; Fig. 17–3). These structures (1) connect the brain with the spinal cord and other sources of information and (2) serve as entrance and exit points for some cranial nerves.

Diencephalon.   The *hypothalamus,* which forms the base of the diencephalon, maintains the constant internal environment and implements behavior patterns. Integrative centers in the hypothalamus also control autonomic nervous systems, and regulate body temperature and endocrine function.

The *hypophysis* is located in the sella turcica of the ethmoid bone and is connected to the hypothalamus by tissue called the hypophyseal (pituitary) stalk. It has two lobes and releases hormones under the control of the hypothalamus (see Fig. 17–2B).

The *thalamus* lies directly above the brainstem and functions as a coordinating center to regulate the activity of the cerebral cortex. It integrates data going to the cortex and transmits motor signals and sensory signals, except smell.

Medulla Oblongata.   The medulla is the lowest section of the brainstem. Motor tracts pass downward through the anterior medulla (pyramidal), and sensory tracts pass upward. Many reciprocal connections exist in the medulla, which transmits continuous data to higher centers of control to initiate changes that maintain homeostasis. Cranial nerves IX (glossopharyngeal), X (vagus), XI (spinal accessory), and XII (hypoglossal) emerge from the medulla, as do portions of cranial nerves VII (facial) and VIII (acoustic) (see Figs. 17–1 and 17–3).

Pons.   The pons contains three tracts (peduncles) to and from the cerebellum. Four cranial nerves originate from the pons: VI (abducens), VII (facial), VIII (acoustic), and V (trigeminal) (see Figs. 17–1 and 17–3).

Midbrain (Mesencephalon).   The midbrain is a small section located between the pons and the diencephalon. It has motor and sensory pathways, plus the inferior and superior colliculi—centers for auditory and visual reflexes. It also contains the small canal located between the third and fourth ventricles called the aqueduct of Sylvius, which transports cerebrospinal fluid. Cranial nerves in the midbrain are III (oculomotor) and IV (trochlear).

Cerebellum

The cerebellum contains both gray matter and white matter, the cortex of which is a thin layer of gray matter arranged in gyri (folia) and separated by sulci (Fig. 7–3). Under the cortex is a white matter core of fibers traveling to and from the cerebellar cortex. The white matter also contains deep cerebellar nuclei whose axons travel to other portions of the brain. Pathways entering the cerebellum originate in the brainstem and spinal cord nuclei and exit to the cerebellar cortex. Output from the cerebellum is produced by the deep nuclei, and axons travel to brainstem nuclei.

The cerebellum controls and coordinates all motor movements by regulating muscle

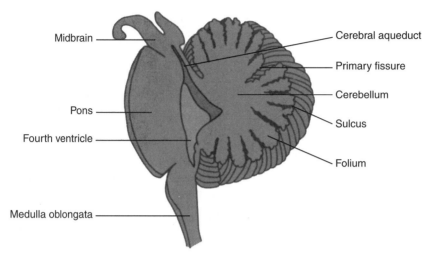

FIGURE 17–3
Sagittal view of the brainstem, fourth ventricle, and cerebellum. (From Black, J. M., & Matassarin-Jacobs, E. [1997]. *Medical-surgical nursing: Clinical management for continuity of care* [5th ed., p. 693.] Philadelphia: W.B. Saunders.)

tension, which prevents tremors and maintains stability (balance) during movement. A client with cerebellar damage displays intention tremor and incoordination.

ASSESSMENT OF COGNITIVE FUNCTION

In any health care setting, the nurse is often the first member of the health care team to assess a patient's or client's cognitive function as a baseline for defining a plan of care. The nurse needs to carefully document all assessment data because the terminology used is subject to a range of interpretations.

A change in level of consciousness is the most sensitive indication of cerebral dysfunction, whether the cause is related to structural, metabolic, or psychogenic elements. Current nursing practice relies on behavioral descriptions and patient responses to stimuli (Table 17–2; Fig. 17–4). In the acute care setting, the nurse may have access to electroencephalogram tracings to augment assessment of brain activity. The Glasgow Coma Scale (GCS) is also used to assess consciousness by evaluating the behavior of eye opening, verbal response, and best motor response. Cognition is usually first demonstrated by the patient's ability to respond to stimuli. No special instrument is necessary to determine cognition at this level.

Assessment Instruments

Overall assessment of the implications of level of consciousness for function is frequently made through the use of the Modified Barthel's Index or the Functional Independence Measure, both of which provide a description of the levels of function and their scores (Mahoney & Barthel, 1965; Grainger & Hamilton, 1986). Periodic reassessment with the same instrument would measure changes and thus provide data to determine interventions and measure rehabilitation outcomes. These instruments measure what the disabled person actually does, not what the person could do. The Functional Independence Measure also indicates the caregiver burden and cost of disability to families and communities.

The assessment instruments just described may be used in clients at all developmental levels except the pediatric population, for whom initial learning of the skills has not occurred. For them, cognition usually means new learning, and the developmental process is complicated. Screening tests used for children include the following:

- Denver II Development Screening Test (DDST)
- Pediatric Evaluation of Disability Inventory (PEDI)
- Vineland Adaptive Behavior Scales (VABS)

Any treatment plan for a child with altered cognitive processes needs to include strategies for promoting age-appropriate development. The inclusion of all family members as well as community caregivers (teachers and clergy) in the plan must be maximized.

TABLE 17–2 ■ LEVELS OF ALTERED CONSCIOUSNESS

Level	Behavior Exhibited
Coma	No verbal or motor response to any external stimuli, even a noxious stimulus such as deep pain. Glasgow Coma Scale Score is less than 7.
Vegetative state	Eyes open and close spontaneously to give the appearance of a sleep-wake cycle; no evidence of verbal responses, perception, or purposeful motor ability.
Minimally conscious state	Eyes open spontaneously; visual tracking often intact; inconsistency in communication ability or purposeful motor activity; unreliable gestures.
Stupor	The person may be aroused from what looks like a deep sleep by vigorous and repeated stimulation, such as bright light. The response frequently is that of withdrawing from or pushing at the stimulus.
Acute confusion or delerium	Abrupt onset; fluctuates in severity; awareness is reduced; person is agitated, restless, uncooperative; disorganized thinking; alertness varies from lethargy to hypervigilance.
Automatism	Obeys simple commands; appears robot-like or gives automatic responses; asks same questions repetitively.
Conscious	Oriented to time, place, and person; cooperative; aware of surroundings; capable of reasoning and reacting to stimuli with purpose.

At the other end of the age continuum, in the geriatric population, aging changes related to cognition must be considered. Research findings show much variation regarding the cognitive changes associated with normal aging. Studies currently being conducted by the National Institute on Aging indicate that cognitive function remains normal unless there are other chronic illnesses, such as the effects of strokes. Small changes in cognition are not noticed by family members, and significant changes go unreported because of myths that all old people undergo some decline in thinking as they age. After the initial general assessment of the patient, more detailed evaluations are carried out by practitioners in the various disciplines.

The instruments designed specifically for measuring cognitive levels of patients are as follows.

Mini-Mental State Examination (MMSE). The MMSE is commonly used because it can be given in any facility or community setting (Table 17–3). It measures orientation, registration, attention, calculation, recall of language, and the ability to follow a three-part command (Folstein, Folstein, & McHugh, 1975). The highest possible score is 30, and the level of cognitive impairment is subdivided into three levels. A score of 23 to 30 is normal; 18 to 24 indicates mild impairment; and 0 to 17 indicates severe impairment. Care must be taken in the use of the MMSE because it is possible to obtain falsely low scores in up to a third of patients assessed (Folstein et al.,

1975). Tombaugh and McIntyre (1992) attribute this to patient age and educational background. The MMSE should not be used in a patient who has less than an 8th-grade education, does not speak English, or is aphasic.

Wechsler Adult Intelligence Scale, Revised (WAIS-R). The Wechsler Adult Intelligence Scale was revised by Kaplan, Fine, Morris, and Dellis (1991) to provide a variety of cognitive and intellectual functions. It may be given to persons aged 16 to 74 years and takes 60 to 120 minutes. It has 11 subtests, six of which statistically contribute to the Verbal Performance Intelligence Quotient and five of which contribute to the Performance Intelligence Quotient. Scores may be combined to give a Full Scale Intelligence Quotient.

Peabody Individual Achievement Test–Revised (PIAT-R). The PIAT-R can be given to persons of low verbal abilities (Markwardt, 1989). The test yields subscores for mathematics, reading recognition, reading comprehension, spelling, and general comprehension.

Halstead-Reitan Battery (HRB). The HRB is made up of five core tests (Reitan & Wolfson, 1986). It measures problem solving, vigilance, attention, abstraction, motor speed, and incidental memory.

Luria-Nebraska Neuropsychological Battery (LNNB). Developed in the Soviet Union, the LNNB emphasizes individual differences (Luria, 1980). This approach allows the examiner

MISSION HOSPITAL
REGIONAL MEDICAL CENTER

ADULT NEURO FLOW SHEET

TIME

			KEY
GLASGOW COMA SCALE	Eyes Open		**MOTOR**
	Best Motor		5+ Normal Power
	Best Verbal		4+ Weakness
	TOTAL		3+ Anti-gravity
VOLUNTARY MOTOR	Right	upper extremity	2+ Not anti-gravity
		lower extremity	1+ Trace
	Left	upper extremity	0 No movement
		lower extremity	
CRANIAL NERVES	**PUPILS** Right	Size	B = Brisk
		Reaction	Pupil S = Sluggish
	Left	Size	Size A = Absent
		Reaction	2mm 3mm 4mm 5mm
	EOMS	Conjugate	● ● ● ●
		Dysconjugate	
		Tracking Right	6mm 7mm 8mm
		Left	● ● ●
	Blink Reflex		✔ = Present
	Gag Reflex		O = Absent
	Facial Symmetry		S = Symmetrical
			A = Asymmetrical

Date

TIME

Speech Patterns:_____

Comments:_____

_____

_____

_____

_____

_____

_____

_____

_____

_____

_____

_____

GLASGOW COMA SCALE	Eyes Open	4 Spontaneously
		3 To verbal command
		2 To Pain
		1 No Response
	Best Motor Response	6 Obeys Commands
		5 Localize Pain
		4 Flexion to pain withdraw
		3 Flexion Decorticate
		2 Extension to pain (decerebrate)
		1 No Response to pain
	Best Verbal Response	5 Oriented
		4 Confused
		3 Inappropriate words
		2 Incomprehensible sounds
		1 No Response

Unit_____

R.N. Signature_____ Shift:_____

R.N. Signature_____ Shift:_____

R.N. Signature_____ Shift:_____

ADDRESSOGRAPH

#408 10/89

Adult Neuro Flow Sheet

FIGURE 17–4
A neurologic observation chart. (Courtesy of Mission Hospital Regional Medical Center, Mission Viejo, CA.)

TABLE 17–3 ■ THE MINI-MENTAL STATE EXAMINATION

Maximum Score	Score	Activity
		Orientation
5	( )	What is the (year) (season) (date) (day) (month)?
5	( )	Where are we (state) (county or neighborhood) (town) (hospital) (floor)?
		Registration
3	( )	Name 3 objects: 1 second to say each. Then ask the patient all 3 after you have said them. Give 1 point for each correct answer. Then repeat them until he/she learns all 3. Count trials and record.
		Trials_____
		Attention and Calculation
5	( )	Serial 7s. 1 point for each correct answer. Stop after 5 answers, if the patient refuses to attempt serial 7s, spell "world" backward.
		Recall
3	( )	Ask for the 3 objects named for registration. Give 1 point for each correct answer.
		Language
2	( )	Name a pencil and a watch. (2 points)
1	( )	Repeat the following. "No ifs, ands, or buts." (1 point)
3	( )	Follow a 3-stage command: "Take a paper in your hand, fold it in half, and put it on the floor." (3 points)
1	( )	Read and obey the following: Close your eyes. (1 point)
1	( )	Write a sentence. (1 point)
1	( )	Copy a design. (1 point)
		Total Score
		Assess level of consciousness along a continuum_____
		Alert→Drowsy→Stupor→Coma

Adapted from Matteson, M. A., McConnell, E. S., & Unton, A. D. (1997). *Gerontological nursing: Concepts and practice* (2nd ed.). Philadelphia: W. B. Saunders.

to learn how the individual performs a task, but it also determines whether the strategy used to fulfill the task results in a successful outcome. The examiner can also manipulate the task to see what changes might help the patient adapt, making the test useful in rehabilitation settings. Results are totally qualitative. The number of times an individual successfully performs a task is counted, then an intervention is provided. Then the number of times a patient successfully performs the task is counted to see if a successful outcome is achieved.

The Galveston Orientation and Amnesia Test (GOAT). The GOAT is invaluable in preventing patients from being discharged in a state of amnesia (Levin, O'Donnell, & Grossman, 1979).

Ranchos Los Amigos Hospital: Scale of Cognitive Functioning (Table 17–4). This scale was developed to sequence the levels of neurobehavioral recovery from traumatic brain injury (TBI). It is useful in decision making about cognitive rehabilitation (Malkmus, Booth, & Kodimer, 1980). Patients were formerly not transferred from acute care settings to tertiary rehabilitation settings until they had reached level II or III. Today it is not unusual, given the current health care delivery system and financial concerns, for patients to be transferred while in an unconscious state to a less intensive care rehabilitation facility or to a skilled nursing facility to await possible further progress. According to Levin, Gary, & Eisenberg: NIH Trauma Coma Data Base Research Group (1990), "About 10–15% of severe TBI patients are discharged from acute care settings while still unconscious." Care must be taken to ensure that the unconscious state is not the result of some correctable medical condition—for example, malnutrition or drug induced. Should improvement or lack of it be observed and documented, the patient is transferred to another appropriate setting. After the initial team assessment based on the

TABLE 17–4 ■ RANCHO LOS AMIGOS HOSPITAL SCALE OF COGNITIVE FUNCTIONING

Level of Response	Behavior
I None	Unresponsive to auditory, visual, or tactile stimuli.
II Generalized	Reacts inconsistently and nonpurposefully to stimuli. Delayed and limited responses.
III Localized	Reacts specifically but inconsistently to stimuli. Responses are related to type of stimuli presented, such as visually focusing on an object or responding to sounds.
IV Confused–agitated	Extremely agitated and in a high state of confusion. Nonpurposeful and aggressive behavior. Unable to fully cooperate with treatments owing to short attention span. Requires maximal assistance with self-care.
V Confused–inappropriate, nonagitated	Alert and can respond to simple commands on a more consistent basis. Highly distractible. Needs constant cuing to attend to an activity. Memory is impaired with confusion regarding past and present. Can perform self-care activities with assistance. May wander, and needs to be watched carefully.
VI Confused–appropriate	Shows goal-directed behavior, but still needs direction. Follows simple tasks consistently, and shows carryover for relearned tasks. More aware of his or her deficits, and has increased awareness of self, family, and basic needs.
VII Automatic–appropriate	Appears oriented in home and hospital, and goes through daily routine automatically. Shows carryover for new learning, but still requires structure and supervision to ensure safety and good judgment. Able to initiate tasks in which he or she has an interest.
VIII Purposeful–appropriate	Totally alert, oriented, and shows good recall of past and recent events. Independent in the home and community.

From Black, J. M., & Matassarin-Jacobs, E. (1997). *Medical-surgical nursing* (5th ed.) Philadelphia: W. B. Saunders.

Rancho Los Amigos Scale, the nurse develops a composite description of the patient with respect to the cognitive processes that are impaired and begins a plan of care based on nursing diagnoses.

Nursing Diagnoses

After the specific cognitive impairments of concern to an individual client have been identified, the nurse, in conjunction with specialists from other health care disciplines, plans and implements interventions for the clinical management of the client. Nursing diagnoses related to cognitive dysfunction, compiled by the North American Diagnosis Association (1994), may be used to organize the plan. Two major nursing diagnoses are related to the cognitive processes:

Altered Thought Processes—state in which an individual experiences a disruption in cognitive operations and activities. As stated earlier in this chapter, it is not possible to witness thinking, but rather the product of thinking, behavior, is seen, usually inferred from a response to a problem.

Knowledge Deficit—state in which specific information is lacking. It has been defined as an inability to state or explain information or demonstrate a required skill related to trauma/disease manage-

ment procedures, practice, or self-care management.

These two diagnoses are major diagnoses, but because of the widespread impact of altered thought processes, other diagnoses may be identified in relation to the individual client. Examples are

Sensory/Perceptual Alterations (visual, auditory, kinesthetic, gustatory, tactile, olfactory)—state in which an individual experiences a change in the amount or patterning of incoming stimuli accompanied by a diminished, exaggerated, distorted, or impaired response to such stimuli.

Risk for Injury—state in which an individual is at risk as a result of environmental conditions interacting with the individual's adaptive and defensive resources. Poor judgment, confusion, impulsivity, and wandering are of concern.

Self-Care Deficit—state in which an individual experiences an inability to perform or complete bathing/hygiene, dressing/grooming, feeding, or toileting.

Altered Role Performance—disruption of the way an individual perceives his or her role performance.

Impaired Adjustment—state in which an individual is unable to modify his or her own lifestyle or behavior in a manner consistent with the change in health status.

Self-Esteem Disturbance—state in which negative self-evaluation and feelings about self develop in response to a loss or change in an individual who previously had a positive self-evaluation.

Social Isolation—state in which an individual has a need or desire for contact with others but is unable to make that contact because of physiological, biological, or sociocultural factors.

Altered Growth and Development—state in which an individual demonstrates deviations from norms of his or her own age group.

Altered Sexuality Patterns—state in which an individual expresses concerns regarding his or her sexuality. These may be actual or perceived difficulties, limitations, or changes in sexual behavior. At times, patients cannot express sexual concerns or are not cognizant of inappropriate sexual behavior.

Altered Parenting—state in which there is an inability of the primary caretaker to create an environment that promotes the optimum growth and development of the child.

Ineffective Family Coping—behavior of significant person (family member or other primary person) that disables his or her capacities and the client's capacities to effectively address tasks essential to either person's adaptation to the health challenge.

Altered Family Processes—a change in family relationships and/or functioning.

NURSING INTERVENTIONS TO BE USED IN PLANNING CARE FOR CLIENTS WITH COGNITIVE DYSFUNCTION

After the acute phase of an illness that involves cognitive impairment, placement of the client, whether in a rehabilitation facility, long-term care unit, or other setting, is often influenced by the level achieved on the Rancho Los Amigos Hospital Scale, which indicates the current stage of recovery and thus the rehabilitation plan. There is consensus that spontaneous recovery occurs from 1 to 2 years after the acute phase of an illness that impairs cognitive function. The nurse may therefore encounter the patient in a nursing home, subacute care unit, comprehensive day care center, residential treatment unit, private residence, or in home care.

Coma

The duration of a coma serves as an indicator of the severity of injury. It is necessary to place the patient in a coma management program with the objectives of preventing complications that will impair more active rehabilitative efforts if the client progresses to a higher level of function. Research is being conducted to assist in the development of guidelines for assessment and management of patients who are in a persistent vegetative state (PVS) and minimally conscious state (MCS) (Brain Injury Update, 1997, December). At a conference in Aspen, Colorado, an attempt was made to discuss the proceedings of the Aspen Workgroup on the Vegetative and Minimally Conscious States conducted since 1994. Some members in the workgroup argued that PVS has become a widely misused term relative to clinical diagnosis and care of the patient with severe impairment following brain injury. Some patients do not persist in this state and go on to make further neurological improvement, some to the point of good functional outcomes as indicated by such measures as the Glasgow Outcome Scale. The use of the guidelines may lead to withholding of care, failure to refer to rehabilitation services, and less aggressive treatment of comorbid factors. Others disagree, suggesting that these terms are too entrenched in the scientific literature to be changed now (Giacino, Zaster, Katz, Kelly, Rosenberg, & Tilly, 1997). It behooves the nurse to follow the current research and discussion in this area because of the impact they have on the counseling of family members of brain-injured patients.

Attempting to improve the level of consciousness by the use of various stimuli, although controversial, is often used. The nurse and other members of the team intervene with controlled stimuli of all the senses, such as (1) the radio, (2) familiar voices, (3) strong odors (cloves, cinnamon, coffee), (4) strong tastes known to have brought enjoyment to the patient (ice cream, honey), (5) tactile stimulation (warm, cold, smooth, rough), and (6) visual stimulation if the eyes are open (family photos, colored cards).

If and when the level of cognitive function improves, further interventions are begun, with the goal of community reintegration. As Braddom (1996) observed, "Most interventions in post acute rehabilitation are based on training patients to use compensatory strategies to overcome their permanent deficits (memory notebooks) or altering the environment so that the patient is more functional (e.g., providing a routine schedule)."

These interventions are based on Cognitive Rehabilitation (CR) as adopted by the Commission on Accreditation of Rehabilitation Facilities (CARF). CARF defines *cognitive rehabilitation* as a systematic, functionally oriented service of therapeutic cognitive activities and an understanding of the person's behavioral deficits. Services are directed to achieve functional changes by (1) reinforcing, strengthening, or establishing previously learned patterns of behavior or (2) establishing new patterns of cognitive activity or mechanisms to compensate for impaired neurological systems. "The efficacy of cognitive retraining, the therapies directed at remediating deficits in memory, attention and other cognitive functions have not been substantially accepted by all professions in the health care field" (Berrol, 1990). Nursing interventions must be related to the individual's level of cognitive functioning, which results from the area of the brain involved.

The nurse also must assist family and friends to cope through education, counseling, and support. Agencies may offer support groups, which may be led by nurses. Families have many decisions to make within the context of the structure and function of the family members, cultural background, ethical concerns, financial constraints, and availability of community resources. The nurse is frequently the health care team member who helps the family to make informed choices.

Posttraumatic Amnesia

If and when consciousness (the ability to follow spoken commands) returns, the patient typically passes through a period of confusion and disorientation. This period is referred to as *posttraumatic amnesia* (PTA) (Levin, Benton, & Grossman, 1982). During PTA, the patient's ability to learn new information is minimal. Patients engage in confabulation or false recall or make up fictitious events and may state that they are at home or are imprisoned, especially if they are in a secured unit. Often after emergence from PTA, a permanent memory gap will exist for events that happened during PTA. Failure to emerge from PTA may indicate a permanent amnesiac disorder.

During PTA, agitation (a neurobehavioral syndrome) may occur. This is manifested by cognitive confusion, extreme emotional lability, motor activity, aggression, poor attention span, frustration, irritability, and inappropri-

ate behavior toward family, staff members, and other patients. The clinical management of patients during PTA requires the use of interventions to prevent the patient from injuring self and others. The nurse must ascertain that the behavior is not the result of reaction to discomfort or to medications, even those used to treat agitation. Environmental management must be directed to lowering the level of stimulation and cognitive complexity. The nurse may plan to use the interventions listed in Table 17–5 (Braddom, 1996).

All efforts should be made to reduce the use of physical and chemical restraints. Continuous efforts should be made to reorient patients to place, date, time, and the structure of a daily schedule. The daily schedule should be posted in the patient's room and often is given in written form to the patient. If the patient requires decreased stimulation, meals may be served in the room or in small supervised feeding groups. The rehabilitation team, family, and friends should avoid making excessive demands on or having unrealistic expectations of the patient. Family members need to be informed that they should

TABLE 17–5 ■ ENVIRONMENTAL MANAGEMENT OF AGITATION

1. Reduce the level of stimulation in the environment:
     Place patient in a quiet private room.
     Remove noxious stimuli if possible (e.g., tubes, catheters, restraints, traction).
     Limit unnecessary sounds (e.g., television, radio, background conversations).
     Limit number of visitors.
     Staff behave in a calm and reassuring manner.
     Limit number and length of therapy sessions.
     Provide therapies in patient's room.
2. Protect patient from harming self or others:
     Place patient in a floor bed with padded side panels (Craig bed).
     Assign 1:1 or 1:2 sitter to observe patient and ensure safety.
     Avoid taking patient off unit.
     Place patient in locked ward.
3. Reduce patient's cognitive confusion
     One person speaks to patient at a time.
     Maintain same staff to work with patient.
     Minimize patient's contact with unfamiliar staff.
     Communicate to patient briefly and simply (e.g., one idea at a time).
     Reorient patient to place and time repeatedly.
4. Tolerate restlessness when possible:
     Allow patient to thrash about in floor bed.
     Allow patient to pace around unit, with 1:1 supervision.
     Allow confused patient to be verbally inappropriate.

Adapted from Braddom, R. L. (Ed.) (1996). *Physical medicine and rehabilitation*. Philadelphia: W. B. Saunders.

avoid unpleasant emotional interactions with the patient. As the patient continues to emerge from PTA, a reduced level of supervision is possible, and the team can begin to plan for longer-term treatment strategies.

Emergence from PTA

Strategies used for loss of cognitive processes and to compensate for the loss are as follows:

- Orientation
  - Put a personal item (ribbon, name, or a wreath) on the door to the patient's room.
  - Keep the environment as unchanged as possible.
  - Ask the patient to verbalize person, place, and time throughout the day.
  - Discuss the daily schedule, and at the end of each therapy session, reorient the patient where to go next and for what activity.
  - Make the patient responsible for getting to activities on time.
  - Place personal photos in the room and query the patient about who is in them.
  - Provide newspaper and discuss articles and other things in it.
  - Try to assign the same caregiving personnel for consistency.
- Memory loss
  - Use maps and memory log books.
  - Repeat information and make verbal and visual connections to promote recall (calendars, clocks, and pictures).
  - Teach the patient to organize activities in a logical sequential way. For example, when brushing teeth, work through the steps of wetting the brush, brushing, flossing, and rinsing the teeth. The steps may be written and posted on the bathroom mirror. If the patient has lost the sense of time, the morning routine can be set up in time increments, and a large clock placed on the wall will help the patient get to breakfast or therapy on time.
  - Give the patient time to encode information in a meaningful way because recall will be easier.
  - Structure opportunities for the patient to recall commonly used skills. For instance, having a pretzel sale gives the patient experience waiting on a customer, wrapping the pretzel in waxed paper, and making change.
  - Rehearse how to get on public transportation and then have the patient actually perform the task.

- Decreased attention span—distractibility
  - Make sure you have the patient's attention before giving instructions.
  - Keep the patient away from distractions such as the television before engaging in an activity.
  - Keep communication short and simple.
  - Cue the patient and gradually reduce cues.
  - Teach the patient simple computer games, and increase the time spent on the computer.
- Problem solving and learning new tasks
  - Label items for visual cues.
  - Use familiar items brought in from the patient's home, and make connections with specific tasks (hairbrush and comb).
  - Take the patient on field trips (supermarket and restaurant) to test specific skills.
  - Take the patient into a kitchen to prepare simple meals. This will enable the team to check on judgment related to safety.
  - Provide positive reinforcement as often as possible.
  - Have the patient tell the story of the illness experience in a monitored group setting.
- Inappropriate behavior
  - Provide training sessions for all staff so they can model behavior problems and practice responses.
  - Approach the patient in a calm and reassuring manner.
  - Keep a behavior log to monitor any behavior that is aggressive or abusive to self or others.
  - Institute a system of behavioral rounds for sharing observations and information.
  - Identify what behaviors of the patient are to be modified or decreased.
  - Construct and communicate a behavioral modification plan for consistency of approach. Be sure to involve family and significant others in the plan.
  - Distract the patient from the cause of the frustration, if possible.
  - Allow the patient as much freedom of movement as is safe in the environment.
  - Avoid overfatigue. Present alternative ideas or tasks to replace the one causing the frustration.
  - Select positive reinforcers, and use them to strengthen desired behaviors. The patient may earn tokens or money to be used for an activity of choice.
  - Provide opportunities for desired behavior to be reinforced and for the patient to be successful.

❑ Give the patient time out to regain control, if necessary.

❑ Keep a behavior log to determine whether desired changes are being achieved. If not, determine why not, and revise the modification plan.

❑ Ignore some behavior; if not receiving the desired attention from staff or family, it may not recur.

❑ Socially unacceptable behaviors (kicking or hitting) may require removal of the patient from the group or event. However, reintegration must occur, or the patient may learn to use the behavior as a means of retreating from socialization.

Pharmacotherapy

Patients who have cognitive impairment may need multiple medications to treat complications or augment recovery. The nurse needs to understand that the drugs used to treat pain, spasticity, agitation, insomnia, decreased arousal, depression, seizures, and hypertension have side effects that alter cognitive performance and behavior. Patients must be monitored closely for such side effects.

Drugs used for pain may have sedating effects or cause confusion, limiting their usefulness. The treatment of spasticity with diazepam (Valium) or baclofen may result in confusion and sedation. The benzodiazepines diazepam and lorazepam (Ativan), which are used for the treatment of agitation, have sedating effects. In small doses, they have been known to actually increase aggressive behavior by decreasing impulse control. These drugs are habit-forming, and their long-term use has been associated with depression (Gaultieri, 1991).

Antihistamines, such as diphenhydramine (Benadryl), are relatively safe when used to treat insomnias, but the nurse needs to monitor the patient for prolonged sedation. Trazodone (Desyrel), which is marketed as an antidepressant, is also used as a hypnotic or sleep-inducing medication. It has short-lived sedating effects and few side effects.

Stimulants are used to improve alertness in patients who are lethargic or have decreased arousal. Methylphenidate (Ritalin) is most commonly used, but the patient must be observed for agitation, because this drug may impair rather than improve performance. Levels of dopamine may be decreased in the central nervous system such that drugs used to increase levels of dopamine (dopaminergics) are sometimes used to assist in recovery of cognitive impairment. Two of these drugs are amantidine (Symmetrel) and bromocriptine (Parlodel). Unwanted side effects include nausea, anorexia, anxiety, and confusion (Gaultieri, 1991).

Some antidepressants increase levels of the neurotransmitters norepinephrine and serotonin. Those that increase norepinephrine are known as noradrenergics; those that increase serotonin are called serotonergics. Serotonergic antidepressants appear to be better tolerated by patients with cognitive impairment. Tricyclic antidepressants such as amitriptyline (Elavil) and desipramine (Norpramin), which decrease the neurotransmitters acetylcholine and histamine, respectively, may cause dry mucous membranes, constipation, and urinary retention. These drugs may also cause orthostatic hypertension, leading to falls.

Tricyclic antidepressants are also used to treat depression. They include fluoxetine (Prozac), paroxetine (Paxil), venlafaxine (Effexor), and sertraline (Zoloft). Fluoxetine tends to be stimulating, whereas sertraline may cause sedation. This makes sertraline useful as a bedtime medication.

Anticonvulsants, drugs used to prevent or treat seizure activity, often have sedating qualities. Phenytoin (Dilantin) and phenobarbital have more sedating qualities than either carbamazepine (Tegretol) or valproic acid (Braddom, 1996). If possible, hypertension in a patient with cognitive impairment should be treated with clonidine, verapamil, or diuretics rather than propranolol, metoprolol, or methyldopa, which have more sedating effects (Braddom, 1996).

Community Resources and Services

Nurses involved in rehabilitation of the client with cognitive deficits must be knowledgeable about the community resources and services that can help clients become reintegrated into the community. Information about supportive agencies and organizations can be compiled from many sources, kept in a file for easy access, and used for referral. Appropriate information can be obtained from such sources as

1. The blue pages of any Bell telephone book (under "Health and Human Services")
2. Federal, state, and county Health Department Offices
3. Services to the aging
4. Church organizations
5. Family service organizations
6. Mental health and mental retardation agencies

7. Advocacy groups
8. Support groups
9. Services to children and adolescents
10. Professional organizations
11. Rehabilitation services
12. The Internet
13. Policy formulation groups
14. American Association of Retired Persons
15. Psychological and counseling services
16. Housing agencies
17. Home care agencies
18. Legal services
19. Education and training agencies
20. Newspapers, magazines, and television programs
21. Networking with health care professionals
22. Textbooks

IMPLEMENTATION OF NURSING INTERVENTIONS

Implementation of nursing interventions for cognitively impaired clients should take into consideration the developmental, psychosocial, and spiritual components of each client's situation. The following case studies illustrate the methodology.

■ CASE STUDY 17–1

Gail, an 18-year-old woman of African-American descent, was a front-seat passenger in a car that struck a tractor trailer on 12/18/99. She was trapped under the dashboard, and it was noted that the extraction was difficult. She arrived in a comatose state at a local community hospital, where a CT (computed tomography) scan showed a large right-sided subdural hematoma plus multiple facial and skull fractures. She was transported to a large metropolitan medical center, where the hematoma was evacuated. On 1/13/00, an MRI (magnetic resonance image) revealed a small residual hematoma overlying a portion of the right cerebral hemisphere and parenchymal hemorrhages in the temporal lobes bilaterally as well as within the inferior frontal region. A midbrain infarction was also seen. A follow-up CT scan showed a very minimal right subdural collection at the operative site. Tracheostomy and gastrostomy tubes had been placed upon admission.

On 2/3/00, Gail was admitted to the brain injury unit in a rehabilitation facility. Initial assessment revealed that she gave no response to verbal commands, opened her eyes spontaneously, and engaged in a sucking and grimacing pattern with her mouth. There was no evidence of eye tracking movement. A reflex withdrawal of the lower extremities occurred when stimulated; the left upper extremity was extended and the right upper extremity was flexed. Tone in the extremities was not increased. Ankle contractions were bilateral. No skin lesions were seen.

The patient was accompanied by her mother, who is employed by a bank but is currently on family leave. Her father is the chief of police in a small town in a neighboring state. Gail has two younger sisters and two aunts, who make up her immediate support system. The family lives in a large home with three steps to enter. There is a bedroom and full bathroom on the first floor. The patient graduated from high school in May 1999 and worked as a retail clerk in a women's fashion store. The family are active members of a Methodist church. The family plans to take Gail home and use community resources to assist in providing care for her. At the time of admission to the brain injury unit, the mother requested that only female nursing staff care for her daughter. The primary nurse noted this request and communicated it to all male staff members, who complied with the request.

From the patient's injuries and resultant pathophysiology described earlier, the nurses expected to see the following cognitive impairments:

1. Changes in arousal
2. Changes in ability to understand speech; loss of long-term memory and the sense of smell
3. Changes in goal-oriented behavior (e.g., ability to concentrate, short-term or recall memory, and the elaboration of thought)
4. Changes in the ability of the eyes to track moving objects in the visual field

The nurses began a plan of care for clinical management of Gail, who was at Level I on the Rancho Los Amigo Scale and had a Modified Barthel Score of 0. Three nursing diagnoses were formulated from the assessment data:

1. Alteration in Knowledge Deficit
2. Alteration in Injury Potential
3. Alteration in Cognitive Thought Processes

The plan of care was organized with the use of the Standards of Care developed by the nursing staff in the Brain Injury Unit at Bryn Mawr Rehabilitation (Fig. 17–5). Because the patient was classified as being at Level 1 on *Text continued on page 262*

Brain Injury: Standards of Care

Nursing Diagnosis/Problem Focus/Date	Date Initiated	Level 1	Expected Patient Outcomes	Met	Date Initiated	Level 2	Expected Patient Outcomes	Met	Date Initiated	Level 3	Expected Patient Outcomes	Met
ALTERATION IN KNOWLEDGE DEFICIT Date Initiated 2/3/00 _____ RN		Assess knowledge base, educational factors, and learning readiness. Distribute educational materials. Initiate BI education.			2/20	Reassess learning readiness in consideration of memory deficit, attention span, thought process, and aphasia.					Pt./SO will demonstrate BI knowledge by D/C, including diet, S/S, and meds.	
		Encourage SO attendance at BI support group.	SO will attend education support group.			Provide pt./SO with learning experience in care.	Pt./SO will demonstrate/verbalize care.			Medication • Provide 1:1 medication education. • Supply pt. with medication teaching cards. Include dosage time, drug, and food interactions.	Pt./SO will verbalize dosage, time, and drug and food interactions of medications.	
		Review with SO need for family participation in pt. care.				Encourage SO to attend and participate in therapies 1x a week.	SO will attend and participate in therapies 1x a week.					

	Orient to unit.	Pt./SO will demonstrate use/understanding of: • Bed controls • Call light • Bathroom • Telephone • TV control • Visiting policy • Smoking policy	
RISK FOR INJURY SEIZURE PRECAUTIONS Date Initiated ___ ___ RN	Implement seizure precautions with known seizure activity: • Pad bedside rails • Suction equipment in pt.'s room • O₂ set in pt.'s room • ___		Pt. will be free of self-sustained injury, aspiration, and inadequate cerebral oxygenation.

Illustration continued on following page

Brain Injury: Standards of Care Continued

Nursing Diagnosis/ Problem Focus/ Date	Date Initiated	Level 1	Expected Patient Outcomes	Met	Date Initiated	Level 2	Expected Patient Outcomes	Met	Date Initiated	Level 3	Expected Patient Outcomes	Met
		Assess falls risk and instruct on safety precautions: • See Falls Prevention Protocol: (ex, BMB, UMP/ Personal Sentry, w/c board, bed alarm). ___ • Evaluate falls prevention program methods for effectiveness and as appropriate Q 7 days and after each fall.	Patient will not sustain a preventable injury.			Implement new interventions according to program.					Pt. will not sustain a preventable injury.	
		Teach SO proper transfer methods prescribed by P.T.	SO will demonstrate proper transfer techniques.			Teach pt. and SO transfer and ambulation techniques prescribed by P.T.					Pt./SO will demonstrate proper transfer methods and ambulation techniques.	
										Reevaluate and provide D/C instructions.	Pt. will verbalize D/C instructions.	
										Discuss home environmental hazards and precautions.	Pt./SO will verbalize environmental hazards.	

ALTERATION IN THOUGHT PROCESSES Date Initiated ___ ___ RN					
• Memory	Assess for memory deficits (short, long, and recent).				Pt./family will participate in the establishment of pt.'s memory/ orientation program.
	Frequent orientation to time and place using calendar, care board, log book, orientaion board.				
	Frequent orientation to personal information— past events, names of significant others, pur- pose for hospi- talization.				
	Orient pt. to names of nurses and therapists, and purpose of therapy.				
	Review orientation information in question/ answer format.				

Illustration continued on following page

Brain Injury: Standards of Care Continued

Nursing Diagnosis/ Problem Focus/ Date	Date Initiated	Level 1	Expected Patient Outcomes	Met	Date Initiated	Level 2	Expected Patient Outcomes	Met	Date Initiated	Level 3	Expected Patient Outcomes	Met
ALTERATION IN BEHAVIOR Date Initiated _____ RN		Assess, monitor, and document early signs of anger, restlessness, agitated aggressive behavior. Implement behavior log PRN.								Assess/ reassess inappropriate behavior: • Attention tactics • Manipulation attempts • Regressive behavior	Pt.'s behavior will be appropriate.	
		Keep pt.'s environment quiet and structured.	Pt. will not escalate out of control.			Assess environment and room, remove hazardous objects that the pt. may use to inflict injury on self or others.	Pt. will cause no injury/harm to self or others.			Encourage independence.	Pt. will demonstrate independent behavior.	
						Keep pt.'s environment quiet when agitated and routinely structured.				Use positive reinforcement when pt. demonstrates inappropriate behavior.	Pt. will self-correct inappropriate dependent behavior.	
						Encourage pt. to verbalize anger. Tell the pt. firmly when he/she behaves inappropriately or has an inappropirate verbal expression.	Pt. will verbalize anger and act appro-priately.			Implement or reevaluate behavior modification plan.		

ALTERATION IN BEHAVIOR					Pt. will remain injury free within appropriate environment.				Behavior guidelines will be followed.
					If the pt. is exhibiting violent or aggressive behavior, do not approach alone (handle with care). Remove pt. from environment/ activity precipitating episode. a. Use private room. b. Holding room PRN for severe agitation to seclude from others. c. Restrain or use restraints only as necessary for safety. d. Keep pt. care at a minimum when violent behavior is evident/ pending. e. Following time-out, reapproach pt. in calm, quiet but firm manner to discuss episode.				
					Refer pt. for Interim Treatment Plan/Behavior Rounds as appropriate. See specific Behavior Guidelines.				

FIGURE 17-5

Standards of Care for Brain Injury. (From Bryn Mawr Rehabilitation Nursing Discipline, Malvern, PA.) BI, brain injury; UMP, Personal Sentry box attached to chair or clothing with Velcro so when pt. moves out of chair, a string pulls out and an alarm is sounded; BMB, Bryn Mawr bed; w/c board/lapboard; alarm, bed; D/C, discharge; pt., patient; P.T., physical therapist; SO, significant other; S/S, signs and symptoms.

the Bryn Mawr Rehabilitation Standards, her mother was designated as the significant other (SO). The medication methylphenidate (Ritalin) was ordered to be administered in 5-mg doses twice a day. This drug, a stimulant, is used in patients who have brain damage. Little is understood about why it appears to work, but its effectiveness may be related to a deficit of neurochemicals active in the reticular activating system. The drug repairs the deficit and allows patients to pay attention (Woolack, Law, & Carter, 1991).

By 2/20/00, perhaps because of her age (which appears to be a predictor of recovery from traumatic unconsciousness, with the best recovery seen in children, followed by adults younger than 40 years [Multi Society Task Force, 1994]), Gail was elevated to Level IV on the Rancho Los Amigos Scale (confused–agitated) and to Level 2 on the Brain Injury Standards (see Fig. 17–4). However, she became impulsive, kicking at the therapists and the table. A behavioral log and a behavioral modification plan were constructed by a neuropsychologist and implemented on 2/27/00. The plan consisted of the following guidelines to be used whenever Gail was uncooperative:

1. Establish contingency that participation will result in a reward of rest for 5 minutes.
2. If Gail "shuts down," attempt to change the treatment activity to reengage, but do not end the session.
3. Maintain the limits, with the contingency to avoid manipulation.
4. Continue to record aggressive behavior for data collection in the behavior log to possibly change the plan.

By 3/7/00, it was noted that Gail was oriented to time, place, and person. She went home for the weekend, where her parents reported observing increased verbalization and improved behavior. Her case manager wrote a letter to the insurance carrier detailing the treatment goals and the progress to date. She pointed out the need to maximize independent function and prevent complications in view of Gail's age. The insurance carrier agreed to a discharge date of 4/11/00.

All efforts were made to make continued improvements and to have Gail reach Level 3 on the Brain Injury Standards. She was being evaluated for an augmentation communication system through assessment of her ability to establish yes/no responses. Gail increased her level of attention, in that she can play solitaire on the computer for 18 minutes. Gail

is fortunate to have good family, community, and church support. Often, the African-American culture is family oriented and does provide care for its family members. Spector (1996) observed that "despite overwhelming hardships and enforced separations, the people [manage] in most circumstances to maintain family and community awareness." The Methodist Church of which she is a member sends Gail cards, flowers, stuffed animals, visitors, and prayers. Her family have a strong faith and believe that she will recover. There does not appear to be spiritual distress with her family, but because of her cognitive impairments, it is not possible to assess whether spirituality is of concern to Gail.

She will be reintegrated into her community by all those involved in her care; this process may take several more years. It will depend on the amount of spontaneous recovery she demonstrates and the successful use of interventions after her discharge. Such interventions include outpatient therapy, special education for the recovery and enhancement of basic skills, and work with the Bureau of Vocational Rehabilitation to assist in job training and placement. Gail is fortunate to have access, through the Rehabilitation Facility and its dedicated staff, to all that is available for the brain-injured.

Gail was discharged on April 28, 2000 after her mother spent 2 full days observing and participating in her care. As the first step in her community reintegration, Gail will spend the day, from 9 AM to 2 PM, 5 days a week, in an Easter Seals outpatient facility located 5 miles from her home.

■ **CASE STUDY 17–2**

Maurice is an 80-year-old Jewish man whose developmental stage would be described as "ego-integrity versus despair" (Erikson, 1963). He is married, a father of four and grandfather of eight. A retired shoe salesman, he lives in Florida 9 months of the year and the other 3 months in a large northeastern city. He and his wife attend services at their synagogue every Saturday morning and are active in the Jewish community.

While in Florida, on December 18, 1999, Maurice experienced flulike symptoms for which he was treated with cough syrup by his physician. Over the next 2 days, he spent much time in bed and had difficulty with balance, falling two times. Observing that his condition was deteriorating, his wife called 911, and he was taken to the local medical center. Maurice required cardiopulmonary resuscitation in the emergency room and then was admitted to the intensive care unit. He was diagnosed as having had a right-sided cerebrovascular accident. The CT scan showed widespread small-vessel disease throughout the cortex and a possible blockage in the right anterior cerebral artery. Clinically, Maurice presented with confusion, dysarthria, and a left-sided hemiparesis. Other contributing medical factors are a history of insulin-dependent diabetes, coronary artery disease (three bypass coronary artery grafts in 1987), hypertension, transurethral prostatectomy in 1990, and glaucoma. The patient's condition was stabilized, and he was flown up north to be admitted on December 29, 1999 to a rehabilitation facility near his home and family. Plans are for him to return home to live with his wife in an apartment located in a high-rise building that has an elevator.

At the time of admission, Maurice and his wife, age 72, shared their concerns about his loss of mobility and use of his left arm and the impact it would have on their daily lives and future together. Because of the widespread nature of the disease processes in this patient, the nursing staff and the interdisciplinary team relied on clinical manifestations to complete their assessments. Developmentally, he is elderly, so the team needed to set goals to achieve as much functional independence as possible and to enhance the quality of his life. Enhancing the quality of life will be especially challenging because of his diffuse brain involvement, leading to altered thought processes and risk for injury. In a survey of literature on rehabilitation after stroke, Johnson, Pearson, and McDivitt (1997) concluded that although the level of independence in activities of daily living improved, the quality of life failed to improve over time for stroke survivors. Difficulties occurred in the areas of leisure activities and major changes in relationships with family, friends, and acquaintances. Thus, more research that addresses stroke survivors' quality of life over an extended time needs to be done.

Nursing diagnoses that were identified for Maurice were as follows:

1. Knowledge Deficit
2. Alteration in Cognitive Thought Processes
3. Injury Potential

The nursing plan for care, which follows the Standards of Care for The Neurology Patient at Bryn Mawr Rehabilitation, was started (Fig. 17–6). Initially Maurice was placed at Level 1, but within a week, he was advanced to Level 2 because he performed at that level 75% of the time. His overall Modified Barthel Score on the Barthel's Index was 38. Maurice reported that his family was his reason for living and that he was, overall, satisfied with his life. He had a rich, full life in the context of his ethnic and religious background.

The nursing staff needed to negotiate a plan of care for this patient and his family and not for themselves (Barry, 1996). Maurice was perceived as being overly demanding of the staff, and some limit setting was necessary. Maurice had already experienced many alterations in his lifestyle because of chronic illness and wanted to participate in the decision-making process. The physicians were concerned because the patient's morning blood sugar levels were elevated to 400 mg/ dl. He expressed frustration because the physicians would not listen to his statements about the amount of his evening insulin dosage. The nurse encouraged him and advocated for him with the physician. The evening insulin dosage was changed, and the blood sugar levels came within normal range. This gave Maurice more energy to participate in his morning therapy program and a feeling of control over his diabetic regimen.

Maurice complained of being unable to sleep at night and frequently rang the bell, asking for something to sleep. He had an order for Xanax, 0.25 mg to be given 3 times a day as needed for anxiety. Xanax (alprazolam), a benzodiazepine, is used for the treatment of panic attacks and anxiety associated with depression. Currently, it is the drug of choice for treating anxiety. Sedation is the most common adverse reaction. It can also impair motor coordination, reaction time, and cognitive reasoning, especially in the elderly patient (Baer & Williams, 1996). Maurice also had an order for Ambien (zolpidem), 5 mg PO HS, PRN for sleep. This agent is a nonbenzodiazepine, nonbarbiturate drug that acts as a hypnotic for short-term treatment of simple insomnia. The drug can produce greater hangover effects, although less than those produced by barbiturates and benzodiazepines, especially in elderly patients (Baer & Williams, 1996).

The patient had received Xanax at 10 PM the evening of January 12, 2000. The nurse gave him Ambien at 1 AM on January 13, 2000. At 6:30 AM, Maurice was difficult to

Neurology: Standards of Care

Nursing Diagnosis/ Problem Focus/Date	Date Initiated	Level 1	Expected Patient Outcomes	Met	Date Initiated	Level 2	Expected Patient Outcomes	Met	Date Initiated	Level 3	Expected Patient Outcomes	Met
KNOWLEDGE DEFICIT Date Initiated ____ ____ RN		Assess knowledge base, educational factors, and learning readiness.				Provide pt./SO with learning experience in care.	Pt./SO will demonstrate/ verbalize care.				Pt./SO will demonstrate stroke knowledge by D/C, including diet, S/S, risk factors and meds.	
		Encourage stroke group series attendance.	Pt./SO will attend education support group.			Reassess learning readiness in consideration of memory deficits, attention span, thought process, and aphasia.				Medication • Provide 1:1 medication education • Supply pt. with medication teaching cards. Include dosage time, drug, and food interactions.	Pt./SO will verbalize dosage, time, drug and food interactions of medications.	
		Instruct on meds/food reaction.				Encourage SO to attend and participate in therapies 1x a week.	SO will attend and participate in therapies 1x a week.					
		Dietary consult for diet.	Pt./SO will be able to select correct menu for diet.									
		Orient to unit.	Pt./SO will demonstrate/ verbalize use of bed control, call bell, BR, telephone, TV, visiting and smoking policies.									

ALTERATION IN THOUGHT PROCESS	Interventions	Expected Outcomes		
Date Initiated ____ ____ RN	Distribute education material.	Pt./SO will verbalize intent of rehab and current knowledge of condition.		
	Assess orientation/ PRN.	Pt. will verbalize communi-cate/ person/ place/time.	Assess pt.'s ability to sequence activities.	Pt. will correctly sequence the steps of a new task with minimal cues.
	Implement reality orientation techniques.	Pt. will utilize en-vironmental orientation props and therapy schedule.	Promote communication that enhances communication skills and clarifies thoughts.	Pt. will hold appro-priate conver-sation with caretakers.
	Schedule pt. with consistent caregivers and maintain environment.	Pt. will address caretaker by name.	Evaluate mastery of ADL skills, moving from simple to complex.	Pt. performs ADL with minimal cues.
	Assess (−) behaviors and implement intervention for (+) coping strategies.		Provide pt. with opportunities for positive social interactions.	Pt. will participate in recreat-ional group activities and social interac-tions.
	Refer to clinical psychologist PRN.		Provide pt./SO with community support group information.	Pt./SO will verbalize available support groups.
	Initiate behavior rounds if assessment warrants.			

Reinforce adaption techniques to cope and deal with memory deficits:
• Memory log

Pt. will demonstrate effective use of memory compensatory techniques.

Illustration continued on following page

Neurology: Standards of Care Continued

Nursing Diagnosis/ Problem Focus/Date	Date Initiated	Level 1	Expected Patient Outcomes	Met	Date Initiated	Level 2	Expected Patient Outcomes	Met	Date Initiated	Level 3	Expected Patient Outcomes	Met
RISK FOR INJURY Date Initiated		Assess falls risk. Instruct safety precautions on admission and q shift.	Pt. will not sustain a preventable injury.			Reassess for fall potential via fall safety scale q 7 days/or PRN fall.				Reevaluate and provide D/C instructions.	Pt. will verbalize D/C instructions.	
RN		See Falls Prevention Protocol. List safety devices: Blue belt-soft restraint-on when in wheelchair				Implement new interventions according to program.				Discuss home environmental hazards and precautions.	Pt./SO will verbalize home environmental hazards.	
		Teach proper transfer methods and ambulation techniques prescribed by PT.	Pt. will demonstrate proper transfer methods and ambulation techniques.			Reinforce program with patient/SO.	Pt./SO will demonstrate safety interventions.					

FIGURE 17-6

Standards of Care for the Neurology Patient. (From Bryn Mawr Rehabilitation Nursing Discipline, Malvern, PA.) ADL, activities of daily living; BR, bathroom; D/C, discharge; pt, patient; P.T., physical therapist; SO, significant other; S/S, signs and syptoms.

arouse but was placed in a chair and pushed into the bathroom to brush his teeth. It had been judged safe to leave this patient alone for short periods. A short time after the nurse left him in the bathroom, a crash was heard, and Maurice was found on the bathroom floor with the wheelchair tipped over onto its side. Maurice did not remember how this occurred, but fortunately, he was not injured. In discussing this incident, the nurse and physician concluded that Maurice may have suffered a hangover effect and that any further sedative should not be given to him so late in the night. Maurice was not to be left unattended again until his level of confusion could be further assessed. Other interventions for addressing his anxiety and his sleeplessness were added to the plan of care.

Maurice's wife also required some support as she tried to find some balance between her role of a traditional wife who waits on her husband and the need to help him achieve more independence. She will need guidance in her role of caregiver, as this new role will determine her quality of life as well as her husband's.

SUMMARY

Clients who are cognitively impaired present unique opportunities in varied settings for nurses to work in multidisciplinary teams. Much more research needs to be conducted on brain function and the cognitive processes to enable identification of interventions and the measurement of outcomes to increase the quality of life while staying within resource constraints. This issue is the challenge of the new century as more individuals survive with cognitive deficits in a society of increasing cultural diversity.

Family members, who are integral parts of care plans for cognitively impaired clients, must understand and accept the cognitive level at which their impaired relatives can function. Family members must be encouraged to discuss their true feelings about the ambiguity of living with a family member who is cognitively impaired. Sometimes they are conflicted by being regarded as "heroes" by friends and health care professionals while they actually harbor feelings of resentment toward the client. Such conflict is very destructive to the caregivers. Failla and Jones (1991) use the term "family hardiness" for the ability to care for a disabled family member. The nurse can encourage the formation of

family hardiness by having discussions with family members designed to (1) enhance their sense of control over the chaotic events they are encountering, (2) increase their commitment, and (3) support them as they grow and develop new abilities (Grzankowski, 1997).

The nurse interested in rehabilitation of cognitively impaired people can gain a solid research base for practice by participating in the Association of Rehabilitation Nurses (ARN). In 1996, the Rehabilitation Nursing Foundation (RNF), which serves as the educational, research, and development foundation of the ARN, developed a research agenda. One of the high priorities identified by the RNF is to focus on effective nursing strategies to promote self-care in people with cognitive and physical impairments, including management of adverse behaviors in people with brain injury (RNF, 1996). Often, it is not the physical deficits that prevent the cognitively impaired individual from returning to and remaining in the family unit or being reintegrated into the community, but the social and behavioral changes that make the individual so different from his or her premorbid self.

REFERENCES

Baer, C. L., & Williams, B. (1996). *Clinical pharmacology and nursing* (3rd ed.). Springhouse, PA: Springhouse.

Barry, P. (1996). *Psychosocial nursing: Care of physically ill patients and their families* (3rd ed.). Philadelphia: Lippincott-Raven.

Berrol, S. (1990). Issues in cognitive rehabilitation. *Archives of Neurology, 47,* 219–272.

Brain injury update (1997, December). HDI 12, 91.

Braddom, R. M. (1996). *Physical medicine and rehabilitation.* Philadelphia: W. B. Saunders.

Corsini, R. (Ed.). (1994). *Encyclopedia of psychology* (2nd ed.). New York: Wiley & Sons.

Erikson, E. (1963). *Childhood and society.* New York: W. W. Norton.

Failla, S., & Jones, L. C. (1991). Families of children with developmental disabilities: An examination of family hardiness. *Research in Nursing and Health, 14*(1), 41–50.

Folstein, M. E., Folstein, S. E., & McHugh, P. R. (1975). Mini-mental state: A practical method for grading the cognitive state of patients for the clinician. *Journal of Psychiatric Research, 12,* 189–198.

Gaultieri, C. T. (1991). *Neuropsychiatry and behavioral pharmacology* (pp. 37–88). New York: Springer-Verlag.

Giacino, J. T., Zasler, N. D., Katz, D. I., Kelly, S., Rosenberg, J., & Tilly, C. (1997). Development of practice guidelines for assessment and management of the vegetative and minimally conscious states. *Journal of Head Trauma Rehabilitation, 12,* 79–94.

Grainger, C. V., Hamilton, B. B., & Sherwin, F. S. (1986). Guide for the use of the uniform data set for medical rehabilitation. Buffalo, NY: Uniform Data System for Medical Rehabilitation Project Office.

Grzankowski, J. (1997). Altered thought processes related to traumatic brain injury and their nursing implications. *Rehabilitation Nursing, 22*(1), 24–31.

Johnson, J., Pearson, V., & McDivitt, L. (1997). Stroke rehabilitation: Assessing stroke survivors' long-term learning needs. *Rehabilitation Nursing, 22,* 243–248.

Kaplan, E., Fine, D., Morris, R., & Dellis, D. (1991). *WAIS-R as a neuropsychological instrument.* San Antonia: The Psychological Corporation.

Levin, H. S., Benton, A. L., & Grossman, R. G. (1982). Neurobehavioral consequences of closed head injury. New York: Oxford University Press.

Levin, H. S., Gary, H. E., Eisenberg, H. M.: NIH Trauma Coma Data Bank Research Group (1990). Neurobehavioral outcome one year after head surgery: Experience of the traumatic coma data bank. *Journal of Neurosurgery, 73,* 699–705.

Levin, H. S., O' Donnell, V. M., & Grossman, R. C. (1979). The Galveston Orientation and Amnesia Test: A practical scale to assess cognition of head trauma. *Journal of Nervous Mental Disorders 167,* 675–684.

Luria, A. R. (1980). *Higher cortical functions in man.* New York: Basic Books.

Mahoney, F. I., & Barthel, D. (1965). Functional evaluation: The Barthel Index. Maryland State Medical Journal, *14,* 56–61.

Malkmus, D., Booth, B. J., & Kodimer, C. (1980). Rehabilitation of head injured adults: Comprehensive cognitive management. Downey, CA: Professional Staff Association of Ranchos Los Amigos Hospital.

Markwardt, F. (1989). Peabody Individual Achievement Test—Revised. Circle Pines, MN: American Guidance Services.

Melvin, J., Graham, P., Graham, L., & Olsen, J. (1997, Fall). Traumatic brain injury: Community-based programs are crucial in limited-resource settings. *Rehab Management,* 7(1), 32–35.

Multi Society Task Force on PVS: Medical aspects of the persistent vegetative state. (1994). New England *Journal of Medicine.* 2, 330, 1572.

North American Nursing Diagnosis Association. (1990). Classification of Nursing Diagnosis. Proceedings of the Tenth Conference. Johnson, R. M., & Pasyette, M. Philadelphia, Lippincott.

Rehabilitation Nursing Foundation (RNF) (1996). A research agenda for rehabilitation nursing. Glenview, IL: RNF.

Reitan, R. M., & Wolfson, D. (1986). Traumatic brain injury: Pathophysiology and Neuropsychological Evaluation I. Tucson: Neuropsychology Press.

Spector, R. E. (1996). *Cultural diversity in health and illness.* Stamford, CT: Appleton & Lange.

Tombaugh, T. N., & McIntyre, N. J. (1992). The Mini-Mental State Examination: a comprehensive review. *Am Geriatr Soc 40,* 922–935.

Woolack, J., Law, N., & Carter, S. (1991). Static encephalopathies. In A. Rudolph (Ed.), *Rudolph's Pediatrics* (19th ed.). Norwalk, CT: Appleton & Lange.

CHAPTER 18

Skin Integrity

Sheila M. Sparks

The maintenance of normal skin integrity protects a person from infection, promotes well-being, and permits the person to participate fully in work, leisure, and personal activities. To have skin integrity means that the individual is free of tears, wounds, incisions, scrapes, scratches, bruises, ulcers, or other indicators of skin breakdown. Often undervalued, the work of maintaining the integrity of the skin is difficult, not very exciting, and extremely time-consuming. Healthy skin is intact and has normal turgor, color, texture, distribution of hair, sebaceous glands, sensation, sweat glands, moisture, and nails. Healthy skin is a reflection of adequate nutritional status, effective hygiene practices, normal psychosocial status, and a general state of well-being. Persons with disabilities may need nursing assistance to accommodate their motor and sensory changes as well as to cope with body image changes and their perceptions of themselves. The nurse is in an ideal position to help persons with disabilities to integrate skin integrity health in their rehabilitation goals. In addition, knowledge of the functions of the skin and the clinical application of preventive, health promotion, therapeutic, and restorative health care practices related to the maintenance of skin integrity will validate the importance of this aspect of nursing practice.

Skin integrity, or the lack of it, has become a major concern for community health nurses, both public and private health care insurers, and health policymakers. The economic burden of managing chronic wounds may be $6 billion (Sorenson, 1997). The personal cost of skin integrity impairment is incalculable; it can only be estimated to negatively affect self-esteem, employment, and personal relationships. To meet these challenges, commissions have been formed and special initiatives have been undertaken. For example, the Agency for Health Care Policy and Research (AHCPR) convened two consensus panels to develop guidelines related to skin care. The first was on the prevention and prediction of pressure ulcers, and the second was on the treatment of pressure ulcers (see the section on AHCPR guidelines). The National Pressure Ulcer Advisory Panel was formed in 1987 as an independent, not-for-profit organization dedicated to the prevention and management of pressure ulcers. It serves as a resource for individuals interested in pressure ulcer issues, conducts national conferences, disseminates educational materials, and supports public policy changes and research.

This chapter provides an overview of the functions, anatomy, and physiology of the skin, reviews common alterations in skin integrity, and discusses preventive, health promotion, therapeutic, and restorative health practices in relation to skin integrity. The chapter concludes with a discussion of relevant quality-of-care issues in skin integrity.

OVERVIEW OF THE FUNCTIONS OF THE SKIN

The skin, the largest organ of the body, has many complex functions. Key functions of the skin include protection, temperature regulation, homeostasis, vitamin synthesis, function as a sensory organ, and maintenance of psychosocial health. These functions are described in more detail in Table 18–1. For persons with disabilities, many of these functions are altered. In some individuals, motor losses contribute to the development of pressure areas; in others, sensory losses add to the risk of being burned or having traumatic injuries. A reduction or an absence of sensation can lead to a loss of intimacy or limit ways in which others can demonstrate caring. Temperature changes or the lack of ability to regulate temperature can lead to hypothermia or hyperthermia. Alterations in skin integrity cause problems in traveling and working, affect the ability to live in one's home, and may limit social interactions.

TABLE 18–1 ■ FUNCTIONS OF THE SKIN

Epidermis	Dermis	Subcutaneous Tissue
Protection		
Keratin provides protection from injury by corrosive materials	Provides fibroblasts for wound healing	Mechanical shock absorber
Inhibits proliferation of microorganisms because of dry external surface	Provides mechanical strength Collagen fibers	
Mechanical strength through intracellular bonds	Elastic fibers Ground substance Lymphatic and vascular tissues respond to inflammation, injury, and infection	
Homeostasis (Water Balance)		
Low permeability to water and electrolytes prevents systemic dehydration and electrolyte loss		
Temperature Regulation		
The eccrine sweat glands allow dissipation of heat through evaporation of sweat secreted onto the skin surface	Cutaneous vasculature, through dilation or constriction, promotes or inhibits heat conduction from the skin surface	Fat cells act as insulators and assist in retention of body heat
Sensory Organ		
Transmits a variety of sensations through the neuroreceptor system	Encloses an extensive network of free and encapsulated nerve endings for relaying sensations to the brain	Contains large pressure receptors
Vitamin Synthesis		
7-Dehydrocholesterol is present in large concentrations in malpighian cells; photoconversion to vitamin D takes place		
Psychosocial		
Body image alterations with many epidermal diseases, such as generalized psoriasis	Body image alterations with many dermal diseases, such as scleroderma	Body image alterations may result from increases, decreases, and redistribution of body fat stores

From Ignatavicius, D., Workman M., Mishler M. (1995). *Medical-Surgical Nursing: A Nursing Process Approach* (2nd ed., p. 1913). Philadelphia: W. B. Saunders.

ANATOMY AND PHYSIOLOGY OF THE SKIN

The skin has three distinct layers: subcutaneous fat, dermis, and epidermis (see Table 18–1). Skin appendages include the hair and the nails. Each of these layers contributes to the maintenance of skin integrity and is depicted in Figure 18–1.

Layers

Subcutaneous Fat

The subcutaneous fat layer covers the bone and muscle and forms the innermost aspect of the skin. Fat cells serve as a thermal insulator, absorb shock, protect against mechanical injury (Ignatavicius, Workman, & Mishler, 1995), and provide for the synthesis of fat-soluble vitamins. The fat layer is vascular and forms capillary networks that supply nutrients and remove waste products; it also contains the hair follicles, sebaceous glands

(which secrete sebum, a substance that lubricates the skin and minimizes water loss), and eccrine and apocrine sweat glands. The eccrine glands aid in regulating body temperature by secreting an isotonic solution; this secretion is evaporated on the skin surface and can lead to excessive water loss and subsequent dehydration and heat stroke. Absence of the ability to sweat occurs in persons with a lack of sympathetic or hypothalamic control. The apocrine sweat glands are near the hair follicles; they are found primarily in the axillae, perineum, nipple areolae, and periumbilicus; their secretions interact with skin bacteria and cause body odor.

Dermis

The dermis is on top of the subcutaneous fat layer. Made of collagen and elastic fibers, the dermal layer gives the skin flexibility and strength. Collagen, a protein, is made by the fibroblasts in the dermis. When tissue is in-

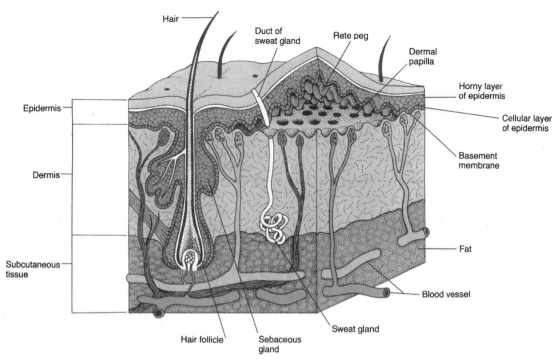

FIGURE 18-1

Anatomy of the hair follicle and sebaceous glands. (From Ignatavicius, D., Workman, M., & Mishler, M. [1995]. *Medical-surgical nursing: A nursing process approach* [2nd ed., p. 1910]. Philadelphia: W. B. Saunders.)

jured, the production of collagen increases and aids in scar formation. The dermal fibroblasts also make ground substance, a material that helps maintain the skin's turgor. Elasticity of the skin is maintained by elastin, the major component of the elastic fibers. Capillaries and lymph vessels in the dermis permit the exchange of oxygen and heat. The dermal layer also contains sensory nerves. Alterations in sensation change the body's response to touch, temperature, pain, pressure, and itch.

Epidermis

The outermost layer of the skin, the epidermis, is attached to the dermal layer by the dermal papillae linking with the rete pegs of the epidermal layer. Although it forms a protective barrier between the body and the environment, the epidermis lacks a blood supply and is less than 1 mm thick. A basement membrane at the dermal-epidermal junction provides the mechanism for the diffusion of nutrients and is the source of the functional cells keratinocytes. Keratinocytes divide to form new cells, and older cells move upward, forming the stratified layer of the epithelium; they also produce a protein called

keratin that helps keep the skin waterproof. This stratified epidermal layer is the site for the final synthesis of vitamin D, in conjunction with exposure to ultraviolet light. The outermost layer of keratinocytes is called the *stratum corneum* and is formed of dead cells. Melanocytes are also found in the basement membrane and give rise to the pigment variations in the color of the skin. The size, distribution, and activity of melanosomes, which contain melanin pigment, determine the color of the skin. Exposure to ultraviolet light stimulates the production of melanin and helps protect the body from the damaging effects of the sun.

Appendages: Hair and Nails

Hair and nails, skin appendages, complete the structures of the skin. Hair is different in structure and rate of growth depending on race, sex, age, and genetic makeup. Hair growth occurs in cycles (growth phase is anagen; resting phase is telogen). Nails are composed of nail keratin. The nail consists of the nail plate (lunula), matrix, nail bed, and cuticle. The nails serve as tools in carrying out many fine motor functions.

KEY COMPONENTS OF SKIN INTEGRITY

Skin integrity involves several components. Healthy skin is intact, supple, elastic, waterproof, and flexible; its functions include the exchange of nutrients, the removal of waste products, the synthesis of vitamin D, temperature regulation, and sensory feelings. Persons with disabilities, both sensory and motor, may have an increased risk of interruption of the skin's normal status.

OVERVIEW OF SKIN ALTERATIONS

Skin alterations occur as a result of infections, trauma, or disease and in response to pressure, to a lack of preventive practices, and to a lack of protection from injury. This section is limited to those skin alterations that commonly occur in persons with disabilities or during the rehabilitative phase of treatment. It does not include discussion of primary skin conditions, cancer of the skin, or dermatological diseases.

Because of the loss of motor and sensory function, the person with a disability is at risk for developing pressure ulcers, arterial ulcers, diabetic/neuropathic ulcers, venous ulcers, skin abrasions, skin tears, dryness, and petechiae or ecchymoses. With a loss of temperature regulation, the disabled person may be subject to hypothermia or hyperthermia; the response of the skin and measures to prevent and manage these temperature changes are discussed. Injury to tissue is another common problem in those with sensory loss; discussion of protective measures and regular skin inspection is included.

Pressure Ulcer

A pressure ulcer, previously called a pressure sore, decubitus ulcer, or bed sore, is defined as "any lesion caused by unrelieved pressure resulting in damage of underlying tissue. Pressure ulcers usually occur over bony prominences and are graded or staged to classify the degree of tissue damage observed" (Bergstrom et al., 1994).

Arterial Ulcer

An arterial ulcer is a clinical condition related to peripheral arterial disease. Arterial ulcers may develop on the toes, between the toes, or on the upper aspect of the foot. They usually are painful, causing intermittent claudication and, in severe cases, rest pain. Other features are hair loss on the lower extremity, dry skin, thickened toenails, coolness of the extremity, and a darkened color. The extremity may have elevational pallor and dependent rubor.

Diabetic/Neuropathic Ulcer

Diabetic ulcers usually develop on the plantar surface of the foot or other surfaces where there is pressure. Because of diabetic neuropathy, there may be numbness or tingling, but such ulcers are not usually associated with pain. About 15% of the 14 million Americans with diabetes will develop foot ulcers. Foot monitoring must be an integral part of the person's daily routine; custom-made shoes or pressure-reducing orthoses may be needed to prevent diabetic foot ulcers.

Venous Stasis Ulcer

The venous stasis ulcer is a chronic nonhealing ulcer that usually occurs in the ankle area and is not very painful. The foot is warm, pulses are palpable, and there is leg or ankle edema. Venous ulcers have an incidence of about 0.2 to 0.4% in the general population, about 500,000 Americans. The average lifetime cost is $40,000 (Sorenson, 1997).

Skin Abrasions

Because of sensory or motor loss, skin abrasions can occur easily from rubbing the skin surface against an abrasive surface or by accidentally scraping or bumping the skin. An abrasion is a localized area of superficial skin loss.

Skin Tears

Skin is subject to tearing in areas that are subject to friction or shearing forces. There is an increased problem in those who already have ecchymotic areas. Risk factors for skin tears include "stiffness and spasticity, sensory loss, limited mobility, poor appetite, polypharmacy, and a history of previous skin tears" (Kopac & McGough-Csarny, 1997). As people age, the skin becomes thin and fragile and is easily torn.

Dryness

Dry skin is a common problem in the winter months, in environments with low humidity, and in individuals with limited circulation. It is intensified with inadequate fluid intake and decreased lubrication of the skin. Dry skin is characterized by scaling, flaking, and, in severe cases, redness and cracking (Sparks, 1997).

Petechiae/Ecchymoses

Bleeding into the tissues causes petechiae and ecchymoses, two types of purpuric lesions. Petechiae are small, nonblanchable vascular lesions. Ecchymoses (bruises) are larger areas of tissue hemorrhage. Persons with chronic venous insufficiency often have stasis dermatitis, clinically characterized by petechiae. Bruises are often the result of striking or hitting an area of the body that is insensate; regular skin inspection is needed to identify problems and initiate preventive measures.

Injury to the Skin

Injury to the skin can occur from trauma, high- or low-temperature exposure, pressure, a lack of cleanliness, or excessive moisture or can be inflicted by weapons or other objects.

CLINICAL PROFILE OF SKIN INTEGRITY PROBLEMS

In rehabilitation nursing, management of skin integrity problems is identified as a high-frequency, high treatment priority (Gordon, 1995). This section provides an overview of the scope of the skin integrity problem.

Incidence

Incidence refers to the number of new cases of a specific disease or disorder during a specified period of time. Venous leg ulcers affect half a million people in the United States (Pontieri-Lewis, 1995). In some populations, the incidence of pressure ulcers is high. For example, elderly persons who sustain femoral fractures and are admitted to hospitals have an incidence reported as high as 66% (Versluyen, 1986). In skilled care facilities and nursing homes, the reported incidence of pressure ulcers ranges from 2.4 to 23%. In the spinal cord injury population, the incidence of pressure ulcers has been reported to range from 7.5 to 85% (Hammond, Bozzacco, Stiens, Buhrer, & Lyman, 1994; Mawson et al., 1988).

Prevalence

Prevalence refers to a cross-sectional count of the number of cases at a specified period of time. The spinal cord injury population has a reported pressure ulcer prevalence of 20 to 66%; in one study, it was 27% (Baggerly & DiBlasi, 1996).

Clinical Implications

For the rehabilitation nurse, the clinical implications for an increased risk of developing a pressure ulcer, the high rates of other types of ulcers, and the magnitude of the skin integrity problem demand focused efforts at preserving the client's skin. Benefits realized from the maintenance of skin integrity and management of skin breakdown are incalculable in terms of increased client self-esteem and ability to participate in work and leisure activities, and in cost savings.

Population at Risk

All clients who have sensory and/or motor changes are at risk to develop skin integrity problems. This includes clients with spinal cord injuries, head injuries, amputations, cerebrovascular accidents (strokes), neuromuscular diseases, congenital conditions, rheumatoid arthritis, and osteoarthritis, as well as other conditions causing weakness, paralysis, or paresthesias.

Cost Data

Estimates for managing skin integrity problems are difficult to summarize. Most reported cost data relate to the prevention and treatment of pressure ulcers. In one study, patients were divided into two groups: those who developed skin breakdown and those who did not. In those who developed skin breakdown, the mean cost of preventive strategies ranged from $0.34 to $0.59 for skin products, $289 for mattresses, $4.66 to $7.71 for bed covers, and zero to $1.37 for other strategies (Bostrom et al., 1996). Pressure ulcer treatment has been estimated to exceed $1.335 billion; implementation of the recommended pressure ulcer treatment guidelines could reduce that amount by $40 million (Bergstrom et al., 1994).

Agency for Health Care Policy and Research Guidelines

In 1989, the federal government established the AHCPR to enhance the quality, appropriateness, and effectiveness of health care services and access to those services. To date,

AHCPR has convened two consensus panels related to skin care, published guidelines for the prediction and prevention of pressure ulcers and the treatment of pressure ulcers, and funded continuing review and research in this area. The guidelines are written in three formats: clinical practice guidelines for health care practitioners, quick reference guides for clinicians, and consumer versions available in English and Spanish. For more information about these guidelines see Table 18–2.

PREVENTION OF SKIN INTEGRITY PROBLEMS

The prevention of skin integrity problems requires regular assessment, the use of pressure ulcer risk screening tools such as the Braden Scale, reassessment through screening, and regular skin inspection. Care must be taken to consider cultural and ethnic variations in the skin.

Skin Integrity Assessment

Assessment of the skin includes obtaining demographic data and a personal and family history of skin problems and performing a physical examination of the skin. Additional data are collected about pressure ulcer risk and the impact of sensory and motor changes that are associated with skin problems.

Demographic data including age, race, nationality, occupation, and hobbies provide information that may be useful in managing skin integrity problems. Normal age-related skin changes occur due to intrinsic aging and photoaging. In intrinsic aging there are decreased immune, vascular, and thermoregulatory responses and a loss of collagen fibers and muscle mass; these changes result in dryness, wrinkling, laxity, and an increase in skin lesions. Photoaging is the result of exposure to sunlight; the changes are unique to the individual. Data on race and nationality can help to differentiate normal from abnormal skin differences in clients of different races or nationalities. Occupation and hobby data may suggest exposure to environmental factors that may lead to skin problems.

A personal and family history of skin problems yields information about genetic skin problems, current and past skin diseases, and responses to skin problems. Data are also collected about medication use and allergy history. A diet history, weight and height measures, and nutritional evaluation are essential.

TABLE 18–2 ■ AGENCY FOR HEALTH CARE POLICY AND RESEARCH GUIDELINES

A fact sheet describing *Online Access for Clinical Practice Guidelines* (Agency for Health Care Policy and Research [AHCPR] Publication No. 94-0075) and copies of the *Quick Reference Guide for Clinicians* and consumer version of each guideline are available through AHCPR's InstantFAX, a fax-on-demand service that operates 24 hours a day, 7 days a week. AHCPR's InstantFAX is accessible to anyone using a facsimile machine equipped with a touchtone telephone handset: Dial (301) 594-2800, push *1*, and then press the facsimile machine's start button for instructions and a list of currently available publications. The full text of guideline documents for on-line retrieval may be accessed through a free electronic service from the National Library of Medicine called HSTAT (Health Services/Technology Assessment Text). To order single copies of guidelines, call the AHCPR Publications Clearinghouse toll free at (800) 358-9295 or write to AHCPR Publications Clearinghouse, P.O. Box 8547, Silver Spring, MD 20907.

Nurses interested in the skin integrity guidelines should request the following:

Panel for the Prediction and Prevention of Pressure Ulcers in Adults. (1992). *Pressure ulcers in adults: Prediction and prevention* (Clinical Practice Guideline No. 3, AHCPR Publication No. 92-0047). Rockville, MD: U.S. Department of Health and Human Services.

This guideline makes specific recommendations to identify at-risk adults and to define early interventions for the prevention of pressure ulcers. Recommendations target four overall goals: (1) identifying at-risk individuals who need prevention and the specific factors placing them at risk; (2) maintaining and improving tissue tolerance to pressure in order to prevent injury; (3) protecting against the adverse effects of external mechanical forces (pressure, friction, and shear); and (4) reducing the incidence of pressure ulcers through educational programs.

Bergstrom, N., Bennett, M. A., Carlson, C. E., (1994). Pressure Ulcer Treatment. Clinical Practice Guideline. Quick Reference Guide for Clinicians, No. 15. Rockville, MD: U.S. Department of Health and Human Services, Public Health Service, Agency for Health Care Policy and Research. AHCPR Pub. No. 95-0653. Dec. 1994.

This guideline addresses the treatment of pressure ulcers. Specific treatment recommendations focus on (1) assessment of the patient and pressure ulcer, (2) tissue load management, (3) ulcer care, (4) management of bacterial colonization and infection, (5) operative repair, and (6) education and quality improvement.

Psychosocial status is assessed, including coping skills, self-concept, and body image.

The physical examination of the skin includes inspection of the skin, nails, and hair. Data are collected about integumentary status, including color, elasticity, hygiene, lesions, moisture, quantity and distribution of hair, sensation, and temperature, texture, and turgor (Sparks & Taylor, 1998). The musculoskeletal status is assessed, including joint mobility, muscular strength and mass, paralysis, and range of motion.

Braden Scale

The Braden Scale is one of two tools recommended by the AHCPR for assessing pressure ulcer risk (Fig. 18–2). It has six subscales: sensory perception, moisture, activity, mobility, nutritional status, and friction/shear. Scoring on each subscale is from 1 (most at risk) to 3 or 4 (least at risk), with a maximal total score of 23. A patient with a pressure ulcer risk score of 16 or less is considered to be at risk for developing a pressure ulcer. Sensitivity, specificity, positive predictive value, and negative predictive value can be calculated. Each facility should evaluate the risk cutoff score for itself and establish standards for the implementation of preventive interventions. Clinically, appropriate interventions should be based on individual risk categories with low scores, for example, reducing friction or shear, rather than on the total score (Harrison, Wells, Fisher, & Prince, 1996).

Screening

All clients should be assessed on admission to rehabilitation facilities and long-term care facilities and assignment to home care agencies. Clients who are bed- or chair-bound or have difficulty with repositioning need to be reassessed on a regular basis (Panel for the Prediction and Prevention of Pressure Ulcers in Adults, 1992). Documentation of findings is essential to monitor the incidence, prevalence, and response to interventions. Regular reassessment can identify clients who require the initiation of preventive strategies or changes in management. Any client who is judged to be at risk for the development of pressure ulcers should have a systematic skin inspection done at least once a day.

Skin Inspection

Regular skin inspections are key to the early identification of problems and the initiation of interventions. Skin surveillance is the collection and analysis of data to maintain skin and mucous membrane integrity (McCloskey & Bulechek, 1996). Clients should be educated in the use of mirrors to visualize skin surfaces; some may require adaptive equip-

ment such as a long-handled mirror to promote independence in this activity.

Cultural/Ethnic Considerations for the Prevention of Skin Integrity Problems

Skin assessment in people with darkly pigmented skin is difficult. It needs to include changes in skin color (red, blue, purple tones), skin temperature (warmth or coolness), skin stiffness (hardness, edema), and/or skin sensation (pain) (Henderson et al., 1997).

EARLY IDENTIFICATION AND TREATMENT OF SKIN INTEGRITY PROBLEMS

Once a client has been classified as at risk, measures should be instituted to minimize irritation, dryness, pressure, shearing force, and friction. The use of mild cleansing agents with warm (not hot) water and washing with a gentle touch as needed helps minimize damage caused by excess force. Dry skin should be treated with moisturizers to promote suppleness. Massage over bony prominences should be avoided—this action can cause additional tissue damage or even deep tissue trauma—and caregivers must be so educated. Skin exposure to moisture should be minimized, and absorbent materials or skin barrier products should be used. Injury from friction and shear forces should be reduced by proper positioning, transferring, and turning techniques. Regular position changes are needed to prevent damage from excess pressure. The nurse should make sure that the client's nutritional intake is adequate to meet energy requirements. A dietary referral and the incorporation of dietary supplements should be initiated, if necessary. The client's mobility status and activity level should be maintained if possible. All nursing interventions performed and client outcomes achieved should be documented.

Prevention of Pressure Ulcers

Prevention of pressure ulcers requires a two-pronged approach: the reduction of risk factors and the use of preventive measures. Reducing risk factors may include the provision of nutritional support, the avoidance of moisture such as from incontinence, or an increase in activity. Preventive measures may include the use of regular repositioning (at least every 2 hours), the application of pressure-relieving

Braden Scale
FOR PREDICTING PRESSURE SORE RISK

Patient's Name _____ Evaluator's Name _____ Date of Assessment

	1	2	3	4		
SENSORY PERCEPTION Ability to respond meaningfully to pressure-related discomfort	**1. Completely Limited:** Unresponsive (does not moan, flinch, or grasp) to painful stimuli, due to diminished level of consciousness or sedation. OR Limited ability to feel pain over most of body surface.	**2. Very Limited:** Responds only to painful stimuli. Cannot communicate discomfort except by moaning or restlessness. OR Has a sensory impairment which limits the ability to feel pain or discomfort over ½ of body.	**3. Slightly Limited:** Responds to verbal commands, but cannot always communicate discomfort or need to be turned. OR Has some sensory impairment which limits ability to feel pain or discomfort in 1 or 2 extremities.	**4. No Impairment:** Responds to verbal commands. Has no sensory deficit which would limit ability to feel or voice pain or discomfort.		
MOISTURE Degree to which skin is exposed to moisture	**1. Constantly Moist:** Skin is kept moist almost constantly by perspiration, urine, etc. Dampness is detected every time patient is moved or turned.	**2. Very Moist:** Skin is often, but not always moist. Linen must be changed at least once a shift.	**3. Occasionally Moist:** Skin is occasionally moist, requiring an extra linen change approximately once a day.	**4. Rarely Moist:** Skin is usually dry. Linen only requires changing at routine intervals.		
ACTIVITY Degree of physical activity	**1. Bedfast:** Confined to bed.	**2. Chairfast:** Ability to walk severely limited or non-existent. Cannot bear own weight and/or must be assisted into chair or wheelchair.	**3. Walks Occasionally:** Walks occasionally during day, but for very short distances, with or without assistance. Spends majority of each shift in bed or chair.	**4. Walks Frequently:** Walks outside the room at least twice a day and inside room at least once every 2 hours during waking hours.		
MOBILITY Ability to change and control body position	**1. Completely Immobile:** Does not make even slight changes in body or extremity position without assistance.	**2. Very Limited:** Makes occasional slight changes in body or extremity position but unable to make frequent or significant changes independently.	**3. Slightly Limited:** Makes frequent though slight changes in body or extremity position independently.	**4. No Limitations:** Makes major and frequent changes in position without assistance.		

NUTRITION *Usual* food intake pattern	1. Very Poor; Never eats a complete meal. Rarely eats more than ⅓ of any food offered. Eats 2 servings or less of protein (meat or dairy products) per day. Takes fluids poorly. Does not take a liquid dietary supplement. OR Is NPO and/or maintained on clear liquids or IV's for more than 5 days.	2. Probably Inadequate: Rarely eats a complete meal and generally eats only about ½ of any food offered. Protein intake includes only 3 servings of meat or dairy products per day. Occasionally will take a dietary supplement. OR Receives less than optimum amount of liquid diet or tube feeding.	3. Adequate: Eats over half of most meals. Eats a total of 4 servings of protein (meat, dairy products) each day. Occasionally will refuse a meal, but will usually take a supplement if offered. OR Is on a tube feeding or TPN regimen which probably meets most of nutritional needs.	4. Excellent: Eats most of every meal. Never refuses a meal. Usually eats a total of 4 or more servings of meat and dairy products. Occasionally eats between meals. Does not require supplementation.	
FRICTION AND SHEAR	1. Problem: Requires moderate to maximum assistance in moving. Complete lifting without sliding against sheets is impossible. Frequently slides down in bed or chair, requiring frequent repositioning with maximum assistance. Spasticity, contractures or agitation leads to almost constant friction.	2. Potential Problem: Moves feebly or requires minimum assistance. During a move skin probably slides to some extent against sheets, chair, restraints, or other devices. Maintains relatively good position in chair or bed most of the time but occasionally slides down.	3. No Apparent Problem: Moves in bed and in chair independently and has sufficient muscle strength to lift up completely during move. Maintains good position in bed or chair at all times.		
				Total Score	

FIGURE 18-2
Braden Scale for predicting pressure ulcer risk. NPO, nothing by mouth; TPN, total parenteral nutrition. (Courtesy of Barbara Braden.)

devices such as heel protectors, and/or the use of pressure-reducing mattresses or wheelchair cushions. The incorporation of regular pressure relief for clients in bed or in chairs is essential; small shifts of body position should be carried out every 15 minutes. The use of lifting devices and lubrication helps to alleviate friction when moving clients.

Nursing Plan of Care

Skin Integrity Impairment Risk: Pressure Ulcer

Definition.   Nonblanchable erythema of intact skin (Makelbust & Sieggreen, 1996).

Desired Client Outcomes

1. The client verbalizes a knowledge of pressure ulcer risk factors and measures to prevent them.
2. The client's nutritional and fluid needs are met.
3. The client and the caregiver understand the importance of implementing a repositioning schedule to prevent the formation of pressure ulcers.
4. Appropriate devices/surfaces are used, for example, mattress consisting of foam, air, water, and gel, as well as low-air-loss overlays in the prevention of the progression of the ulcer (Adamson, 1996).
5. The client verbalizes the importance of doing a skin integrity assessment, practices appropriate hygiene procedures, and carries out routine skin inspection.
6. The client and the caregiver verbalize the importance of proper lubrication as a way of promoting skin integrity.
7. The client and the caregiver identify activities that cause friction and shearing of the skin.
8. Infection does not occur.
9. The client has a healthy image of his or her body.

Nursing Interventions

1. Relieve the pressure on skin that is causing the stage 1 pressure ulcer. Follow a repositioning schedule; turn at least every 2 hours, do minor position changes every 15 minutes.
    Use special support surfaces (e.g., heel protectors).
2. Ensure that the nutritional needs of the client are being met; clients with a pressure ulcer risk need 30 to 35 kcal and 1.25 to

1.50 g of protein per kilogram of body weight daily (Himes, 1997).
    Consult a nutritionist and incorporate suggestions into meals and snacks.
    Watch laboratory data, especially if the serum albumin level is less than 3.5 g/dL or there is a decrease in total body weight of more than 5%.
    Establish nutritional learning needs and educational goals with both the client and the caregiver.
    Record the weight of the client daily.
3. Document findings in order to monitor the progression of the potential pressure ulcer.
4. Minimize skin exposure to moisture due to incontinence, perspiration, or wound drainage.
5. Spend time with the client discussing feelings that she or he may be having regarding self-image.

Evaluation of Outcomes

1. The client does not have further progression of a pressure ulcer and does not form any new ones.
2. The client verbalizes an understanding of pressure ulcer risk factors and the measures to prevent them.
3. Skin integrity is restored to a healthy status: it is intact and has normal skin turgor, color, texture, distribution of hair, sebaceous glands, sensation, sweat glands, and moisture.
4. There is no evidence of infection.
5. A daily inspection of the skin is done by either the client or the caregiver.
6. Nutritional and fluid requirements are met.
7. The client verbalizes a healthy body image.

PROMOTION OF SKIN INTEGRITY

One of the goals of rehabilitation is to prevent skin integrity problems. However, the maintenance of skin integrity may not help the client achieve high-level wellness or meet personal client goals. Promoting skin integrity includes the use of lubricants, positioning, and adaptive equipment and may enable the client to achieve a sense of well-being and self-satisfaction.

Lubricants

A lubricant works by sealing in the moisture on the skin after bathing or showering; however, lubricants can act as drying agents when applied to dry skin. Emollient creams or lotions applied to damp skin rehydrate the stratum corneum and make the skin feel soft and supple. After an emollient containing urea or lactic acid is applied, the skin should be blotted but not wiped completely dry.

Positioning

In addition to the therapeutic effects of positioning, proper positioning can prevent skin breakdown in areas where two body surfaces rub together or cause excess pressure. Care must be taken to uncross toes and fingers, pad surfaces that come in contact with one another, and remove wrinkles and seams in fabrics contacting areas that are under pressure. Sitting or lying on a crease or wrinkle can cause enough pressure to create a pressure ulcer. The same care and attention to avoiding wrinkles should be paid to socks and shoes.

Use of Adaptive Equipment and Devices

Adaptive equipment to aid in providing skin care and regular inspection of the skin includes a range of products. A long-handled mirror may be needed to see all skin surface areas during daily skin inspection. Pump handles on lotions or soaps may permit independence. A wash mitt can often be used when using a washcloth might be difficult. The occupational therapist should be consulted and will be able to suggest specific adaptive equipment to meet the client's needs.

Nursing Plan of Care

Potential for Enhanced Skin Integrity

Definition. A state of healthy skin.

Desired Client Outcomes

1. The client's skin is soft, supple, and without redness, dryness, or breakdown.
2. The client verbalizes an understanding of preventive measures that promote skin integrity.
3. The client carries out a regimen of enhancement of skin integrity.

Nursing Interventions

1. Educate the client to perform skin inspec-

tion on a regular basis to detect skin problems early.
2. Educate the client in the use of lubricants, proper positioning, and adaptive equipment.
3. Apply lubricants to moist skin to enhance lubricating action.

Evaluation of Outcomes

1. The client has intact skin that is soft and supple.
2. The client can perform a skin care regimen.
3. The client verbalizes measures that promote skin integrity.

TREATMENT OF SKIN INTEGRITY IMPAIRMENTS

Measurement of Wound Healing

Normal wound healing occurs in phases: the inflammatory, or lag, phase; the fibroblastic, or connective tissue repair, phase; and the maturation, or remodeling, phase (Ignatavicius, Workman, & Mishler, 1995). Figure 18–3 provides a summary of the wound-healing phases (Black & Matassarin-Jacobs, 1997). Pressure ulcers do not heal in the same predictable way as other wounds. Although there is general agreement about the staging of pressure ulcers for the purpose of classification and treatment, there is also consensus that reverse staging does *not* describe pressure ulcer healing (National Pressure Ulcer Advisory Panel, 1995). Several tools are available for assessing pressure ulcer healing. The Pressure Sore Status Tool (Bates-Jensen, 1999; Fig. 18–4) was developed by Bates-Jensen to indicate wound healing. The Pressure Sore Status Tool consists of 13 rated items and 2 nonrated items. The rated items are summed and reported as a total score that represents overall wound status. It is intended to be used over time (repeated measures) by indicating regeneration or degeneration of the wound. It can be automated to provide computerized tracking. Reports about validity and reliability are ongoing.

The National Pressure Ulcer Advisory Panel is developing a tool, the Pressure Ulcer Scale for Healing (Bergstrom et al., 1994; Fig. 18–5), to simplify the evaluation of pressure ulcer healing. It consists of three categories: surface area, exudate, and appearance. The categories are weighted and given a numerical score. The pressure ulcer is evaluated over time, and the scores are plotted on a graph to show healing or nonhealing. The Pressure

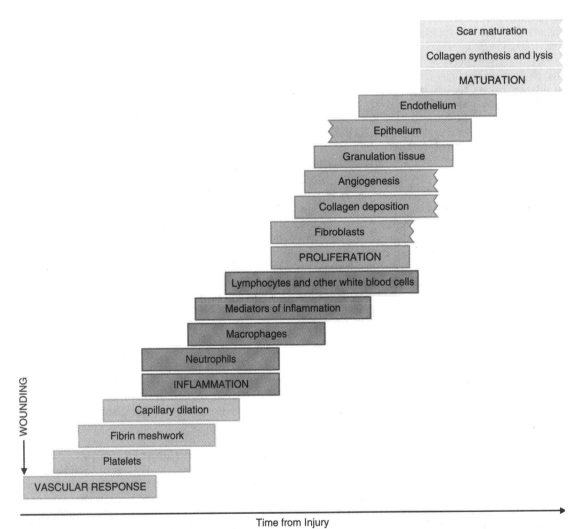

FIGURE 18–3
Phases of normal wound healing. (From Black, J. M., Matassarin-Jacobs, E. [1997]. *Medical-surgical nursing: Clinical management for continuity of care* [5th ed., p. 427]. Philadelphia: W. B. Saunders.)

PRESSURE SORE STATUS TOOL
Instructions for use

General Guidelines:

Fill out the attached rating sheet to assess a pressure sore's status after reading the definitions and methods of assessment described below. Evaluate once a week and whenever a change occurs in the wound. Rate according to each item by picking the response that best describes the wound and entering that score in the item score column for the appropriate date. When you have rated the pressure sore on all items, determine the total score by adding together the 13-item scores. The HIGHER the total score, the more severe the pressure sore status. Plot total score on the Pressure Sore Status Continuum to determine progress.

Specific Instructions:

1. **Size:** Use ruler to measure the longest and widest aspect of the wound surface in centimeters; multiply length × width.

2. **Depth:** Pick the depth, thickness most appropriate to the wound using these additional descriptions:

   1 = tissues damaged but no break in skin surface.
   2 = superficial, abrasion, blister or shallow crater. Even with and/or elevated above skin surface (e.g., hyperplasia).
   3 = deep crater with or without undermining of adjacent tissue.
   4 = visualization of tissue layers not possible due to necrosis.
   5 = supporting structures include tendon, joint capsule.

3. **Edges:** Use this guide:

Indistinct, diffuse	= unable to clearly distinguish wound outline.
Attached	= even or flush with wound base, <u>no</u> sides or walls present; flat.
Not attached	= sides or walls <u>are</u> present; floor or base of wound is deeper than edge.
Rolled under, thickened	= soft to firm and flexible to touch.
Hyperkeratosis	= callus-like tissue formation around wound and at edges.
Fibrotic, scarred	= hard, rigid to touch.

4. **Undermining:** Assess by inserting a cotton tipped applicator under the wound edge; advance it as far as it will go without using undue force; raise the tip of the applicator so it may be seen or felt on the surface of the skin; mark the surface with a pen; measure the distance from the mark on the skin to the edge of the wound. Continue process around the wound. Then use a transparent metric measuring guide with concentric circles divided into 4 (25%) pie-shaped quadrants to measure.

5. **Necrotic tissue type:** Pick the type of necrotic tissue that is <u>predominant</u> in the wound according to color, consistency, and adherence using this guide:

White/gray nonviable tissue	= may appear prior to wound opening; skin surface is white or gray.
Nonadherent, yellow slough	= thin, mucinous substance; scattered throughout wound bed; easily separated from wound tissue.
Loosely adherent, yellow slough	= thick, stringy, clumps of debris; attached to wound tissue.
Adherent, soft, black eschar	= soggy tissue; strongly attached to tissue in center or base of wound.
Firmly adherent, hard/black eschar	= firm, crusty tissue; strongly attached to wound base <u>and</u> edges (like a hard scab).

6. **Necrotic tissue amount:** Use a transparent metric measuring guide with concentric circles divided into 4 (25%) pie-shaped quadrants to help determine percent of wound involved.

7. **Exudate type:** Some dressings interact with wound drainage to produce a gel or trap liquid. Before assessing exudate type, gently cleanse wound with normal saline or water. Pick the exudate type that is <u>predominant</u> in the wound according to color and consistency, using this guide:

Bloody	= thin, bright red
Serosanguineous	= thin, watery pale red to pink
Serous	= thin, watery, clear
Purulent	= thin or thick, opaque tan to yellow
Foul purulent	= thick, opaque yellow to green with offensive odor

© 1990 Barbara Bates-Jensen

FIGURE 18–4
Pressure sore status tool. (Courtesy of Barbara Bates-Jensen.)

Illustration continued on following page

8. **Exudate amount:** Use a transparent metric measuring guide with concentric circles divided into 4 (25%) pie-shaped quadrants to determine percent of dressing involved with exudate. Use this guide:

None = wound tissues dry.
Scant = wound tissues moist; no measurable exudate.
Small = wound tissues wet; moisture evenly distributed in wound; drainage involves ≤25% dressing.
Moderate = wound tissues saturated; drainage may or may not be evenly distributed in wound; drainage involves >25% to ≤75% dressing.
Large = wound tissues bathed in fluid; drainage freely expressed; may or may not be evenly distributed in wound; drainage involves >75% of dressing.

9. **Skin color surrounding wound:** Assess tissues within 4 cm of wound edge. Dark-skinned persons show the colors "bright red" and "dark red" as a deepening of normal ethnic skin color or a purple hue. As healing occurs in dark-skinned persons, the new skin is pink and may never darken.

10. **Peripheral tissue edema:** Assess tissues within 4 cm of wound edge. Nonpitting edema appears as skin that is shiny and taut. Identify pitting edema by firmly pressing a finger down into the tissues and waiting for 5 seconds; on release of pressure, tissues fail to resume previous position and an indentation appears. Crepitus is accumulation of air or gas in tissues. Use a transparent metric measuring guide to determine how far edema extends beyond wound.

11. **Peripheral tissue induration:** Assess tissues within 4 cm of wound edge. Induration is abnormal firmness of tissues with margins. Assess by gently pinching the tissues. Induration results in an inability to pinch the tissues. Use a transparent metric measuring guide with concentric circles divided into 4 (25%) pie-shaped quadrants to determine percent of wound and area involved.

12. **Granulation tissue:** Granulation tissue is the growth of small blood vessels and connective tissue to fill in full-thickness wounds. Tissue is healthy when bright, beefy red, shiny; and granular with a velvety appearance. Poor vascular supply appears as pale pink or blanched to dull, dusky red color.

13. **Epithelialization:** Epithelialization is the process of epidermal resurfacing and appears as pink or red skin. In partial-thickness wounds it can occur throughout the wound bed as well as from the wound edges. In full-thickness wounds it occurs from the edges only. Use a transparent metric measuring guide with concentric circles divided into 4 (25%) pie-shaped quadrants to help determine percent of wound involved and to measure the distance the epithelial tissue extends into the wound.

PRESSURE SORE STATUS TOOL   NAME _____

Complete the rating sheet to assess pressure sore status. Evaluate each item by picking the response that best describes the wound and entering the score in the item score column for the appropriate date.

Location: Anatomic site. Circle, identify right (R) or left (L) and use "X" to mark site on body diagrams:

_____ Sacrum and coccyx   _____ Lateral ankle
_____ Trochanter   _____ Medial ankle
_____ Ischial tuberosity   _____ Heel   Other site _____

Shape: Overall wound pattern; assess by observing perimeter and depth.
Circle and <u>date</u> appropriate description:

_____ Irregular   _____ Linear or elongated
_____ Round/oval   _____ Bowl/boat
_____ Square/rectangle   _____ Butterfly   Other shape _____

© 1990 Barbara Bates-Jensen

FIGURE 18–4 *Continued*

Item	Assessment	Date	Date	Date
		Score	**Score**	**Score**
1. Size	1 = Length × width <4 sq cm 2 = Length × width 4–16 sq cm 3 = Length × width 16.1–36 sq cm 4 = Length × width 36.1–80 sq cm 5 = Length × width >80 sq cm			
2. Depth	1 = Nonblanchable erythema on intact skin 2 = Partial thickness skin loss involving epidermis and/or dermis 3 = Full-thickness skin loss involving damage or necrosis of subcutaneous tissue; may extend down to but not through underlying fascia; and/or mixed partial- and full-thickness and/or tissue layers obscured by granulation tissue 4 = Obscured by necrosis 5 = Full-thickness skin loss with extensive destruction, tissue necrosis or damage to muscle, bone or supporting structures			
3. Edges	1 = Indistinct, diffuse, none clearly visible 2 = Distinct, outline clearly visible, attached, even with wound base 3 = Well-defined, not attached to wound base 4 = Well-defined, not attached to base, rolled under, thickened 5 = Well-defined, fibrotic, scarred or hyperkeratotic			
4. Undermining	1 = Undermining <2 cm in any area 2 = Undermining 2–4 cm involving <50% wound margins 3 = Undermining 2–4 cm involving >50% wound margins 4 = Undermining >4 cm in any area 5 = Tunneling and/or sinus tract formation			
5. Necrotic Tissue Type	1 = None visible 2 = White/gray nonviable tissue and/or nonadherent yellow slough 3 = Loosely adherent yellow slough 4 = Adherent, soft, black eschar 5 = Firmly adherent, hard, black eschar			
6. Necrotic Tissue Amount	1 = None visible 2 = <25% of wound bed covered 3 = 25% to 50% of wound covered 4 = >50% and <75% of wound covered 5 = 75% to 100% of wound covered			
7. Exudate Type	1 = None or bloody 2 = Serosanguineous: thin, watery, pale red/pink 3 = Serous: thin, watery, clear 4 = Purulent: thin or thick, opaque, tan/yellow 5 = Foul purulent: thick, opaque, yellow/green with odor			

Illustration continued on following page

FIGURE 18–4 *Continued*

Item	Assessment	Date	Date	Date
		Score	Score	Score
8. Exudate Amount	1 = None 2 = Scant 3 = Small 4 = Moderate 5 = Large			
9. Skin Color Surrounding Wound	1 = Pink or normal for ethnic group 2 = Bright red and/or blanches to touch 3 = White or gray pallor or hypopigmented 4 = Dark red or purple and/or nonblanchable 5 = Black or hyperpigmented			
10. Peripheral Tissue Edema	1 = Minimal swelling around wound 2 = Nonpitting edema extends <4 cm around wound 3 = Nonpitting edema extends ≥4 cm around wound 4 = Pitting edema extends <4 cm around wound 5 = Crepitus and/or pitting edema extends ≥4 cm			
11. Peripheral Tissue Induration	1 = Minimal firmness around wound 2 = Induration <2 cm around wound 3 = Induration 2–4 cm extending <50% around wound 4 = Induration 2–4 cm extendng ≥50% around wound 5 = Induration >4 cm in any area			
12. Granulation Tissue	1 = Skin intact or partial-thickness wound 2 = Bright, beefy red; 75% to 100% of wound filled and/or tissue overgrowth 3 = Bright, beefy red; <75% and >25% of wound filled 4 = Pink, and/or dull, dusky red and/or fills ≤25% of wound 5 = No granulation tissue present			
13. Epithelialization	1 = 100% wound covered, surface intact 2 = 75% to <100% wound covered and/or epithelial tissue extends >0.5 cm into wound bed 3 = 50% to <75% wound covered and/or epithelial tissue extends to <0.5 cm into wound bed 4 = 25% to <50% wound covered 5 = <25% wound covered			
TOTAL SCORE				
SIGNATURE				

PRESSURE SORE STATUS CONTINUUM

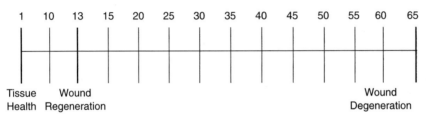

Plot the total score on the Pressure Sore Status Continuum by putting an "X" on the line and the date beneath the line. Plot multiple scores with their dates to see-at-a-glance regeneration or degeneration of the wound.
© 1990 Barbara Bates-Jensen

FIGURE 18–4 *Continued*

PUSH Scale

Patient Name: _____

Ulcer Location: _____

Patient ID#: _____

Date: _____

DIRECTIONS:

Observe and measure the pressure ulcer. Categorize the ulcer with respect to surface area, exudate, and appearance and record in the column labeled "Ulcer Category." Multiply the Ulcer Category times the appropriate Weight Factor for each subscale and record in the column labeled "Weighted Sub-score." Add the Weighted Sub-scores to obtain the Total Score. A comparison of Total Scores measured over time provides an indication of the improvement or deterioration in pressure ulcer healing.

	1	2	3	4	5	Ulcer category (1–5) _____	Weight factor ×2	Weighted sub-score
Surface Area	< 0.3 cm²	0.3–0.9 cm²	1.0–1.9 cm²	2.0–5.0 cm²	>5.0 cm²			
	1	2	3	4		Ulcer category (1–4) _____	Weight factor ×3	Weighted sub-score
Exudate	≤ ¼	¼ to ½	½ to ¾	>¾				
	1	2	3	4		Ulcer category (1–4) _____	Weight factor ×3	Weighted sub-score
Appearance (predominant tissue)	Epithelial tissue	Granulation tissue	Slough	Necrotic eschar				
							Total Score	

Surface Area: Measure the greatest length (head to toe) and the greatest width (side to side) using a centimeter ruler. Multiply these two measurements (length × width) to obtain the surface area in square centimeters (cm²).
    Caveat: Do not guess! Always use a centimeter ruler and always use the same method each time the ulcer is measured.

Exudate: Estimate of the portion of the pressure ulcer bed covered by drainage following removal of all dressings, but prior to any cleansing. Divide the ulcer into four imaginary quadrants each representing about ¼ of the ulcer surface. Estimate the portion of the ulcer covered by exudate.

Appearance: Divide the pressure ulcer into four imaginary quadrants each representing about ¼ of the original ulcer surface. Estimate the portion or amount of each tissue type on the ulcer. Identify the predominant tissue type on the ulcer and record the predominant tissue type in the space provided.
    Epithelial tissue: New pink or red skin that covers the original ulcer surface, growing in at the edges or in spots on the ulcer surface.
    Granulation tissue: Pink or beefy red tissue with a shiny, moist, granular appearance.
    Slough: Yellow or white tissue that adheres to the ulcer bed in strings or thick clumps.
    Necrotic eschar: Black or brown tissue that adheres firmly to the wound bed or ulcer edges and may be either firmer or softer than surrounding skin.

Illustration continued on following page

FIGURE 18–5
Pressure ulcer scale for healing.

PRESSURE ULCER HEALING CHART
(use a separate page for each pressure ulcer)

Patient Name: _____   Patient ID#: _____

Ulcer Location: _____   Date: _____

Directions: Observe and measure pressure ulcer wounds at regular intervals using the PUSH scale. Date and record PUSH Weighted Sub-scale and Total Scores on the Pressure Ulcer Healing Record below.

	PRESSURE ULCER HEALING RECORD													
DATE														
Surface Area														
Exudate														
Appearance														
Total Score														

Graph the PUSH Total Score on the Pressure Ulcer Healing Graph below.

PUSH Total Score	PRESSURE ULCER HEALING GRAPH												
34													
31													
29													
26													
23													
20													
17													
14													
11													
Healed 8													
DATE:													

Version: 1/31/97

Figure 18–5 *Continued*

Ulcer Scale for Healing is undergoing tests for reliability and validity. More information can be obtained from Nancy Stotts, Department of Physiological Nursing, N611Y, Box 0610, University of California, San Francisco, CA 94143-0610.

Nursing Plans of Care

Skin Integrity Impairment: Pressure Ulcer Stage II

Definition. "Loss of partial thickness skin, which includes the epidermis, dermis, or both. A Stage II ulcer is superficial and presents clinically as an abrasion, blister, or shallow crater" (Sparks & Taylor, 1998).

Desired Client Outcomes

1. The client verbalizes a knowledge of pressure ulcer risk factors and measures to prevent them.
2. The client's nutritional and fluid requirements are met.
3. The client verbalizes the importance of maintaining a repositioning schedule to prevent the formation of new pressure ulcers.
4. Appropriate devices/surfaces, such as air flotation beds and alternating pressure mattresses (Adamson, 1996), are used.
5. The client verbalizes the importance of doing a skin integrity assessment and carrying out routine skin inspection on a daily basis.
6. The client verbalizes the importance of proper lubrication as a way of promoting skin integrity.
7. The client recognizes actions that cause friction and shearing of the skin.
8. Infection does not occur.
9. The client has a healthy body image regarding the pressure ulcer.

Nursing Interventions and Evaluation of Outcomes (see under next plan)

Skin Integrity Impairment: Pressure Ulcer Stage III

Definition. "Full thickness skin loss involving damage or necrosis of subcutaneous tissue that may extend down to, but not through, underlying fascia. The ulcer presents clinically as a deep crater with or without undermining of adjacent tissue" (Bergstrom et al., 1994).

Desired Client Outcomes

1. The client verbalizes a knowledge of pressure ulcer risk factors and measures to prevent their occurrence.
2. The client's nutritional and fluid requirements are met.
3. The client verbalizes understanding of the repositioning schedule.
4. Appropriate pressure-relieving devices/surfaces are used.
5. The client or the caregiver carries out regular skin inspection.
6. The client or the caregiver carries out measures to reduce friction and shear.
7. Pressure ulcer healing is occurring (document size, appearance, and exudate using an established tool).
8. No signs of infection occur in the pressure ulcer.

Nursing Interventions

1. Relieve pressure on skin surfaces through the use of a repositioning schedule and special support surfaces.
2. Provide adequate nutrition and fluid. AHCPR guidelines suggest the ingestion of 30 to 35 kcal and 1.25 to 1.5 g of protein per kilogram of body weight daily. Monitor laboratory values such as serum albumin regularly (Bergstrom et al., 1994).
3. Weigh the client weekly and report a decrease of total body weight of more than 5%.
4. Clean the pressure ulcer at each dressing change using an isotonic solution such as 0.9% sodium chloride.
5. Minimize skin exposure to moisture due to incontinence, perspiration, or wound drainage.
6. Carefully remove unwanted debris from the pressure ulcer surface while protecting viable tissue.
7. Maintain a moist, clean site with minimal bacterial colonization.
8. Use a dressing that has properties to promote optimal healing, that is, does not adhere to the wound surface and does not remove epithelial cells when changed. Two main types of dressings are
   a. Hydrophobic dressings—nonabsorbent, waterproof
   b. Hydrophilic dressings—absorbent
9. If healing does not occur, biological skin substitutes may be applied during surgery. These include
   a. Homograft skin
   b. Heterograft skin

c. Amniotic membranes
10. If infection occurs, antibiotics may be ordered. Monitor the client for side effects.
11. Encourage the client to discuss feelings and concerns associated with the pressure ulcer and changes in body image.

Evaluation of Outcomes

1. There is no further progression of the existing pressure ulcer and no incidence of new ulcers.
2. Skin integrity is restored.
3. There is no evidence of infection.
4. Skin inspections are carried out by the client or the caregiver.

Skin Integrity Impairment: Pressure Ulcer Stage IV

Definition. Loss of full-thickness skin with extensive "destruction, tissue necrosis, or damage to muscle, bone, or supporting structures" (Bergstrom et al., 1994).

Desired Client Outcomes

1. The client verbalizes a knowledge of pressure ulcer risk factors and measures to prevent their occurrence.
2. The client's nutritional and fluid requirements are met.
3. The client verbalizes an understanding of the repositioning schedule.
4. Appropriate pressure-relieving devices/surfaces are used.
5. The client or the caregiver carries out regular skin inspection.
6. The client or the caregiver carries out measures to reduce friction and shear.

Nursing Interventions

1. Place the client on an air-fluidized bed.
2. Débride necrotic tissue; chemical débridement uses enzymes, and surgical débridement uses a scalpel and can be carried out only by a wound care specialist.
3. Apply dressings, moist saline gauze, hydrocolloid, or Gelfoam.

Evaluation of Outcomes

1. The pressure ulcer is healed.
2. The client or caregiver carries out the skin care regimen.
3. No further evidence of skin breakdown occurs.

RESTORATIVE TREATMENT OF SKIN INTEGRITY IMPAIRMENTS

Rehabilitation clients may require care for skin problems other than pressure ulcers. This section provides plans of care for clients with skin tears, dryness, venous ulcers, arterial ulcers, and diabetic foot ulcers.

Nursing Plans of Care

Skin Integrity Impairment: Skin Tears/Abrasions

Definition. A traumatic wound that separates the epidermis from the dermis that occurs primarily on the extremities (Kopac & McGough-Csarny, 1997).

Desired Client Outcomes

1. The client verbalizes a knowledge of risk factors that cause skin tears.
2. The skin tear heals without infection.
3. The client and the caregiver verbalize an understanding of preventive measures to prevent a further occurrence of skin tears.

Nursing Interventions

1. Educate the client and the caregiver to reduce friction and shearing force and to lift the extremities with care to prevent skin tears.
2. Cleanse the skin tear with mild soap, rinse well, and cover with a loose dressing if necessary to prevent further skin breakdown.
3. Monitor the skin tear closely for signs of infection and report redness, purulent drainage, or other signs of infection.
4. Educate the client and the caregiver on proper positioning and moving techniques.

Evaluation of Outcomes

1. The client and the caregiver state the risk factors for skin tears.
2. No infection occurs.
3. The skin tear is healed.
4. The client and the caregiver demonstrate correct positioning and moving techniques.

Skin Integrity Impairment: Dryness

Definition. Areas of scaling, flaking, redness, or cracking skin.

Desired Client Outcomes

1. The client identifies dry skin on regular skin inspection.
2. The client or the caregiver applies lotions or emollients to dry skin areas.
3. The client consumes adequate fluids.
4. The client lives in an environment with adequate humidity.

Nursing Interventions

1. Educate the client about regular skin inspection.
2. Demonstrate the application of lotion or emollients to damp skin to rehydrate the skin. Blot the skin but do not wipe completely dry.
3. Ensure an adequate intake of fluids.
4. Modify the environment to provide adequate humidity; the client may need to use a humidifier.

Evaluation of Outcomes

1. The skin is soft and supple.
2. The fluid intake is adequate.
3. The humidity is adequate.

Skin Integrity Impairment: Venous Ulcer

Definition. Skin breakdown over the medial aspect of the leg.

Desired Client Outcomes

1. The venous ulcer heals.
2. The client verbalizes an understanding of preventive and therapeutic measures: meticulous foot care, elevation of the feet, compression stockings, the Unna boot, nutritional therapy, and control of systemic diseases such as anemia and diabetes mellitus.
3. The client or the caregiver demonstrates the correct application of dressings and occlusive therapy.

Nursing Interventions

1. Educate the client about proper foot care and the use of aseptic technique.
2. Apply compression stockings; remove them at least every 8 hours and inspect the skin for areas of redness or breakdown.
3. Consult with a nutritionist to provide a diet adequate in vitamin C and zinc.
4. Follow the institutional protocol for cleansing the ulcer and applying the steroid ointment; cover the ulcer with an occlusive dressing and apply an Unna zinc paste boot. Arrange for weekly follow-up care for the dressing and Unna boot changes. As an alternative therapy, synthetic occlusive dressings may be used. As this dressing can fill with exudate and have an unpleasant odor, instruct the client *not* to remove the dressing; changes are done about every 2 to 3 weeks (Black & Matassarin-Jacobs, 1997).

Evaluation of Outcomes

1. The venous ulcer is healed, with no signs of infection.
2. The client carries out prevention and treatment regimens.

Skin Integrity Impairment: Arterial Ulcer

Definition. Skin breakdown over the lateral aspect of the leg or the malleoli (ankles). Characterized by pallor; patchy, bluish-purple mottling of the skin; and cold, clammy skin.

Desired Client Outcomes

1. Peripheral vascular disease risk factors are minimized.
2. The client stops smoking.
3. The arterial ulcer is healed.

Nursing Interventions

1. Educate the client about smoking-cessation programs and control of diseases (hypertension, diabetes mellitus, hyperlipemia, and obesity).
2. Instruct the client on a meticulous foot care regimen.
3. Maintain a clean environment and minimize pressure and irritation over the areas of ulceration.
4. Follow institutional protocols for the use of wet-to-damp saline dressings or moist occlusive dressings. Whirlpool treatments may enhance healing.
5. If arterial bypass surgery is necessary because of a lack of healing, provide preoperative education and postoperative care according to policy.
6. If conservative medical and surgical management fails, educate the client about limb amputation and follow institutional protocols for postoperative management.

Evaluation of Outcomes

1. The arterial ulcer is healed.
2. The client stops smoking.

3. The client follows recommended skin care regimen.

Skin Integrity Impairment: Diabetic/Neuropathic Ulcer

Definition. Leg and foot ulcers occurring in the client with diabetes mellitus.

Desired Client Outcomes

1. The blood glucose level is under control.
2. The client verbalizes an understanding of the relationship between good foot care, cessation of smoking, maintenance of good nutrition, early treatment for skin problems, and occurrence of diabetic ulcers and possible amputation.
3. The client carries out regular foot inspection and hygiene.
4. There are no foot infections or skin breakdown.
5. The ulcer is healed.

Nursing Interventions

1. Educate the client about the control of hyperglycemia, smoking cessation, foot inspection, signs and symptoms to report, and the foot care regimen.
2. Instruct the client not to walk barefoot, to select properly fitting shoes made of materials that breathe (avoid synthetics), and to check footwear daily for rough spots or areas of breakdown.
3. Demonstrate and have the client give a return demonstration of foot care: bathe the feet with mild soap in warm (not hot) water, pat the skin dry, and apply mild moisturizer.
4. Instruct the client to avoid crossing the legs when sitting, using chemicals to remove calluses or corns, and using heating pads or hot water bottles. Inform the client of the benefit of regular exercise and the need to cut the toenails along the curve of the toe and to file the nails to prevent rough spots. The client with thick nails or with fungal infections should be referred to a podiatrist for toenail cutting.
5. Follow the institutional protocol for cleansing the ulcer and applying the steroid ointment; cover the ulcer with an occlusive dressing and apply an Unna zinc paste boot. Arrange for weekly follow-up care for dressing and Unna boot changes. As an alternative therapy, synthetic occlusive dressings may be used. As this dressing can fill with exudate and have an unpleasant odor, instruct the client *not* to remove the dressing; changes are done about every 2 to 3 weeks (Black & Matassarin-Jacobs, 1997).

Evaluation of Outcomes

1. The diabetic ulcer is healed.
2. The client can carry out the foot care regimen and seek help when appropriate.

QUALITY-OF-CARE ISSUES IN THE MAINTENANCE OF SKIN INTEGRITY

A coordinated, comprehensive skin care program is the first step in ensuring the maintenance of skin integrity. It must, however, be combined with quality-improvement activities in order to monitor results and take remedial action when necessary. Ethical issues such as in recurrent skin breakdown and nurse-versus-client accountability complete the steps necessary to promote and enhance skin integrity in the disabled population.

Monitoring

An interdisciplinary team is recommended to develop pressure ulcer prevention and treatment guidelines. Members of the skin integrity management team should include a skin integrity expert (enterostomal therapist or clinical nurse specialist), staff nurses, a nutritionist, a physical therapist, an occupational therapist, a physiatrist, and a quality-improvement coordinator. Other consultants such as dermatologists or plastic surgeons may be used when needed. At a minimum, data should be collected about the prevalence and incidence of pressure ulcers at the facility on a regular basis. Data collected from these monitors should be used to develop and implement educational programs directed at care providers such as nurses, nursing assistants (unlicensed assistive personnel), families, and personal care attendants.

Ideally, skin care protocols for the management of pressure ulcer risk, pressure ulcers of various stages, and other skin care problems should be developed and evaluated. Through regular evaluation of client outcomes, changes and improvements in the protocols can be made. The continuous quality improvement approach to skin care promotes a proactive approach to remedial action when measured indicators fall below threshold levels.

Remedial Action

If monitoring of pressure ulcer incidence and prevalence reveals a problem, remedial action must be initiated. Actions are directed at the underlying cause and should be targeted to the groups most involved in the management of the problem. Baseline data from monitors are used to establish goals for improvement. Protocols are developed and used for a specified period of time, and outcomes are then evaluated.

Ethical Issues in Recurrent Skin Breakdown

Clients with motor and sensory changes frequently have recurrent problems with skin breakdown. These physiological changes combined with technological advances and consumers' right to make decisions about their health care have led to moral and ethical dilemmas. With the passage of the Patient Self-Determination Act, patients can specify their wishes about life-prolonging technology and authorize a delegate to make decisions on their behalf.

Nurse-Versus-Client Accountability

Traditionally, nurses have been held accountable for the care provided to clients. Today, we recognize the interrelationship of the nurse's role with the client's and the caregiver's roles. Responsibility for the maintenance of skin integrity is a shared one. The nurse has an obligation to assess, diagnose, intervene, and evaluate all aspects of skin management. Clients and their caregivers, on the other hand, have a corresponding obligation to carry out regular skin inspections, seek professional advice for the management of potential or actual problems, and perform the skin care regimens necessary to correct or alleviate problems.

Because of this shared responsibility, it is difficult to hold either party totally accountable. For this reason, it is essential that managers and administrators evaluate the maintenance of skin integrity in a sensitive and comprehensive manner.

In a clinical situation, a client may be assessed to be at high risk for the development of a pressure ulcer, have preventive protocols followed precisely, and still develop a pressure ulcer. This situation must be evaluated in terms of both the performance of the nursing staff and the adherence to the skin preventive protocol on the part of the client. In some cases, it may be determined that despite excellent nursing care, the client developed the pressure ulcer. The nursing staff should not be punished or otherwise penalized for the care they provided. In another situation, it may be determined that the nursing staff did not carry out preventive measures; in this case they would be held accountable.

SUMMARY

Nursing management of skin integrity problems is, for the most part, in the domain of independent nursing action. Nurses should assert the full measure of their ability to maintain and enhance the skin integrity of their clients, and they should be given full credit for positive outcomes. It is hard and time-consuming work to prevent pressure ulcers, treat skin breakdown, and enhance a positive self-image. The maintenance of a client's skin integrity may make the difference in whether the client will be able to participate fully in the daily activities of a normal life.

REFERENCES

Baggerly, J., & DiBlasi, M. (1996). Pressure sores and pressure sore prevention in a rehabilitation setting: Building information for improving outcomes and allocating resources. *Rehabilitation Nursing, 21,* 321–325.

Bates-Jensen, B. M. (1999). Chronic wound assessment. *Nursing Clinics of North America, 34,* 799–845.

Bergstrom, N., Bennett, M. A., Carlson, C. E., et al. Pressure Ulcer Treatment. Clinical Practice Guideline. Quick Reference Guide for Clinicians, No. 15. Rockville, MD: U.S. Department of Health and Human Services, Public Health Service, Agency for Health Care Policy and Research. AHCPR Pub. No. 95-0653. Dec. 1994.

Black, J., & Matassarin-Jacobs, E. (1997). *Medical-surgical nursing* (5th ed., p. 427). Philadelphia: W. B. Saunders.

Bostrom, J., Mechanic, J., Lazar, N., Michelson, S., Grant, L., & Nomura, L. (1996). Preventing skin breakdown: Nursing practices, costs, and outcomes. *Applied Nursing Research, 9,* 184–188.

Gordon, M. (1995). Report of an RNF study to determine which nursing diagnoses have high frequency and high treatment priority in rehabilitation nursing: Pt. 2. *Rehabilitation Nursing Research, 4,* 38–46.

Hammond, M. C., Bozzacco, V. A., Stiens, S. A., Buhrer, R., & Lyman, P. (1994). Pressure ulcer incidence on a spinal cord injury unit. *Advances in Wound Care, 7,* 57–60.

Harrison, M. B., Wells, G., Fisher, A., & Prince, M. (1996). Practice guidelines for the prediction and prevention of pressure ulcers: Evaluating the evidence. *Applied Nursing Research, 9,* 9–17.

Henderson, C. T., Ayello, E. A., Sussman, C., Leiby, D. M., Bennett, M. A., Dungog, E. F., Sprigle, S., & Woodruff, L. (1997). Draft definition of Stage I pressure ulcers: inclusion of persons with darkly pigmented skin. NPUAP Task Force on Stage I definition and darkly pigmented skin. *Advances in Wound Care, 10,* 16–19.

Himes, D. (1997). Nutritional supplements in the treatment of pressure ulcers: practical perspectives. *Advances in Wound Care, 10,* 30–31.

Ignatavicius, D., Workman, M., & Mishler, M. (1995). *Medical-surgical nursing: A nursing process approach* (2nd ed., Vol. 2). Philadelphia: W. B. Saunders.

Kopac, C., & McGough-Csarny, J. The epidemiology of skin tears in the institutionalized elderly. Presented at 1997 Symposium on Advanced Wound Care and Medical Research Forum on Wound Repair, New Orleans, LA, 1997.

Makelbust, J., & Sieggreen, M. (1996). *Pressure ulcers: guidelines for prevention and nursing management* (2nd ed.). Springhouse, PA: Springhouse Corporation.

Mawson, A., Biundo, J., Neveille, P., Linares, H., Winchester, Y., & Lopez, A. (1988). Risk factors for early occurring pressure ulcers following spinal cord injury. *American Journal of Physical Medicine and Rehabilitation, 67,* 123–127.

McCloskey, J. C., & Bulechek, G. M. (1996). *Nursing interventions classification (NIC)* (2nd ed.). St. Louis: Mosby–Year Book.

National Pressure Ulcer Advisory Panel. (1995). NPUAP position on reverse staging of pressure ulcers. *NPUAP Report, 4,* 1.

Panel for the Prediction and Prevention of Pressure Ulcers in Adults. (1992). *Pressure ulcers in adults: Prediction and prevention.* (Clinical Practice Guideline, No. 3, AHCPR Publication No. 92-0047). Rockville, MD: Agency for Health Care Policy and Research.

Pontieri-Lewis, V. (1995). Focus on wound care: Venous leg ulcers. *Medsurg-Nursing, 4,* 492–493.

Sorenson, J. C. (1997). Healing the wound in a managed care environment. *Biomechanics: Special Podiatry Issue.*

Sparks, S. M., & Taylor, C. M. (1998). *Nursing diagnosis reference manual* (4th ed.). Springhouse, PA: Springhouse Corporation.

Sparks, S. M. (1997). Integument. In M. M. Burke & M. B. Walsh (Eds.), *Gerontologic nursing: Wholistic care of the older adult* (2nd ed.). St. Louis: C. V. Mosby.

Versluyen, M. (1986). How elderly patients with femoral fractures develop pressure sores in hospital. *British Medical Journal of Clinical Research Education, 292,* 1311–1313.

CHAPTER 19

Assistive Devices

Judith A. Hines and Susan Christie

Rehabilitation professionals are challenged by today's health care industry to set standards for the delivery of client services that are outcome based. A model for assistive technology services for children with disabilities already exists. This is primarily due to Pub. L. No. 94-142 and the Education for All Handicapped Children Act of 1975, which support the adaptation, accommodation, and socialization of all handicapped children within the public school systems. The new challenge for the health care professional in the 21st century is to address the issues of assistive technology in a more diverse population, justifying the need and qualifying the outcomes.

It is well established that advances in medical technology and surgical procedures have enhanced longevity. The art of medicine is such that as individuals in our society age, the probability of encountering multiple diseases and multiple system failures increases. Assistive technology offers all individuals throughout their lives greater independence and improved function. It also offers individuals the ability to surpass their physical limitations: to continue to be valuable assets in the workforce, to attend school, and to participate in activities that may previously have been off-limits.

In light of increasing statistics on disability and longevity and society's quest for functional independence, we need to focus on a client-centered model of care. We must also quantify our services using outcome data to justify the needs and benefits a client will receive from the use of assistive technology services. School nurses continue to be in a unique place as they function in many ways within client-centered teams. Their professional practice contributes to the development and implementation of creative approaches to the delivery of assistive technology services for children. Case managers have continually a high profile in the field of assistive technology. Their primary role is to be involved in assisting patients and families in practical strategies that encourage functional independence. Case managers are client focused. They use their clients' goals to assess, evaluate, and gather documentation that affords them the power to advocate for their clients and families.

Rehabilitation is now in a unique position as patients are being triaged to various levels of service. The rehabilitation nurse who practices in either a hospital or a community setting brings value to the team when an assistive equipment prescription is initiated. The primary role of the rehabilitation nurse is to assess the client's values, interests, goals, and problems. The second role in the process is implementation. Implementation means reinforcing the education and training required to meet the client's goal of an optimal level of function and proficiency in accomplishing activities of daily living.

One challenge the professional team has in the emerging health care system is to evaluate, recommend, and document that the prescribed assistive equipment improves the client's function, maximizes the client's strength, allows compensatory techniques, and meets the goals of the client, the caregivers, and the rehabilitation team. Critical documentation provides the support to justify reimbursement.

DEFINITION OF ASSISTIVE TECHNOLOGY

Assistive technology can be defined as any item or piece of equipment that is used to increase, maintain, or improve a person's ability to act independently when carrying out activities of daily living such as eating, dressing, talking, walking, driving, working, and engaging in leisure activities. Assistive technology devices vary immensely from items as simple as an instrument to help hold a pencil to something as complex as a computer system to allow communication or to control an individual's environment through eye movements. The challenge of choosing the appropriate device or devices is based on many factors including functional abilities, goals, and resources available.

ACTIVITIES OF DAILY LIVING

"Activities of daily living" encompasses everything that a person does in order to function as an independent person. On a basic level, this includes feeding, dressing, grooming and hygiene, bowel and bladder management, skin management, menstrual care, bathing, and toileting. The next level, instrumental activities of daily living, includes cooking, cleaning, using tools and appliances appropriately, shopping, and managing finances. Mobility and communication are also addressed.

Feeding

Feeding is a basic need of all creatures, and feeding oneself is begun early in life. The act of feeding requires an ability to grasp the food or utensil, to maneuver it to the mouth, and then to chew and swallow. A poor grasp or no grasp may require the use of utensils with built-up handles or straps or the use of a universal cuff or mitt to hold a utensil (Fig. 19–1). This device may be applied by the person with the disability, or the person may require assistance. With the aging of America's population, utensils with built-up handles are becoming commonly available for purchase in kitchen and specialty stores, but such adaptations can be made simply through the use of hollow cylindrical foam tubing, cut to size and placed over the handle of a conventional fork or spoon. This type of handle can also be made with the use of a

moldable foam or putty that hardens after exposure to air and can be custom-molded to an individual.

A loss of range of motion may mean that a person is unable to hold a utensil or is unable to bring the utensil to the mouth. In this case, an extended handle, straight or hinged, may allow the person to self-feed as long as the person has sufficient strength (Fig. 19–2). A long straw enables a person to drink from a standard cup or mug. Numerous inexpensive drinking cup and straw combinations are available.

Those who have the use of only one hand, through amputation, stroke, or another loss of function of the hands, may have difficulty stabilizing a plate of food and/or may not be able to cut food with a standard knife. Nonskid material placed under the plate aids in holding it in place, and the use of a bowl with steep sides helps keep food from spilling over the edge. A plate guard, a strip of washable stiff plastic, can be clipped onto the edge of a plate to prevent spillage. Clients can use rocker knives with serrated curved blades to cut items by rocking back and forth rather than using a sawing motion.

In addition to the devices mentioned, there are custom-made splints to stabilize the hand or wrist that allow some people to use utensils and to feed themselves. Splints or cuffs may be used in conjunction with a balanced forearm orthosis that supports the distal arm and is controlled by shoulder movements. In extreme cases, a powered feeding device such as the Winsford Self Feeder or a robotic arm operated by switch or voice can be used to scoop food and place it into a person's mouth without human assistance. Barriers to the use of such devices include cost, the slow speed of operation, and the user's concerns about

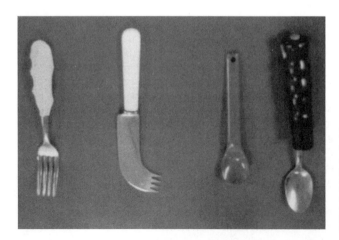

FIGURE 19–1
Adapted utensils (*left to right*); a utensil used by a person with decreased stability; a rocker knife used by an individual with functional use of one hand; a spoon with a plastic shallow bowl; a custom-made putty handle. (From Braddom, R. [Ed.]. [1996]. *Physical medicine and rehabilitation* [p. 515]. Philadelphia: W.B. Saunders.)

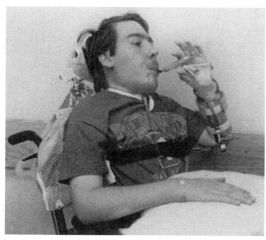

FIGURE 19–2
Mobile arm support used with a long opponens splint and vertical holder to aid in feeding: the mobile arm support and the upper extremity function when the shoulder or forearm strength is weak. The client also has a long opponens splint with a utensil and a vertical holder for a spoon for feeding. (From Braddom, R. [Ed.]. [1996]. *Physical medicine and rehabilitation* [p. 516]. Philadelphia: W.B. Saunders.)

appearance when eating in the presence of other people.

Dressing

Dressing is a complex activity that involves sequencing and perception as well as the physical act of donning and doffing clothing. A person must be mobile enough to adjust the clothing and to manage buttons, snaps, zippers, and other closures. As with feeding, a person must have a sufficient range of motion, strength, and coordination to perform all the tasks.

For those with limited range, such as immediately after hip replacement, various devices that extend the reach are available. A reacher that has a pincer at the end of a long handle can be used to don socks or pants (Fig. 19–3). A dressing stick that is nothing more than a dowel with a hood on the end may also work. Sock and pantyhose donners can be used for hose.

Closures can be managed in several ways (Fig. 19–4). A standard zipper can be made easier to handle by adding a ring or ribbon to the pull so that a weak or uncoordinated hand can pull it up and down. A button hook, popular in the days of high-button shoes, can be used by those with limited hand strength or a prosthesis to close buttons of all sizes. An original fastener can be replaced with a strip of hook-and-loop material (Velcro) with a cosmetic button sewn on top so that the change is not obvious. In some cases, clothing that is already adapted is available for purchase. These items may have wider openings for ease of dressing and have simple closures such as Velcro. They may be cut specifically to fit a wheelchair user who sits all day, or someone who wishes to conceal a catheter bag, braces, or other medical appliances.

Shoes are often hard for people with disabilities to don and doff. Standard shoelaces can be replaced with elastic ones that allow

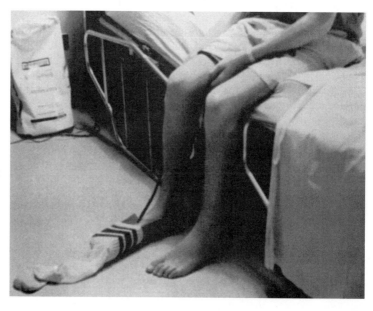

FIGURE 19–3
Stocking aid used when a person is limited in reaching down to the feet or when lower extremity mobility limits bringing the foot near the hands. A person places a stocking over the sock holder, places the holder in front of the foot, and pulls at the rope to pull up the stocking. (From Braddom, R. [Ed.]. [1996]. *Physical medicine and rehabilitation* [p. 518]. Philadelphia: W.B. Saunders.)

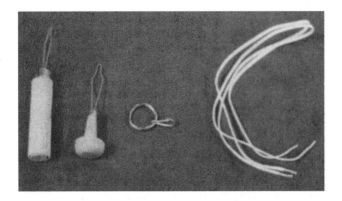

FIGURE 19–4
Fastener adaptations (*left to right*): button aid, knob handle button aid, zipper pull, and elastic laces. (From Braddom, R. [Ed.]. [1996]. *Physical medicine and rehabilitation* [p. 517]. Philadelphia: W.B. Saunders.)

the shoe to be put on and taken off without untying it. Shoes can also be modified by adding a flap of Velcro to replace the laces. A long-handled shoehorn can make the donning process easier.

Grooming and Hygiene

Physical skills needed for grooming and hygiene are similar to those needed for self-feeding. Adequate range of motion, strength, coordination, and an ability to grasp a tool or utensil are necessary. A person must have sufficient balance and trunk control to free the arm for skilled use and the ability to reach all body parts from the top of the head to the tips of the toes.

Areas of grooming and hygiene management include washing the face and hands, tooth or denture care, shaving, combing or brushing hair, nail care, and makeup application. Independent function in these areas requires some degree of fine motor control, alternative strategies, or adaptive equipment.

For people with a limited range of motion, an extended handle on a comb or brush may allow them to reach the top or back of the head, and a long-handled back brush or sponge can be used for the extremities. A person with a weak grasp may use a built-up handle or universal cuff to hold a tool such as a toothbrush. Powered devices such as electric toothbrushes and razors may make up what is lacking in fine motor skills. For tasks such as applying toothpaste to a toothbrush, which requires stabilizing one or both items, a holder for either the brush or the tube may work. A person with visual difficulties may be able to apply makeup using a lighted close-up mirror. The balanced forearm orthosis is also useful in tasks such as makeup application and tooth brushing but usually requires setup. For those with poor

grasp or coordination, a washing mitt and/or soap on a rope can be used.

Nail care, especially for the toes, is difficult. An emery board or stone can be mounted on a board to stabilize it, and a side-mounted clipper is available. Many people choose to have a podiatrist or a helper assist with foot care.

Bathing

Bathing must be performed in a wet and slippery environment, which poses safety concerns. In addition to reaching and bending, the person may need to perform tub or shower transfers and maintain a sitting or standing posture to bathe.

If a person is able to stand, the addition of grab bars and a hand-held shower may improve safety and independence. Nonskid surfaces glued to the tub floor or rubber mats provide additional security. Several types of tub stools and benches, with and without backs, are available for those who need to sit rather than stand. Some people use a seat that fits into the tub, and others use an extended tub bench that has two legs in the tub and two legs out on the bathroom floor. The person sits down on the bench, slides partway over, lifts the legs into the tub, and slides the rest of the way in. This bench can also be used by a wheelchair user who can transfer to the bench directly from a wheelchair. Grab bars and a hand-held shower can be very useful here.

If a roll-in shower is available, a person may use a wheeled shower chair. This resembles a wheelchair, although it may either have four small wheels or be self-propelled with large wheels in the rear. The roll-in shower must have minimal dimensions of 5 feet by 5 feet so the shower chair can be turned in it and sloped so that it does not need a lip to contain the water. A hand-held showerhead provides easy access to water for the user and/or attendant.

If a roll-in shower is not feasible because of space limitations, a lift for the tub may be appropriate. Usually this consists of a chair-type seat that raises and lowers a person in and out of the tub with a mechanical or water-powered lift.

A lack of ability to sense temperature may be a problem for some people with disabilities. An automatic temperature control that presets the water temperature to a specific point prevents burns or injury for people with impaired sensation. The maximal water temperature can also be controlled by a setting on the hot water heater.

Toileting and Bowel and Bladder Management

Toileting requires transferring onto and off of the seat, managing clothing, and wiping. If a standard toilet is inaccessible or on another floor, a portable bedside commode can be used. A raised toilet seat and rails may be useful for people who have difficulty getting up from a standard-height toilet or who have limited hip range or strength. A hydraulically powered toilet seat is available to help someone rise to a standing position.

For small children with poor trunk control, potty chairs are available with a chest strap and a head support as well as smaller seat openings for proper fit.

Managing toilet tissue and wiping may require a toilet tissue holder for someone with limited reaching ability or someone who is unable to manipulate the toilet tissue.

A person with impaired bladder control may use diapers or absorbent pads or a condom, suprapubic, or indwelling catheter. The use of a mirror and/or grasping device may help in self-catheterization for those with limited hand function, and a knee separator may be used in a bed or wheelchair to help with positioning.

Various clamps are available for people who use a leg bag, including a battery-operated, switch-controlled valve to empty into a urinal or toilet once the leg bag is positioned. Velcro straps can secure the bag to a leg or wheelchair.

The placement of suppositories for bowel management or digital stimulation can be accomplished with a long-handled tool for those with limited reach and finger dexterity. Hand and wrist splints may also be used to improve function. The placement of menstrual products such as tampons can also be assisted with such devices.

Skin Management

Prevention of pressure sores requires constant attention by a person with poor or absent sensation, and assistive technology is only one component of a good skin management program. The use of a long-handled mirror allows a person to visually check the back and buttocks daily for skin breakdown. Pressure relief ("wheelchair pushups") or some type of weight shifts should be done frequently throughout the day, and a person should turn or be turned periodically throughout the night. A low-pressure mattress or mattress overlay and a pressure-relieving wheelchair cushion complement a good positioning program. For people with memory or attention deficits, the use of a timer or alarm wristwatch set to beep periodically may help to make weight shifts more regular. See Chapter 18 for additional information.

Transfers

Transfers refer to any action that permits a person to get from one point to another. Common transfers assessed are between a wheelchair and a bed, a toilet, a tub, a floor, and a car. Rising from a sitting to a standing position is a transfer.

Types of transfers include stand-pivot, in which an individual shifts to the edge of a chair, comes to a full or partial standing position, pivots on the feet, and sits down. In a lateral transfer, a person uses a similar action but does not actually come to standing and may bear little or no weight on the feet, but instead uses the arms and upper body to move the trunk. This works best using a wheelchair with one of the armrests removed. A lateral transfer may also be performed with the help of a transfer board (also called a sliding board) (Fig. 19–5). One end of the board is placed under the buttocks and the other end on the surface to which the person is transferring. The person slides across using the arms and upper body. A transfer board may also be used to lessen the work done by a caregiver in a situation in which the person requires assistance.

For dependent transfers, various devices make it easier and safer for both the person and the caregiver. A portable lifting device

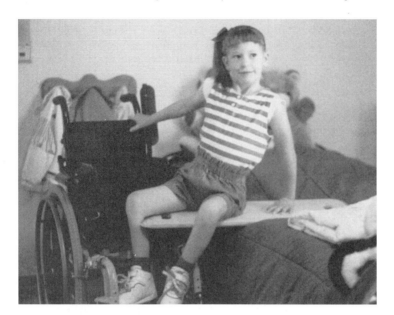

FIGURE 19–5
Sliding board transfer. The sliding board bridges the gap between the wheelchair and the bed. The person uses upper extremities to scoot across the surface from the wheelchair to the bed. (From Braddom, R. [Ed.]. [1996]. *Physical medicine and rehabilitation* [p. 520]. Philadelphia: W.B. Saunders.)

consists of a base and sling and allows a single caregiver to transfer a dependent person (Fig. 19–6). The caregiver places the sling under the person while he or she is in bed by rolling the person from side to side. The base is rolled so that the lifting arm is directly over the person to be transferred, and the sling is attached to the arm of the lifting device with straps or chains. The caregiver then operates the lift until the person is clear of the bed. The entire device is rolled over to a wheelchair, commode, or other destination, and the person is then lowered. Modifications of this concept have an overhead track or a fixed base for an application such as a pool lift. Other dependent lifting systems are available.

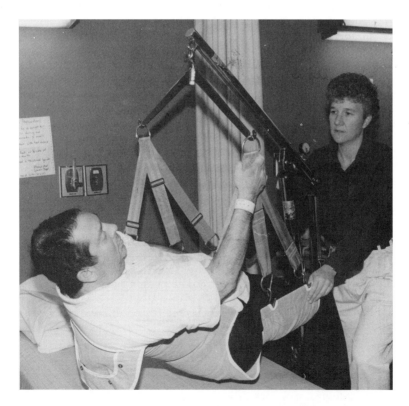

FIGURE 19–6
Portable lifting device.

Bed Mobility

Bed mobility includes rolling, moving up and down in bed, coming to a sitting from a supine position, going from sitting to supine, and getting one's feet on and off the bed. An electric hospital bed may allow some people to be independent through raising and lowering the head and foot or by the use of the side rail. Straps or loops attached to the side rail can be added to customize the setup for a person with a weak grasp. A rail can be attached to a standard bed frame with a handle or bar that is sturdy enough to pull on, or an overhead trapeze may allow someone with good upper body strength to move weak or paralyzed lower extremities. A "leg lifter," a strap with a loop on the end, enables an individual with lower body weakness to raise one leg at a time onto the bed.

Control of the Environment

In order to function independently, a person needs to have control over the immediate environment, including lights, appliances, telephone, heat or air conditioning, doors, and windows. For those people who cannot physically manage some or all of these areas, an environmental control unit is useful. Environmental control units range from a simple remote control for a stereo or television set to a complex computer-driven voice-activated system that operates lights and appliances and even calls 911 in an emergency.

MOBILITY

Mobility is the act of moving from one place to another over level surfaces, elevations, and rough terrain. Walking, wheelchair use, driving, and public transit are all components of mobility.

Walking

Walking, or ambulating, usually begins around 1 year of age and lasts a lifetime. Skills needed for walking are good strength and range of motion, coordination, and balance, as well as sufficient judgment and cognition. More Americans report walking disabilities than any other disability.

There are many types of ambulation aids, and they may be needed at any time in life for short-term or long-term use. A cane is often used to provide balance for a one-sided problem, such as an arthritic hip or weakness

from a stroke. Crutches and walkers are used when weight bearing is limited or when more support is needed and both arms are available to bear the body's weight. Walkers may be equipped with wheels for those who are unable to lift the walker's weight, or with platforms that are used when the hands and wrists are not strong enough to support a person. Canes and crutches can be used on all types of surfaces including curbs, ramps, and stairs, but walkers are not safe on stairs and may be difficult to use on steep ramps or uneven surfaces. Some people choose to use a wheelchair for long distances or outdoor use even if they are able to walk.

Wheelchairs

A person who is unable to walk may find that a wheelchair allows a great deal of independence. Lightweight folding wheelchairs have been around since World War II, and advances in design and materials have continued to improve them. Manual wheelchairs are generally made of steel or aluminum with two small casters on the front and two large wheels on the back that allow the user to self-propel. Various styles of armrests and footrests are available, as well as different rims, wheels, and other accessories. A seating system including a back support and a seat cushion may be used on a wheelchair frame where positioning and/or skin protection are needed.

Protective seat cushions may be made of foam, air, gel, or a combination and may be flat or contoured. The weight of the cushion, ease of transferring on and off, and simplicity of use are all factors in choosing the proper one for any individual. Improper cushion use can lead to pressure sores.

For people who cannot propel a manual wheelchair, powered mobility may be indicated. Good cognition and judgment are needed, but almost any motion can be used to operate the controls of the power chair. The standard controller is a joystick, similar to those used in a video game. It functions as both "gas" and "brake" and is operated with one hand. If the user lacks strength, range of motion, or motor control in the upper extremities, systems available to operate the chair include a chin control, pneumatic switches, or other specialized configurations. A power chair can also be equipped with a tilt or recline system for pressure relief, bladder management, or blood pressure control.

Another type of powered mobility is the

three- or four-wheeled scooter, like those found in malls and supermarkets. These are operated with a tiller similar to the handlebars of a bicycle, and thumb levers for forward and reverse. The seats do not generally offer much support, but the scooters are useful for part-time users, and many people feel they are more cosmetically acceptable.

Transporting a power wheelchair usually requires a van and a lift, although a few light-duty power chairs and most scooters can be disassembled and put into a car. Most power chairs are transported intact because of their weight and because the user would have a very difficult time transferring it to a car.

Driving

Losing the ability to drive is devastating to most people. In any area without a good, accessible public transit system, driving may mean the difference between living independently and requiring assistance, or may mean the ability to get to and from a job.

Driving requires good vision, cognitive function and judgment, reaction time, and endurance. Drivers need sufficient range of motion and strength to operate controls and may need to be able to transfer themselves and equipment both into and out of a vehicle.

For drivers who have lost the function of both legs, hand controls can substitute for foot pedals. A left-side gas pedal can be in-

stalled for someone who cannot use the right foot. Extensions for the gear shift or turn signals may be needed in addition to a spinner knob if the driver can use only one hand. Wheelchair users with good upper body strength may be able to load a wheelchair into a car behind the driver's seat. A car-top carrier that folds, lifts, and loads a manual wheelchair into a box mounted on a car's roof is available.

Power chair users generally ride in the chair and require a van with a lift for transport (Fig. 19–7). A van can be equipped with hand controls, low-effort steering, and sophisticated switches as needed to allow independence in driving. Some minivans even "kneel down" to allow the user to enter via a ramp rather than a lift.

ARCHITECTURAL ACCESSIBILITY

The Americans with Disabilities Act of 1990 provides federal accessibility standards for public buildings and programs including places of lodging, restaurants, entertainment and exhibit halls, retail operations, schools, recreation areas, social service centers, and medical care facilities. The Americans with Disabilities Act includes standards for ramps (Fig. 19–8), parking, entrances, rest rooms, elevators, telephones, assembly areas, and other facilities. Private homes do not fall un-

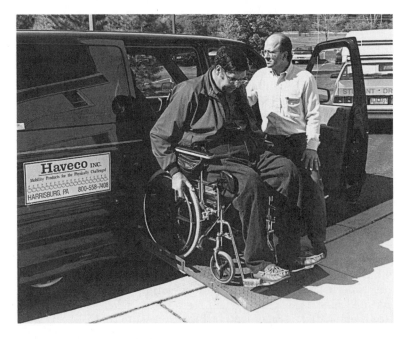

FIGURE 19–7
Van with lift for transport.

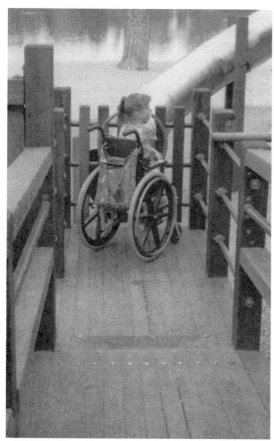

FIGURE 9–8
Playground equipment accessible by wheelchair with platforms and ramps. (From Braddom, R. [Ed.]. [1996]. *Physical medicine and rehabilitation* [p. 530]. Philadelphia: W.B. Saunders.)

der the Americans with Disabilities Act, but the guidelines are useful when making renovations or building a new home for a person with a disability. Specific areas to be addressed are entrances and exits from the home, access between floors, and the use of the bathroom and kitchen.

COMMUNICATION

Communication is a basic need usually met by the spoken and written word. People with good literary skills can use a paper and pencil or letter board to spell out their needs, especially if the need is short term. For long-term need, a keyboard-operated voice-output device may be appropriate. These are usually computer based and can be programmed for the individual user. For those who cannot use a keyboard, other access methods are avail-

able including a head switch, eye-blink switch, or mouth switch. These devices require evaluation and training with a specially trained speech therapist.

For those who cannot use a paper and pencil, written communication can be addressed several ways. A tape recorder can be used for note taking at school or work. A computer-based word processor, accessed by keyboard or switches, provides a means of written output. There are several voice-activated word processors that require no physical input.

COGNITIVE AND MEMORY PROBLEMS

All people can think of a time when they misplaced an item and could not find it, yet it turned out to be in an obvious place. Occasional memory problems are annoying but not usually life-threatening. Significant memory loss or a poor ability to learn new routines can be a serious barrier to independent living. Causes vary, from lifelong issues such as mental retardation and learning disabilities, to acquired neurological problems such as stroke and head injury, to age-related decreases in mental acuity. A combination of compensatory strategies and assistive technology may lessen the effect of memory problems.

The simplest device is a paper and pencil to keep a logbook and lists of tasks to be completed. Pocket electronic devices can keep appointments handy and can sometimes be set to beep or ring on a preset schedule. Pill bottles with timers and pop-up lids are helpful for someone who has trouble remembering a medication schedule. For someone who might leave the electric stove on, there is a timer that will shut it off automatically.

SENSORY DISABILITIES

People with loss of vision or hearing have long been assistive technology users, through corrective lenses (glasses) and hearing aids, but advances in electronics have created new devices.

People with hearing loss can often use devices with visual output to alert them. A doorbell can be hooked up so that a light flashes when the button is pushed, and a baby monitor can work the same way. All new television sets with screens larger than 13 inches are equipped with closed-captioning devices that print text at the bottom of the screen for programs that are captioned. This allows viewers who are deaf and hard of hearing to follow the program without having to depend on lip reading (only about 40% of the English language is visible on the lips). In public places such as lecture and concert halls, an assistive listening system may be available for those with some hearing.

Telecommunication is another area in which assistive technology can help. A text telephone allows the user to type back and forth over the telephone line to another text telephone user. If the other party is hearing, telephone companies in the United States offer a relay service, with a trained operator acting as a liaison between the text telephone user and the hearing or speaking user. A fax machine at home can also be a useful tool for a person who is deaf to communicate with businesses and other places where fax is available. For those with some hearing, many pay telephones and private lines are equipped with an adjustable hearing aid–compatible volume control.

Persons with low vision may use various types of magnifiers, either hand held or desk mounted, in addition to glasses. Computer screens can be fitted with a full-screen magnifier as well. If that is not enough, the text on the screen can be made larger through software installed in the system. For someone who has no functional vision, there are software programs that read the text on the screen. Other reading systems accept papers and books and read the text to the user. On a smaller scale, many home appliances such as clocks and wristwatches actually "tell" time out loud or have braille or raised numbers so they can be manually checked.

The white cane is a traditional mobility device for a person who is blind, and the canes are now made with electronic sensors for enhanced feedback. Although not strictly an assistive technology device, guide dogs serve long and faithfully for many people who are blind or physically disabled, providing significant mobility and independence within the community.

NEW ERA FOR ASSISTIVE TECHNOLOGY SERVICES

Assistive technology, in conjunction with a team approach, is a key element that assists clients in maintaining their optimal level of independence. Four case studies demonstrate

to the reader how clients' values and roles in their life affect the use of adaptive equipment. The importance of the client as a member of the team, to direct and interact with the professional, is clear. These case studies demonstrate the rehabilitation professional's role in assessing a client's goals and planning for equipment that is practical and medically justified according to the client's lifestyle. Outcomes can then be measured using the associated cost and the client's successful training and mastery of the skills necessary to increase functional independence.

■ CASE STUDY 19–1

Jeff is a 33-year-old newly married man who was employed as a chemist for a large pharmaceutical company. He and his wife own a small condominium in a suburban area with good access to community services. Jeff was diagnosed with anoxic encephalopathy after an accidental chemical exposure at work. After a lengthy acute hospitalization, Jeff was transferred to a rehabilitation center and made gradual improvement during his inpatient stay. He had limitations in feeding that included cutting his meat. His ambulation improved to the point that he was using a walker for short distances and a wheelchair for long distances. The team recognized that home safety was a critical issue because Jeff's judgment was impaired. The discharge plan included continued therapy that would be provided at a nearby outpatient day-treatment program. The adaptive prescriptions were based on needs and benefits that could be achieved to enable Jeff to move to a high level of self-care and manage safely within his home. Before any equipment prescription was implemented, the team assessed the following:

■ What is Jeff's current status?
■ What will Jeff's and his wife's new roles be?
■ Can the device or devices improve his function?
■ Is Jeff able to use the equipment from a cognitive standpoint?
■ Is independence realistic for this client?
■ Is the equipment safe and appropriate?
■ Is the equipment economical?

It was determined through practice and a home trial that the following equipment and community-based services would meet this client's needs and be beneficial in reestablishing a sense of control, introducing independence, and enhancing safety within his environment:

- A custom-made splint to stabilize the wrist to allow increased independent function in eating
- A walker and a wheelchair, both on a short-term basis
- Public transportation as a means of getting to and from the day-treatment program
- Safety products for bathroom activities, including grab bars, a hand-held shower, a shower seat, and an automatic temperature control

In conclusion, the long-range rehabilitation plan and equipment needs were established by the outpatient team with Jeff and his wife. They worked together to determine what was necessary for Jeff's long-term equipment use, his satisfaction, and the potential for his community reentry and vocational retraining. ■

■ CASE STUDY 19–2

Sharon was diagnosed with multiple sclerosis 5 years ago. She is married, lives in a one-story home in the city, and works in the city. She is employed as a secretary in a large corporation.

Sharon felt threatened about her continued employment because she was experiencing a decrease in functional mobility. It became apparent to Sharon that powered mobility was her best option to maintain active employment. She also needed to conserve her energy because it was taking her too long to prepare herself for work each morning. To match Sharon's equipment needs, a client- and family-centered team assessment helped to establish her equipment goals as well as understand

- Her lifestyle
- Her attitude toward her disability
- Techniques that could be used instead of a device
- Characteristics and limitations of each device for her
- Her desire to use self-help devices
- Cost issues

An outpatient program was initiated, and in occupational therapy Sharon learned dressing techniques in combination with a reacher.

The occupational therapist made suggestions for modifications in clothing, shoes, and hosiery to improve the ease of dressing and to maximize Sharon's energy and efficiency. The decision to use powered mobility was complicated by a home with barriers, that is, no ramp to the house, and narrow doorways. The physical therapist made a home visit to assess Sharon's home environment and then made recommendations to Sharon and her husband. Sharon's insurance nurse case manager was then contacted to discuss funding for a scooter to maintain functional mobility outside of her home, and to allow her to continue to work. A standard wheelchair was also available for in-home use. ■

ELDERLY PERSON WITH A DISABILITY

One health care challenge of the 21st century is to address the issues of assistive technology with elderly persons with a disability so that they, too, may effectively achieve or maintain maximal functional independence. Many medical problems that in the past resulted in death no longer do so but may cause limitations or disability.

According to Daniel Perry, director of the Alliance for Aging Research, cited by Sheredos (1995), "There is a noticeable lack of urgency in training and preventing the health and rehabilitation problems of older people." Yet assistive technology can range from something as simple as an instrument to help hold a pencil to as complex as a computer system that allows communication. Assistive technology has many benefits and is used by many disciplines. These disciplines include physical, occupational, and speech therapies, therapeutic recreation, vocational rehabilitation, and psychology, and they play an important part of a client's rehabilitation treatment plan. Examples include custom wheelchairs to maximize mobility, devices that assist communication, adaptive driving education and devices, and memory devices. Also, environmental control units can offer freedom, independence, and security at home, and recreational and leisure devices enhance the quality of life. Community- and hospital-based rehabilitation nurses are becoming increasingly important participants on the transdisciplinary team to assess the provision of assistive technology, reinforce learning, and educate clients and families on safety issues.

■ **CASE STUDY 19–3**

Louise is a 78-year-old woman who fell while shopping and fractured her right hip. She underwent surgery and a hip pinning and is now partial weight bearing. Her past medical history includes type 2 diabetes controlled by diet; poor vision; and peripheral neuropathy. Because of her neuropathy, Louise has difficulty maintaining her weight bearing and requires assistance with a walker for ambulation. She is independent in wheelchair propulsion and management, feeds herself independently, and grooms and dresses herself independently from the wheelchair. Toileting is accomplished with assistance to manage her clothing, and bathing requires assistance. Louise is alert and cooperative, is very social, and takes responsibility for her own care whenever possible. She is currently in a skilled nursing facility (subacute unit) because she lives alone and cannot be discharged home until she is able to care for herself. She states that she would like to be as self-sufficient as possible.

During her stay in the subacute unit, the team that worked with Louise met to plan a course of treatment that would help her become more independent. With her occupational therapist, she tried several tub benches and a hand-held showerhead. She performed best with an extended tub bench that allowed her to transfer onto the bench, then slide over into the tub while lifting her legs over the side. The nursing staff worked with her until she was independent with this and the hand-held showerhead. With instruction from the nursing staff and practice with toilet safety rails, she became independent in toileting.

Louise continues to have difficulty maintaining her partial weight bearing. In physical therapy, the therapist tried a limb-load monitor as a training tool. The monitor was set so that it made a beeping noise when she exceeded a set amount of pressure on a sensor placed in her shoe, but this did not help her to judge her weight bearing accurately. The team hopes that when Louise is allowed to increase her weight bearing, she will be able to be independent with her ambulation.

In this case, it is clear that the assistive technology has helped Louise achieve some of her goals of independence. She was able to articulate these goals, and her team of caregivers responded, using a combination of client education and assistive devices. When it is time for Louise to be discharged home, the entire team will be involved in making recommendations for services and equipment that she will need. Louise's case manager is to arrange for the prescribed devices and document the justification. This case study shows that elderly people can continue to grow and learn and have the potential and promise for connection with their own independent destiny. ■

CHILD WITH A DISABILITY

The passage of Pub. L. No. 94-142 and the Education for All Handicapped Children Act of 1975 has had a major impact on the design and implementation of programs for children with disabilities (Parette & Parette, 1992). Nurses have become an integral part of the multidisciplinary professional team to develop and implement creative approaches to the delivery of services for young children.

Today's school nurses have a unique role as they function independently in many roles in their day-to-day performance of nursing to the population they serve. This includes everything from specific nursing tasks such as performing tracheostomy care to working as part of an assessment team in developing a student's educational plan. School nurses influence the use and management of assistive technologies within the school system. Proactive school nurses are aware of the public law amendments and the constant modifications and changes that are driven by litigation and case law.

■ **CASE STUDY 19–4**

John is a 10-year-old boy with a diagnosis of spina bifida and hydrocephalus. He has a complicated medical history that includes multiple surgeries for repair of his myelomeningocele, shunt placement and revision, and repair of a left club foot; a flaccid bladder; and a history of urinary tract infections. He lives with his parents and two brothers in a one-story home. He attends public school and participates in a regular fourth-grade class.

John is not conscious of the fact that he uses assistive technology as it has been a part of his entire life, but he has limitations in the following areas:

- Mobility
- Self-care
- Bowel and bladder management
- Accessibility

John uses a wheelchair for his morning care routine and for long-distance travel. He is beginning to be interested in wheelchair sports, particularly tennis, and his parents have encouraged him in this area. He uses braces and crutches for shorter distances within his home and within the classroom. At school, he has had occasional problems with pressure areas caused by the braces, and the school nurse has been helpful to him.

John is independent with bathing at home once his mother transfers him into the tub. He uses a hand-held showerhead. He is beginning to value his privacy and to want to be independent. He manages his bladder via clean intermittent catheterization, which is done by a parent or the nurse. He wants to learn to do it himself, and the nurse is working with him on this skill. Once he learns, he will be able to leave home for longer periods of time with his friends. His bowel program is managed by diet with occasional use of laxatives.

John's environment is very accessible as he lives in a one-story house with a ramp at the front door, and his school is also accessible. Both places have large bathrooms and the necessary equipment.

One issue John and his family face is the fact that children grow! He has had many sets of braces and will need a new wheelchair as soon as he has grown too heavy and tall for the present one. In a few years, he and his parents will also encounter the reality that he will want to obtain a driver's license. At that time he will likely require hand controls and will need to learn to load his wheelchair into the car, too. ■

FUNDING ASSISTIVE TECHNOLOGY

There are many sources of funding for assistive technology, depending on the individual's needs and goals. For medical needs such as walking and self-care activities, funding may be through Medicare, Medicaid, or private health insurance. Medicare is a federal program providing hospitalization and related services to people older than 65 years and to people with permanent disabilities. It is administered by regional carriers, and the guidelines are the same in every state. Medicaid is a similar program for low-income adults and children funded by both state and federal dollars. Services covered vary from state to state. Recipients of both programs are served in a variety of financial models including a traditional fee-for-service or fee-schedule model and a newer managed care model. The lack of funding for assistive devices and support services is a persistent problem for persons with disabilities. Communities need to partner closely with state agencies and public and private funding sources to help reshape outdated policies. Even devices such as wheelchairs can be too expensive for many clients.

Private insurance may cover assistive technology for people who have injuries or illnesses and who were covered under such a plan at the time of onset. Coverage varies widely from basic equipment such as a walker to extensive home renovations if included on the insurance policy. Someone who is injured on the job may be covered under a workers' compensation plan for equipment and services related to the injury. Also, if the person is of working age, all states have a vocational rehabilitation program for people with disabilities seeking to enter or return to the workforce. School-aged children may be eligible for devices and services through the educational system or through various agencies such as the United Cerebral Palsy Association, which serves people with a specific diagnosis. Many community service clubs, churches, and civic organizations give financial assistance to people with disabilities. In addition, funding may be available through employers, the Department of Veterans Affairs, work incentives, low-interest loans, and the use of some tax options.

SUMMARY AND CONCLUSION

One of our main goals as rehabilitation professionals working in the area of assistive technology funding is to be able to justify the expenses in time and dollars of advocating for and providing equipment and services on the basis that they contribute to an improvement in the client's functional outcome. This means being aware of the goals of the client, family, school, residence, employer, and any other stakeholders in this process. It also means an awareness of the cost and value of the equipment and a look at the "bigger picture" to ensure that all areas of the person's life have been considered.

The field of assistive technology and related services is huge, ranging from simple to complex, from low cost to major expense, from basic activities of daily living to leisure activities. The Technology Assistance Act of 1988 ("Tech Act") mandated that all states begin building statewide networks of resources to help citizens with disabilities identify appropriate assistive technologies. Today's clients can try hundreds of devices at assistive technology centers. Each year, awareness and training sessions are provided for thousands of people who want to learn more about the benefits of assistive technology.

The rehabilitation case manager nurse now has an important role in triaging clients to various levels of health care service. This requires assessment, planning, and creative decision making that is driven by cost containment. There are many nursing roles such as skilled care provider, case manager, school nurse, geriatric specialist, and community and long-term care nurses who validate and support the benefit of assistive technology. The primary goal is for the lives of sick, elderly, and disabled clients to be enhanced through the use of equipment designed to make tasks easier. Factors that influence the abandonment of assistive devices are the lack of client involvement in the selection process, difficulty in obtaining the item, poor device performance, and changes in the client's needs for the device. Effective equipment use means that the equipment is necessary, it will be useful over a period of time, and it enables the client to be more functional. The third-party payer's goal is to see the value of an assistive device in the recipient's daily life with home use in mind. A professional understanding of the system can best be demonstrated by the documentation that quantifies and qualifies the cost benefit. The ability to enhance clients' level of independence in making their own decisions and maintaining productivity at work, school, and home is the most successful measurement of the cost benefit of clients' quality of life within their lifestyles and their communities.

REFERENCES

Parette, H. P., Parette, P. C. (1992). Young children with disabilities and assistive technology: The nurse's role on multidisciplinary technology teams. *Journal of Pediatric Nursing Care of Children and Families, 7*(4), 237–245.

Sheredos, C. A. (1995). Technology in long term care. *Rehabilitation Management* Feb-Mar, 39–44.

BIBLIOGRAPHY

Giltin, L., Schemm, R. (1996). Assistive device use among older adults. *Team Rehab Report, 7*(4):25–28.

Guerette, P., Moran, W. (1994). ADL awareness. *Team Rehab Report, 5*(6):41–44.

Harrison, B. S., Faircloth, J. W., Yaryan, L. (1995). The impact of legislation on the role of the nurse. *Nursing Outlook, 43*(2), 57–61.

Mix, C. M., & Specht D. P. (1996). Achieving functional independence. In R. L. Braddom (Ed.), *Physical medicine and rehabilitation.* Philadelphia: W. B. Saunders, 514–530.

Parette, H. P. (1993). High risk infant case management and assistive technology funding and family enabling perspective. *Maternal-Child Nursing Journal, 21*(2), 53–64.

Sanford, J., Arch, M., Megrew, M. B. (1995). An evaluation of grab bars to meet the need of elderly people. *Assistive Technology, 7*, 36–44.

Smith, R., Giltin, L. (1995). Issuing assistive devices to older patients in rehabilitation: An exploratory study. *American Journal of Occupational Therapy, 49*(10), 994–1000.

Smith, R. (1995). A client-centered model for equipment prescription (clients' values and roles, effective use of adaptive equipment). *Occupational Therapy in Health Care, 9*(4), 39–52.

Steele, S. (1988). Young children with meningomyelocele, with special reference to handling, positioning, and child-adult play interactions. Issues in *Comprehensive Pediatric Nursing, 11*(4):213–225.

Watson, P.G. (1992). The optimal functioning plan key in cancer. *Cancer Nursing, 15*(4), 254–263.

PART III

Nursing Management of Selected Diagnostic Populations

Nursing Management of the Patient with a Cerebrovascular Accident

Nancy M. Youngblood

Cerebrovascular disease is the most common cause of neurological disability in Western countries. Its incidence has fallen in recent decades, but evidence suggests that the decline has now leveled off, and it remains a major source of disability. Although vascular injury to the brain can occur as part of a number of diseases, most cerebrovascular illness is secondary to atherosclerosis, hypertension, or both.

The major specific types of cerebrovascular disease are (1) cerebral insufficiency due to transient disturbances of blood flow or, rarely, to hypertensive encephalopathy; (2) infarction, due to either embolism or thrombosis of the intra- or extracranial arteries; (3) hemorrhage, including hypertensive parenchymal hemorrhage and subarachnoid hemorrhage from congenital aneurysm; and (4) an arteriovenous malformation, which can cause symptoms of a mass lesion, infarction, or hemorrhage.

The vernacular term *cerebrovascular accident* (CVA) lacks specificity; it is commonly applied to the syndromes that accompany either ischemic or hemorrhagic lesions. *Stroke*, by common usage, designates ischemic lesions. The most current term used to describe vascular alterations that affect brain function is *brain attack*. This term has become popular because it denotes the urgency necessary to treat the cerebral injury because rapid treatment can limit tissue distruction, prevent complications, and preserve or restore function. The terms *stroke*, *CVA*, and *brain attack* are used interchangeably to refer to the cerebral injury that results from altered cerebrovascular function.

This chapter is concerned with the most common types of CVA, which are ischemic stroke and cerebral hemorrhage. Both ischemic stroke and cerebral hemorrhage tend to develop abruptly, but hemmorrhage generally has the more catastrophically acute onset. Symptoms and signs in cerebrovascular disease reflect the damaged area of brain and not necessarily the specific artery affected. Occlusion (e.g., of either the middle cerebral artery or the internal carotid artery) can produce a similar clinical neurological abnormality. Nevertheless, cerebrovascular injuries generally conform to fairly specific patterns of arterial supply; a knowledge of these distributions is important to distinguish stroke from a space-occupying lesion (e.g., brain tumor or abscess).

The most important step in treatment is to identify a potential or impending stroke or brain hemorrhage so that brain damage may be prevented.

INCIDENCE AND COST

Strokes remain the third leading cause of death (U.S. Department of Health and Human Services, 1991) and a major cause of disability in the United States today. Because the occurrence of brain attacks is not required to be reported for statistical purposes, it is unknown to what extent strokes truly exist. It is estimated that about 500,000 new cases occur yearly, with 25% of these being recurrent strokes. The incidence has declined over the past 35 years because of increased awareness of risk factors, especially increased efforts to control hypertension. Statistics differ according to the data from various studies, but according to the Howard Stroke Registry, 53% are thrombotic strokes, with 31% caused by emboli and 16% caused by hemorrhage (Schnell, 1997)

More than 2 million people in the United States are disabled from brain attacks; the annual cost for their care is $15.6 billion. Brain attack survivors represent 75% of all patients in long-term care facilities, 60% in rehabilitation facilities, and 50% of hospitalized neurological patients (Flannery, 1997). Approximately 150,000 survive yearly; 0.07% have another stroke in 1 year, and 42% in 5 years (Barker, 1994; Macabasco & Hickman, 1995; Slide, 1995).

Incidence of both ishemic and hemorrhagic types of brain attacks is currently rising related to cocaine use among the younger population. It is thought that cocaine potentates neurotransmission of serotonin and blocks its reuptake. Serotonin is the most potent vasoconstrictor in the cerebral circulation (Hickey, 1992). People may have a stroke at any age; however, the incidence rises sharply in those older than 65 years. The risk factors can be grouped into those that can be modified and those that cannot be changed.

RISK FACTORS FOR BRAIN ATTACK

Modifiable Risk Factors

Modifiable risk factors are those factors that can be changed or controlled. When these risk factors are modified, the pathological lesion underlying a brain attack is less likely to occur. The modifiable factors are as follows:

- *Smoking:* Cigarette smoking has been clearly established as a biologically plausible independent determinant of increased stroke risk (Higa & Davanipour, 1991).
- *Obesity:* Obese persons have higher levels of blood pressure, blood glucose, and atherogenic serum lipids and on that account alone could be expected to have an increased stroke incidence. Studies have suggested that the pattern of obesity is also important, with central obesity and abdominal deposition of fat more strongly associated with atherosclerotic disease (Folsom, Prineas, Kaye, & Munger, 1990)
- *Hypercholesterolemia:* Abnormalities in the levels of serum lipids, including triglycerides, cholesterol, low-density lipoprotein, and high-density lipoprotein, are regarded as risk factors, more for coronary artery disease than for cerebrovascular disease (Smith, Shipley, Marmont, & Rose, 1992).
- *Oral contraceptives:* Risk increases if patient smokes: an increased risk of stroke has been reported in users of oral contraceptives, particularly in older women—that is, older than 35 years—and predominantly in those with other cardiovascular risk factors, par-

ticularly hypertension and cigarette smoking (Barnett, Mohr, Stein & Yatsu, 1992).
- *Diabetes mellitus:* Diabetes has also been associated with an increased stroke risk. People with diabetes are known to have an increased susceptibility to coronary, femoral, and cerebral artery atherosclerosis.
- *Hypertension:* After age, hypertension is the most powerful stroke risk factor. It is prevalent in the U.S. population in both men and women and is of even greater significance in blacks. The risk of stroke rises proportionately with increasing blood pressure.
- *Cardiac disease:* Cardiac disease, particularly atrial fibrillation, valvular heart disease, myocardial infarction, coronary artery disease, and congestive heart failure, has been clearly associated with increasing the risk of ishemic stroke.
- *Alcohol consumption:* The impact of alcohol consumption on stroke risk is related to the amount of alcohol consumed (Wolf, Cobb, & D'Agostino, 1992). Heavy alcohol use, either habitual daily alcohol consumption or binge drinking, seems to be related to an excess of stroke and stroke deaths.
- *Sedentary lifestyle:* Leisure time and work-associated vigorous physical activity have been linked to lower cardiac disease incidence. Vigorous exercise may exert a beneficial influence on risk factors for atherosclerotic disease by reducing elevated blood pressure as a result of weight loss, reducing pulse rate, raising high-density lipoprotein and lowering low-density lipoprotein cholesterol levels, improving glucose tolerance, and promoting a lifestyle conducive to favorably changing detrimental health habits such as cigarette smoking (Wolf, Cobb, & D'Agostino, 1992).

Nonmodifiable Risk Factors

There are inherent risk factors that cannot be modified. Nonmodifiable risk factors are as follows:

- *Male gender:* Stroke incidence is greater among men. However, because women often outlive men, many studies have found a greater prevalence in women than in men.
- *Advanced age:* Advanced age is the strongest determinant of stroke. Stroke incidence rises exponentially with age, with the majority of strokes occurring in persons older than 65 years. Clearly, as the population ages, the burden of stroke becomes even more apparent.

- *Black race:* A decline in stroke mortality has occurred in each race and gender group, but the relative difference between the races has remained fairly uniform, with a nearly twofold increased stroke mortality in blacks. Blacks may have an increased burden of stroke risk factors to account for their increased incidence of stroke.
- *Family history of stroke*: The hereditability of cerebrovascular disease has, perhaps, been underemphasized (Fisher, 1995; Post-stroke Rehabilitation Guideline Panel, 1995).

A combination of several risk factors intensifies the likelihood of having a stroke. Control of the modifiable factors can significantly reduce the probability of having a stroke. If a person has nonmodifiable risk factors, it is of utmost importance that the modifiable factors be controlled so that the person is less likely to have a stroke. It is important to consider that even though more men have strokes than women, 60.7% of the women who have strokes die at the time of the stroke; therefore all the risk factors that apply to women are potentially fatal. Strokes are less likely to be fatal in men.

PATHOPHYSIOLOGY OF STROKE SYNDROME

Blood to the brain is supplied by the right and left common carotid arteries, which branch to form the internal and external carotid arteries. Within the cranial vault, the internal carotid arteries branch to form the ophthalmic, posterior communicating, anterior choroidal, and anterior and middle cerebral arteries. These arteries and their numerous branches supply blood to most of the cerebral hemispheres. The external carotid arteries, together with their branches, supply blood to the face, the orbits, and the dura matter. An important function of the external carotid arteries is their ability to supply blood to the brain in the event of occlusion or blockage of the internal carotid arteries.

The two vertebral arteries arise from the subclavian artery and join at the base of the brain to form the basilar artery. Anatomically, the basilar artery is located near the pons, the middle structure of the brainstem. Branches of the basilar artery provide blood to the brainstem. The two posterior cerebral arteries, which branch from the basilar artery, provide blood to the temporal and occipital lobes of the brain.

An important area at the base of the brain is the circle of Willis, a network of blood vessels composed of the two anterior cerebral, one anterior communicating, two posterior cerebral, and two posterior communicating arteries. The circle of Willis functions as a type of collateral circulation between the blood vessels of the two cerebral hemispheres and between the carotid and vertebrobasilar circulations. Branches of the basilar artery supply the diencephphalon and the basal ganglia.

If blood flow through the cerebral vessels is interrupted, the brain is often able to receive an adequate blood supply through collateral circulation or the shunting of blood via other pathways. Although this is helpful, it does not entirely eliminate the problems of inadequate cerebral profusion.

The brain must receive a constant flow of blood for normal function, as it is unable to store oxygen or glucose. In addition, blood flow is important for the removal of metabolic waste, carbon dioxide, and lactic acid. If deprived of its blood flow, the brain can be damaged irreparably within a few minutes.

Through the processes of cerebral autoregulation, blood flow is maintained at a fairly constant rate of 750 mL/min. In response to blood pressure changes or to changes in carbon dioxide tension, the cerebral arteries dilate or constrict. Cerebral autoregulation is impaired after a cerebral insult, both at the site and in distal arteries, and the brain cannot regulate cerebral blood flow according to metabolic needs of cerebral tissue. Instead, cerebral blood flow and cerebral perfusion pressure depend on the systemic systolic blood pressure. If hypotension develops, collateral circulation may be inadequate and cerebral perfusion pressure decreases, which can result in a brain attack. Further problems resulting from loss of autoregulation occur with the loss of sensitivity of the vessels to hypercapnia and hypoxemia. The usual vasodilation that occurs may be altered, further aggravating existing ischemia.

Once autoregulation is disturbed, increasing cerebral edema occurs with increased systemic arterial pressure. Cerebral blood flow is increased, and plasma proteins leak from the congested, distended capillaries, pulling fluid from the intravascular space into the interstitial space. This swelling is at its worst from days 2 to 4 after the insult, during which time ischemia and infarction are also worsened; the ventricular system may become obstructed, and herniation may occur.

The signs and symptoms of a CVA are the

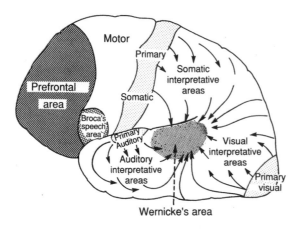

FIGURE 20–1
Organization of the somatic, auditory, and visual association areas into a general mechanism for interpretation of sensory experience. All these feed into *Wernicke's area*, located in the posterosuperior portion of the temporal lobe. Note also the prefrontal area and Broca's speech area. (From Guyton, A. C., & Hall, J. E. [1997]. *Human physiology and mechanisms of disease* [6th ed.]. Philadelphia: W. B. Saunders.)

result of a narrowing or complete closure of one of the arteries that supply the brain tissue with nutrients and oxygen. The narrowing or blockage of the vessels is most commonly the result of thrombosis or emboli formation. Hemorrhage, vascular compression, and arterial spasm are less frequent causes of a CVA. The blockage, regardless of the cause, results in a decrease in the blood supply to the brain tissue. The outcome of the progressive tissue ischemia is changes in the functioning of the neurological system. Figure 20–1 depicts the areas of the brain that seem to be responsible for specific function.

CLASSIFICATION OF BRAIN ATTACK

Classification of brain attack is based on the underlying problem that is created within the blood vessels of the brain. The brain attack is divided into two major categories: ischemic and hemorrhagic. The predisposing pathophysiological factors causing the two basic mechanisms of brain attacks are listed in Table 20–1.

Each of these categories can be further subdivided. Ischemic brain attacks may be classified as either thrombotic or embolic, and hemorrhagic brain attack may be classified into intracerebral hemorrhage and subarachnoid hemorrhage. Although the cause and pathophysiology of these two are different, the outcomes are the same.

Ischemic

Thrombotic. A thrombotic brain attack is most commonly associated with the development of atherosclerosis of the blood vessel wall. Arteriosclerosis is a noninflammatory degenerative disease affecting almost any ce-

rebral blood vessel. Atheroslerosis is a thickening of the intimal layer of the arteries by a buildup of a cholesterol-based fatty plaque. The plaque buildup occurs over a period of 20 to 30 years. As the plaque builds, the intima becomes progressively hypertrophied and fragmented, which results in an intimal surface that is roughened. The enlarging plaque decreases the diameter of the blood vessel. Platelets adhere to the roughened surface of the blood vessel and a thrombus forms, further narrowing the vessel lumen. This process continues until the blood vessel is completely occluded, resulting in ischemia to the brain tissue supplied by the vessel.

Embolic. An embolus is a thrombus that breaks loose from distant sites, migrates to the vessels in the brain, and blocks lumina of these blood vessels, causing ischemia of the brain tissue that they supply. These strokes occur suddenly, usually during waking activities. A large embolus can occlude the internal carotid artery, resulting in severe hemiplegia.

TABLE 20–1 ■ **PREDISPOSING PATHOPHYSIOLOGICAL FACTORS CAUSING BRAIN ATTACKS**

Ischemia	Hemorrhage
Atherosclerosis	Hypertension
Emboli	Aneurysms
Vasospasm	Bleeding disorders
Smoking	Arteriovenous malformations
High-fat diet	Neoplasms
Erythrocyte disorders	Amphetamine and intranasal cocaine use in younger persons
Crack cocaine smoking	
Thrombosis	

If arising from the heart, as most cerebral emboli do, the fragments are likely to be small and travel through either the carotid or the vertebral arteries. The embolus may fragment and move, allowing symptoms to clear, but the fragments will eventually occlude another smaller branch and produce symptoms from the area of the brain affected. The mortality is approximately 20%, with many patients having recurrent strokes if the underlying problem is not corrected.

Hemorrhagic

Intracerebral. Intracerebral hemorrhagic stroke is caused by a rupture of a blood vessel, causing blood to enter brain tissue. The rupture generally occurs in a deep and small vessel that penetrates deep inside brain tissue. Brain damage in the hemorrhagic stroke is the result of compression of the brain tissue, which compromises cerebral perfusion and also may result in brain herniation. The hemorrhage may be a small, localized, necrotic disruption of the arteriolar wall with 1 or 2 mL of blood lost and a subsequent cystic wall (less than 1 cm) called a *lacuna* formed around the space. These infarcts are often multiple and are commonly in the thalamus, pons, and cerebellum. Depending on the location, they produce various mild and often transient clinical findings, including hemiparesis, hemiplegia, ataxia, dysarthria, clumsiness, and facial weakness.

There is a major difference between a lacuna and an extensive hemorrhage. In an extensive intracerebral hemorrhage, extravasated blood forms a hematoma, producing pressure on the brain and perhaps causing increased intracranial pressure. The onset is sudden, with headache and steady development of neurological deficits over minutes to hours with progressive deepening coma within the maximum of 24 hours. A massive hemorrhage (ranging from 50 mL or less) probably will be fatal. If the patient survives, the patient's condition persists until the clot is resolved, which takes weeks to months. An optimistic point is that if the patient survives this critical period, the prognosis may be better than the symptoms would indicate because the brain tissue is usually dysfunctional from compression of the hematoma rather than from being infarcted.

Subarachnoid. A subarachnoid hemorrhagic stroke is the result of bleeding into the subarachnoid space. A subarachnoid hemorrhage most often occurs when there is a rupture of an aneurysm or arteriovenous malformation.

The mechanisms that cause brain tissue destruction are different. These differences explain the course of the disease and the potential outcome of the brain injury. The ischemic attack may progress slowly. On the other hand, the hemorrhagic attack can be very dramatic and quickly result in death. The mechanisms of brain attack are listed in Table 20–2.

Regardless of the cause of the brain attack, the brain tissue responds in the same manner. A space-occupying lesion eventually develops, and this lesion increases intracranial pressure. The increased pressure in turn causes the neurological signs that are seen in a person with a stroke. The localizing signs may be permanent or reversible depending on the type of brain attack, the part of the brain that has been injured, and the length of time that the brain tissue has been hypoxic. The effects of the brain attack on brain tissue are listed in Figure 20–2.

TABLE 20–2 ■ MECHANISMS OF BRAIN ATTACK

Ischemia	Hemorrhage
Infarction	Subarachnoid or intracerebral hemorrhage
Destruction of brain substance	Destruction of brain substance
	Expanding mass from arterial hemorrhage
Marked edema of surrounding brain	Edema of surrounding brain

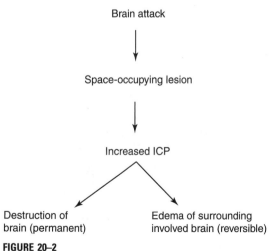

FIGURE 20–2
Effects of brain attack on brain tissue. ICP, intracranial pressure.

CLINICAL FINDINGS OF A BRAIN ATTACK

Generalized clinical findings can occur with any brain attack. These generalized symptoms are incontinence, altered level of consciousness, amnesia, vertigo, gray vision (as if looking through a fuzzy glass or with the light being dimmed), syncope, and confusion. Such nonfocal symptoms may indicate a cardiac origin (inadequate cardiac output resulting in cerebral ischemia) of the brain attack. For the diagnosis of brain attack the neurological deficits must last for 24 hours or longer.

Syndromes Leading to Completed Stroke

There are other syndromes that can lead to a completed stroke. These are transient ischemic attack (TIA), reversible ischemic neurological deficit, and stroke-in-evolution.

Transient Ischemic Attack

These episodes of ischemia usually last from 5 to 30 minutes and occasionally up to 24 hours but never longer. The symptoms clear completely when the ischemia resolves. When multiple TIAs recur with the same symptoms, a thrombotic origin is suggested. The recurrence of different symptoms implies recurrent emboli. Clinical findings are related to the involved arteries.

TIAs are forewarnings of an impending stroke in 75% of cases. The transient symptoms seen with TIAs may become permanent deficits when a stroke develops. There may be only one TIA or as many as 100 before a stroke occurs. Hours, weeks, months, or years may lapse between the TIA and the stroke. Sometimes patients have only one TIA and a subsequent stroke does not occur. The number of recurrences of TIAs is not predictable and is not directly related to the number or severity of risk factors.

The subclavian steal syndrome is a form of TIA. It is a vascular syndrome caused by an occlusion or stenosis that impairs the vertebrobasilar cerebrovascular system. Blood that was destined for the brain is shunted into another area because the normal flow is obstructed; therefore, the blood flows to the area that is not obstructed, usually the left arm, thus depriving the cerebral tissue of adequate circulation. The deprived area has a decreased blood pressure. The most common location for this obstruction is in the left subclavian artery. Atherosclerosis is the most frequent cause of the obstruction. To compensate for the occlusion, blood flow is diverted from the right vertebral artery down the left vertebral artery to supply the distal portion of the subclavian artery beyond the obstruction. Although this diversion improves circulation to the left arm, the patient experiences symptoms of vertebrobasilar insufficiency because the blood is prevented from flowing into the basilar artery. The degree of resulting cerebral ischemia depends on the amount of blood that can perfuse the brain through the intracerebral collateral circulation furnished by the circle of Willis.

Clinical findings develop when this collateral circulation cannot compensate for an excessive diversion of blood to the affected arm. Such a situation is likely to occur during exercise of the upper extremities, which may occur during work or recreation. The patient develops numbness, tingling, and claudication in the affected arm on elevation or exercise. A difference in the radial pulses and as much as a 20-mm Hg difference in arterial blood pressure between the two arms is common. The patient may also experience transient visual loss, vertigo, nausea, ataxia, syncope, or typical TIA episodes. Diagnosis is confirmed by angiography. Treatment is removal of the obstruction by surgery with an endarterectomy, grafting of the damaged subclavian artery, or a bypass graft to provide adequate collateral circulation to the basilar artery. Without treatment, cerebral infarction can occur if the basilar circulation becomes severely compromised; if it is totally occluded, coma and death result (Fisher, 1995).

Reversible Ischemic Neurological Deficit

Also called a *small stroke*, this condition is like a TIA except that the signs persist for longer than 24 hours. Reversal is usually evident within 48 hours. Multiple small infarctions may occur over a period of years with complete recovery. Usually the same area of the brain is involved, commonly a result of arteriosclerotic carotid artery stenosis. The definition of this syndrome may be of little clinical value, because in reality the patient may be experiencing a stroke-in-evolution (Mohr, Gautier, & Pessin, 1992).

Brain Attack (Stroke)-in-Evolution

This progressive stroke may also result from emboli or hemorrhage. Generally, large-artery disease exists. Symptoms develop stepwise over a period of hours or days until permanent deficits are manifested, although the more common pattern is for the entire syndrome to evolve over a period of more than 24 hours. The symptoms may occur without change for a varied length of time. As the stroke progresses, the symptoms become more severe and the deficits may extend to a much greater degree. The patient may have remained at home during this phase, coming to the hospital only when the symptoms continue to worsen or do not resolve.

Completed Brain Attack (Stroke)

This produces a stable syndrome of neurological deficits within a short time from the beginning of the attack. It may have reached this point within minutes or may take longer than 3 days for the neurons to die from delayed metabolic factors or cerebral edema. Approximately 60% of thrombotic strokes occur during sleep. When a completed stroke occurs, which is common, the full impact of the damage is exhibited on first awakening. Most patients survive the initial insult; the mortality is 30 to 40%. The poorest prognosis exists with infarctions of the brainstem and cerebellum. Clinical findings vary according to the location. They may include deviation of the eyes, pupillary changes, gaze paralysis, and various hemisensory deficits. When the cerebellum is affected, there is severe ataxia, the cerebrospinal fluid is bloody in 90% of cases, and immediate mortality is high.

The dominance or nondominance of the hemisphere involved also affects the manifestations. The speech center is usually in the dominant hemisphere. More than 90% of the population is right-handed, which indicates that the left cerebrum is dominant. More than half of the left-handed people also have the speech center on the left. When it is determined in which cerebral hemisphere damage has occurred, general assumptions regarding deficits can be made.

Signs and Symptoms of Stroke According to the Involved Vessel or Hemisphere

The presenting signs and symptoms of stroke depend on the extent and location of the insult. Middle cerebral artery syndrome is by far the most common of all cerebral occlusions. If the main stem of the middle cerebral artery is occluded, a massive infarction of most of the hemisphere results. Initially, there may be vomiting and a rapid onset of coma; the coma may last a few weeks. The anterior cervical artery is least often occluded. If the occlusion occurs proximal to a patent anterior communicating artery, the blood supply will not be compromised. If the occlusion is distal, or if the communicating artery is inadequate, there will be infarction of the medial aspect of one frontal lobe. Bilateral medial frontal lobe infarction occurs if one anterior cervical artery is occluded and the other artery is small and dependent on blood flow. Cerebral edema is extensive.

Occlusion of the vessel within the vertebrobasilar system produces unique syndromes. The vertebral and basilar arteries and their branches supply the brainstem and cerebellum. The posterior cerebral arteries are the terminal branches of the basilar artery and supply the medial temporal and occipital lobes, as well as part of the corpus callosum.

Occlusion of the anterior cerebellar artery is also known as the *lateral inferior pontine syndrome*. Symptoms of the anterior inferior cerebellar artery syndrome include vertigo, nausea, vomiting, tinnitus, and nystagmus.

Few strokes involve the posterior cerebral artery. The usual consequence of the superficial occlusion of a posterior cerebral artery is contralateral homonymous hemianopia. If the penetrating branches are occluded, the cerebral peduncle, thalamus, and upper brainstem are involved. There is wide variation in the manifestations of the syndrome. If the thalamus is involved, there is sensory loss of all modalities; spontaneous pain; intentional tremors; and mild hemiparesis. If the cerebral peduncle is involved, Weber's syndrome (oculomotor nerve palsy with contralateral hemiplegia) occurs. If the brainstem is involved, there are deficits involving conjugate gaze, nystagmus, and pupillary abnormalities, with the other possible symptoms of ataxia and postural tremors.

When a cerebral artery is occluded by a thrombus or embolus, classic syndromes are said to develop, although in reality, syndromes frequently overlap one another rather than appearing in their "pure" form. Table 20–3 compares the signs and symptoms when the carotid and vertebrobasilar circulation are compromised. In addition to these signs and symptoms, there are common findings associated with the side of the brain that is involved. The patient who has a left-sided CVA has signs and symptoms different from those in the person who has a right-sided CVA. The

TABLE 20–3 ■ **SIGNS AND SYMPTOMS OF STROKE**

Carotid Region	Vertebrobasilar Region
Impaired gait	Pain in face, nose, or eye
Abulia (inability to perform acts voluntarily or make decisions)	Ipsilateral numbness and weakness of face
Flat affect, lack of spontaneity, slowness, distractibility, and lack of interest in surroundings	Dizziness
Mental impairment, such as perseveration and amnesia	Clumsiness
Paralysis of contralateral face, arm, and leg	Quadriplegia
Sensory deficits of contralateral face, arm, and leg	Weakness of facial, tongue, and pharyngeal muscles
Aphasia, if dominant hemisphere is involved	Possibly, "locked-in" syndrome
Apraxia, agnosia, and unilateral neglect, if nondominant hemisphere is involved	Paresis of lateral conjugate gaze
	Horner's syndrome
Contralateral homonymous hemianopia	Cerebellar signs (ataxia, nystagmus)
Urinary incontinence (usually lasts for weeks)	Impaired pain and temperature sensation in trunk and limbs (may also involve face)
Looking toward side of lesion	Nausea and vomiting
Mild Horner's syndrome	Loss of pain and temperature sensation on contralateral side of trunk and limbs
	Several visual deficits, such as color blindness, lack of depth perception, failure to see objects that are not centrally located, visual hallucinations
	Memory deficits
	Perseveration
	Dysphasia and dysarthria

From Burrell, K., Gerlach, M. J., & Pless, B. (Eds.). (1997). *Adult nursing: Acute and community care* (2nd ed.). Stanford, CT: Appleton & Lange; and Hickey, J. (1992). *The clinical practice of neurological and neurosurgical nursing* (3rd ed.). Philadelphia: J. B. Lippincott.

person with a left-sided CVA generally has visual deficits, impulsive behavior, right-sided weakness, spatial impairment, decreased insight into deficits, and sensory loss. The person with a right-sided CVA has speech and language deficits, slow and cautious behavior, left-sided weakness, sensory loss, and motor planning problems.

ASSESSMENT OF PATIENTS WITH ALL TYPES OF BRAIN ATTACKS (STROKES)

To determine the extent of deficits, one must obtain a complete history of any previous vascular events and the general state of health. Assessment must also include physical and neuropsychological examinations. The patient may not be able to provide accurate information; therefore, a reliable family member may be the historian to provide the necessary information. The elements of a historical assessment are listed in Table 20–4.

During the acute admission, the history taking is brief and focused on the current symptoms, any history of TIAs, and other diagnosed conditions. The purpose of this history is to provide enough information to

facilitate emergency treatment. Once the patient is stabilized, a second, detailed history is taken to enlarge and corroborate the database obtained during the acute admission. This second history includes a review of information about the present episode because information may have been forgotten by the patient or family during the acute admission. Questions should be carefully worded so that

TABLE 20–4 ■ **HISTORICAL ELEMENTS OF THE PATIENT WITH A BRAIN ATTACK**

Patient and/or family history of hypertension, coronary heart disease, diabetes, thyroid disease, valvular heart disease, atherosclerosis, stroke, seizures, vascular disease, transient ischemic attacks

Presence of risk factors: smoking, use of excessive alcohol, illegal drugs, birth control pills

Present episode: time of onset of symptoms, number and pattern of previous attacks, loss of consciousness, changes in mood or behavior, changes in speech and other neurological deficits, current medications, recent acute medical and/or surgical illness, concurrent illness, presence of pain

Social and family constellation: financial arrangements, recent losses, family aggregation, primary relationships, community activities, hobbies, work and leisure activities the patient or family can provide concise information in relation to the CVA. For example, questions should be asked in a manner that helps the patient or family to distinguish among seizures, syncopal episodes, and the symptoms of a TIA. Seizures and syncopal episodes may or may not be related to the onset of the stroke; however, they need to be evaluated because they may herald other important medical problems that need to be investigated. Additionally, this is a good time to assess the coping skills of family members and give them any information that will help them understand the situation. The family members should also be apprised of the patient's prognosis as it is known at the time.

The physical assessment should be done serially to ensure that every system is included in the assessment, and all systems should be assessed, with particular focus on the nervous and cardiovascular systems. The initial physical assessment begins with an evaluation of the level of consciousness, airway patency and respiration, and safety measures. The vital signs are monitored and a neurological examination is done. Symptoms suspected of being caused by ischemia must be evaluated and other causes ruled out. A rapid serial assessment, often called a "neuro check," is instituted, mainly to identify a rapid decline that indicates an increase in intracranial pressure. The first neurological check is considered to be the baseline assessment; changes from this baseline are documented and the physician notified if necessary.

A neurological examination is an assessment of the status of the nervous system; this assessment must establish both anatomical and functional status. Data are collected on reflex activity, functional status, and cognitive function. These assessments are repeated frequently for the first few days after a stroke but are then tapered as the patient becomes consistently more stable. Evaluation of cognitive and physical functioning is important to determine the resolution of the brain damage suffered during the brain attack. Evaluation of function determines when the stroke is completed. Also, it is necessary to monitor the progress of rehabilitation and the return of function as the nervous system heals. The elements of a physical examination are found in Table 20–5.

In addition to the physical assessment, Black and Matassarin-Jacobs (1997) suggest that neuropsychological assessment also be carried out and include the following areas:

TABLE 20–5 ■ ELEMENTS OF A PHYSICAL ASSESSMENT

Cardiac examination: Include all major vessels for pulse pressure and bruits; heart for murmurs, enlargement, arrhythmias

Chest and lungs: Include breath sounds, quality and depth of respirations, adventitious sounds, dullness

Vital signs: Blood pressure (include right and left measurement, attention to all three positions), temperature, respirations

Neurological examination: Include all cranial nerves, fundoscopy, range of motion and mobility, motor strength, sensation, balance, abnormal movements, reflexes and pathological reflexes, mental status, speech, bowel and bladder function

Skin integrity: General and areas of dependent pressure, edema, rashes

Pain: Presence, location, and effects of drug therapy and comfort measures

(1) level of consciousness, (2) orientation, (3) memory, (4) mood and affect, (5) intellectual performance, (6) judgment and insight, and (7) language and communication. Although some of these functions can be monitored in daily interaction with the patient, it is difficult to obtain reliable results without the use of mental status examinations that can be performed serially and used consistently.

DIAGNOSTIC STUDIES

Diagnostic studies are paramount to the management of a patient who has had a brain attack. The goals of initial studies are to confirm that the patient has had a stroke, to determine the extent of the stroke, and to determine if the patient has had an ischemic or a hemorrhagic brain attack so that appropriate therapy can begin. Additional testing should be performed to rule out other types of abnormality that may complicate treatment and patient outcomes. Testing can also monitor the patient's response to treatment and can determine the prognosis. With these diagnostic expectations, the following tests may be appropriate for the patient:

- Chest x-ray will detect an enlarged heart.
- Cranial computed tomography (CT) with a contrast medium, commonly used, will outline the extent of cerebral damage and detect the presence of hemorrhage or other space-occupying lesions. A CT scan is most useful in identifying hemorrhagic stroke. It is extremely accurate in assessing the location and extent of damage caused by blood collecting in the subarachnoid space or

within the brain substance. These areas show up in CT images as areas of higher density. CT scans do have some limitations. The CT scan is not as precise in assessing the location and extent of damage in ischemic strokes as in hemorrhagic strokes. Even large ischemic strokes do not show up for several hours. They also cannot differentiate between embolic and thrombotic occlusions. This procedure is noninvasive.

- Magnetic resonance imaging can visualize infarcts and detect the extent of ischemic damage not seen on CT. The data available from magnetic resonance imaging combine high sensitivity with excellent spatial resolution. Magnetic resonance imaging can distinguish between infarcted and ischemic tissue. This procedure is noninvasive.

- Positron-emission tomography shows a larger area of metabolic dysfunction than is possible on CT and can identify how different parts of the brain are metabolizing glucose and oxygen after injury. The patient is injected with a radiographic oxyglucose. The isotope emits activity in the form of positrons, which are scanned and converted into an image by computer. The image is displayed in color. The more active a given part of the brain, the greater the glucose uptake. One problem at present is that radioisotopes have such a short life that there must be a cyclotron on the premises to prepare them, which limits the number of medical centers able to offer the test. This is an invasive procedure.

- Cerebral angiography (arteriography) illuminates cerebral circulation by injecting contrast medium into an artery (usually the femoral) and taking x-ray films sequentially as the contrast medium flows with the blood to visualize carotid, vertebral, and cerebral circulations. The purpose is to diagnose vascular aneurysms, malformations, displacements, and occluded or leaking vessels. Arteriography is an invasive procedure. There are two types of arteriography:

  □ *Contrast medium method*: Contrast medium (usually 40 to 50 mL) is injected, and a series of x-ray films is taken automatically as the contrast material moves through the circulation.

  □ *Digital subtraction method*: A large angiocatheter is threaded into the brachial vein (usually) and positioned in the superior vena cava near the right atrium. Intravenous fluid is given via catheter. An initial film is taken; the image is placed in a computer to be used as a reference for the subsequent images. The contrast medium is injected. As subsequent images appear on the screen and are transferred to the computer, the original reference image is subtracted from the later images, producing a heightened image. Although not quite as satisfactory as the contrast method because details may not be as clear, digital subtraction angiography is the best choice for some patients.

MEDICAL TREATMENT IN THE ACUTE PHASE

Thrombolytic therapy is the currently accepted medical treatment of an ischemic stroke. This therapy uses a thrombolytic agent to dissolve a clot and restore circulation to an ischemic portion of the brain. In 1994, a panel of the American Heart Association Stroke Council wrote guidelines on the management of patients with acute ischemic stroke. They cautioned against the use of the thrombolytic drugs because of the high rate of intracranial bleeding that continued to complicate their use. However, in 1996, the Food and Drug Administration approved the first thrombolytic drug to be used specifically for brain attack—recombinant tissue plasminogen activator (r-TPA [Activase]) or urokinase (Brott, 1996). r-TPA has been shown to improve the outcome after a stroke when given within 3 hours of the onset of stroke. The benefit of the administration of r-TPA for an ischemic stroke beyond 3 hours from the onset of symptoms is not established. Additionally, this drug is not recommended for treatment if the time of onset of the stroke cannot be reliably ascertained, including strokes recognized on awakening. Thrombolytic therapy is not recommended unless the diagnosis of ischemic stroke can be made by a physician with expertise in the diagnosis of stroke and CT of the brain confirms the diagnosis. If CT demonstrates edema or hemorrhage, thrombolytic therapy should be avoided. The major complication with the administration of a thrombolytic agent is the potential for hemorrhage. If an artery has ruptured and a clot has formed, thereby preventing further blood loss, a thrombolytic agent may dissolve the clot. Once the clot has been dissolved, it no longer acts as a plug and the patient may hemorrhage.

Thrombolytic agents reduce an occlusion by activating the conversion of plasminogen to plasmin, the enzyme that breaks down clots (Macabasco & Hickman, 1995). The plasmin lyses fibrin and releases fibrin degradation products, which inhibit clot formation.

SURGICAL TREATMENT

In general, surgery is considered a mode of prevention rather than a specific treatment after a stroke. The surgical techniques for brain attack prevention are carotid endarterectomy (CEA) and extracranial-intracranial (EC-IC) bypass. A decision to operate is influenced by the risk/benefit ratio in a specific surgical candidate. The probability of a positive outcome for the patient should be determined before the operation is attempted. A number of risk factors must be considered, such as age, the general state of health, chronic health conditions, and previous ischemic incidents. The patient's age, however, should not be a determining factor in the decision to perform an operation. CEA appears to be most beneficial in appropriately chosen symptomatic patients. Medical and surgical factors that increase the risk of surgery must also enter into the decision whether to perform CEA or to treat the patient medically.

Surgery for vertebrobasilar insufficiency is performed occasionally and with some increasing frequency, but the precise indications for its use and proof of its efficacy remain to be determined. Carotid atherosclerosis commonly occurs in asymptotic elderly patients, and an anatomical irregularity in itself is not an indication for surgical therapy (Fisher, 1995). Despite the unproven nature of surgical therapy, it is frequently the only option in caring for symptomatic patients threatened with the risk of stroke.

Surgical procedures to reperfuse the ischemic area, such as angioplasty, embolectomy, recanalization, and evacuation of hemorrhagic material, are performed when other treatments are less likely to have a positive outcome.

Carotid Endarterectomy

At the present time, a CEA of symptomatic common carotid bifurcation lesions offers the most direct and efficient mechanism for removing the source of cerebral emboli and for restoring blood flow when a lesion produces a critical stenosis. The decision to perform CEA must rely on an accurate correlation of clinical symptomatology and angiographic findings.

The primary indication for CEA is the angiographic demonstration of a stenotic or ulcerated lesion in the extracranial carotid artery that is compatible with the patient's cerebrovascular symptomatology. The symptoms most often seen are transient monocular blindness, carotid distribution TIAs, prolonged reversible ischemic neurological deficits, and mild to moderate fixed neurological deficits. These symptoms are found in a spectrum of diseases. The decision to do a CEA is based on the hope that the outcome of the surgery will be to prevent a devastating stroke. The specific risk of stroke in an individual patient should be determined. Those patients at greatest risk, including patients with TIAs, stuttering stroke symptomatology, or an acute onset of mild to moderate neurological deficit, should be evaluated on an urgent basis. Patients having infrequent cerebral episodes are at unknown risk but should be evaluated without undue delay. The evaluation of each patient should include an assessment of surgical risk factors for CEA. The decision to do surgery is often made on a clinical basis because there is no noninvasive test that can reliably detect all the conditions that are responsible for cerebral symptomatology. Cerebral angiography is the only reliable study that will accurately demonstrate extracranial and intracranial vascular lesions and therefore must be performed on a person displaying symptoms rather than waiting to do a series of inconclusive noninvasive testing.

The indications for surgical therapy in those with asymptomatic cervical bruits and asymptomatic angiographic lesions associated with carotid artery stenosis are controversial (Fisher, 1995).

The long-term outcome of CEA is difficult to evaluate. Wide variation in the severity of preoperative neurological deficits and the natural history of improvement of stroke without treatment make it difficult to assess the role of endarterectomy in neurological recovery. In selected patients with mild, stable strokes, CEA appears to lower the incidence of recurrent strokes and may be responsible for improvement in neurological function beyond that expected from the natural course of the disease. CEA is effective in relieving the symptoms of TIAs and in lowering the incidence of stroke in selected patients. Symptomatic patients who have less than 30% narrowing of the internal lumen of the carotid artery do not benefit from surgery (Glaser, 1997) The effect of CEAs on survival rates of surgical patients compared with control patients is controversial; however, it is believed that if CEA helps to prevent stroke, the quality of life is significantly improved.

Extracranial-Intracranial Bypass Surgery

A number of significant atherosclerotic lesions responsible for cerebral ischemia involve the internal carotid artery at sites inaccessible to extracranial surgical approaches. Although many of these lesions are generally insignificant, they are at risk for occlusion by emboli from other sources. These emboli occlude vessels and obstruct blood flow to the cerebral hemispheres.

During the past 2 decades, neurosurgeons have developed increasingly sophisticated microvascular surgical techniques that should logically lead to the effective treatment of cerebrovascular lesions previously not amenable to surgical correction. The most popular of these operations has been the EC-IC arterial bypass procedure. When successful, this procedure has added collateral blood flow and has been demonstrated to be capable of returning diminished cerebral flow and deranged cerebral oxidative metabolism to normal. However, the natural history of specific anatomical cerebral vascular lesions is poorly understood, and the indications for EC-IC bypass remain to be fully defined. Clear indications for this operation exist only in certain cases of vascular trauma or surgically planned vascular occlusion, where the augmentation of blood supply to the brain by an EC-IC anastomosis may provide an added degree of safety. This technique has been successfully used in the treatment of giant aneurysms at the base of the skull and arteriovenous malformations. Although it remains logical to assume that some patients will require added blood flow to diminish the risk of stroke, this procedure has been used with caution in the management of TIAs and other cerebral symptomology. It is usual to treat this patient as any other craniotomy patient. Therefore, the patient is maintained on anticoagulants for 3 to 6 months after surgery (Hickey, 1997).

NURSING APPROACHES TO CARE

The patient experiencing a stroke will require intense nursing care for long periods of time. The goals of care and the nursing responsibilities will change as the patient progresses from the acute phase to the rehabilitation phase. The care needs of the patient depend on the deficits that are manifested. The functional deficits exhibited by the patient depend on the part of the brain that has been injured. Although brain cells do not reproduce in the adult, there are some dynamic characteristics that make it possible to use techniques that facilitate recovery to a greater or lesser degree.

Several programs exist, such as the Bobath System and the Motor Relearning Program (Carr & Shepherd, 1991). These programs provide the rationale and methods that support the nursing care and management of the person who has had a stroke during the acute and rehabilitation phases. The Bobath principle, or neurodevelopmental therapeutic approach, and the Motor Relearning Program build on the ideas that because of the plasticity properties of the brain, relearning can occur after the brain is damaged. Three theories of brain plasticity are as follows:

1. The level of excitability of nerve cells is changeable. Thus, when a cell dies, the remaining cells function more efficiently.
2. When neural connections are impaired, there is degeneration of inhibitions that had previously masked unused connections that were laid down in excess in the embryo; this unmasking provides avenues for impulses through damaged areas.
3. Although the damaged nerve cannot regenerate itself, it appears that collateral sprouting occurs. This theory suggests that previously unconnected axons develop attachments to the dendrites of cells deprived of input because of cell deaths, providing new input. This sprouting is described as similar to the growth that takes place during learning (Bachman, 1992).

Both the Motor Relearning Program and the neurodevelopmental approach build on the theory that the brain can be retrained and that previously impaired function can be restored when the brain is reprogrammed to transfer function to different areas. This restoration can be accomplished through specific positioning and patterned exercise of normal automatic postural reactions. The recovery process from the stroke is linear, with each new action building on the previous behavior. Therefore, the function is restored by stimulating basic motions. Once the basic motions are restored, they can be used to support the next level of functioning. The return of function may not be possible for all stroke patients; however, even minimal improvement can contribute to the patient's quality of life.

If any aspect of posture, tone, movement, or function is abnormal, all other components of motor function are modified negatively and the patient cannot compensate for the deficits. Because of the inability to compensate for a loss of function, each movement must be analyzed so that future activity will be normalized for this patient. The process is cyclical. For example, during the acute phase, the nurse focuses first on normal bed posture to obtain adequate tone before movement can be expected. Movement is necessary for the development of the ability to function, which once again affects posture (Borgman & Passarella, 1991).

When organizing the principles of nursing care, it is helpful to divide nursing treatment into phases that reflect the type of care needed at a particular point in the disease process. The first phase is the acute phase, and the presenting symptoms reflect the initial insult to the brain, which is generally a medical emergency. During this phase, care is directed at the need for immediate emergency attention and is prescribed by the nature of the symptoms. As the patient begins to recover, the focus of care shifts from life support to the recovery of normal functioning or adaptation to the existing deficits, which occurs during the rehabilitation phase. The underlying principle of care in both phases is that rehabilitation must begin as soon as the patient is diagnosed with a stroke. The care that is provided during the acute phase must be based on rehabilitation principles so that the patient recovers from this phase with the preservation of function that will support the rehabilitation phase.

ACUTE PHASE

Nursing Care

When the patient begins to exhibit the signs and symptoms of a brain attack the patient is admitted to the hospital, generally through the emergency room. The patient may then be admitted to an intensive care unit or a special stroke unit. The goal of nursing care during this phase is the maintenance of vital functions to ensure the patient's survival. The patient may die during the initial emergency event or may begin to stabilize. Once the patient's vital functions have been stabilized and survival is apparent, nursing care is di-

rected at maintaining a steady state and preventing complications that can hamper recovery and interfere with the rehabilitation process. This phase may last for 1 to 2 days, or longer in severe cases. The patient is most commonly unconscious during this time and begins to slowly regain consciousness as the physiological functions are stabilized. When the patient regains consciousness or has been conscious from the onset of symptoms, the patient will be very confused and frightened. The confusion and fear are compounded by the changes in mental status resulting from the loss of normal cognitive function. The loss of motor function is very upsetting to the patient who does not understand the changes in perception and motor ability. The nurse must be aware of the cognitive changes and confusion that occur in every patient who has had a stroke.

Psychological Support

An essential component of nursing care must be the provision of psychological support for the patient and family members, who are in a state of shock related to the dramatic event. This is a challenge when the patient is unable to communicate. The emphasis in psychological support is the provision of information through an open channel of communication. The nurse must provide information to the patient and help the patient express feelings and concerns by using the cognitive, sensory, and motor function that remain. Family members must be informed, and this is particularly important when the patient's level of consciousness is altered. At this time, family members are in particular need of much psychological support and education.

Physiological Monitoring

During the acute phase, the patient is placed on extensive monitoring. All systems are monitored so that vital functions can be kept within the normal ranges, with the major attention paid to the cardiovascular and respiratory systems, as well as renal function. When vital functions are maintained within normal ranges, normal function is likely to be the desired outcome. Fluid and electrolyte balance is a critical component of the monitoring agenda. The patient is frequently assessed for neurological deficits to identify changes in neurological function.

Nurses should be aware that patients with left-hemisphere damage recover more readily than those with right-hemisphere damage. This an important fact to process as the nursing care plan is developed, because the patient with left-hemisphere damage and resulting motor impairment is generally more severely affected than the patient with right-hemisphere damage. If nurses are not aware of the differences in function or recovery, the tendency is to underestimate the ability of the left-hemisphere–damaged patient because of aphasia and to overestimate capabilities of patients with right-hemisphere damage because they are cheerful and eager to try and they believe that they can do anything. It is easy to give the patient with right-hemisphere damage too much freedom, which can result in a fall or high-risk behavior.

Support Return to Independence

A basic goal of treatment is to support the return of independence in the patients. Therefore, the nurses must always foster the independence that the patient is capable of demonstrating. The nurse should also encourage family members to encourage independence in the patient by allowing the patient to do tasks, even though it may take a much longer time and the struggle may cause a great deal of emotional pain in the family member witnessing the activity. The nurse and family members need to have the patience necessary to allow the patient to make mistakes, recognize the errors, and try to correct them. Nurses can guide and assist and take over a task when it becomes apparent that the patient cannot handle it. Praise for any step accomplished is given readily, just as correction for inappropriate actions is given. It is extremely important for nurses not to become frustrated when the patient must start at the same point over and over. Perceptual and spatial deficits take time to overcome and require constant practice.

Rehabilitation Principles

The rehabilitation principles that need to be started from the time of admission are those that maintain proper positioning and those that reduce spasticity and the disability that results from spasticity.

Positioning

From the onset of the stroke, positioning is a nursing priority. A specific plan is necessary for each patient so that the patient's remaining function is maximized. Positioning involves more than raising or lowering the head to prevent changes in intracranial pressure, stabilizing blood pressure, or turning the patient from side to side to prevent respiratory complications and skin breakdown. In a patient with a stroke, the neurological deficits quickly result in physical disabilities. In order to minimize the progression of long-term disabilities, careful attention is given to positioning the affected limbs, particularly the hip and shoulder joints, 24 hours a day; this provides the patient with a chance of returning to normal living by reducing spasticity and the subsequent development of contractures.

Neurogenic shock begins with the onset of hemiplegia; the affected muscles are flaccid because of a loss of reflex activity. As the shock resolves, over a period of days to weeks, depending on the degree of neural damage, reflex activity begins to return, some degree of muscle tone develops, and spasticity usually occurs. As the patient begins to recover, the spasticity can be diminished if the patient receives rehabilitation treatment that involves stretching, weight bearing, range-of-motion exercises, and the maintenance of normal posture. The patient with hemiplegia has four problems: (1) a loss of balance on the affected side, (2) sensory disturbance that inhibits movement, (3) developing extensor spasticity, and (4) loss of precision movements. Additional changes or variables may include (1) the head laterally flexed toward the affected side but rotated away from the affected side, (2) internal rotation of the leg, and (3) hip and knee extension (Borgman & Passarella, 1991; Gee & Shandera, 1985). The rehabilitation goals that are geared toward maintaining function and supporting the return of function are to

- Normalize muscle tone through proper positioning, weight bearing, trunk rotation, and carefully graded stimulation
- Facilitate normal movements
- Provide sensory experiences
- Facilitate normal automatic postural reactions
- Avoid effort that results in untoward reactions

These goals are achieved through the use of positioning principles, stretching, and range-of-motion exercises. Specific positioning begins when the patient is first placed in a bed, and attention is paid to positioning when the patient begins sitting and walking.

Principles for Bed Positioning

Principles for bed positioning include the following:

- Position the spine in alignment
- Position the hips straight without rotation
- Position the upper extremities away from the body
- Support the superior extremities when the patient is side-lying
- Keep the knee joints flexed 15 degrees when the patient is supine
- Turn the patient from side to side and prone on a scheduled basis
- Support the head and slightly flex the neck
- Teach quadriceps and gluteal setting exercises to strengthen muscles for better gait retraining

Principles for Positioning in Sitting Balance

Principles for positioning in sitting balance include the following:

- Teach the patient to evenly distribute weight on both buttocks
- Teach the patient to keep the feet flat on the floor and close together
- Teach the patient to keep the spine in alignment with the shoulders over the hips and the head balanced on level shoulders
- Nurse should adjust the position frequently to maintain proper alignment
- Nurse should enhance sitting balance by keeping the head of the bed rolled high; frequent upright positions help overcome vasomotor deficits, which lead to dizziness and orthostatic hypotension

Principles for Positioning in Standing Balance

Standing balance is learned using assistive devices such as walkers, four-point canes, splints, braces, and slings to help the patient accomplish this goal. Principles for positioning in standing balance include teaching the patient to

- Position the feet a few inches apart
- Position the hips in front of the ankles
- Position the shoulders over the hips
- Keep the head balanced over the shoulders
- Keep the spine straight

Passive Stretching

In addition to positioning, passive stretching and range-of-motion exercises should be begun as soon as the patient's condition is stabilized. Each joint is moved regularly through its full range of motion in a careful, slow, and steady manner. Jerky or rapid movements are avoided because they provoke spasticity. The extremities need support, and to prevent joint dislocation, traction should not be applied. Dislocation occurs easily in a paralyzed limb. When the affected arm and leg are being moved, the elbow and ankle are supported below the joints to prevent traction on the shoulder and hip, respectively, and also to prevent friction burns caused by rubbing against the sheet during exercises. The hand and wrist may be kept in extension with the thumb abducted by a splint that keeps the extremity in anatomically correct positioning and reduces spasticity. No transient pressure should be applied to the palm (i.e., hand roll) because it provokes a spastic grasp reflex and increases tone in the hand, resulting in a contracted fist. Excessive stress, effort, and fatigue are prevented because each can precipitate spastic responses. The nurse reinforces the practice of activities exactly as they were taught in therapy, always encouraging weight bearing and proper positioning of the affected side.

Care for the prevention of problems may extend for months. The hazards of immobility must always be considered, from the onset of neurological deficits through the long-term care, and measures to maintain and regain normal function should be ongoing.

The nursing care should include activities and reminders that focus the patient's attention on the affected side with the goal of helping the patient to become a bilaterally functioning individual again. This approach is used during positioning and practices that involve the overlearning of functional movements and automatic posture reactions (procedural memory) to regain normal muscle tone, posture, movement, and function.

Until the 1980s, treatment used an approach that focused on the movement of the unaffected side and had little expectation for function of the affected side. The patient was taught to compensate for the functional disabilities of the affected side by increasing the movement of the functioning side. The strain produced by the excessive effort in the unaffected side intensified spasticity in the affected side. Proper posture and balance were inhibited, fear of falling could never be overcome, and little or no functional movement was encouraged in the affected side. The affected limbs were traditionally supported, braced, or placed in slings, limiting any residual activity. Although a certain degree of function can be accomplished through compensatory learning to "do for" the affected side, the approach suggested that there were limited expectations for the return of function of the affected side and that there was a limited period of time during which the patient had any hope of improvement. It was suggested that no improvement could be expected 6 months after the stroke.

On the other hand, the therapeutic approach used from the rehabilitative perspective offers continued hope and reason to try to persevere for the patient with a stroke. The positive attitude that the patient will relearn gives not only the patient but also the family higher expectations.

REHABILITATION PHASE

Rehabilitation Principles

The goal of rehabilitation is to help the patient reach that person's maximal level of functioning. Care is provided by interdisciplinary health team members who develop a plan of care that ensures the quality of rehabilitation so that the patient can reach maximal functioning or maintain residual function. There are a number of principles that underlie a program that ensures successful outcomes for the patient. These include the following:

- Rehabilitation should be started as soon as the patient is medically stable, which is usually 24 to 36 hours after the acute care admission. This should involve the principles of positioning. The patient should be getting out of bed and standing a day or so after vital signs are stable.
- A positive mental attitude should be fostered by encouragement toward normal activities and interests. Encouragement should begin from the time of admission in order to prevent a secondary mental deterioration.
- The program plan should include a clinical pathway for all patients so care will be consistent. The general program plan is concerned with the way the patient spends the day and the type of treatments that the patient will receive. The pathway also needs to be flexible enough allow the addition of specific plans for particular problems. Specific treatments are planned for each person's needs and may include a motor training program with a physical therapist and self-care management with an occupational therapist. The speech pathologist plans the means by which communication can be established and stimulated in a dysphasic patient. The psychologist plans programs for the management of cognitive and emotional changes. General relaxation training may need to be organized for the anxious or tense patient.

- The patient should be active, both physically and mentally, for most of the day and must not spend long periods doing nothing, in isolated or depressing surroundings. Restriction of activity is known to cause impaired intellectual functioning. The patient's day is planned, therefore, to avoid both helplessness and disorientation in time and place. Activities are planned carefully so they are enjoyable and not passive or meaningless. They should stimulate cognitive functioning and require from the patient responses to challenges similar to those the patient would normally receive in daily life.
- Consistency of practice is an important concept to the rehabilitation setting. The patient needs to be able to practice the behaviors developed in the therapy. Time spent in individual therapy sessions without further practice throughout the rest of the day should be considered time wasted. Additionally, if the patient is provided the opportunity to practice but the behaviors are practiced in a different and contradictory way to the original plan, the patient will not only be confused but will actually be prevented from regaining effective motor behavior.
- Motivation is critical to patient recovery. One of the objectives of the treatment plan is to provide an enriched physical and emotional environment that will motivate the patient toward recovery. It may be lacking if the patient is fearful, anxious, apathetic, or depressed. To benefit from and be involved in the rehabilitation program, the patient must be able to learn, and it is well known that little learning takes place in the absence of motivation. Many stroke patients need closer personal contact with staff than is usual in the hospital or rehabilitation setting in order to participate fully in their treatment program.

After a stroke, all patients have two major objectives: to walk and to use both hands. Part of the effectiveness of a rehabilitation program may be attributable to the motivating effect of the emphasis on directly training the patient for these tasks, in contrast to exercises and activities that are assumed by the therapist to carry over into function but that have no apparent relevance.

To make the best possible recovery, patients need to have people around them from whom they can draw courage. Nursing staff who are uncaring, silent, aloof, or too protective may actually prevent patients from tapping their personal resources. Patients need reassurance and encouragement. Positive reinforcement encourages patients to persist with the treatment plan and overcome the barriers with which they are surrounded. It is the therapeutic relationship, established between the nurse, the patient, and the family, that provides success through reward, positive reinforcement such as praise or an attitude of pleasure, and immediate feedback about a performance.

Success in treatment sessions has the added benefit of counteracting the tendency toward depression after stroke. As the patient is successful, the tendency for eager participation in rehabilitation leads to a more rapid development of skill.

Rehabilitation Program

After a stroke, once patients are stable and ready for an intense rehabilitation program they may be admitted to a stroke unit or a rehabilitation unit (a disability-oriented unit) or receive rehabilitation at home. The decision for placement is based on the patient's and family's resources, third-party payment, and the degree of disability. Regardless of the site of rehabilitation, the rehabilitation principles are the same. If rehabilitation occurs in a rehabilitation unit, the unit should be staffed with specially trained nurses and other health care workers who are members of an interdisciplinary team and experts in the management of the special needs of a patient with a stroke. Specialized stroke units are recommended for patients who have moderate to severe functional deficits. Stroke units have the advantage of providing the specialized care that ensures a better quality of patient care and improved patient outcome.

During the rehabilitation phase of care, nursing management begins with assessment on the admission of the patient and continues until the patient has reached the maximal level of functioning and has adapted successfully to this level, and the patient and family have learned treatment routines that may still be required. A comprehensive program may be begun, using many transdisciplinary health team members. The team generally consists of a physiatric physician, rehabilitation nurse, physical therapist, occupational therapist, social worker, and member of any other discipline that is necessary for the rehabilitation of the patient. The patient and family are also members of the team. In fact, they are the most important members because they need to agree to the plan if it is to be successful.

The patient's family must be aware of the patient's needs and participate actively in helping the patient reach the established goals. Unless the family has cohesiveness and caring for each member, with understanding of how to use each other's strengths and accommodate each other's limitations, the stress of attending to the needs of the patient as slow improvement occurs will overwhelm them. The nurse coordinating the patient's rehabilitative care is responsible for assessing these family needs and referring the members to the appropriate health care team members and support groups.

The plan is changed as the patient's needs change and new goals are set. In order to keep the plan up to date, frequent assessments are made by the members of the team with a focus on the area of their expertise. The assessments provide the information that is reviewed at transdisciplinary conferences. The transdisciplinary conferences are held to establish and evaluate interventions to be followed and supported by all. Patients and family members are included in the conferences. The patient's goals as well as the goals of the team are identified. The goals may reflect the patient's need to learn to communicate, walk, and use the hands, among other tasks. The team designs a treatment plan that states the interventions that will enable the patient to reach goals. The interventions must begin one step at a time. The treatment begins at a basic level and progresses to a higher level as soon as the patient is able. The patient continues to be monitored for progress and the development of any complications.

Rehabilitation Issues

As the rehabilitation treatment plan evolves for the patient, several issues must be taken into consideration. The patient assessment and evaluation should be conducted to review the following issues:

- Swallowing
- Total (urinary) incontinence; bowel incontinence

- Sensory/perceptual alterations
- Painful shoulder
- Spasticity
- Impaired speech and language
- Discharge planning
- Home care preparation
- Patient and family education
- Psychosocial preparation

Swallowing

Positioning the patient to facilitate the swallowing process is the most important element to be considered for successful and safe swallowing. The patent should eat all meals sitting in a chair or sitting straight up in bed. The patient's head and neck are positioned slightly forward and flexed to open the airway and avoid aspiration. Generally, patients with swallowing problems are able to tolerate or swallow soft or semisoft foods and fluids better than thin liquids or table food. The feeding should begin with instructing the patient to place food in the back of the mouth on the unaffected side to prevent trapping food in the affected cheek. This technique can also prevent aspiration. The patient should be taught to sweep the affected cheek with the tongue to prevent food pocketing in the affected cheek.

Some patients are able to swallow without difficulty, but because they are easily distracted and impulsive, they are at risk for aspiration. These patients require a distraction-free environment with minimal disruption from television, visitors, or other environmental noise. The nurse needs to keep the patient's head facing forward and focused on the act of eating. The nurse observes the patient for indications of fatigue, as this can significantly interfere with the desire and ability to eat.

Total (Urinary) Incontinence; Bowel Incontinence

Urinary incontinence occurs in 75% of patients with completed brain attack, but most are able to achieve continence within 3 to 6 months. Those that do not achieve continence by this time frequently do so within the next 6 months. Reaching the goal of continence and the independence it brings requires the development of an intense bowel and bladder training program that should be followed by every member of the treatment team, starting immediately after stabilization while in the acute phase. Incontinence has been deter-

mined to be a good predictor of outcome, because it reflects disturbance in the frontal lobes, brainstem, cerebellum, basal ganglia, thalamus, hypothalamus, and limbic system (areas that control voiding and social continence) rather than a focal deficit. Patients with cognitive deficits in memory, problem solving, and orientation to time need the greatest number of nursing measures and take the longest time to improve in the area of bladder training (Owen, Getz, & Bulla, 1995).

Patients may be incontinent of urine and stool owing to an altered level of consciousness, cognitive deficits, muscle weakness, or the inability to communicate the need to urinate or defecate. Before beginning a training program to correct these problems, the nurse must first establish the cause or causes. To begin a bladder training program, the nurse places the patient on the bedpan or commode, or offers the urinal, every 2 hours. Unless it is contraindicated, the nurse encourages the patient to have a total fluid intake of 2000 mL or more per day. If the patient is given a substantial amount of fluids, the use of the bathroom is imperative so that the patient can empty the bladder before incontinence occurs.

Before establishing a bowel training program, the nurse determines the patient's normal time for bowel elimination and any routine that helps to ensure an acceptable evacuation. If possible, this routine is followed, and the patient is placed on the bedpan or commode at the same time as normal evacuation occurs. A diet high in bulk and fiber is provided. The nurse encourages the patient to drink apple or prune juice to help promote bowel elimination.

Sensory/Perceptual Alterations

The sensory/perceptual changes depend on the part of the brain that has been damaged. Patients with right-hemisphere brain damage have difficulty with visual-perceptual or spatial-perceptual tasks. They have problems with depth and distance perception and with discriminating right from left or up from down. Because of these problems, they have difficulty performing routine activities of daily living. The nurse can help the patient adapt to these disabilities by using frequent verbal and tactile cues and by breaking tasks down into small steps. The patient should be approached from the nonaffected side. The patient who has experienced a stroke may have difficulties ambulating and may lack depth perception and proprioception. The nurse teaches the patient with visual field deficits to turn the head from side to side and scan with the eyes to compensate for the disability. Objects should be placed within the patient's field of vision; a mirror may be helpful to assist the patient to see more of the environment. If the patient has diplopia, a patch may be placed over the affected eye. The nurse ensures a safe environment by removing clutter from the room.

The patient with a left-hemisphere lesion generally experiences memory deficits and may show significant changes in the ability to carry out simple tasks. To assist the patient with memory problems, the nurse should reorient the patient to the month, year, day of the week, and circumstances surrounding admission to the hospital. The nurse establishes a routine or schedule for the patient that is structured, repetitive, and consistent. Information should be presented in a simple, concise manner. A step-by-step approach is often most effective because the patient can master one step before moving to the next. When possible, the family should bring in pictures and other objects that are familiar to the patient. The patient may be unable to plan and execute tasks in an organized manner. Typically, the patient exhibits a slow, cautious, and hesitant behavior. Neglect syndrome places the patient at additional risk for injury owing to an inability to recognize the physical impairment or to a lack of proprioception.

Painful Shoulder

A common impairment for the patient who has had a CVA is pain in the hemiplegic arm. It is the result of depressed motor activity around the shoulder and the surrounding musculature. The glenohumeral joint is not a stable joint, even when there is normal function. The loss of nervous control results in total instability. The instability that occurs when the joint is inactive causes a soft tissue injury with resultant pain, stiffness, and subluxation (Carr & Shepherd, 1991). There are four mechanical factors that may be responsible for the injury: (1) pinching of soft tissue against the acromion, (2) friction of soft tissue against bone, (3) traction of soft tissue, and (4) soft tissue contracture (Carr & Shepherd, 1991). The mechanical factors that cause painful shoulder are frequently iatrogenic and can occur during routine care and treatments as a result of pulling on the arm during dressing and activities of daily living. The shoulder

may also become subluxed when the arm is allowed to hang without support. Treatment is often ineffective, so preventive measures are important. Every staff member who has contact with the patient should be educated about the syndrome and the general measures that can prevent the problem. The staff members need to know how to support the arm and keep it supported at all times. Besides elevating the arm, the staff should be educated on the proper way to handle the arm—for example, how to dress the patient without pulling on the arm (Warlow, Dennis, van Gijn, Hankey, Sandercock, Bamford, & Wardlaw, 1996).

Another syndrome that frequently occurs in the hemiplegic arm is the shoulder-hand syndrome. The overall incidence of shoulder-hand syndrome is 41% (Ozer, Materson, & Caplan, 1994). In this syndrome, the shoulder is painful, especially on movement. Additionally, the forearm and hand are often swollen, red, and shiny. The most severe manifestation of this syndrome is reflex sympathetic dystrophy. The signs of this level of the syndrome reflect vasomotor instability such as erythema and sweating in addition to edema and pain. If these signs persist for a period of time, the skin, hair, and nails may become atrophic. The relationship between pain and edema remains unclear. The edema may result from a reduction in the drainage of fluid via lymphatics and veins from the hand, shoulder, or both. The edema tends to be most severe on the dorsum of the hand. The underlying process may be immobilization of the shoulder and hand, which limits the pumping action of movement and finger flexion that normally move fluids back into circulation.

Spasticity

Patients who have experienced a stroke may exhibit hypotonia and/or spasticity. The nurse performs passive range-of-motion exercises at least once during each shift for involved extremities and teaches the patient to do active range-of-motion exercises for the unaffected areas. Careful positioning is necessary to maintain proper alignment of the body and to decrease spasticity or increased muscle tone in flaccid extremities. The affected hand or lower leg may need splinting to prevent contractures. The nurse collaborates with therapists (physical and occupational) to determine the most appropriate positions for lying, sitting, and transferring from bed to chair. As soon as patients are able, they should begin to sit and ambulate. If the spasticity becomes progressively worse, the patient may need to be placed on medications such as diazepam (Valium) and baclofen to control spasticity.

A major complication of immobility that results from functional losses and spasticity is the development of deep vein thrombosis. If the nurse suspects the development of thrombosis, the physician should be notified and the findings documented in the patient's chart. Immobile patients should have weekly measurements of their thighs and calves; an abnormal increase in the size of the leg or a Homans' sign may indicate venous stasis.

Impaired Speech and Language

Language or speech problems are usually the result of a stroke involving the dominant hemisphere. In all but 15 to 20% of the population, the left cerebral hemisphere is the speech center. Language problems may be the result of aphasia, an inability to use or comprehend language or dysarthria; problems with the rate or rhythm of speech or with articulation. Although aphasia is caused by hemispheric damage, dysarthria is due to a loss of motor function to the tongue or muscles of speech.

Aphasia is classified as expressive, receptive, or global (mixed). An expressive (Broca's or motor) aphasia is due to damage in Broca's area of the frontal lobe. Broca's aphasia is a motor speech problem—the patient has not lost the ability to understand what is said but is unable to coordinate muscles controlling speech. This is also called *expressive aphasia*. More often, the patient exhibits language dysfunction in the areas of both expression and reception; this is known as a *global*, or *mixed*, *aphasia*. Broca's area is seen in Figure 20–1.

The receptive aphasic patient does not understand spoken or written language and usually requires repetitive directions to understand or complete a task. Each task should be broken down into component parts and given to the patient one step at a time. The nurse should face the client and speak slowly and clearly in order to give the patient a chance to understand what is being said. The patient should be given sufficient time to understand and process the information and to respond. The nurse encourages the patient to communicate, and when attempts are successful, positive reinforcement should be given for this behavior. Family members or

the nurse repeats the names of objects used on a scheduled basis. If necessary, a picture board or communication board should be developed for the patient who has Broca's aphasia. It consists of a picture of an activity, with the printed description below. The patient can point to the activity or object desired.

It is difficult to understand the patient who is dysarthic and has difficulty forming words. The same techniques used by the nurse for the patient with aphasia can be used for the individual with dysarthria. Facial muscle exercises may be performed to strengthen the muscles used for speech. Many patients who are dysarthric are also aphasic. The patient with communication impairments is usually referred to a speech-language pathologist.

Discharge Planning

Discharge planning implies that the patient will be returning home or to a community agency for care and follow-up. Many patients experience slight to moderate neurological dysfunction as the result of their stroke and are able to return home and live independently or with minimal support. Other patients are able to return home but require ongoing assistance with activities of daily living, as well as supervision to prevent accidents or injury. Speech, physical, or occupational therapy is conducted in the home or on an outpatient (ambulatory) basis. When patients are admitted to a rehabilitation or long-term care facility, they usually require continued or more complex nursing care, as well as extensive physical, occupational, recreational, and speech or cognitive therapy

Preparation for returning home involves a home visit for the patient to assess whether any adjustments of the house are necessary. A weekend leave will help prepare for the permanent return home. The patient with restricted mobility should have access to a list of shops and other buildings free from architectural barriers. An introduction to community support services such as Meals on Wheels or the visiting nurse helps the patient develop social and personal confidence and makes the return into the community easier. A member of the rehabilitation team should visit the patient at home to see if the patient is maintaining the appropriate level of performance, to solve any unforeseen problems, and to ensure that the patient is happy, active, and still improving.

Home Care Preparation

When the patient is discharged to the home setting, needs for adaptive or safety equipment must be identified. A home visit and evaluation are necessary. The extent of this assessment depends on the disabilities experienced by the patient. Home safety is an important component of the home evaluation. The home of the patient with hemiparesis should be free of scatter rugs or other obstacles in the walking pathways. The bathtub and toilet should be equipped with grab bars. Antiskid patches or strips should be placed in the bathtub to prevent the patient from slipping. The physical or occupational therapist works with the patient and the family to obtain all needed assistive devices before discharge from the hospital. The home is assessed for the difficulty of using assistive devices there. If such barriers are identified, the plan or the home must be altered so that the patient can use assistive devices in the home. Appointments for outpatient speech, physical, and occupational therapy must also be arranged before discharge.

Patient and Family Education

The teaching plan for the patient with a stroke includes the medication schedule, mobility transfer skills, and self-care skills. The patient must take the prescribed medication to prevent another stroke and to keep hypertension under control. The nurse teaches the patient and the family the name of the drug, the dosage, the timing of administration, how to take it, and possible side effects. In collaboration with the physical and occupational therapists, the nurse reinforces the teaching plan with the patient and family so that the patient can safely climb stairs, transfer from bed to chair, get into and out of the car, and use any aids to mobility. Finally, the patient and family members are taught how to use any adaptive equipment recommended to increase independence in self-care skills. The most important information the nurse provides the patient concerns what to do in an emergency, signs of recurring brain attack, and whom to call for nonemergency questions.

Psychosocial Preparation

It is not unusual for patients to become depressed within 6 months after discharge from the hospital. This depression may represent the grieving that the patient must experience because life has changed and the patient has experienced a loss of control. Generally, this is self-limiting, although the patient may require antidepressants, such as amitriptyline (Elavil), for a short period of time. If the depression does not change after 6 months of therapy, the patient should begin treatment for severe depression.

Families need to know that they may feel overwhelmed by the continuing demands placed on them by the patient. Depending on the location of the lesion, the patient may be anxious, slow, cautious, hesitant, and lacking in initiative (left hemisphere), or impulsive and seemingly unaware of any deficit. The family members need to spend time away from the patient on a routine basis to continue to provide full-time care without sacrificing their own physical and emotional health. Family members need to know that self-care is necessary. If the family member becomes excessively stressed, adequate patient care will be impossible. The family needs to be informed that asking for help is appropriate and that they should not feel guilty about obtaining support.

CONCLUSION

The patient who has had a brain attack may have severe neurological damage. Function can be returned through the development and application of a rehabilitation plan that addresses the patient's physical and cognitive functioning. The rehabilitation nurse plays a significant role in facilitating positive patient outcomes. The nurse is an important member of the rehabilitation team and can offer the patient and family support and encouragement. It is through the nurse-patient relationship that the patient develops the trust and confidence to perform the difficult activities needed to complete the rehabilitation program.

REFERENCES

Bachman, D. (1992). The diagnosis and management of common neurologic sequelae of closed head injury. *Journal of Head Trauma Rehabilitation, 7,* 50.

Barker, E. (1994). *Neuroscience nursing.* St. Louis: C. V. Mosby.

Barnett, H. J., Mohr, J. P., Stein, B. M., & Yatsu, F. M. (Eds.). (1992). *Stroke: Pathophysiology, diagnosis and management* (2nd ed.). New York: Churchill Livingstone.

Black, J. M., & Matassarin-Jacobs, E. (1997). *Medical-surgical nursing: Clinical management for continuity of care* (5th ed.). Philadelphia: W. B. Saunders.

Borgman, M., & Passarella, P. (1991). Nursing care of the stroke patient using Bobath principles: An approach to altered movement. *Nursing Clinics of North America, 26*, 1019.

Brott, T. (1996). Thrombolysis for stroke. *Archives of Neurology, 53*, 1305–1306.

Carr, J. H., & Shepherd, R. B. (1991, p. 49). *A motor relearning program for stroke.* Rockville, MD: Aspen.

Fisher, M. (1995). *Stroke therapy.* Boston: Butterworth-Heineman.

Flannery, J. (1997). Disruption of circulation in the brain and spinal cord. In K. Burell, M. J. Gerlach, & B. Pless (Eds.), *Adult nursing: Acute and community care* (2nd ed.). Stamford, CT: Appleton & Lange.

Folsom, A. R., Prineas, R. J., Kaye, S. A., & Munger, R. G. (1990). Incidence of hypertension and stroke in relation to body fat distribution and other risk factors in older women. *Stroke, 21*, 701.

Gee, E., & Shandera, W. (1985). *Nursing care of the stroke patient: A therapeutic approach based on Bobath principles.* Pittsburgh: AREN.

Glasser, V. (1997). Who can benefit from carotid endarterectomy? *Patient Care, 31*, 58–75.

Hickey, J. (1992). *The clinical practice of neurological and neurosurgical nursing* (3rd ed.). Philadelphia: J. B. Lippincot.

Hickey, J. V. (1997). *Clinical practice of neurological and neurosurgical nursing.* Philadelphia: Lippincott.

Higa, M., & Davanipour, Z. (1991). Smoking and stroke. *Neuroepidemiology, 10*, 211–221.

Macabasco, A., & Hickman J. (1995). Thrombolytic therapy for brain attack. *Journal of Neuroscience Nursing, 27*, 138–149.

Mohr, J. P., Gautier, J. C., & Pessin, M. S. (1992). Internal carotid artery disease. In H. J. Barnett, J. P. Mohr, B. M. Stein, & F. M. Yatsu (Eds.), *Stroke: Pathophysiology,* *diagnosis, and management* (2nd ed.). New York: Churchill Livingstone.

Owen, D., Getz, P., & Bulla, S. (1995). A comparison of characteristics of patients with completed stroke: Those who achieve continence and those who do not. *Rehabilitation Nursing, 20*, 197.

Ozer, M. N., Materson, R. S., & Caplan, L. R. (1994). *Management of persons with stroke.* St. Louis: Mosby–Year Book.

Passarella, P., & Lewis, N. (1987). Nursing application of Bobath principles in stroke care. *Journal of Neuroscience Nursing, 19*, 106.

Post-stroke Rehabilitation Guideline Panel. (1995). Post-stroke rehabilitation: Clinical practice guidelines. *American Family Physician, 52*, 461–470.

Schnell, S. (1997). Nursing care of clients with cerebrovascular disorders. In J. M. Black & E. Matassarin-Jacobs (Eds.), *Medical-surgical nursing: Clinical management for continuity of care* (5th ed.). Philadelphia: W. B. Saunders.

Slide, C. (1995). Management of the acute ischemic stroke in the first six hours. *Cardiogram, 7*, 1.

Smith, G. D., Shipley, M. J., Marmont, M. G., & Rose G. (1992). Plasma cholesterol concentration and mortality. *Journal of the American Medical Association, 267*, 70–76.

U.S. Department of Health and Human Services. (1991). *Healthy people 2000: National health promotion and disease prevention objectives.* U.S. Department of Health and Human Services Publication No. 91-50212 (Public Health Services). Washington, DC: U.S. Government Printing Office.

Warlow, C. P., Dennis, M. S., van Gijn, J., Hankey, G. J., Sandercock, P. A., Bamford, J. M., & Wardlaw J. (1996). *Stroke: A practical guide to management.* Cambridge, MA: Blackwell Science.

CHAPTER 21

Nursing Management of the Patient with Head Trauma

Joanne Baggerly and Nancy Le

The complexity of physical, cognitive, and neurobehavioral consequences of traumatic brain injury creates a dysequilibrium that permeates the life of the injured person. Changes in roles, goals, and relationships that occur as a consequence of traumatic brain injury present challenges for the individual and family members that are rivaled by few other life circumstances. Recovery is a process occurring over an extended period and requiring collaboration of and commitment from all involved. Rehabilitation nurses, by virtue of their presence in each setting along the continuum of care, are in a position to assist brain-injured individuals and families from onset of care through community reintegration.

An understanding of where the person is in the recovery trajectory and what neuropathological process or processes the person is recovering from is essential for assessment, planning, and intervention throughout the continuum of care. The goal of this chapter is to provide a foundation to enhance this understanding. The scope and significance, neuropathology, recovery, and rehabilitation nursing assessment and management considerations pertaining to traumatic brain injury and each stage of recovery will be shared. The discussion focuses primarily on problems unique to clients during the acute rehabilitation period and assumes that the potential for recovery exists. The reader is referred to basic nursing textbooks for information on the general aspects of caring for clients with altered consciousness.

SCOPE AND SIGNIFICANCE

Incidence

Precise brain injury statistics are difficult to determine because of a variety of variables, including (1) how the injury is defined, (2) how individuals with brain injury are identi-

fied (for example, by diagnostic codes, emergency room visits, or late follow-up in physician offices), and (3) how severity is measured (Jennett, 1996; Sorenson & Kraus, 1991). According to the National Center for Injury Prevention (1997) the average traumatic brain injury incidence rate (combined hospitalization and mortality rate) is 95 per 100,000 population. There are 5.3 million Americans living with traumatic brain injury–related disability (Thurman, Alverson, Dunn, Guerrero, & Sniezek, 1999). If ethnic, racial, and socioeconomic factors are considered, the incidence in specific populations is even higher, with rates of 262 and 278 per 100,000 per year reported for Hispanic Americans and African Americans, respectively (Cooper, Tabaddor, Hauser, Shulman, Feiner, & Factor, 1983). Brain injury accounts for roughly 40% of all trauma deaths, a figure that translates to a brain injury death rate of 22 per 100,000 per year.

It is estimated that 300,000 persons were hospitalized with a brain injury in 1992 (Kraus & McArthur, 1996). Of those admitted to the hospital who survive, nearly 80% have mild injuries, and, conversely, 20%, or roughly 50,000, incur long-term disability. In terms of estimating the need for rehabilitation services, Kraus and Sorenson (1994) indicate that nearly 80,000 persons annually in the United States require some type of rehabilitation services for neurological involvement following brain injury. Figure 21–1 compares rates of brain injury with those of other neurological disorders; Figure 21–2 illustrates the number and ratio of brain injury deaths in comparison with nonfatal injuries.

Causes and Risk Factors

The causes of traumatic brain injury include vehicular accidents (crashes involving cars, trucks, bicycles, motorcycles, and road and farm equipment, and pedestrians' being hit

331

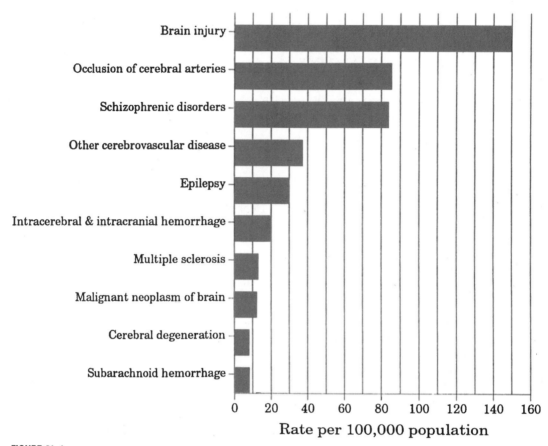

FIGURE 21–1
Brain injury discharge rates compared with rates of nine leading neurological diagnoses. (From Kraus, J. F., & McArthur, D. L. [1996]. Epidemiology of brain injury. In R. W. Evans [Ed.], *Neurology and trauma*. Philadelphia: W. B. Saunders.)

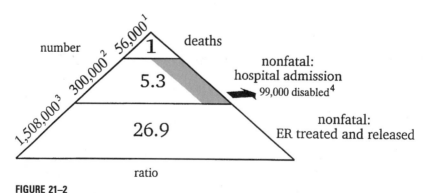

FIGURE 21–2
Number and ratio of brain injury deaths to nonfatal brain injuries. (From Kraus, J. F., & McArthur, D. L. [1996]. Epidemiology of brain injury. In R. W. Evans [Ed.], *Neurology and trauma*. Philadelphia: W. B. Saunders.)

TABLE 21-1 ■ CAUSE OF INJURY IN SEVEN TRAUMA DATABASES

Data Source	% Vehicular	% Assaults	% Falls
TBI Model Systems	56	30	10
Traumatic Coma Data Bank	63	20	14
SCI Model Systems	45	17	18
Missouri TBI Surveillance	53	19	20
Oklahoma TBI Surveillance	43	22	24
Utah TBI Surveillance	54	18	20
Washington TBI Surveillance	55	9	27

From Harrison-Felix, C., Newton, N., Hall, K. M., & Kreutzer, J. S. (1996). Descriptive findings from the Traumatic Brain Injury Model Systems National Data Base. *Journal of Head Trauma Rehabilitation, 11* (5), 1–14.

by moving vehicles); falls; assaults; sports; and recreational activities (Kraus & McArthur, 1996). Table 21–1 summarizes data from several studies on the incidence of brain injury according to cause. Both risk and cause vary by age, gender, ethnic or racial background, socioeconomic status, and demographic factors. People between 15 and 24 years of age are at greatest risk, with males incurring injury at a 2:1 ratio in comparison with females. The cause most commonly associated with this group is vehicular accidents. People younger than 5 years and people 60 years or older are at moderate risk for brain injury, with falls as a predominant cause (Max, MacKenzie, & Rice, 1991; Vollmer et al., 1992). Although vehicular accidents rank first regardless of ethnicity, assaults account for more injuries in minority populations. One source reports that gunshot wounds accounted for 2% of injuries in nonminority patients and for 8% in minority groups (Cavallo & Saucedo, 1995). Urban residents, in general, are more likely to be involved in interpersonal violence that results in a brain injury (Whitman, Coonley-Hoganson, & Desai, 1984).

Alcohol use is often implicated in trauma, with head injuries and fractures being the two most common types of injury (Jernigan, 1991). It is estimated that between one-third and one-half of the persons who sustain a head injury are intoxicated at the time of injury (Corrigan, 1995). Alcohol use at the time of injury, along with heavy preinjury or postinjury drinking, can adversely affect postinjury outcomes.

Prevention

Preventive measures, such as seat belts, airbags, and helmets, contribute to a reduction in deaths and injuries (Sosin, Sniezek, & Waxweiler, 1995). Seat belts have been shown to reduce injury severity, and it is estimated that the universal use of seat belts would reduce vehicular fatalities by 50% and injuries by 65% (Vollmer et al., 1992). Nurses and other health care professionals have a significant role in the development and implementation of prevention strategies at several levels. During assessment of health perception and health management issues, asking about the use of seat belts and other safety devices can reinforce the value of such behaviors. Providing information on the use and effectiveness of safety devices such as seat belts and helmets and the implications of alcohol-impaired driving serves to raise consciousness. Materials containing such information can be left in waiting rooms and included in discharge teaching packets, particularly for patients or clients in vulnerable age groups. Community outreach is another important aspect of nurses' role in prevention. The results of one nurse-initiated community outreach program aimed at adolescents demonstrated significant changes in driving behaviors at 1 month after program completion (Kuthy, Grap, Penn, & Henderson, 1995).

Health care providers can contribute to the social and cultural environmental influences that de-emphasize risk taking by modeling appropriate behaviors themselves (Jernigan, 1991). Broader public health endeavors can be supported through participation in organizational efforts. Mothers Against Drunk Driving (MADD) and Remove Intoxicated Drivers (RID) have been influential in promoting the passage of laws aimed at deterring driving under the influence of alcohol. The National Brain Injury Foundation (NBIF) has been instrumental in promoting public awareness of causes; addressing prevention issues; influencing public policies; and providing information, referrals, support, and education to people who have experienced brain injury and their families.

Human Consequences

A review of statistics, risks, causes, and costs cannot capture the ultimate significance of traumatic brain injury for the individual and family. As the crisis of the initial event subsides, new concerns arise, and the individual and family are confronted with impairments that underscore disruptions in integrated brain functions. Behaviors and cognitive skills that were taken for granted prior to the injury may be lost or may need to be relearned. The impact on the quality of life for the individual and family in the areas of social interaction, work, and leisure activities is enormous.

The internal and external resources a person needs to deal with such major life changes are considerable. Even for those with a mild injury, an initial response of gratitude for having escaped potentially deadly consequences may be replaced by feelings of disappointment or frustration, particularly when recovery takes longer than expected, interferes with work and leisure activities, or is complicated by lingering symptoms.

Costs

The costs associated with brain injury are substantial, with the average charge for hospitalization, adjusted for 1995 dollars, being $105,823 for acute care and $58,415 for rehabilitation (Harrison-Felix, Newton, Hall, & Kreutzer, 1996). According to the Centers for Disease Control and Prevention (1997), acute care, rehabilitation, chronic care, and indirect injuries impose an estimated annual economic burden of $37 billion in direct and indirect costs. In one study, less than half of people with moderate to severe brain injury with a successful work history had returned to work 2 years after injury, and only 10% of those who did return to work were financially independent (Dikmen, Machamer, & Tempkin, 1993).

Although the sequelae of traumatic brain injury are varied and complex, characteristic impairments in the areas of behavior, cognition, and emotion are observed in all injuries. Understanding the mechanisms of traumatic brain injury and the subsequent disorders that lead to these impairments facilitates appropriate assessment and intervention for injuries at all levels of severity.

NEUROPATHOLOGY

Relating the clinical picture to the specific disorder involved facilitates treatment planning and outcome prediction, because the various pathological processes influence recovery differently. *Diffuse injury* implies widespread and scattered damage throughout the brain and results from diffuse axonal injury and diffuse hypoxic-ischemic injury. *Focal injury* refers to discrete localized damage, such as contusions, deep hemorrhages, and focal hypoxic-ischemic injury. Secondary processes associated with extracerebral hematomas and herniation syndromes cause further damage and contribute to the overall clinical picture.

Diffuse Axonal Injury

Diffuse axonal injury is the major neuropathological process of brain injury. It is best understood when conceptualized as a continuum of injury from very mild to severe (Fig. 21–3). The injury mechanism is qualitatively the same along the continuum; it is the quantity or severity of injury that varies (Hayes, Povlishock, & Singha, 1992; Katz & Alexander, 1994). When subjected to inertial forces, the brain, which usually rests immobile within the skull, responds to mechanical forces by moving forward and back within the skull. At the same time, the brain rotates or twists upon itself. The pathological process is shearing of axons resulting from the inertial forces associated with sudden deceleration and leading to diffuse axonal injury. Rotational forces damage axons and small blood vessels running along the axis of the brain, from the hemispheres of the cortex to the brainstem, with subcortical white matter and deep structures disrupted most (Figs. 21–4 and 21–5). The cascade of events that follows comprises cellular transport failures, edema and often lysis, and subsequent degeneration of axons (Hayes et al., 1992).

The degree of force and extent of strain determine the severity of injury: the greater the force, the greater the injury. With the very mildest level of injury, there may be only transient functional impairment, not actual disruption of axons, whereas at the upper limit of a mild injury, there is scattered axonal damage and loss (Katz & Alexander, 1994). It is postulated that the pattern of white matter axonal damage is responsible for the attentional deficits demonstrated even after mild traumatic brain injury (Alexander, 1995). Immediate coma without lucid interval was formerly considered the hallmark of diffuse axonal injury; however, later studies have suggested that there may be a lucid period with milder diffuse axonal injuries (Graham & McIntosh, 1996).

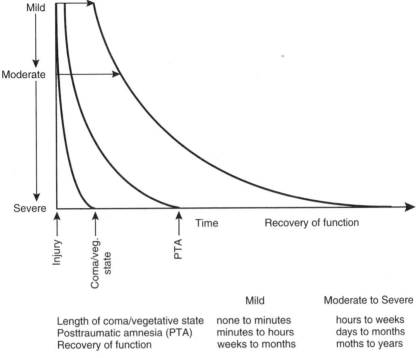

	Mild	Moderate to Severe
Length of coma/vegetative state	none to minutes	hours to weeks
Posttraumatic amnesia (PTA)	minutes to hours	days to months
Recovery of function	weeks to months	moths to years

FIGURE 21–3
Recovery curves for mild, moderate, and severe diffuse <u>axonal</u> injury.

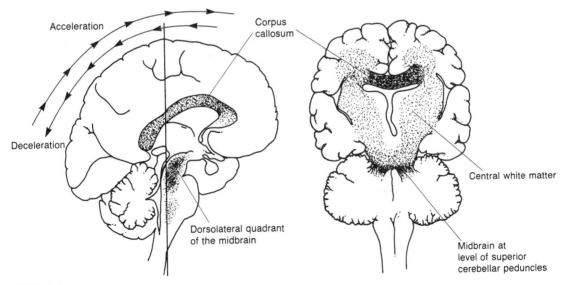

FIGURE 21–4
Diffuse axonal injury. Diffuse axonal injury results from acceleration-deceleration and shearing force on the brain. Depending on the severity of the injury, the areas of the brain most often affected are the corpus callosum, the dorsolateral area of the midbrain, and the parasagittal white matter. (From Hickey, J. [1992]. *Neurological and neurosurgical nursing* [3rd ed., p. 362]. Philadelphia: J. B. Lippincott.)

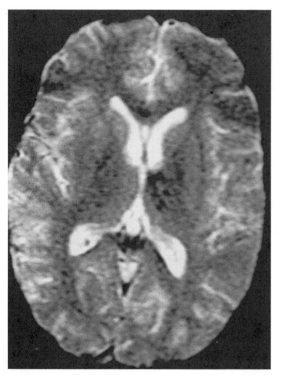

FIGURE 21–5
Magnetic resonance imaging scan demonstrating lesions typical in diffuse axonal injury.

Individuals with diffuse axonal injury have remarkably similar clinical courses of recovery. There is an initial period of coma followed by stages of (1) increasing arousal, (2) confusional or posttraumatic amnesic state, and (3) clearing of confusion. With mild injury, progression through these stages is rapid, but with moderate or severe injury, progression occurs over a longer time (Table 21–2). With moderate or severe injury, cognitive and behavioral problems emerge as confusion and *posttraumatic amnesia* (the period of disorientation and inability to register and recall ongoing events [Capruso & Levin, 1996]) clear. Because of the disruption of frontal connections, behavioral issues are similar to those seen with contusions. Other clinical effects associated with moderate and severe diffuse axonal injury are far more variable; they include potential changes in tone, coordination, balance, gait, swallowing, and continence. Extraocular movements and vision may be impaired because of cranial nerve damage. Nutritional deficits related to swallowing problems and negative nitrogen balance are not uncommon, particularly in the early recovery period.

Diffuse Hypoxic-Ischemic Injury

Diffuse hypoxic-ischemic injury is a consequence of severe, sustained increased intracranial pressure or cardiovascular and/or respiratory compromise. The hypoxia associated with increased intracranial pressure results in diffuse neuronal loss, infarction, or both. The areas of the brain most vulnerable to the lack of oxygen are the hippocampus, basal ganglia, and cerebellum. Impairment of oxygenation due to cardiovascular or respiratory compromise also causes diffuse neuronal loss. The cortical areas supplied by the distal arterioles, referred to as border-zone areas, are most sensitive to hypoperfusion; the consequence is commonly referred to as a *watershed infarction*.

In the context of traumatic brain injury, diffuse hypoxic-ischemic injury often accom-

TABLE 21–2 ■ HEAD TRAUMA CLASSIFICATION

Category	Acute Glasgow Coma Scale Score (GCS)	Clinical Features
Mild	13–15	Loss of consciousness is <20 minutes, no deterioration of GCS, no focal neurological deficit or complication (e.g., hypotension), no intracranial mass lesion or intracranial surgery
Moderate	9–12	Includes GCS >12, with complication or focal brain lesion seen on CT scan, and may include patients rapidly recovered from coma
Severe	3–8	Coma duration must be ≥6 hours

From Capruso, D. X., & Levin, H. S. (1996). Neurobehavioral outcome of head trauma. In R. W. Evans (Ed.), *Neurology and trauma* (pp. 201–221). Philadelphia: W. B. Saunders.

panies diffuse axonal injury and can be difficult to distinguish. It is postulated that people who take longer than anticipated to progress from either coma or the confusional state may have suffered some hypoxic injury (Katz & Alexander, 1994). The clinical parameters most often implicated in producing diffuse hypoxic-ischemic injury are a critical drop in systemic blood pressure (systolic pressure <80 mm Hg) and a sustained rise in intracranial pressure (>20 mm Hg) (Katz, 1997; Marmarou, Anderson, Ward, et al., 1991). The nature and distribution of the damage are the same as for classic anoxic hypoxia as would be seen following cardiac arrest or status epilepticus (Graham & McIntosh, 1996).

The clinical effects extend beyond attention problems and "minor" memory problems to memory deficits and persisting amnesia as a consequence of damage to the hippocampus. Tone and movement abnormalities, which are present to varying degrees, include spasticity, ataxia, choreoathetoid movements, and dystonic posturing related to the predilection for damage to the basal ganglia and cerebellum. Border-zone ischemia or watershed infarctions occur because of low flow in the most distal vascular territories, and the resulting clinical manifestations correspond to the cortical areas affected. Proximal limb weakness, visual-spatial deficits, and transcortical aphasia are examples of the deficits that may be seen.

Focal Cortical Contusions

Because the frontal and temporal lobes of the cortex are situated over the irregular, jagged, bony undersurface of the cranial base, these areas are particularly vulnerable to contusions as a result of inertial or contact forces (Figs. 21–6 and 21–7). Contusions are characterized by localized hemorrhage, edema, and tissue distortion, evolving over time to areas of scarring and retraction (Katz, 1992). Contusions and the associated edema can cause brain ischemia. The term *laceration* is usually applied to a contusion in which there is also tearing of the pial layer of the meninges, which is sometimes referred to as a "burst lobe" (Graham & McIntosh, 1996).

A variety of deficits are associated with frontal lobe dysfunction. The person may (1) lack impulse control, (2) demonstrate disinhibited behaviors, (3) lack insight and social judgment, and (4) offer tangential and verbose responses. Irritability and easy frustration may be seen. Disturbances in planning,

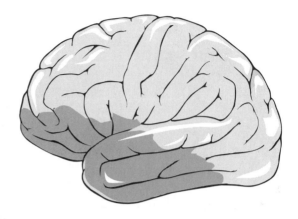

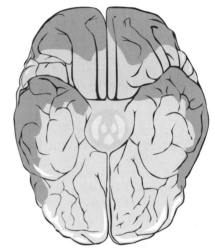

FIGURE 21–6
Areas predominantly affected by cortical contusions.

organizing, and sequencing events may also be evident. Conversely, depending on the precise portion of the frontal lobe that is disrupted, findings may include a flat affect, slow mental processing, decreased initiation, or paucity of motor activity and verbalizations.

A brief explanation of frontal lobe functions helps to clarify the reason for these clinical manifestations. The frontal lobes are involved with regulation of affect and emotion, higher-level cognitive functions, and complex behaviors that are the basis for goal-directed behavior (Katz & Alexander, 1994). Deficits result from impairments in the regulation of drive or initiation, information processing, self-awareness, and the ability to anticipate, select, or inhibit behavior (executive functions) (Stuss, 1987).

The temporal lobes, with connections to

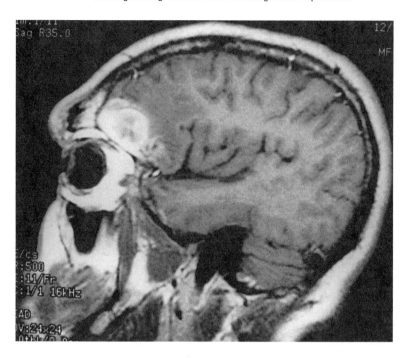

FIGURE 21–7
Magnetic resonance imaging scan depicting large cortical (frontal) contusion.

other areas of the brain, regulate aspects of emotion, memory, and learning. Language functions, particularly comprehension and word recognition, are associated with the dominant temporal lobe (the left lobe in most people). Behavioral manifestations include sudden changes in mood and verbal or physical outbursts. Cognitive deficits related to temporal lobe involvement include severe learning and memory deficits. Anomia with impaired word finding is the common language deficit. Specific aphasia syndromes are not common with contusions, but when aphasia does occur, the presentation is consistent with a Wernicke or transcortical sensory aphasia.

Deep Hemorrhages

Deep hemorrhages, although relatively rarer, can occur in the basal ganglia, invariably in the context of diffuse axonal injury (Katz, 1992). The clinical effects reflect the size of the hemorrhage and extension to surrounding structures. Common findings in deep hemorrhages are contralateral motor weakness and, possibly, sensory loss if the thalamus is also involved.

Focal Hypoxic-Ischemic Injury

Focal hypoxic-ischemic injury refers to ischemia or infarction in a particular vascular territory that is most commonly a consequence of the secondary processes of trauma, such as brain

swelling, increased intracranial pressure, and herniation. Brain swelling may occur as a consequence of (1) an increase in brain water content or cerebral blood volume or (2) expansion of a mass lesion, such as an intracerebral hematoma. Increased intracranial pressure occurs in 75% of cases of severe head injury, particularly when mass lesions are present. Increased intracranial pressure occurs when the volume of the brain, blood, and cerebrospinal fluid exceeds the ability of the craniospinal cavity to displace volume; the consequence is compression of blood vessels and subsequent ischemia (Mitchell, 1986; Vollmer et al., 1992).

A displacement or shift in brain tissue also causes what is referred to as *herniation* of the brain. Temporal lobe–tentorial herniation occurs when a portion of the medial temporal lobe known as the uncus is forced into the oval tentorial opening through which the midbrain passes. When a hematoma expands, for example, the temporal lobe stretches the tentorium (a thick fold of dura that separates the medial temporal lobe from the neighboring midbrain) downward and inward. The third cranial nerve, which passes through this area, is compressed, resulting in a dilated pupil. Direct neural damage from this type of herniation involves the medial temporal lobe, the midbrain, the third cranial nerve, and the hypothalamus.

Vascular compression most commonly involves compromise of the posterior cerebral artery related to uncal or tentorial herniation, followed by compromise of the anterior cerebral artery from a subfalcine herniation. Focal ischemic injury may also occur in a border-zone distribution related to low flow, such as in cardiovascular compromise. The clinical effects are consistent with the vascular territory affected. When the posterior cerebral artery, which supplies the occipital lobe, is involved, hemianopia might be present as well as visual-perceptual and visual-spatial problems if ischemia is extensive. Reading and visual recognition may be impaired. If a segment of the posterior cerebral artery supplying the thalamus is affected, amnesia and dementia may occur. Ischemia in the territory of the anterior cerebral artery supplying the frontal lobe is associated with contralateral limb paresis, with the leg weaker than the arm, and impairments in visual tracking. If damage is bilateral, there are frontal release signs, such as a grasp reflex. The cognitive profile may include confusion, decreased memory, perseveration, and distractibility. Depending on the precise area of damage, the patient may have either psychomotor agitation or delayed responses and a paucity of movement. (See Table 21–3 for a summary of focal lesions and their consequences.)

Extracerebral Hematomas

Extracerebral hematomas occur outside the brain, between the layers of the meninges. Their clinical manifestations relate to pressure effects as the size of a hematoma increases within the closed space of the cranial vault. *Epidural* hematomas are often seen in association with a temporal bone fracture and laceration of the middle meningeal artery. Rupture of the artery leads to a bleed on the outside of the dural layer of the meninges.

Subdural hematomas represent bleeding into the potential space between the dura and arachnoid layer of the meninges either in association with tearing of bridge veins or damage to pial arteries or after a brain laceration (Figs. 21–8 and 21–9). Subdural hematomas can result from contact or acceleration injuries and may occur immediately or later after trauma. *Hygroma* is slowly accumulating subdural fluid, which can occur from tears in the arachnoid membrane. Acute subdural hematomas treated within 4 hours are associated with good outcomes, whereas those for which treatment is delayed can have poor outcomes related to secondary hypoxic damage (Vollmer et al., 1992).

TABLE 21–3 ■ FOCAL LESIONS: TYPICAL LOCATIONS AND CONSEQUENCES

Lesion	Location	Consequences
Focal cortical contusions	Frontal polar and orbital frontal	Alterations in affect and behavior (apathy or disinhibition) Higher level intellectual abilities (processing, executive functions, self-awareness)
	Anterior-inferior temporal	Alterations in affect and behavior Auditory association deficits (e.g., aphasia) Visual association deficits (e.g., agnosia)
Deep hemorrhages	Basal ganglia area	Hemiparesis Discoordination Hypertonia Movement disorders Aphasia (left) Neglect Visuospatial problems (right)

Focal hypoxic-ischemic artery infarct	Posterior cerebral	*Left side*
		    Hemianopia
		    Amnesia
		    Aphasia (alexia and anomia)
		 Right side
		    Hemispatial neglect
		    Topographic disorientation
		    Prosopagnosia

From Katz, D. I. (1997). Traumatic brain injury. In V. M. Mills, J. W. Cassidy, & D. I. Katz (Eds.), *Neurological rehabilitation: A guide to diagnosis, prognosis, and treatment planning.* Malden, MA: Blackwell Scientific.

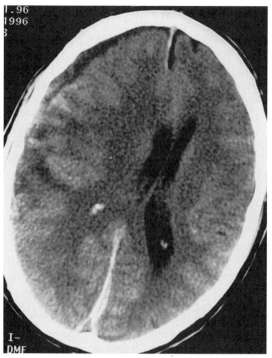

FIGURE 21–8
Computed tomography scan depicting an acute subdural hematoma, cerebral edema, and marked midline shift.

COMPLICATIONS

Although many complications can result from trauma to the brain, this discussion is limited to two. The first, hydrocephalus, although relatively rare, has functional implications. The second, seizures, warrants discussion because many brain-injured clients are started on prophylactic antiseizure medications.

Dilation of the ventricular system as a physiological response to brain atrophy is a phenomenon seen as a late effect of severe brain injury for which there is no treatment. A relatively rare type of symptomatic hydrocephalus may occur, however, that is amenable to treatment. The presentation, which can be subtle, consists of (1) slower than anticipated recovery, (2) failure to improve, or (3) regression. When this type of hydrocephalus is suspected, a neurosurgical evaluation should be considered to determine whether a shunt would be beneficial (Bachman, 1992).

Posttraumatic epilepsy is categorized as early (occurring within the first week) or late (occurring after the first week). The incidence for both types is roughly 5%. The risk for early seizures is greater in people with severe injury, intracranial hematomas, depressed skull fractures, and posttraumatic amnesia lasting more than 24 hours. Early posttrau-

matic epilepsy increases the likelihood of persistent seizure disorder; however, the occurrence of a seizure within the first hour of trauma does not increase the risk for development of late seizures (Vollmer et al., 1992). Prophylactic anticonvulsant treatment is considered to be effective in preventing seizures during the first week after brain injury, but not thereafter. Of the 5% of clients who have late seizures, half experience their first seizure within the first year, but one-fourth do not have their first seizure until 4 years or longer after the trauma. The factors associated with risk of development of late seizures include: (1) a period of posttraumatic amnesia longer than 24 hours, (2) depressed skull fracture, (3) intracranial hematoma, and (4) missile injury (Vollmer et al., 1992).

SEVERITY, RECOVERY, AND OUTCOMES

The Glasgow Coma Scale is one method of delineating severity in the acute period after brain injury (Jennett & Teasdale, 1981). Scores lower than 8 indicate coma and severe injury; scores ranging from 9 to 12 are consistent with moderate injury; and scores of 13 to 15

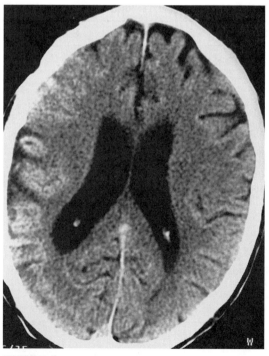

FIGURE 21–9
Late (4 months) follow-up computed tomography scan of same patient shown in Figure 21–8, depicting post–subdural hemorrhage ischemia.

indicate mild injury (Rimel, Giordani, Barth, Boll, & Jane, 1981).

As the course progresses, severity is reassessed, with both the length of coma and the duration of posttraumatic amnesia taken into account. Serial Glasgow Coma Scale scores are a means of recording the duration of coma. The presence of posttraumatic amnesia is determined by assessing orientation and memory through objective measurement with an instrument such as the Galveston Orientation and Amnesia Test (GOAT) (Levin, O'Donnell, & Grossman, 1979) or the Orientation Group Monitoring System (OGMS) (Corrigan, Arnett, Houck, & Jackson, 1985). The presence or absence of lesions on neuroimaging scans, such as computed tomography (CT) or magnetic resonance imaging (MRI), contributes to an assessment of severity and adds a further dimension to outcome prediction (Katz & Alexander, 1994).

Predicting recovery, however, is not as straightforward when other disease is present. Frontal behavior that is due to diffuse axonal injury demonstrates gradual improvement over time, whereas recovery from frontal behavior related to contusions may plateau earlier. The extent of deficits depends on whether the contusions are unilateral or bilateral as well as on their size and precise location. Tissue damage associated with secondary processes also complicates recovery and recovery prediction. Other variables, including age, premorbid personality, previous injury, and drug or alcohol abuse, also influence recovery (Reeder, Rosenthal, Lichtenberg, & Wood, 1996; Rimel et al., 1981; Webb, Rose, Johnston, & Attree, 1996).

A number of measurement tools are used to assess different aspects of recovery. For the individual client, these outcome measures are helpful for tracking progress and changes over time and allow for meaningful communication, in that the descriptions are standardized. Research studies employing such measures are important for aggregating data and for building outcome profiles linked to specific variables and conditions. Table 21–4 lists

TABLE 21–4 ■ MEASUREMENT TOOLS COMMONLY USED IN BRAIN INJURY

Instrument	Description	Purpose
Glasgow Coma Scale (GCS) (Jennett & Teasdale, 1981)	15-point scale with cumulative scoring for eye movement, motor and verbal responses Minimum score 3, maximum 15 Score ≤8 indicates coma Severity of injury indicated by score: 3–8: severe injury 9–12: moderate injury 13–15: mild injury	Standardize terminology for communicating level of consciousness Score at 6 hours after injury/ resuscitation useful in predicting severity When linked with other variables such as age and pupillary responses, is best early predictor of recovery
Glasgow Outcome Scale (GOS) (Jennett & Bond, 1975)	Categorizes recovery in broad terms: Good = functioning at or near pre-injury level Moderate = disability sufficient enough to preclude a return to pre-injury level Severe = dependence during at least some part of a 24-hour period Vegetative state = condition in which there is no cerebral cortical functioning as judged behaviorally (Jennett & Teasdale, 1981)	Assessment of recovery at 3 months after injury may provide a realistic picture of the anticipated long-range outcome Takes into account the effects of mental and neurological deficits Broad scope of categories limits sensitivity
Galveston Orientation and Amnesia Test (GOAT) (Levin, O'Donnell, & Grossman, 1979)	Evaluates orientation and estimates the duration of retrograde amnesia and duration of anterograde amnesia Can be performed at the bedside and completed in 5–10 minutes Scores range from 0 to 100, with 75 or more on consecutive days consistent with clearing of posttraumatic amnesia	Assess progress through PTA

Table continued on following page

TABLE 21-4 ■ MEASUREMENT TOOLS COMMONLY USED IN BRAIN INJURY *Continued*

Instrument	Description	Purpose
Orientation Group Monitoring System (Corrigan, Arnett, Houck, & Jackson, 1985)	Structured to gather data from observed responses in a daily 30-minute reality orientation group Areas examined include: Orientation to time and place Orientation to person, group members, and staff Ability to attend to tasks and respond appropriately Associative learning Episodic memory Use of environmental cues Scoring for each response ranges from 1 to 3, with 1 representing an incorrect response, 2 a partially correct response, and 3 a correct response Mean of the daily scores is tabulated weekly (Mysiw, Bogner, Arnett, Clinchot, & Corrigan, 1996)	Assesses progress through PTA Helps in understanding how the person progresses through PTA Helps clinicians to more accurately determine type, density, and duration of programming that will benefit client (Mysiw et al., 1996)
Disability Rating Scale (DRS)	Derivative of the GOS	Captures quality-of-life issues Has more sensitivity than GOS
Neurobehavioral Rating Scale (NRS) (Levin, High, Goethe, Sisson, Overall, Rhoades, et al., 1987)	Frequently used outcome measures in traumatic brain injury research that target specific areas such as behavior, social, family functioning, and adjustment Based on the Brief Psychiatric Rating Scale Consists of 27 items and seven rankings, ranging from not present to extremely severe Takes 30 minutes to complete and subsequent ratings based on structured interview and observation	Captures quality-of-life issues and broadens the scope of outcome considerations Useful for defining a range of affective disturbances and behaviors, screening for presence of psychiatric disturbances after brain injury, and demonstrating improvement over time (Sandel & Mysiw, 1996)
Agitated Behavior Scale (ABS) (Corrigan, 1989)	Ratings based on behavioral observations after 30 minutes of treatment/therapy session or after 8 hours of nursing care Consists of 14 items or behaviors on a scale of 1 (absent) to 4 (present in the extreme) Scores range from 14 to 56; score below 21 considered normal; 22–28 represents mild agitation; 29–35 represents moderate agitation; and 36–56 represents severe agitation	Provides objective, serial assessment for presence and degree of PTA
Overt Aggression Scale–Modified for Neurorehabilitation (OAS-MNR) (Alderman, Knight, & Morgan, 1997)	Observational questionnaire that records the frequency and severity of four categories of aggression (verbal, against objects, against others, against self) Severity rated on a scale from 1 to 4 Includes a range of categories to describe antecedents, a range of interventions used to manage the aggressive behaviors, and a method for recording findings	Offers a method to measure, quantify, and facilitate analysis of aggressive behavior following brain injury Attempts to standardize classification of aggressive behavior and provides a means of recording the behaviors, antecedents, and interventions

the common measurement tools and provides a brief explanation of each.

Recovery from diffuse axonal injury occurs in a generally predictable pattern. The levels of cognitive functioning developed by Hagen, Malkmus, and Durham (1979) constitute the most widely known description of recovery from diffuse axonal injury. Another model that incorporates neurological concepts and a functional recovery perspective is offered by Katz and Alexander (1994). Tables 21–5 and 21–6 outline these two models.

Mild Diffuse Axonal Injury

There is no universally accepted definition of *mild brain injury*, but the characteristics most often used are as follows (Alexander, 1995):

- Trauma due to contact forces or acceleration/deceleration forces
- Unconsciousness for seconds or minutes; in some cases, no actual loss of consciousness
- Glasgow Coma Scale score of 13 to 15 at the scene or in the emergency room, with no subsequent decline
- A period of confusion or posttraumatic amnesia lasting minutes or only a few hours
- No focal neurological signs
- No evidence of focal or space-occupying lesions on neuroimaging studies

A Glasgow Coma Scale score of 13 or 14 reflects the upper end of the mild injury category, and when coma lasts longer than 10 minutes and posttraumatic amnesia lasts 4 to 6 hours, recovery may require months or years (Alexander, 1995). Some sources, however, consider a period of confusion and posttraumatic amnesia of up to 24 hours to be consistent with mild injury (Mild Traumatic Brain Injury Committee, 1993).

Concussion is the prototypical example of mild brain injury, and the pathology consists of diffuse axonal injury. Typically, consciousness is lost for less than a minute and posttraumatic amnesia lasts 30 to 60 minutes, with rapid recovery and no symptoms beyond the first few days (Katz & Alexander, 1994). In the immediate postinjury period, pallor, diaphoresis, nausea and vomiting, and ataxia are common symptoms. In the first few days following a concussion, the person may complain of headache, dizziness, drowsiness, and memory or concentration problems. Over the next few days and weeks, other subjective

TABLE 21–5 ■ RANCHO LOS AMIGOS SCALE: COGNITIVE LEVELS ASSOCIATED WITH TRAUMATIC BRAIN INJURY*

	Levels	Descriptive Characteristics
I	No response	No response to any stimuli
II	Generalized response	Responses are nonpurposeful and inconsistent; posturing and reflex responses may be evident
III	Localized response	Localized and purposeful responses; follows commands inconsistently; responses often related to discomfort, i.e., pulls tubes
IV	Confused, agitated-inappropriate	Severely impaired information processing; responding to internal confusion; attention span very limited; behavior often bizarre; short-term memory impaired; dependent in all aspects of care; safety of major concern
V	Confused, nonagitated-inappropriate	Remains distractible; with direction and assistance, can perform previously learned tasks; performance deteriorates when structure decreases or complexity increases
VI	Confused, appropriate	Less concrete; memory problems persist, but more aware of not knowing correct answer; completes previously learned tasks with supervision
VII	Automatic-appropriate	Oriented consistently; initiates tasks and carries out routines; more awareness of self and others, but lacks insight, judgment, and problem-solving ability
VIII	Purposeful-appropriate	Demonstrates more responsibility for self; able to learn new tasks; new situations, variations in routines can be stressful; more aware of deficits

*The scale was originally developed by C. Hagen, D. Malkmus, and P. Durham and was revised in 1974 by D. Malkmus and K. Stenderup. From Baggerly, J. (1986). Rehabilitation of the adult with head trauma. *Nursing Clinics of North America, 21*(4), 581.

TABLE 21–6 ■ STAGES OF RECOVERY FROM DIFFUSE AXONAL INJURY AS DESCRIBED BY KATZ AND ALEXANDER

Stage of Recovery	Description
Coma	Unresponsive
	Eyes closed
Vegetative state	No cognitive responsiveness
	Gross wakefulness
	Sleep-wake cycles
Minimally conscious state	Purposeful wakefulness
	Responses to commands (inconsistent)
Confusional state	Posttraumatic amnesia (PTA) evident
	Speech ability recovered
	Severe attentional deficits
	Agitation, hypoarousal, labile behaviors
Evolving independence/postconfusional state	Resolution of PTA
	Cognitive improvement
	Achievement of independence in self-care activities
	Improving social interaction
	Developing independence in home environment
Social competence/community reentry	Recovering cognitive abilities
	Goal-directed behaviors, social skills, personality
	Developing independence in community
	Returning to vocational and/or academic activities

Adapted from a table in Katz, D. I. (1997). Traumatic brain injury. In V. M. Mills, J. W. Cassidy, & D. I. Katz (Eds.), *Neurological rehabilitation: A guide to diagnosis, prognosis, and treatment planning* (p. 116). Malden, MA: Blackwell Scientific, which is based on a model developed by Alexander, M. P. (1982). Traumatic brain injury. In D. H. Benson & H. Blumer (Eds.), *Psychiatric aspects of neurological disease* (pp. 251–278). New York: McGraw-Hill.

symptoms may emerge, including one or more of the following: difficulty concentrating; poor memory; fatigue; irritability; headache (particularly when attempting to work); emotional lability; anxiety; depression; forgetfulness or memory loss; sleep disturbance (insomnia); and increased sensitivity to noise. It is postulated that these symptoms are not apparent initially because the stresses and strains of life activities are not encountered during the immediate recovery period. Once the person attempts to resume normal activities, symptoms are noticeable because of a reduced ability of the brain to respond to them (Alexander, 1995; Alves, Macciocchi, & Barth, 1993; Cicerone, 1992; Gronwall & Wrightson, 1974, 1980; Rutherford, 1989).

The forces responsible for the brain injury have the potential to cause injury to other areas of the body, leading to symptoms related to musculoskeletal, cranial, or facial trauma (Zasler, 1993). Conceptualizing the symptoms as belonging to neurological, peripheral, and psychological categories helps illuminate the etiology of specific symptoms as well as guide treatment and the selection of interventions (Katz & Alexander, 1994).

The primary *neurological* injury of mild brain trauma, which is reversible, is impaired attention, leading to deficits in information processing ability, reaction time, and memory difficulties. The neurological symptoms dissipate by 1 to 3 months, depending on the degree of mild injury. *Attention deficit*, or inability to process information, is a stage in the recovery process, not a complication (Gronwall & Wrightson, 1974). Other complaints associated with neural injury are poor concentration, forgetfulness, and disturbances in sleep-wake cycles. It is likely that these mild and often clinically undetectable deficits render the person unable to perform tasks at the preinjury level. During the first few weeks after injury, these subjective cognitive or neurologically based attention impairments can be measured by neuropsychological tests focused on aspects of attention. Decreased performance is expected for 4 to 6 weeks after the trauma event.

Symptoms indicative of *peripheral* or musculoskeletal injury are referable to specific areas of injury and have a more variable recovery time frame. Neck pain is often related to cervical soft tissue injury. Headache can be related to scalp injury, neck injury, or a mixture of causes, including neuronal injury. Dizziness may be due to peripheral vestibular injury or cervical injury. Altered sensations, such as numbness and hyperesthesia, in the distribution of the peripheral nerve injury may occur (Alexander, 1995; Zasler, 1993). Recovery time frames are linked to the specific problem.

Emotional responses such as anxiety, lability, and irritability may be related to neural injury, pain, or *psychological* factors (Alexander, 1995). At what point in the recovery trajectory such symptoms occur offers clues about etiology. Irritability in the first few days following injury is likely neurological in origin. Irritability, frustration, or anxiety related to decreased performance during the recovery period is likely to be psychological in origin, but the decreased performance stems from the neurological attention impairment. Inadequate understanding of or preparation for the recovery period is postulated as contributing to the client's emotional reactions (Gronwall, 1986; Hinkle, Alves, Rimel, & Jane, 1986; Kay, 1992). Anxiety and frustration may be exhibited or compounded (1) when complaints are dismissed by the provider or (2) when the help needed to manage recovery is not available. Other client variables, including concussion severity, the presence of peripheral musculoskeletal problems, age, psychological status and history, and previous trauma, also influence recovery.

Although the literature reflects overlapping and inconsistent terminology, *postconcussion syndrome* generally refers to recovery from concussion or mild head injury with a recovery time frame of 3 months as the outer limit. Some sources reserve the term for recovery extending beyond 35 days (Gronwall & Wrightson, 1974). *Persistent postconcussion syndrome* is used when symptoms are present well beyond the 3-month mark; this condition occurs in a minority of clients with concussion.

Moderate and Severe Diffuse Axonal Injury

The stages of recovery are clinically the same for moderate and severe diffuse axonal injury; it is the intensity and duration that differ. Residual cognitive and behavioral dysfunctions may persist for years with moderate and severe injury. Clients with moderate injury, indicated by a brief coma or a Glasgow Coma Scale score from 9 to 12, who pass through the stage of posttraumatic amnesia relatively quickly (hours to a few days), require careful monitoring and screening, as they may appear to be intact, leading to their being misclassified as having a "mild" injury. Individuals at the low end of the continuum of moderate injury may show slower improvement. The presence of focal injuries or mass lesions adversely influences the outcome. Severe injury is associated with coma usually lasting days to weeks and posttraumatic amnesia lasting weeks to months.

Coma and Emergence from Coma

Arousal is the predominant problem during the period of coma and emergence from coma. The person exhibits no meaningful response, movement, or verbalization, and the eyes remain closed. Motor responses that do occur reflect brainstem or spinal cord activity and are automatic and reflexive. Abnormal posturing may be seen, particularly in those with severe injury. During unresponsive periods, there is no evidence of cognitive responsiveness, but gross wakefulness and sleep-wake cycles are seen.

The distinguishing characteristic of the mute or low-level responsive stage is rudimentary cognitive responsiveness, demonstrated as purposeful movement that initially is inconsistent, such as localizing to stimuli or following a simple, one-step command. This occurs before any spontaneous speech output is evident. The neuropathology of diffuse axonal injury in this case may have interrupted the supplementary motor area fiber projections that are responsible for initiation of speech (Katz & Alexander, 1994). The presence of focal left-hemisphere contusions may also contribute to delays in verbal responsiveness. Some people remain in this stage for an extended period. Individuals with severe injury are most likely to have a number of physical problems, such as increased muscle tone or spasticity as a result of disease involving facilitory and inhibitory motor control areas in the brain and brainstem regions.

Confusional Stage

In the stage marked by confusion and posttraumatic amnesia, cognitive operations are severely limited as a result of profound attention deficits. The individual is disoriented and exhibits obvious memory deficits. Verbalization may be incoherent or confused, with a tendency to confabulate. Neurological problems such as cranial nerve deficits become more evident as the individual becomes more active, but full evaluation is likely to be precluded by the marked confusion. Arousal and motor skills are greatly improved, but the main cognitive problem is the inability to focus and sustain attention. Attention reflects the ability to be aware of internal and external stimuli and forms the basis of mental functions such as thinking, communicating, and performing tasks. Examples of internal stimuli are thoughts and memories; those of external stimuli are sights and sounds in the environment (Weber, 1990).

The likely pathological substrates for the development of posttraumatic amnesia and confusional state are injuries to the frontotemporal system and related subcortical and brainstem regions that subserve arousal, attention, memory, and behavioral functions (Mysiw & Sandel, 1997). Precise anatomical localization of the neurophysical disruption is not possible; it is likely the result of the combined effects of multiple lesions, as is typical of diffuse axonal injury.

The overwhelming memory and attention problems, coupled with a global lack of insight regarding the circumstances and the inability to reason, leave the client dependent in all aspects of daily living. Often, the magnitude of these deficits is such that the person cannot tolerate even routine care activities. Behavior is often labile, ranging from hyperactive to hypoactive. Most clients exhibit some degree of agitation or motor restlessness, frustration, and distractibility. Disinhibited behavior is common. Combativeness, aggressiveness, and paranoia may occur. During this period, structure, environmental engineering, and behavioral interventions are essential and occur in the context of interdisciplinary collaboration.

Agitation

Although agitation is a behavior frequently associated with the confusional stage of recovery, there are few data to quantify the occurrence and extent of the problem. The rates of agitation noted in the literature range from 11 to 50% (Brooke, Questad, Patterson, & Bashak, 1992; Levin & Grossman, 1978; Reyes, Bhattacharyya, & Heler, 1981). Interpretation of these figures is difficult because the definition of *agitation* is not consistent among studies, nor are the data stratified by diagnoses or pathological processes. Cross-study comparisons are not possible, and the evaluation of interventions and advancement of practice standards is hampered.

In one study, Reyes et al. (1981) defined the agitated person as one who exhibits constant uninhibited movement and defined the restless person as one who is constantly active but capable of briefly inhibiting movement. Agitation was a clinical feature at the time of admission to rehabilitation in nearly 14% of cases, and restlessness was present in nearly 37%. Brooke et al. (1992), however, defined agitation as episodic motor or verbal behavior that interfered with care or clearly required physical or chemical restraints to prevent injury to persons or property. These researchers defined restlessness as behavior that required some action, such as redirection, but was not severe enough to interfere with care, therapy, or safety. Using these definitions, they identified agitation as present in 11% of their subjects and restlessness in 35%.

Work on clarifying the definition of agitation has been advanced by Sandel and Mysiw (1996) and Fugate, Spacek, Kresty, Levy, Johnson, and Mysiw (1997). On the basis of a comprehensive review of the literature, Sandel and Mysiw (1996) propose the following definition of agitation: "a subtype of delirium occurring during the period of posttraumatic amnesia characterized by excessive behaviors, including some combination of aggression, akathisia (motor restlessness), disinhibition, and emotional lability." The clinical implication of this definition is the potential for development of research-based practice for the management of posttraumatic amnesia and agitation. The first component, posttraumatic amnesia, can be assessed and quantified through valid and reliable instruments, such as the GOAT or the OGMS (Mysiw, Bogner, Arnett, Clinchot, & Corrigan, 1996). The behavioral excesses—aggression, disinhibition, motor restlessness, and emotional lability—can be quantified through an instrument such as the Agitation Behavior Scale (ABS), which is considered to have acceptable reliability and validity in the traumatic brain injury population (Corrigan, 1989; Corrigan & Bogner, 1994; Sandel & Mysiw, 1996).

Bowel and Bladder Management

During the emergence from coma and confusional stages, the individual remains dependent in bladder and bowel management. It is important to assess for adequate hydration, emptying, and patterns of elimination. Care is directed at preventing iatrogenic complications, such as urinary retention and fecal impaction. Incontinence is most often a transient problem during the confusional stage related to cognitive issues, specifically, lack of awareness of or inability to process information regarding toileting needs or to initiate toileting (Grinspun, 1993). When incontinence does not respond to behavioral techniques such as scheduled toileting or persists beyond the confusional stage, further investigation is warranted. Frontal lesions, particularly bifrontal lesions, may lead to a hyperreflexive bladder and urge incontinence similar to that associated with poststroke incontinence (Oostra, Everaert, & Van Laere, 1995). Pudendal nerve damage as a result of a pelvic fracture may lead to urinary retention or overflow incontinence.

Stage of Evolving Independence

As posttraumatic amnesia resolves, attention skills improve, and the stage of evolving independence begins. The person is more aware of the environment and able to participate in the treatment program. During the period of posttraumatic amnesia, all activities of daily living are performed by the caregiver, but as the stage of evolving independence progresses, the client assumes some responsibility. Disinhibition, agitation or motor restlessness, and lability are likely to persist, but their intensity and frequency decline. Formal evaluation of focal deficits is possible because of the improvement in participation and cooperation.

Behavioral and social problems are more apparent as the person progresses through the stage of evolving independence. These problems are predominantly the sequelae of damage to the frontal lobes and the associated complex connections to other areas of the brain because of diffuse axonal injury or contusions. The cognitive processes, or executive functions, that are primarily affected are information processing, initiation, planning, execution, and regulation of behavior. When these processes are impeded, thought processes are disorganized, motivation is impaired, insight and self-appraisal are inaccurate, and planning skills are limited (Capruso & Levin, 1996). Lack of impulse control, disinhibition, perseveration, easy frustration, and irritability are behaviors that disrupt social interactions.

Stage of Intellectual and Social Competence

During what is often the longest part of recovery, the stage of intellectual and social competence, the person begins to recognize that problems are present. Physical deficits may still be present, but the cognitive, behavioral, and psychosocial issues are more limiting and translate into problems with interpersonal relationships, social interactions, and vocational pursuits. Because of the duration of this stage of recovery, it is often the most challenging for clients and families.

NURSING CARE THROUGHOUT RECOVERY

This section first deals with considerations for general assessment of a client with brain injury. It then turns to assessment and interventions specific to various injury severity levels and specific stages of recovery.

General Assessment Considerations

Culturally Competent Care

Assessing, planning, intervening, and evaluating care are predicated on knowledge of the neuropathology and functional issues that occur during recovery from brain injury. To individualize care, the nurse also must be able to take on the perspective of the client and understand ethnic and cultural influences that may affect the client's relationship with and response to the health care situation. The interpretation of the injury, the etiology, symptoms, beliefs about causation, and expectations regarding recovery and rehabilitation are subject to cultural and language influences. If the nurse and client speak different languages, subtle inaccuracy or misrepresentation during the initial assessment and data collection period can be avoided through the use of a bilingual professional; nonprofessional third parties and family members should not be asked to serve as translators (Cavallo & Saucedo, 1995; Fitzgerald, 1992).

Information regarding the client's world prior to the event offers important insights into how to prepare him or her for return to the community. Examination of how the person with a brain injury might be able to contribute to social exchanges and to social roles once back in the community is important to determining the type of assistance needed once the person leaves the rehabilitation setting (Spencer, 1993).

Knowledge of how and when people ask

for help and how reciprocity is managed in the particular community is important when one is considering the client's community resources. Spencer (1993) describes the work that she and others have done in exploring the use of neighborhood environments by elderly persons of African-American, white, Chinese, Hispanic, and Vietnamese descents. The following three adaptive patterns have been identified:

- Independent/autonomous
- Interdependent with family
- Interdependent with neighbors

The general characteristics of the *independent/autonomous* pattern are (1) living alone or with spouse, (2) self-reliant coping style, (3) driving own car, and (4) minimal social support or contact with family or neighbors. This style, consistent with the values and expectations in American rehabilitation settings that independence be achieved in all activities, was prevalent among white participants. Many participants from Chinese, Hispanic, and Vietnamese cultures were involved in extended family households consisting of two and sometimes three generations, and their pattern was described as *interdependent with family*. Daily activities and household management were conducted in an interdependent manner. When queried about how difficulties were managed, many of the participants in these groups indicated that they seek assistance or advice from others. African Americans were found to use both of these adaptive patterns, as well as the *interdependent with neighbors* pattern.

Family Needs During Assessment

Offering a context for the information being sought during the assessment, acknowledging the misfortune of the situation, and encouraging questions are strategies that rehabilitation nurses can use to build alliances and rapport with clients and their families. Entering a health care system is intimidating enough, but when it is coupled with the devastating situation precipitated by the traumatic event, families and clients can be overwhelmed. Simple explanations, such as "This information will help us identify strengths and possible areas we will be monitoring," provide a context. Age-specific assessment data are important, particularly in light of the fact that with impaired consciousness, the client's roles, functions, and developmental goals are disrupted.

An adequate discussion of family needs and concerns is beyond the scope of this chapter, but key points for assessment and intervention are offered. Rosenthal and Young (1988) advocate the use of the PLISSIT model, which was originally developed by Anon for use in sexual counseling. The acronym PLISSIT describes four levels of intervention, with *P* standing for permission, *LI* standing for limited information, *SS* designating specific suggestions, and *IT* indicating intensive therapy. In the *permission* stage, relatives or significant others are encouraged (given permission) to ask questions and express their fears, hopes, and concerns with respect to the client's recovery and the treatment program. The team member to whom questions are directed should listen in a supportive and uncritical way and direct questions to the appropriate resource. At the *limited information* level, basic information about brain injury and the brain injury program is provided through verbal, written, or audiovisual material. At the next level, specific suggestions are provided to enhance sexual function, with detailed and concrete responses to questions to meet the family's educational needs. *Intensive therapy* involves psychological counseling to assist families in the process of coping with the uncertainty, emotional distress, and changes precipitated by the brain injury. Although all members of the team may be able to provide assistance at the first two levels of this model, the third and fourth levels of intervention are most appropriately conducted by the core treatment team involved with the client.

Assessment and Intervention Related to Severity and Stage of Recovery

Table 21–7 summarizes the assessments and interventions discussed here.

Mild Head Injury

Nurses are likely to encounter individuals with mild head injury in the emergency room, in a community setting, or during hospitalization for other injuries sustained in the traumatic event, such as fractures. The key assessment parameter in the immediate posttraumatic period is monitoring for neurological deterioration from undetected focal or space-occupying lesions. People who are discharged from emergency rooms and hospitals routinely receive full information on the signs and symptoms of neurological deterioration but little on what to expect during recovery. Many people experience no symptoms following concussion until after discharge, because only when they attempt or resume normal activities do they note problems. Information about the recovery period prepares the person for the possibility of such symptoms and may help avert psychological distress associated with not knowing how to interpret them. Early intervention, in terms of information, reassurance about recovery, and support, has been identified as an effective way to help prevent the development of chronic or persistent problems after mild head injury (Alexander, 1995; Cicerone, 1992; Gronwall, 1986; Gronwall & Wrightson, 1974; Kay, 1992).

Gradual resumption of activities is recommended to help manage fatigue, poor concentration, and cognitive inefficiency. Support in coping and providing printed information that can be read later are helpful in decreasing anxiety and preventing emotional complications precipitated by lack of information and understanding of symptoms and perceived changes in performance. If the client is experiencing problems, providing his or her employer with the rationale for gradual resumption of work activities can alleviate unnecessary distress associated with mismatched expectations for work performance and work output (Hinkle et al., 1986; Kay, 1992).

The literature and anecdotal accounts from clinicians indicate that a significant number of people with mild brain injury experience considerable distress. Several researchers link the inadequate care received during the acute phase of recovery, particularly a lack of information, reassurance, and support, with delayed recovery or the development of persistent symptoms or secondary neurosis after mild head injury (Alexander, 1995; Alves, Colohan, O'Leary, Rimel, & Jane, 1986; Gronwall, 1986; Hinkle et al., 1986; Kay, 1992). Risk factors for neurobehavioral complications after mild injury are as follows (Alexander, 1995; Dicker, 1989; Gronwall & Wrightson, 1974):

- History of previous concussion
- Age greater than 40 years
- Preexisting emotional or psychiatric problems
- High-stress or high-demand occupation
- Substance abuse
- Evidence of posttraumatic amnesia indicative of a more severe injury

The standard of care most often advocated for the person with mild brain injury is some type of monitoring and both oral and written information regarding what to expect during recovery. At a minimum, a follow-up phone call is recommended. For the client who is symptomatic or has a diagnosis of "mild" injury more accurately resembling "moderate" injury, follow-up is essential.

When information has not been provided and the person enters the health care system some time after the mild injury with symptoms of a more chronic nature, it is important to validate the person's reason for struggling and to explain the deficits (Kay, 1992). Identifying symptoms and time frames for recovery from neurological, peripheral, and psychological categories of problems serves as a guide for referral, testing, and intervention (Katz & Alexander, 1994).

Moderate and Severe Injury

Nurses are likely to encounter clients with moderate or severe brain injury at various points in the recovery trajectory, from acute care and acute and subacute rehabilitation units to home and community environments. Knowledge of expected patterns of recovery and progression forms the foundation of the nurse's role in providing care, contributing to interdisciplinary planning and evaluation, and advocating for clients and families.

Initial Rehabilitation Stages: Coma and Emergence from Coma (Rancho Los Amigos Scale Levels I, II, and III)

Arousal

From a functional perspective, arousal is the predominant issue during coma and emergence from coma. The goals of treatment are preventing deterioration, preventing complications, and providing stimulation. From a nursing perspective, impaired consciousness renders the person dependent in all aspects of care. Monitoring neurological status and physiological responses to the trauma and to treatment regimens is the assessment priority, which is accomplished through evaluation of serial neurological vital signs, Glasgow Coma Scale scores, and physiological assessment data. From a rehabilitation perspective, the specific neurological indicators of progression from coma to vigilance are the return of sleep-wake cycles and spontaneous eye opening.

Text continued on page 356

TABLE 21–7 ■ ASSESSMENTS AND INTERVENTIONS RELATED TO SEVERITY OF BRAIN INJURY AND STAGE OF RECOVERY

Problem or Nursing Diagnosis	Stage of Recovery			
	Emergence from Coma	Mute/Low Level	Confused	Evolving Independence and Intellectual and Social Competence
Arousal problem	Provide sensory input through all senses Monitor responses and for changes in level of responsiveness	Continue as previous stage	(Resolved)	
	Assess level of consciousness, neurological vital signs	Assess level of consciousness		
		Assess ability to respond to 1-step commands Assess purposeful versus nonpurposeful movement		
		Anticipate needs to minimize restlessness (full bladder, bowel, pain, noxious stimuli from tubes, casts, positioning devices)		
		If pharmacological intervention for arousal initiated, monitor responses		
High Risk for Injury	Protect airway	Assess for onset of confusional stage, restlessness in response to noxious stimuli, discomfort	Continue as needed with interventions per previous stage	Assess and monitor responses and safety as supervision decreased and self-responsibility increased
		Initiate safety and protective measures (i.e., prevent decannulization of tracheotomy, injury from orthopedic devices, and perseverative physical movement, such as banging extremities, constant rubbing of elbows/heels)	Assess/monitor behavior with frequent observation	
			Provide safe environment (modify stimulation, simplify, provide structure, remove all external solutions, objects that could be used inappropriately during confusional state; structure)	
			Implement fall prevention interventions (bed check, frequent observation) as mobility improves	
			Anticipate needs to minimize agitated or aggressive responses	

Impaired Thought Processes	Assess for onset of restlessness, stage of confusion
	Provide consistent caretakers
	Facilitate routine
	Provide visual and verbal orientation information cues (clocks, calendar, signs, subtle conversation cues)
	Facilitate gradual increase in client responsibility
	Assess and monitor responses
	Collaborate with interdisciplinary team in planning day outings and community visits
	Debrief families upon return
	Assess specific behaviors and deficits, social interactions that impact discharge and discharge planning
Posttraumatic amnesia	Initiate preventive measures:
	Make calming interactions
	Minimize environmental factors
	Remove person from situations that escalate behaviors
	Provide structured psychomotor activities
	Reinforce self-control
	Assess for and minimize cognitive and physical fatigue
	Provide structure, consistency, repetition, and positive re-inforcement
	Collaborate with interdisciplinary team and establish clear goals and plans

Table continued on following page

TABLE 21–7 ■ ASSESSMENTS AND INTERVENTIONS RELATED TO SEVERITY OF BRAIN INJURY AND STAGE OF RECOVERY *Continued*

Problem or Nursing Diagnosis	Stage of Recovery			
	Emergence from Coma	*Mute/Low Level*	*Confused*	*Evolving Independence and Intellectual and Social Competence*
Agitation			Verbally redirect	
			Keep interactions brief, simple, direct	
			Model behavior with calm, controlled approach and interaction	
			Provide feedback that reassures, establishes boundaries, reinforces positive behaviors	
			Avoid confrontation; redirect inappropriate behaviors and confusional beliefs	
			Redirect	
			Provide structure and boundaries	
			Protective/pharmacological interventions:	
			Use when external controls not sufficient and safety is threatened	
			Initiate restraint standards if used	
			Monitor responses to pharmacological interventions	
			Provide care activities in a flexible manner (when person is calm, able to tolerate activities)	
			Monitor/document PTA through validated, reliable instruments	
			Collaborate with team	
			Assess day-to-day memory (i.e., can now remember what was consumed/offered for breakfast)	

For specific deficits/problems			Redirect when behaviors inappropriate (attempts to correct or provide feedback not possible in confused state)	Feedback and alternatives for behaviors; Reinforce correct responses, use verbal and gestural cues to give feedback for inappropriate comments, answers; Use strategies to enhance judgement; Rehearse, role play, simulate situations, collaborate with team; Praise, encourage, remind of progress
Sleep-wake disturbance	Monitor for return of gross sleep-wake cycles	Monitor for return of sleep-wake cycles (day/night); organize care activities to allow for periods of sleep without interruption as permitted by medical condition	Monitor fatigue; provide environment conducive to sleep; incorporate relaxation, therapeutic touch; comfort measures at hour of sleep; assess need for pharmacological intervention if conservative measures ineffective	Continue per previous stage as needed; Teach relaxation strategies if appropriate/needed
Impaired Communication	Monitor for response to commands	Establish y/n communication	Address in a clear, calm manner, establish eye contact; avoid extraneous communication and excess verbiage to facilitate processing	Assess for specific problems: word finding, comprehension problems; Assess for hypophonation, monotone
High Risk for Disuse Syndrome	Develop plans to ensure all activities of daily living, hygiene, elimination needs are met	Continue as per previous stage	Continue as per previous stages; Encourage client participation as tolerated	Resolve and initiate specific self-care diagnoses, teaching learning program as the person or significant other is able to assume at least partial responsibility for care

Table continued on following page

TABLE 21–7 ■ ASSESSMENTS AND INTERVENTIONS RELATED TO SEVERITY OF BRAIN INJURY AND STAGE OF RECOVERY *Continued*

Problem or Nursing Diagnosis	Stage of Recovery			
	Emergence from Coma	*Mute/Low Level*	*Confused*	*Evolving Independence and Intellectual and Social Competence*
Impaired Physical Mobility	Frequent repositioning Minimize positions that increase tone problems Monitor for complications (DVT, pneumonia, infection, atelectasis, heterotrophic calcification) Initiate collaborate interventions ROM Monitor for decreases in ability to range	Increase frequency of monitoring for positioning problems, tone as restlessness evolves Assess tone management; intervene as appropriate	Continue as in previous stages Manage as per disuse syndrome	Assess impact of impaired mobility on toileting, and hygiene needs, and intervene as indicated Begin discharge teaching as indicated
Self-care deficits	(see High Risk for Disuse Syndrome)			Assess limitations of neurological versus functional barriers Collaborate with team recompensatory techniques and equipment to maximize client's level of independence
Pain	Administer analgesics as indicated for procedures ROM	Assess nonverbal indicators (grimace, autonomic signs, moaning, increased restlessness) Assess and monitor responses to splinting, positioning devices, positioning and tone problems Administer analgesics as indicated	As per previous stage Assess impact on behavior	Collaborate with client/family to ensure pain is addressed and does not decrease mobility/ disuse, or reduce participation in care and activities
Nutrition/impaired swallowing		Continue as per previous stage Initiate swallowing evaluation and oral feedings with supervision and interdisciplinary collaboration as needed Initiate calorie count as indicated	Supervise meals, structured environment to facilitate attention to the activity Continue to monitor intake and nutritional/metabolic status Initiate intervention for specific problems (i.e., impulse control problems, self-feeding deficits related to paralysis, altered appetite)	Assess and monitor as supervision decreased

Nursing Diagnosis				
Coping: individual and family	Engage family in care activities and have them bring in objects from home Provide information on condition Implement PLISSIT model Provide information on support groups, brain injury foundation, team and team functions Advocate and assist family in navigating systems	Change the focus of support and information (no longer life-threatening) Focus on behavior and how to interact with/respond to client	Continue as per previous stage Role model interactions for families Address concerns, provide opportunity for feedback, and observe client-family interactions Continue educational process Assess, monitor responses Initiate referrals for formal counseling, support as warranted Schedule time with family for open communication and incorporation of family perspective	Feedback and role modeling re specific cognitive and behavior deficits Assess intimacy concerns for client and family; intervene and refer as indicated Include teaching re anticipated problems/concerns Ongoing teaching for physical care issues after discharge Assess for depression and substance abuse; refer as indicated
Knowledge deficit	Begin assessment of family teaching learning needs Collaborate with other disciplines to determine best approach for client learning and family/client teaching Initiate PLISSIT model	Provide information on stage of recovery Continue as per previous stage Provide feedback/encouragement on family's interactions and responses Formal educational offerings (usually interdisciplinary)	As above	Establish resources for continuing care Begin teaching for specific deficits, problems; include safety awareness; evaluate postdischarge referral and services needed
Incontinence (specify type) or inability to self-manage risk for constipation, functional incontinence	(see High Risk for Disuse Syndrome)	Discontinue indwelling catheters as soon as possible Monitor through intake and output, auscultation of bowel sounds, postvoid residuals Add dietary fiber fluids as indicated Assess voiding, defecation patterns	Monitor intake, emptying, residuals as indicated by assessment Provide cues, structure, scheduled times Incorporate toileting/transfers into therapy schedules Praise and reinforce successes Initiate interventions for specific problems if indicated	

DVT, deep venous thrombosis; PTA, posttraumatic amnesia; ROM, range-of-motion exercises.

Progression from vigilance to low-level responsiveness is evidenced by purposeful responses and movement.

Sensory Stimulation

Although sensory input is important for maintaining arousal, the benefit of formal sensory stimulation programs aimed at *hastening* arousal in clients with low-level responsiveness has yet to be demonstrated (Sandel, Horn, & Bontke, 1992). Sensory input, at a minimum, provides a means by which changes in the level of responsiveness can be monitored and a way for families to participate in care and the assessment of changes. Sensory stimulation is incorporated into activities of daily living and treatment activities through tactile, visual, gustatory, auditory, olfactory, and kinesthetic modalities (Grzankowski, 1997; Sosnowski & Ustik, 1994).

Touch, an integral component of all aspects of care, can be provided through innumerable actions, such as hand holding and applying heat or cold. Having family members bring in familiar objects for the client's room serves the dual purpose of involving the family and providing meaningful visual stimulation. Even when oral feeding is not possible, gustatory stimulation can be provided through tooth brushing and the use of oral swabs. Auditory input is provided by talking to the person, giving brief explanations and information throughout the performance of care activities. The use of radios or cassettes with favorite music or favorite television shows should be scheduled into daily routines as appropriate.

Olfactory stimulation is accomplished through the introduction of inoffensive aromas, such as those of coffee, chocolate, or citrus fruit. In addition, positioning, stretching, and range-of-motion activities can augment sensory stimulation by providing proprioceptive feedback and vestibular input. When any of these interventions is employed as a means of evaluating changes in neurological response, it is important to observe and document the responses.

Communication

Once it is clear that the person is at the mute low-level responsive stage, establishing some reliable form of communication becomes a priority. This usually involves setting up a "yes/no" response system through any appropriate modality, such as nodding the head, raising a finger, or blinking the eyes.

Restlessness and Safety

A further component of the neurological assessment is focused on monitoring for restlessness and the concomitant safety implications. This is a particularly serious issue if the person still requires airway support via an endotracheal tube or tracheotomy, because he or she will attempt to eliminate noxious stimuli by pulling at tubes and catheters. If there are precautions related to orthopedic injuries, such as external fixtures or casts, the frequency of assessment and monitoring must be increased to ensure that no iatrogenic complications occur. Making sure the plan of care includes anticipatory interventions for problems that contribute to restlessness, such as pain or a full bladder or bowel, is an important preventative strategy.

Drugs

Pharmacological treatment is considered when improvement in arousal is slow or has reached a plateau. Although there are no clear guidelines for the selection of a specific agent, dopamine or dopamine agonists, such as amantadine, methylphenidate, and bromocriptine, may be used alone or in combination to capitalize on their synergistic effects (Wroblewski & Glenn, 1994). A period of trial and error may be required to find an effective regimen. Nursing considerations include understanding the desired effect, dosage, mechanism of action, and side effects of the agents used in order to monitor client responses.

Tone, Spasticity, and Pain

Tone problems and spasticity change or evolve as recovery progresses, complicating positioning, range of motion, and mobility. Severe traumatic brain injury may involve upper motor neuron lesions in the cerebral, subcortical, or brainstem areas, leading to increased muscle tone. Primitive reflexes that are normally not seen after the central nervous system matures may return. These reflexes are often stimulated by head and trunk positions that deviate from the midline (Habel, 1997). As is true for all aspects of care, the assessment and management of tone problems involves ongoing interdisciplinary collaboration. Therapists may recommend splints, which are generally most effective for spasticity of a mild or moderate severity. Ankle contractures may be better managed with serial casting (Ferido & Habel, 1988). Often, specific muscle groups and target areas require special stretching and positioning, which are carried out as part of the therapy program. Whatever modality is selected, monitoring for treatment response, pain, and skin integrity is essential.

For clients unable to communicate, the behavioral responses indicative of pain might consist of moaning or increased restlessness, whereas physiological indicators might be autonomic signs, such as tachycardia or diaphoresis. Premedication to prevent or minimize pain during range-of-motion activities, stretching, or casting is an important aspect of the nurse's role in management of spasticity and tone. Positioning and range-of-motion activities, whether part of a prescribed therapy regimen or part of general nursing care, are most effective if a slow, smooth stretch is used and positions and movements that increase spastic responses are avoided (Ferido & Habel, 1988). Other nursing interventions advocated for the management of tone problems are noted in Table 21–8.

When conservative interventions for spasticity management prove ineffective, systemic or local pharmacological approaches are considered. Phenol nerve blocks and intramuscular botulinum toxin are two types of local modalities that are effective. Phenol blocks have an immediate onset and long duration of effect, possibly permanent. Therefore, if recovery is expected, a phenol block may not be the appropriate first choice. The effects of botulinum toxin may take several weeks to become evident, but the duration of action is shorter, making it a good option when motor recovery and improvement in spasticity are expected (Grazko, Polo, & Jabbari, 1995; Pierson, Katz, & Tarsy, 1996). Systemic agents, such as baclofen and dantrolene, are used only as a last resort because the spasticity and increased tone associated with brain injury do not generally respond to them. In addition, the central nervous system side effects of such agents preclude their use when arousal is already impaired.

Metabolic Needs

Metabolic needs during early recovery are extreme, particularly for people with severe injuries. Hypermetabolism increases caloric utilization to the level that resembles that of clients with burns over 30% of the body (Anderson, 1987; Clifton, Robertson, Grossman, Foltz, & Garza, 1984). Assessment of metabolic and nutritional status is accomplished through calorie counts, evaluation of laboratory parameters such as serum albumin and protein levels, body weight measurement, and collaboration with the registered dietitian. The frequency of reassessment and the level of monitoring required are determined from the results of these clinical indicators.

Because the hallmark of the low-level responsive stage is the evolution of purposeful and responsive movement, nursing and speech therapy personnel may collaborate to assess the client's swallowing ability.

Airway protection and the prevention of aspiration are the paramount concerns. As the client exhibits enough initiation and attention to cooperate, the motor aspects of swallowing are examined through a bedside screen and, possibly, a modified barium swallow radiography study. Supervision and structure are essential components of early oral feeding programs. Whenever the transition to oral feedings occurs, assessment focuses on monitoring for adequate hydration and nutrition through collaboration with the dietitian, attention to calorie counts, body weight measurements, and monitoring of metabolic parameters reflective of nutritional status.

TABLE 21–8 ■ NONINVASIVE NURSING INTERVENTIONS FOR MUSCLE TONE PROBLEMS

Keep the head in a neutral, midline position to avoid abnormal limb postures and spasticity.

Provide range of motion with sustained stretch, and slow, rhythmic motion.

Use gentle, steady touch when moving spastic extremity; avoid rapid movement.

Provide noninvasive pain management (therapeutic touch, guided imagery, distraction, massage).

Manage physical and environmental stimuli (avoid rapid movement, room temperature too hot or cold, bumping of bed or wheelchair).

Provide a calm environment to increase the threshold to nociceptive stimulation.

Employ therapeutic use of self (i.e., calming, soothing tone and touch, reassurance) to avoid fear, anxiety, and anger responses that may increase tone.

Incorporate behavioral interventions to redirect or minimize fear, anxiety, and agitation responses that may increase tone.

Adapted from Habel, M. (1997). Muscle tone abnormalities. *Rehabilitation Nursing, 22* (3), 118–123.

Family Concerns

Common concerns or emotions expressed by families during the acute recovery period from a brain injury are (1) needing to relive the incident, particularly the "unexpected" nature of the event, (2) dealing with the unpredictability, (3) anger and guilt, (4) grief over the possible loss of the person as he or she was, (5) changes in roles, (6) feelings of inadequacy in communicating with the person, and (7) disruption of life (Richmond, Metcalf, & Winterhalter, 1987).

Confusional Stage (Rancho Los Amigos Scale Levels IV and V)

As arousal problems resolve with the return of the client's alertness and responsiveness, attention problems emerge, heralding the onset of the confusional stage. The profound confusion that marks this stage of recovery is predominantly a reflection of attention deficits. Attention or information processing difficulties manifest as impaired concentration, the inability to take in more than one piece of information at a time, and diminished retention of immediate events (posttraumatic amnesia). Inconsistent performance is common, and despite obvious improvement in verbal expression and purposeful motor activity, the person remains functionally dependent as a result of confusion.

Behavior

The major goals revolve around ensuring safety and supporting the individual through this period, mainly via a behavior program. The neurological assessment priorities include continuing to monitor neurological status, monitoring responses to behavioral management and treatment, and assessing the impact of behavior on other essential treatments. From a rehabilitation perspective, neurological indicators of progress include (1) resolution of posttraumatic amnesia, as indicated by improved GOAT or OGMS scores, and (2) participation in self-care and rehabilitation activities.

The confusion, restlessness, and agitation observed in the person in the confusional stage of recovery reflects a world of inner turmoil, in which the person is responding to and overwhelmed by internal stimuli. This turmoil highlights the need to regulate external stimuli through manipulation of the environment and behavioral interventions (Malec & Basford, 1996). A successful behavioral management plan begins with a comprehensive interdisciplinary team assessment, clear plans and goals linked to specific targeted behaviors oriented to prevention and outcome, and a caring environment. The fundamental tenets of interventions performed by all disciplines are structure, consistency, repetition, and positive reinforcement (Howard, 1988).

The person's physical fatigue is often obvious, and endurance is limited. Cognitive or mental fatigue, especially in the early postarousal period, may manifest as behavior changes, such as increased irritability, greater confusion, or diminished performance on tasks. Indicators of physical and mental fatigue guide team members in determining the amount of stimulation and activity the person can tolerate. Some interventions aimed at avoiding fatigue are providing frequent rest periods, keeping tasks simple, and minimizing environmental stimuli.

Consistent caregivers, daily routines, orientation information, and modulation of the type and amount of input and stimulation facilitate information processing. When a particular interaction or activity appears to increase confusion, the person should be redirected or removed from the situation. Caregivers' interactions with patients should be brief, simple, and direct. Calm, controlled behavior modeling, in the context of a familiar environment, is therapeutic in this situation. Caregivers interact as role models and provide feedback that reassures, establishes boundaries, and reinforces positive aspects of the client's behavior (Howard, 1988). Confronting inappropriate behaviors and confusional beliefs is not helpful because the profound memory and attentional deficits of the person in the confusional stage preclude the ability to incorporate such higher-level feedback. People in this stage are often bewildered and afraid. In addition to a calm approach, the setting of limits in a firm, simple way provides structure, boundaries, and security. Even if the person cannot respond to the limits, caregivers are offering reassurance and communicating that they are in control.

Orientation

Assessing the client's orientation status and providing accurate information to help with orientation are achieved through subtle references to clocks, calendars, and events rather than through the conventional approach of soliciting the answers to place, date, and time questions. The aims of this intervention are to provide reassurance and support during confusion and to avoid interactions that may be interpreted as confrontational and may therefore have an ego-defeating impact on the client.

Agitation

Agitation and behavioral outbursts are common during this period, with overstimulation and misinterpretation of the environment being common precipitants. The primary intervention is prevention, which is accomplished through recognition of the early signs of escalating behavior, increasing confusion, or growing restlessness. Attempts to avert the progression of agitation and behavioral outbursts include (1) calming interactions, (2) removal of contributing environmental factors, (3) removal of the person from the situation, (4) acknowledgment of feelings expressed by the client, and (5) reinforcement of self-control (Howard, 1988). Structured psychomotor activities are important strategies used to channel excess energy into appropriate outlets, thus helping reduce agitated and restless behavior.

Assessment of behavior, particularly of episodic agitation or outbursts, involves more than identification of the specific action of the client. What occurs before (the antecedent) and after (the consequence) the target behavior is critical to effective management. A useful approach is focused observation and documentation of antecedent, behavior, and consequence, commonly referred to as *ABC charting* (Howard, 1988). The approach requires the collaboration of all disciplines working with the client and is usually coordinated by a neuropsychologist. Once patterns of behavior are identified, interventions can be used to (1) modify or avoid specific antecedents, (2) prevent the formation of behavioral patterns that are maladaptive, and (3) promote reinforcement of appropriate behaviors and responses. The Agitated Behavior Scale (ABS) offers a means to quantify the presence and extent of behaviors (Corrigan, 1989; Corrigan & Bogner, 1994; Sandel & Mysiw, 1996). ABC charting is more specific, in that the antecedent behavior is documented in order to gain insight regarding possible patterns and thereby identify specific triggers. The goals are to develop behavioral interventions that will minimize unwanted responses and to elicit responses that will allow the person to participate in rehabilitation activities.

Restraint

When clients exhibit signs of irritability and physical combativeness but are able to respond to reduced environmental stimulation, redirection, and limit setting, the behavioral interventions are sufficient. When external controls are no longer sufficient and the safety and well-being of the client or staff are threatened, additional environmental manipulation or protective restraint interventions are implemented. Chemical restraint, which is generally avoided because it may impede recovery by slowing or dulling already impaired cognition, is also considered.

The elements of a protective environment are (1) a private or "quiet" room, with sparse furnishings, minimal stimulation, and maximal comfort measures, and (2) brief interactions with one person at a time, with great attention given to providing reassuring, calming communications (Patterson & Sargent, 1990; Rehabilitation Nursing Foundation, 1989). A bed such as the Craig bed or Vale bed may be used; such beds afford freedom of movement while providing security and safety. Close supervision and monitoring are necessary. Physical restraints tend to increase agitation and are employed only as a last resort. Their use should be short-term, criteria-driven, and supported by a specific standard of care.

Research available to direct the selection of appropriate chemical restraints is limited, but anticonvulsants, antidepressants, β-blockers, benzodiazepines, and neuroleptics are commonly used. Lithium, buspirone, and even stimulants may have a role in the management of agitation. Medications may be used alone or in combination (Cassidy, 1994; Mysiw & Sandel, 1997; Rose, 1988). The nursing role in the use of such agents consists of (1) understanding the desired effect, dosage, mechanism of action, side effect profile, and potential interactions of the agent used and (2) monitoring and documenting client responses, with attention to quantifying and qualifying behaviors and improvements.

When the extreme interventions of physical or chemical restraint are implemented, families need information, education, and ongoing communication with the team to understand the goals, evaluate progress, and learn how to interact with and support the client.

Sleep-Wake Regulation

Sleep-wake disturbances interfere with progress by worsening confusion, decreasing participation, and contributing to the development of agitation. Regulating the sleep-wake cycle is an integral part of behavior management and is governed by the principles of the overall program. Environmental manipulation and comfort measures are the first interventions, with the introduction of pharmacological agents only when it is evident that conservative measures are not effective. Sedating antidepressants or short-acting benzodiazepines are reasonable choices because they have less propensity to dull cognition or interfere with daytime wakefulness.

Bowel and Bladder Management

The approach to bowel and bladder continence during this period of recovery revolves around fluid management, assessment of voiding patterns, attention to dietary intake, and behavioral interventions. Early in this stage, a toileting schedule is the most appropriate behavioral strategy because of the limited ability of the client to identify and act on needs. Assessment of voiding patterns through observation may reveal the times most likely to lead to success in toileting. Praise at the time of success serves to positively reinforce the individual's efforts. Ultrasonographic assessment of postvoid or postincontinence residual should be obtained to ensure adequate emptying (Grinspun, 1993). A consistent approach is necessary for success in any continence program, making interdisciplinary collaboration and participation essential.

Assessing Progress

There is no sharp transition from one stage of recovery to another, but by the end of the confusional stage, posttraumatic amnesia has resolved. The client remembers what is happening from moment to moment and then from day to day and is consistently oriented. For example, he or she can remember the names of caregivers or what therapy activities he or she participated in that day. Completion of some aspect of activities of daily living with less cuing, coaxing, and refocusing is an indicator of improved attention skills and progression from the confusional state. The GOAT is a more formalized and standard instrument for assessing posttraumatic amnesia; the responsibility of completing the assessment at specified intervals is assigned to a particular discipline.

Evolving Independence (Rancho Los Amigos Scale Level VI)

The functional limitations of the person in the stage of evolving independence are related to cognitive issues. As the global inattention that characterized the confusional state clears, simple attention skills are improved to the point that the person can attend to tasks within the framework of a structured environment. Specific underlying cognitive issues become apparent and manifest as deficits in the areas of complex attention, concentration, memory, perception, insight and judgment, orientation, comprehension, language, and self-awareness (Stratton & Gregory, 1994). Persisting physical problems, such as paralysis and fractures, also contribute to functional limitations.

The goal during this stage is preparation for discharge, which consists of (1) promoting independence in activities of daily living, (2) facilitating awareness of functional limitations and safety, and (3) coaching for the resumption of personal responsibilities and social competence. Because the lingering cognitive problems influence all aspects of planning and intervention, the neurological and rehabilitation assessment priorities often converge. The neurological assessment priorities are screening for specific deficits and monitoring behavioral responses, whereas rehabilitation assessment comprises the evaluation of self-care ability, safety, and social issues that might impede discharge.

Functional problems must be understood in the context of the underlying neurological cause in order for appropriate treatment approaches to be determined. Deficits in self-care, for example, are often due to a combination of cognitive and physical factors. Decreased attention and impulsivity may not be major impediments to the performance of activities of daily living but, when coupled with balance problems, may compromise the person's safety. The inability to organize and sequence, although improved by the simplified environment and cuing that served as the main interventions in the previous stage, may emerge as a serious limitation to discharge once the structure and environmental supports are decreased.

Behavior

The behavioral interventions during this phase of recovery reflect the improved ability to process and retain information and include providing feedback and presenting acceptable alternatives in a nonjudgmental manner. Client responsibility increases and supervision decreases, often starting with overlearned tasks, such as activities of daily living. Situations or tasks that are novel or complex present a challenge for the person, and responses serve as a guide for advancing both the type of activity and the setting in which therapy occurs, with movement from the narrow confines of the room to the unit, facility, surrounding grounds, and, finally, community.

Although routine and structure remain important props for behavioral performance, the client's clearing sensorium does allow for gradual withdrawal of these supports. The ability to lay down day-to-day memories and the capacity for basic problem solving also allow the client to incorporate feedback and behaviors modeled by staff. The use of aids, such as written schedules, memory logs, and frequent reference to clocks and calendars, may remain a mainstay. However, the client can now begin to assume responsibility for managing and maintaining logs and schedules.

Family Education

Family education at this stage focuses on providing information about the person's cognitive deficits. Observation of family involvement in care activities, role modeling, and feedback with regard to client-family interactions are components of the teaching-learning strategies.

Bowel and Bladder Management

The incontinence that may have been present during the confusional period should now be resolved. Behavioral interventions, such as cuing and scheduling, may continue to be necessary, but there is a shift from caregiver to client responsibility and involvement in bowel and bladder management. Persistent incontinence warrants further investigation to determine whether the cause is neurological, functional, or an iatrogenic complication such as an infection. As mentioned previously,

frontal lesions, particularly bifrontal lesions, may lead to a hyperreflexive bladder and urge incontinence similar to that associated with poststroke incontinence (Oostra et al., 1995). Pudendal nerve damage as a result of pelvic fracture may lead to urinary retention or overflow incontinence. Assessment of intake, output, and frequency of voiding, as well as questions directed to the client regarding the presence of any symptoms, will help determine the cause. Ultrasonographic bladder assessment for postvoid residual is a noninvasive means for gathering the necessary information to direct appropriate strategies or referrals.

At this stage of recovery, underlying physical or cognitive issues result in a *functional incontinence*. For example, paralysis with limited mobility can lead to incontinence when the client is unable to physically meet his or her own toileting needs. The person may be too slow or clumsy to be efficient in managing clothing, a urinal, or transfers. Interventions for such problems include physical assistance and collaborating with practitioners of other disciplines to provide appropriate adaptive techniques and equipment. Cognitive deficits related to frontal lobe damage, however, can result in a disinhibited state in which the individual lacks adequate judgment and restraint. This state leads to voiding at times or in settings that are inappropriate. For example, despite the awareness of the need to void, the disinhibited individual may void in an immediate and primitive manner with indifference to the social inappropriateness of these actions. Interventions for this problem include providing feedback and appropriate alternatives.

Promoting Community Integration

Therapeutic day passes, community visits, and group activities serve as the general format through which rehabilitation interventions occur. The goals revolve around providing real-life and postdischarge situations to enable (1) assessment of functional, cognitive, and psychosocial skills that will facilitate the person's successful transition to the community and (2) identification of areas that require follow-up after discharge. Therapeutic day passes allow the staff and family to evaluate the client's family interactions, carryover of skills to the home environment, and awareness of limitations and allow the client to practice working with existing limitations

(Capruso & Levin, 1996). Community visits are structured outings with professional staff in which the client can practice specific skills, including social interactions and money and time management. Group activities, such as meal preparation, recreational outings, and social encounters, allow for the practice of specific skills. An additional benefit of group activities is the opportunity for peer support and feedback, which can be more compelling than feedback from caregivers and families.

Intimacy and Sexuality

Assessment of intimacy and concerns about sexuality are part of the ongoing evaluation of the person's psychological and interpersonal functioning. A decrease in both libido and frequency of intercourse following brain injury has been reported (Garden, Bontke, & Hoffman, 1990). Hypersexual behavior may also occur in relation to disinhibition. Proactive interventions include discussion and education prior to discharge. The availability of sexual counseling is an important component of the postdischarge rehabilitation program.

Discharge Planning

When discharge to home is planned, the priorities include ensuring that (1) services and equipment are in place, (2) supervision is arranged, and (3) the person who will assume primary responsibility for the client at home demonstrates competence and a level of comfort in providing care. Strategies for accomplishing the third goal include hands-on involvement of and direct observation by the responsible person during the client's hospitalization.

A formal community reentry program or transitional living center may be effective in reducing the client's need for supervision and improving his or her domestic and community skills (Johnston & Lewis, 1991). McLaughlin and Peters (1993) found that people who participated in transitional living for the last few weeks of rehabilitation showed more independence in the activities of daily living than those who remained in the traditional rehabilitation setting until discharge. Some clients evolve slowly or remain dependent in some areas, necessitating alternative considerations for discharge, such as day hospital programs and specialized behavioral disorder units. Client needs, along with the availability of resources, influence the type of program selected.

Intellectual and Social Competence (Rancho Los Amigos Scale Levels VII and VIII)

Once established in a community setting with some degree of independence, the person enters what is often the longest phase of recovery. The major concerns of clients in the first year after brain injury revolve around physical functioning, return to work, and the ability to live independently (Dikmen et al., 1993). Personal, social, or vocational competence may be impeded as a result of a range of persisting cognitive, behavioral, or psychosocial issues. Cognitive impairments may persist in specific domains, such as memory, high-level attention, insight, and organization and planning skills. From a functional perspective, deficits in these areas may impede performance in personal and household management as well as vocational and educational pursuits. For example, the person may be able to prepare a simple meal, but the full spectrum of tasks involved in planning beyond one meal—that is, organizing a grocery list, obtaining the groceries, and having meals ready at certain times—may be overwhelming.

The goals of interventions at this stage are to help the client adapt and achieve a level of independence commensurate with his or her skills and abilities in the areas of personal, social, and vocational or educational endeavors. Assessment priorities include monitoring for behavioral and emotional responses that may interfere with roles, relationships, and activities. Premorbid functioning in each of these areas must be considered. Treatment plans are organized around specific residual problems, such as cognitive and vocational needs, refractory behavioral problems, and psychological adjustment. Availability of resources in the community setting, as well as the values and personal preferences of the client, guides the selection of programs (Racino & Williams, 1994). Ambulatory care rehabilitation and vocational programs, in conjunction with other supportive services, provide the format for ongoing interventions.

Vocational, Rehabilitation, and Behavioral Programs

There is some evidence that cognitive rehabilitation programs, even late in recovery, can improve the function of people with brain injury. Treatment in structured settings, with professional attention and psychosocial group support, uses one of two possible approaches. *Cognitive remediation* focuses on improving information processing and attention, whereas *functional skills retraining* involves teaching compensatory strategies that target specific behaviors in real-life settings (Malec, 1996; Malec & Basford, 1996; Mills, Nesbeda, Katz, & Alexander, 1992).

Models for vocational reentry programs for people with traumatic brain injury range from supportive employment techniques to more cognitively based retraining programs. When return to gainful employment is not realistic, goals are directed toward other meaningful or productive activities, such as volunteer or assisted-work programs. Specialized behavior management programs are appropriate for the small group of people with behavior problems too severe to be managed with less intense approaches.

Long-term Needs

The long-term needs of clients and families are significant and indicate the need for continued alliances and follow-up with health care professionals specializing in brain injury. Residual behavior problems, such as lack of impulse control, disinhibition, perseveration, easy frustration, and irritability, result in impaired social skills that interfere with interpersonal relationships and further limit the ability to engage in or complete tasks. Psychological adjustment is an ongoing process.

Even when a person's functional status continues to improve, emotional difficulties may emerge. Krefting (1989) has documented the struggles and strategies families and clients used to deal with a loss of self-identity and personhood experienced as a result of injury. Concealment of less visible deficits, denial, and redefining or reframing situations were the strategies most often employed by the subjects of the study. Acorn (1993), in a study mainly of women who had been caring for their brain-injured sons for an average of 6 years, identified a number of perceived stressors, such as memory impairments, problems with decision making, mood swings, and dependency. Major concerns the participants had about the future were (1) anxiety about what would happen to the brain-injured person if something happened to the caregiver, (2) availability of community resources, and (3) worry about financial resources. Participants also expressed the need for education, information, and honest communication from health care providers.

Depression and Suicide

Depression may emerge as a person's insight improves, as demands on the patient increase, or both. Gomez-Hernandez, Max, Kosier, and Paradiso (1997) suggest that vocational concerns and difficulties with interpersonal relationships are two psychosocial factors associated with depression. A 3-year follow-up of a transitional living program found that loneliness and depression were the two problems most commonly reported by clients (Harrick, Krefting, and Johnston, 1994). Tate, Simpson, Flanagan, and Coffey (1997), after examining a cohort of 896 people with traumatic brain injuries, demonstrated the suicide rate to be less than 1% (8 suicides). They concluded that psychosocial failures were more compelling than severity of neuropsychological impairments as a risk factor for suicide. Klonoff and Lage (1995) followed the progress of 111 people with traumatic brain injury for 8 years and found that 1.8% (2 subjects) committed suicide; another 21.8% (24) reported significant depression, with 12.6% (14) having suicidal ideation.

A history of alcohol and drug abuse, depression, and other psychiatric disturbances, along with feelings of helplessness, hopelessness, despair, worthlessness, and loss of the sense of integrity, are identified as risk factors for suicide. Limited coping abilities, suicidal ideation, and acute emotional distress in combination with the problems of impulse control, cognitive inflexibility, and social isolation are additional risk factors for suicide (Klonoff & Lage, 1995). When a person's risk for suicide is found to be present or escalates to the level of suicidal ideation, treatment and assessment should be conducted jointly by psychiatric and brain injury professionals. Family members need education about identification of risk factors and intervention when such factors are present (Tate et al., 1997).

Substance Abuse

Drugs and alcohol adversely affect postinjury outcomes, and abstinence is recommended. When a substance abuse problem is identified, education, prevention, and treatment programs are long-term considerations. The results of one study indicate that there is a pattern of risk for higher alcohol consumption after brain injury in young people and in people with preinjury alcohol problems (Kreutzer et al., 1996).

The limited research available indicates that traditional approaches to substance abuse, such as Alcoholics Anonymous and Narcotics Anonymous, must be modified to meet the needs of brain-injured clients (Malec & Basford, 1996). Bogner, Corrigan, Spafford, and Lamb-Hart (1997) endorse a treatment philosophy incorporating substance abuse resources with other services aimed at stabilizing the client's overall situation, including health, financial, and social areas.

CONCLUSION

This chapter has focused on the characteristics and patterns demonstrated by a majority of clients with traumatic brain injury during the first few months after injury. The neurological aspects of assessment, the implications of various injuries, and the interpretation of behaviors are emphasized to help the nurse understand the markers of progress and the focus of interventions. Rehabilitation, of course, encompasses much more than the limited perspective offered here. It takes place in a milieu of interdisciplinary collaboration and in the context of complex and rich human conditions and circumstances that require the efforts, energies, and courage of all involved.

A major challenge for nursing is to focus our research efforts to continue to develop knowledge in the area of traumatic brain injury rehabilitation in a systematic fashion. We suggest that this chapter serve as a starting point for inquiry. In closing, we offer some of the questions we believe need to be answered:

What are the needs of clients and families during each stage of recovery? at the time of transitions from one stage to the next and from one care setting to another?

What are the current standards of practice?

How are transitions of care best managed?

What interventions promote positive outcomes? under what circumstances?

How are cognitive and behavioral symptoms best managed?

How do systems of care delivery affect the processes and outcomes of care?

What are the best approaches to delivering care?

What does the traumatic brain injury mean to the client? to the family?

REFERENCES

Acorn, S. (1993). Head-injured survivors: Caregivers and support groups. *Journal of Advanced Nursing, 18*(1), 39–45.

Alexander, M. P. (1982). Traumatic brain injury. In D. H. Benson & H. Blumer (Eds.), *Psychiatric aspects of neurological disease* (pp. 251–278). New York: McGraw-Hill.

Alexander, M. P. (1995). Mild traumatic brain injury: Pathophysiology, natural history, and clinical management. *Neurology, 45*(7), 1253–1260.

Alves, W. M., Colohan, A. R. T., O'Leary, T. J., Rimel, R. W., & Jane, J. A. (1986). Understanding posttraumatic symptoms after minor head injury. *Journal of Head Trauma Rehabilitation, 1*(2), 1–12.

Alves, W. M., Macciocchi, S. N., & Barth, J. T. (1993). Post-concussive symptoms after uncomplicated mild head injury. *Journal of Head Trauma Rehabilitation, 8*(3), 48–59.

Anderson, B. J. (1987). The metabolic needs of head trauma victims. *Journal of Neuroscience Nursing, 19*(4), 211–215.

Anon, J. S. (1976). The PLISSLT Model: A proposed conceptual scheme for behavioral treatment of sexual problems. *Journal of Sex Education Therapy, 2*, 1–15.

Bachman, D. L. (1992). The diagnosis and management of common neurologic sequelae of closed head injury. *Journal of Head Trauma Rehabilitation, 7*(2), 50–59.

Bogner, J. A., Corrigan, J. D., Spafford, D. E., Lamb-Hart, G. L. (1997). Integrating substance abuse treatment and vocational rehabilitation after traumatic brain injury. *Journal of Head Trauma Rehabilitation, 12*(5), 57–71.

Brooke, M. M., Questad, K. A., Patterson, D. R., & Bashak, K. J. (1992). Agitation and restlessness after closed head injury: A prospective study of 100 consecutive admissions. *Archives of Physical Medicine and Rehabilitation, 73*, 320–323.

Capruso, D. X., & Levin, H. S. (1996). Neurobehavioral outcome of head trauma. In R. W. Evans (Ed.), *Neurology and trauma* (pp. 201–221). Philadelphia: W. B. Saunders.

Cassidy, J. W. (1994). Neuropharmacological approaches to the patient with affective and psychotic features. *Journal of Head Trauma Rehabilitation, 9*, 43–60.

Cavallo, M. M., & Saucedo, C. (1995). Traumatic brain injury in families from culturally diverse populations. *Journal of Head Trauma Rehabilitation, 10*(2), 66–77.

Centers for Disease Control and Prevention (1997). Traumatic Brain Injury—Colorado, Missouri, Oklahoma, and Utah, 1990–1993. *MMWR, 46*(1), 8–11.

Cicerone, K. D. (1992). Psychological management of post-concussive disorders. *Physical Medicine and Rehabilitation: State of the Art Reviews, 6*(1), 129–141.

Clifton, G., Robertson, C., Grossman, R., Hodge, S., Foltz,

R., & Garza, C. (1984). The metabolic response to severe head injury. *Journal of Neurosurgery, 60,* 687–696.

Cooper, K. D., Tabaddor, K., Hauser, W. A., Shulman, K., Feiner, C., & Factor, P. R. (1983). The epidemiology of head injury in the Bronx. *Neuroepidemiology, 2,* 70–78.

Corrigan, J. (1995). Substance abuse as a mediating factor in outcome from traumatic brain injury. *Archives of Physical Medicine and Rehabilitation, 76,* 302–309.

Corrigan, J. D. (1989). Development of a scale for the assessment of agitation following traumatic brain injury. *Journal of Clinical and Experimental Neuropsychology, 11,* 261–277.

Corrigan, J. D., Arnett, J. A., Houck, L. J., & Jackson, R. D. (1985). Reality orientation for brain injured patients: Group treatment and monitoring of recovery. *Archives of Physical Medicine and Rehabilitation, 66,* 626–630.

Corrigan, J. D., & Bogner, J. A. (1994). Factor structure of the agitated behavior scale. *Journal of Clinical and Experimental Neuropsychology, 16,* 386–392.

Dicker, B. G. (1989). Preinjury behavior and recovery after minor head injury: A review of the literature. *Journal of Head Trauma Rehabilitation, 4,* 73–81.

Dikmen, S., Machamer, J., & Temkin, N. (1993). Psychosocial outcome in patients with moderate to severe injury: 2 year follow-up. *Brain Injury, 7,* 113–124.

Ferido, T., & Habel, M. (1988). Spasticity in head trauma and CVA patients: Etiology and management. *Journal of Neuroscience Nursing, 20,* 17–22.

Fife, D. (1987). Head injury with and without hospital admission: Comparison of incidence and short term disability. *American Journal of Public Health, 77,* 810–812.

Fitzgerald, M. H. (1992). Multicultural clinical interactions. *Journal of Rehabilitation, 58,* 38–42.

Fugate, L. P., Spacek, L. A., Kresty, L. A., Levy, C. E., Johnson, J. C., & Mysiw, W. J. (1997). Definition of agitation following traumatic brain injury: I. A survey of brain injury special interest group of the American Academy of Physical Medicine and Rehabilitation. *Archives of Physical Medicine and Rehabilitation, 78,* 917–923.

Garden, F. H., Bontke, C. F., & Hoffman, M. (1990). Sexual functioning and marital adjustment after traumatic brain injury. *Journal of Head Trauma Rehabilitation, 5*(2), 52–59.

Gomez-Hernandez, R., Max, J. E., Kosier, T., & Paradiso, S. (1997). Social impairment and depression after traumatic brain injury. *Archives of Physical Medicine and Rehabilitation, 78,* 1321–1326.

Graham, D. I., & McIntosh, T. K. (1996). Neuropathology of brain injury. In R. W. Evans (Ed.), *Neurology and trauma* (pp. 53–90). Philadelphia: W. B. Saunders.

Grazko, M. A., Polo, K. B., & Jabbari, B. (1995). Botulinum toxin A for spasticity, muscle spasms, and rigidity. *Neurology, 45*(4), 712–717.

Grinspun, D. (1993). Bladder management for adults following head injury. *Rehabilitation Nursing, 18,* 300–305.

Gronwall, D. (1986). Rehabilitation programs for patients with mild head injury: Components, problems, and evaluation. *Journal of Head Trauma Rehabilitation, 1,* 53–62.

Gronwall, D., & Wrightson, P. (1974). Delayed recovery of intellectual function after minor head injury. *Lancet, 2,* 605–609.

Gronwall, D., & Wrightson, P. (1980). Duration of post-traumatic amnesia after mild head injury. *Journal of Clinical Neuropsychology, 1*(1), 51–60.

Grzankowski, J. A. (1997). Altered thought processes related to traumatic brain injury and their nursing implications. *Rehabilitation Nursing, 22,* 24–31.

Habel, M. (1997). Muscle tone abnormalities. *Rehabilitation Nursing, 22*(3), 118–123.

Hagen, C., Malkmus, D., & Durham, P. (1979). *Levels of cognitive functioning: Rehabilitation of the head injured adult: Comprehensive physical management.* Downey, CA: Professional Staff Association of Rancho Los Amigos Hospital.

Harrick, L., Krefting, L., Johnston, J., Carlson, P., & Minnes, P. (1994). Stability of functional outcomes following transitional living programme participation: 3 year follow-up. *Brain Injury, 8,* 439–447.

Harrison-Felix, C., Newton, N., Hall, K. M., & Kreutzer, J. S. (1996). Descriptive findings from the Traumatic Brain Injury Model Systems National Data Base. *Journal of Head Trauma Rehabilitation, 11,* 1–14.

Hayes, R. L., Povlishock, J. T., & Singha, B. (1992). Pathology of mild head injury. *Physical Medicine and Rehabilitation: State of the Art Reviews, 6,* 9–20.

Hinkle, J. L., Alves, S. M., Rimel, R. W., & Jane, J. A. (1986). Restoring social competence in minor head-injured patients. *Journal of Neuroscience Nursing, 18*(5), 268–271.

Howard, M. E. (1988). Behavior management in the acute care rehabilitation setting. *Journal of Head Trauma Rehabilitation, 3,* 14–22.

Jennett, B. (1996). Epidemiology of head injury. *Journal of Neurology, Neurosurgery and Psychiatry, 60*(4), 362–369.

Jennett, B., & Teasdale, G. (1981). *Management of head injuries* (pp. 77–80). Philadelphia: F. A. Davis.

Jernigan, D. H. (1991). Alcohol and head trauma: Strategies for prevention. *Journal of Head Trauma Rehabilitation, 6,* 48–59.

Johnston, M. V., & Lewis, F. D. (1991). Outcomes of community reentry programmes for brain injury survivors: Part 1. Independent living and productive activities. *Brain Injury, 5,* 141–154.

Katz, D. I. (1992). Neuropathology and neurobehavioral recovery from closed head injury. *Journal of Head Trauma Rehabilitation, 7,* 1–15.

Katz, D. I. (1997). Traumatic brain injury. In V. M. Mills, J. W. Cassidy, & D. I. Katz (Eds.), *Neurological rehabilitation: A guide to diagnosis, prognosis, and treatment planning.* Malden, MA: Blackwell Scientific.

Katz, D. I., & Alexander, M. P. (1994). Traumatic brain injury. In D. C. Good & J. R. Couch (Eds.), *Handbook of neurorehabilitation* (pp. 493–549). New York: Marcel Dekker.

Kay, T. (1992). Neuropsychological diagnosis: Disentangling the multiple determinants of functional disability after mild traumatic brain injury. *Physical Medicine and Rehabilitation: State of the Art Reviews, 6*(1), 109–127.

Klonoff, P. S., & Lage, G. A. (1995). Suicide in patients with traumatic brain injury: Risk and prevention. *Journal of Head Trauma Rehabilitation, 10*(6), 16–24.

Kraus, J., & Sorenson, S. (1994). Epidemiology. In J. Silver, S. Yudofsky, & R. Hale (Eds.), *Neuropsychiatry of traumatic brain injury.* Washington, DC: American Psychiatric Press.

Kraus, J. F., & McArthur, D. L. (1996). Epidemiology of brain injury. In R. W. Evans (Ed.), *Neurology and trauma* (pp. 3–17). Philadelphia: W. B. Saunders.

Krefting, L. (1989). Reintegration into the community after head injury: The results of an ethnographic study. *Occupational Therapy Journal of Research, 9,* 67–83.

Kreutzer, J. S., Witol, A. D., Sandler, A. M., Cifu, D. X.,

Marwitz, J. H., & Delmonico, R. (1996). A prospective longitudinal multicenter analysis of alcohol use patterns among persons with traumatic brain injury. *Journal of Head Trauma Rehabilitation, 11*(5), 58–69.

Kuthy, S., Grap, M. J., Penn, L., & Henderson, V. (1995). After the party's over: Evaluation of a drinking and driving prevention program. *Journal of Neuroscience Nursing, 27,* 273–277.

Levin, H. S., & Grossman, R. G. (1978). Behavioral sequelae of closed head injury: A quantitative study. *Archives of Neurology, 35,* 720–727.

Levin, S. L., O'Donnell, M., & Grossman, R. G. (1979). The Galveston Orientation and Amnesia Test: A practical scale to assess cognition after head injury. *Journal of Nervous and Mental Disease, 167,* 675–684.

Malec, J. F. (1996). Cognitive rehabilitation. In R. W. Evans (Ed.), *Neurology and trauma* (pp. 231–248). Philadelphia: W. B. Saunders.

Malec, J. F., & Basford, J. S. (1996). Postacute brain injury rehabilitation. *Archives of Physical Medicine and Rehabilitation, 77,* 198–207.

Max, W., MacKenzie, E. J., & Rice, D. P. (1991). Head injuries: Costs and consequences. *Journal of Head Trauma Rehabilitation, 6,* 76–91.

McLaughlin, A. M., & Peters, S. (1993). Evaluation of an innovative cost effective programme for brain injury patients: Response to a need for flexible treatment planning. *Brain Injury, 7,* 71–75.

Mild Traumatic Brain Injury Committee of the Head Injury Interdisciplinary Special Interest Group of the American Congress of Rehabilitation Medicine. (1993). Definition of mild traumatic brain injury. *Journal of Head Trauma Rehabilitation, 8,* 86–87.

Mills, V. M., Nesbeda, T., Katz, D., & Alexander, M. P. (1992). Outcomes for traumatically brain-injured patients following post-acute rehabilitation programs. *Brain Injury, 6,* 219–228.

Mitchell, P. H. (1986). Intracranial hypertension: Influence of nursing care activities. *Nursing Clinics of North America, 21,* 563–576.

Mysiw, W. J., Bogner, J. A., Arnett, J. A., Clinchot, D. A., & Corrigan, J. D. (1996). The orientation group monitoring system for measuring duration of post-traumatic amnesia and assessing therapeutic interventions. *Journal of Head Trauma Rehabilitation, 11,* 1–8.

Mysiw, W. J., & Sandel, E. (1997). The agitated brain injured patient: Part 2. Pathophysiology and treatment. *Archives of Physical Medicine and Rehabilitation, 78,* 213–220.

National Head Injury Foundation. (1980). Facts about traumatic brain injury (Interagency Head Injury Task Force Reports). Bethesda, MD: National Institute of Neurological Disorders and Stroke.

Oostra, K., Everaert, K., & Van Laere, M. (1995). Urinary incontinence in brain injury. *Brain Injury, 10,* 459–464.

Patterson, T., & Sargent, M. (1990). Behavioral management of the agitated head injury client. *Rehabilitation Nursing, 15,* 248–249.

Pierson, S. H., Katz, D. I., & Tarsy, D. (1996). Botulinum toxin A in the treatment of spasticity: Functional implications and patient selection. *Archives of Physical Medicine and Rehabilitation, 77,* 717–721.

Racino, J. A., & Williams, J. M. (1994). Living in the community: An examination of the philosophical and practical aspects. *Journal of Head Trauma Rehabilitation, 9,* 35–48.

Reeder, K. P., Rosenthal, M., Lichtenberg, P., & Wood, D. (1996). Impact of age on functional outcome following traumatic brain injury. *Journal of Head Trauma Rehabilitation, 11*(3), 22–31.

Rehabilitation Nursing Foundation. (1989). *Head injury: Nursing management of agitated/aggressive behavior* [Video]. Skokie, IL: Author.

Reyes, R. I., Bhattacharyya, A. K., & Heler, D. (1981). Traumatic head injury: Restlessness and agitation as prognosticators of physical and psychologic improvement in patients. *Archives of Physical Medicine and Rehabilitation, 62,* 20–23.

Richmond, T. S., Metcalf, J. A., & Winterhalter, J. (1987). Support group for families of acute neurological patients. *Journal of Neuroscience Nursing, 19,* 40–43.

Rimel, R. W., Giordani, B., Barth, J. T., Boll, T. J., & Jane, J. A. (1981). Disability caused by minor head injury. *Neurosurgery, 9,* 221–228.

Rose, M. (1988). The place of drugs in the management of behavior disorders after traumatic brain injury. *Journal of Head Trauma Rehabilitation, 3,* 7–13.

Rosenthal, M., & Young, T. (1988). Effective family intervention after traumatic brain injury: Theory and practice. *Journal of Head Trauma Rehabilitation, 3,* 42–50.

Rutherford, W. H. (1989). Postconcussion symptoms: Relationship to acute neurological indices, individual differences, and circumstances of injury. In H. S. Levin, H. M. Eisenberg, & A. L. Benton (Eds.), *Mild head injury* (pp. 217–228). New York: Oxford University Press.

Sandel, M. E., Horn, L. J., & Bontke, C. F. (1992). Sensory stimulation: Accepted practice or expected practice: Controversies. *Journal of Head Trauma Rehabilitation, 7,* 115–120.

Sandel, M. E., & Mysiw, W. J. (1996). The agitated brain injured patient: Part 1. Definitions, differential diagnosis, and assessment. *Archives of Physical Medicine and Rehabilitation, 77,* 617–623.

Sorenson, S. B., & Kraus, J. F. (1991). Occurrence, severity, and outcomes of brain injury. *Journal of Head Trauma Rehabilitation, 6,* 1–10.

Sosin, D. M., Sniezek, J. E., & Waxweiler, R. J. (1995). Trends in death associated with traumatic brain injury, 1979 through 1992: Success and failure. *JAMA, 273,* 1778–1780.

Sosnowski, C., & Ustik, M. (1994). Early intervention: Coma stimulation in the intensive care unit. *Journal of Neuroscience Nursing, 26,* 336–341.

Spencer, J. C. (1993). The usefulness of qualitative methods in rehabilitation: Issues of meaning, of context, and of change. *Archives of Physical Medicine and Rehabilitation, 74,* 119–126.

Stratton, M. C., & Gregory, R. J. (1994). After traumatic brain injury: A discussion of consequences. *Brain Injury, 8,* 631–645.

Stuss, D. T. (1987). Contribution of frontal lobe injury to cognitive impairment after closed head injury: Assessment and recent findings. In H. S. Levin, H. M. Eisenberg, & J. Grafman (Eds.), *Neurobehavioral recovery from head injury* (pp. 166–177). New York: Oxford University Press.

Tate, R., Simpson, G., Flanagan, S., & Coffey, M. (1997). Completed suicide after traumatic brain injury. *Journal of Head Trauma Rehabilitation, 12,* 16–28.

Thurman, D. J., Alverson, C. A., Dunn, K. A., Guerrero, J., & Sniezek, J. E. (1999). Traumatic Brain injury in the United States: A public health perspective. *Journal of Head Trauma, 14,* 602–615.

Vollmer, D. G., Dacey, R. G., & Jane, J. A. (1992). Craniocerebral trauma. In R. J. Joynt (Ed.), *Clinical neurology* (Vol. 3, pp. 1–80). Philadelphia: J. B. Lippincott.

Webb, C., Rose, F. D., Johnston, D. A., & Attree, E. A. (1996). Age and recovery from brain injury: Clinical opinions and experimental evidence. *Brain Injury, 10,* 303–310.

Weber, A. M. (1990). A practical clinical approach to understanding and treating attentional problems. *Journal of Head Trauma Rehabilitation, 5,* 73–85.

Whitman, S. T., Coonley-Hoganson, R., & Desai, B. T. (1984). Comparative head trauma experiences in two socioeconomically different Chicago-area communities: A population study. *American Journal of Epidemiology, 119*(4), 570–580.

Wroblewski, B. A., & Glenn, M. B. (1994). Pharmacological treatment of arousal and cognitive deficits. *Journal of Head Trauma Rehabilitation, 9,* 19–42.

Zasler, N. D. (1993). Mild traumatic brain injury: Medical assessment and intervention. *Journal of Head Trauma Rehabilitation, 8,* 13–29.

BIBLIOGRAPHY

Baggerly, J. (1986). Rehabilitation of the adult with head trauma. *Nursing Clinics of North America, 21*(4), 581.

Rehabilitation Nursing Foundation: Nursing Diagnoses Publications Task Force. (1995). *Rehabilitation nursing diagnoses: A guide to intervention and outcome.* Glenview, IL: Author.

CHAPTER 22

Nursing Management of the Patient with Spinal Cord Injury

Dianne.Mahoney

Spinal cord injury (SCI) is a profound disability whose impact begins immediately, whether the damage is from trauma or disease. Records of spinal cord injury date back to prehistoric times. Evidence of vertebral injury has been found in skeletons of people of the Paleolithic age, who lived more than 750,000 years ago.

Historical descriptions of people with SCI depict injury to the spine as one of the most totally maiming and lethal human injuries. Sir Ludwig Guttmann stated that "of the many forms of disability which can beset mankind, a severe injury or disease of the spinal cord undoubtedly constitutes one of the most devastating calamities in human life" (cited in Pires & Adkins, 1996).

During the two decades following World War II, there was significant progress in treatment of people with SCI. Advances in treatment have led to higher survival rates and improved prognoses. Morbidity and mortality rates associated with SCI have improved dramatically over the past two decades. The rate of early death from complications such as respiratory failure and pulmonary emboli has been reduced with advances in acute care technology, although pulmonary complications are the most common cause of death during the first year after injury and again in later years. Mortality from renal failure and other urinary tract complications, once the leading causes of death among long-term survivors, have been dramatically reduced as well.

Much of the credit for these improvements belongs to Guttmann in England and Monroe, Bors, Comarr, and Talbot in the United States, who demonstrated that dedicated centers with specially trained staff could most effectively address the extensive medical, psychological, social, and vocational needs of individuals with SCI. In the early 1960s a federal initiative by the Rehabilitation Services Administration resulted in funding for an innovative and experimental service delivery model for SCI. Known as the Model Spinal Cord Injury (SCI) Systems, these centers provided a centralized, multidisciplinary program designed to meet the acute and lifetime needs of those with spinal cord injury. Dr. Donald Munro, a neurosurgeon, is credited with starting the first civilian spinal cord injury unit, a 10-bed unit at Boston University Hospital. By the early 1990s, there were 13 accredited Model SCI Care Systems in the country, which treated about 20% of all spinal cord injury cases (Thomas, 1995, p. 2). Today there are 24 Model SCI Care Systems.

The rest of the cases are treated in SCI units accredited by the Commission on Accreditation of Rehabilitation Facilities (CARF), rehabilitation hospitals, or community hospitals. Wherever treatment is given, care of the spinal cord–injured patient is complex and demanding. The rehabilitation nurse must understand the effects of SCI in all its phases to provide comprehensive care to this patient population. The lifelong effects of SCI are physical, psychological, financial, and social. Few injuries result in more profound and long-term disability than traumatic SCI. Less than 10% of patients die of the acute injury, but those who survive are disabled for life. Data for 1998 estimated the expense for "the first year post-injury to be $251,885 with the yearly costs of $30,676 thereafter" (NSCISC, January, 2000).

ANATOMY

The spinal cord is about 18 inches (46 cm) long and extends from the base of the brain to the waist (Fig. 22–1). The upper end of the spinal cord is located at the foramen magnum of the skull. The cord ends at the first lumbar vertebra (L1) in adults. Approximately 1 cm in diameter, the spinal cord is wider in the cervical and lumbar areas. The spinal (vertebral) column, which serves to protect the

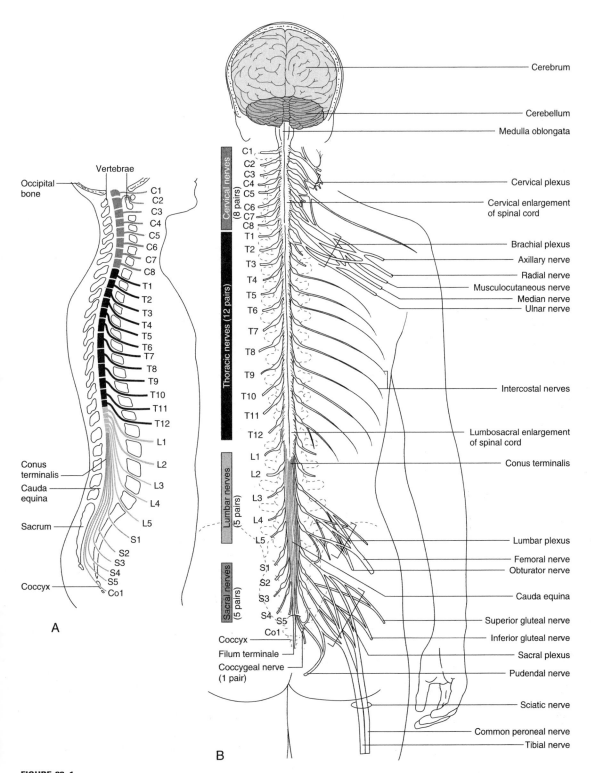

FIGURE 22–1

Spinal cord, spinal nerves, and vertebral column. *A,* Right lateral view of the spinal cord and vertebral column, showing the various spinal segments and the emergence of spinal nerves from the vertebral column. *B,* Posterior view. (Redrawn from National American Spinal Cord Injury Association, 1992.)

cord, is composed of four sections (Table 22–1):

- Cervical section with 7 vertebrae
- Thoracic section with 12 vertebrae
- Lumbar section with 5 vertebrae
- Sacral section with 5 vertebral bones fused into one

The C1 vertebra is called the *atlas*—a bony ring modified to articulate the cerebral condyles, allowing flexion and extension of the occiput. The C2 vertebra, called the *axis*, articulates with the atlas and rotates around the odontoid. It forms the transitional level with the mobile midpart of the cervical spine. About 50% of cervical rotation occurs at the atlantoaxial articulation.

"The spinal cord is the structure through which information is channeled from the brain to the muscles in the periphery of the body and through which sensations from the body tissues are sent to the brain" (DePace, 1994).

Cross-Section of the Spinal Cord

A cross-section of the spinal cord displays gray and white matter. The gray matter consists of nerve cell bodies, dendrites of association, efferent neurons, sensory and motor neurons, and the axon terminals of neurons. The gray matter, which forms an H shape, is composed of three pairs of columns of neurons going up and down the length of the spinal cord. These columns are called the *dorsal*, *ventral*, and *lateral horns*. Nerve fibers run across the columns and function in cross-reflexes.

The white matter of the spinal cord is composed of myelinated nerve fibers divided into three pairs of columns running the length of the spinal cord. The fibers within the columns are divided into tracts that carry sensory and motor impulses to and from the brain.

The major sensory (ascending) tracts are as follows (Emick-Herring, 1993):

Posterior column: Large area in the posterior cord that relays information about conscious proprioception, localization of touch, two-point tactile discrimination, and vibration.

Dorsal spinocerebellar: Found in the posterior and lateral cord; conveys reflex, proprioceptive information from the arms and/or legs.

Ventral spinocerebellar: Lies anteriorly and laterally in the cord and transmits reflex proprioceptive information from the legs.

Lateral spinothalamic: Found in the lateral part of the cord; conducts impulses for pain, heat, and cold; crosses in segments of the cord near the entry level and ascends to the thalamus.

Ventral spinothalamic: Found in the anterior lateral part of the cord; conducts impulses for coarse touch and pressure.

TABLE 22–1 ■ THE SPINAL COLUMN: FUNCTIONS SERVED BY SPINAL NERVE MOTOR ROOTS

Root Segment	Function Served
C1 and C2	Aid in head control
C3 and C4	Inspiration (breathing in)
C5 and C6	Shoulder flexion, abduction (arm forward, out to side) Elbow flexion (elbow bent)
C6 and C7	Wrist dorsiflexion (back of hand up) Wrist pronation (palm down)
C7 and C8	Elbow extension (elbow straight) Finger extension ("knuckles" straight)
C8 and T1	Finger flexion (fist clenched) Thumb opposition (thumb brought to little finger) Spreading and closing the fingers
T2–T6	Forced inspiration (breathing in) Expiration (breathing out, coughing)
T6–T12	Forced inspiration (breathing in) Aid in expiration (coughing) Aid in trunk flexion (sitting up)
L1, L2, L3	Hip flexion (thigh to chest) Hip adduction (thigh to midline, legs together)
L3 and L4	Knee extension (knee straight)
L4, L5, S1	Hip abduction (thigh out to side, legs apart) Foot dorsiflexion (foot up, walk on heels)
L5, S1, S2	Hip extension (thigh in line with trunk, hips straight, e.g., standing) Foot plantar flexion (foot down, walk on toes)
S2, S3, S4	Bowel function (fecal continence) Bladder control (urinary continence)

From National Spinal Cord Injury Association, Chicago, 1992.

The major motor (descending) tracts are as follows (Emick-Herring, 1993):

Lateral corticospinal: Lie in the lateral cord and transmit impulses for voluntary movement, especially in the limbs.
Ventral corticospinal: Lie in the anterior and medial part of the cord and control voluntary movement in the neck and trunk.
Extrapyramidal: Control involuntary muscle movement; modify muscle tone; integrate motor activity with vestibular and visual input.
Corticospinal (pyramidal): Start from pyramid-shaped neurons in the motor area of the cortex and descend within the pyramid of the medulla and control most voluntary movements.

Emerging from the spinal cord are the spinal nerves. There are 31 spinal nerves within the spinal cord: 8 cervical, 12 thoracic, 5 lumbar, 5 sacral, and 1 coccygeal. "The spinal nerves course outward from the spinal cord to innervate the muscles and skin of the body below the neck. Each spinal nerve and spinal cord segment is responsible for the innervation of muscles and skin in a corresponding body segment" (DePace, 1994). There is a pair of spinal nerves for each vertebra. In the area of the spinal cord, each spinal nerve divides into a ventral (anterior, motor) root and a dorsal (posterior, sensory) root. Dorsal roots contain afferent nerve fibers, which carry sensory information. Ventral roots contain efferent nerve fibers, which carry motor information. The axons of cell bodies of motor neurons located within the anterior horn of the gray matter emerge from the spinal cord to form the ventral roots.

Spinal Reflex Arc

The spinal reflex arc is a protective involuntary response to a stimulus. It consists of afferent and efferent neurons carrying signals from the initiation of a noxious or painful stimulus to the completed action or reaction to it. The reflex action protects the body from serious tissue damage.

The stimulus is detected by sensory endings in the skin, which then generate impulses in the afferent neurons and conduct them toward the spinal cord. These impulses enter the dorsal horn of the gray matter in the spinal cord through the dorsal root of the spinal nerve. The afferent neurons synapse on an interneuron, which modifies the signal and sends it on to the neurons in the ventral horn

of gray matter, where it activates the motor (efferent) neurons to the skeletal muscles to complete the reflex arc.

Upper and Lower Motor Neurons

Upper motor neurons (UMNs) are long tracts that travel from the brain to the spinal cord, whose cell bodies are located in the motor strip of the cerebral cortex. UMNs synapse with lower motor neurons (LMNs) in the anterior horn cell of the spinal cord at each segmental level. UMNs exert supraspinal control over LMNs by suppressing reactions to local stimuli at the spinal cord reflex level.

LMNs originate in the anterior horn cell in the ventral spinal cord at each segmental level and exit from the spinal cord to form the spinal nerves and branches of the peripheral nervous system. They transmit efferent (motor) messages to muscles and afferent (sensory) messages back to the spinal cord. The sensory-motor loop of the LMN constitutes a reflex arc.

LMN lesions occur when the reflex arc is destroyed and communication with the UMN is lost. UMN lesions occur when the reflex arc is intact but supraspinal control over spinal reflexes is destroyed or damaged.

EPIDEMIOLOGY AND PREVENTION

Traumatic SCI occurs primarily in young adults, with more than half of all people with SCI being between 16 and 30 years old at the time of injury (Table 22–2). The "typical" person with an SCI is a young, single man who was injured in a motor vehicle collision. SCI occurs more frequently in the summer and on weekends.

Nontraumatic SCI disorders are those caused by internal disease rather than the sudden external forces causing traumatic injury. Nontraumatic SCI is less common and generally less acute than traumatic injury. Early diagnosis and treatment often lead to a favorable outcome. According to Hinkle (1994), the major causes of nontraumatic spinal cord disorders are tumor, infection, arteriovenous malformations, disc disease, syrinxes, and infarctions; because the spinal canal is fixed in size, tumor growth, edema, or inflammation from a spinal cord disorder quickly causes symptoms. "The epidemiology of nontraumatic spinal cord disease is not well examined. Cancer alone may be a more common cause of cord disease than trauma.

TABLE 22–2 ■ STATISTICS ON SPINAL CORD INJURY (SCI)

Number of new injuries per year

Per million	32
Total number in United States	7800

Total number of people with SCI

Sex distribution:	
Male	82%
Female	18%
Age at injury:	
Average age	33.4 years
Median age	26 years
Mode (most frequent) age	19 years
Causes of injury:*	
Motor vehicle accidents	44%
Acts of violence	24%
Falls	22%
Sports	8% (⅔ from diving)
Other	2%
Marital status at time of injury†	
Single	53%
Married	31%
Divorced	9%
Other	7%

*Falls overtake motor vehicle accidents as the leading cause of injury after age 45; acts of violence and sports account for fewer injuries as age increases.

†At 5 years after injury, 88% of people who had been single at the time of the SCI were still single, versus 65% of the population without SCI; and 81% of the people of the people who had been married at the time of SCI were still married, versus 89% of the population without SCI.

Data from National Spinal Cord Injury Statistical Center (1995). *Factsheet #2: Spinal cord injury statistical information.* Birmingham, AL: University of Birmingham.

Traumatic injury is more common in persons younger than 40 years of age, while nontraumatic disease may be more common in those over age 40" (Stass, Formal, Gershkoff, Hirschwald, Schmidt, Schultz, & Smith, 1993).

Prevention efforts must be multifaceted and must address the variations in causes associated with age, race, and sex. Prevention programs focusing on white men should focus on motor vehicle accidents, whereas those targeting blacks must address violence issues. Programs for older adolescents and young adults should address risk-taking behaviors, such as alcohol and drug use, diving, motor vehicle accidents, and violence. Prevention programs for older adults should target motor vehicle collisions and falls. Mandatory wearing of helmets while riding motorcycles and bicycles has reduced the incidence of head injury, which is often associated with SCI. The much more common use of seat belts, although not mandatory in all states, has reduced the incidence of severe injury in motor vehicle accidents.

MECHANISMS OF INJURY

Overall, 10 to 14% of spinal fractures and dislocations result in SCI. Traumatic injuries to the cervical spine cause SCI in 40% of cases, whereas injuries to the thoracic spine and thoracolumbar junction cause SCI in 10% and 4% of cases, respectively. SCI is commonly associated with head injury (Stass et al., 1993).

Spinal cord injury results from compression, contusion, or transection of the spinal cord. The major mechanisms of injury are (1) flexion (Fig. 22–2); (2) flexion-rotation; (3) hyperextension (Fig. 22–3); and (4) compression (axial loading) (Fig. 22–4). Flexion injury with tearing of the posterior ligaments and dislocation is the most unstable injury and is often associated with severe neurological deficits. Hyperextension injury is the most common mechanism of cord injury (Walleck, 1994).

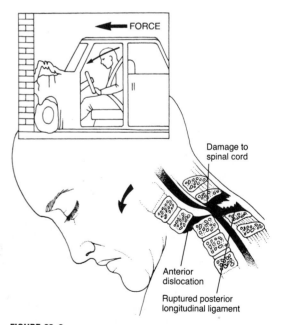

FIGURE 22–2

Hyperflexion injury of the cervical spine. (From Ignatavicius, D. D., Workman, M. L., and Mishler, M. A. [Eds.]. [1999]. *Medical-surgical nursing across the health care continuum* [3rd ed., p. 1065]. Philadelphia: W. B. Saunders.)

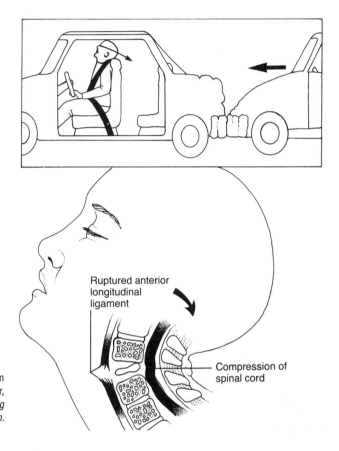

FIGURE 22–3
Hyperextension injury of the cervical spine. (From Ignatavicius, D. D., Workman, M. L., and Mishler, M. A. [Eds.]. [1999]. *Medical-surgical nursing across the health care continuum [3rd ed., p. 1065]. Philadelphia: W. B. Saunders.)*

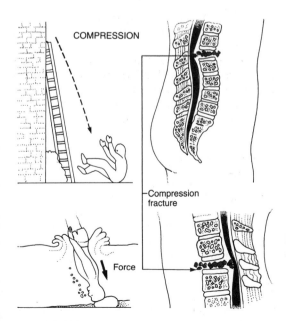

FIGURE 22–4
Axial loading (vertical compression) injury of the cervical spine and the lumbar spine. (From Ignatavicius, D. D., Workman, M. L., and Mishler, M. A. [Eds.]. [1999]. *Medical-surgical nursing across the health care continuum* [3rd ed., p. 1066]. Philadelphia: W. B. Saunders.)

Vertebral Fractures

"Of the estimated 162,000 Americans hospitalized annually for vertebral fractures, one fourth have an associated injury to the spinal cord" (Fletcher, Taddonio, Byrne, Wexler, Cayten, Nealon, & Carson, 1995).

Fractures, dislocations, and fracture-dislocations of the occiput and C1 and C2 vertebrae either are fatal, because of the location of the injury above the innervation of the diaphragm, or have no neurological consequences.

The *Jefferson fracture* is a bursting of the ring of C1 (atlas) resulting from axial compression. It is typically without neurological deficit because the fracture itself decompresses the canal. The most common complaint is pain in the cervical area.

The *hangman's fracture* is a fracture through the arch of vertebra C2 caused by flexion or extension or both and axial compression (Fig. 22–5). An abrasion of the forehead or chin may be present. Typically, this fracture does not cause SCI (Stass et al., 1993).

Odontoid fractures involve the odontoid process (dens) of vertebra C2 (Fig. 22–6). These fractures are poorly understood. There are three types of fractures at this site. Shearing may be present. Death occurs if the odontoid process is driven into the spinal cord,

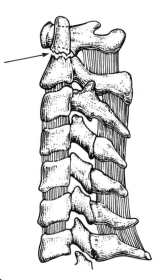

FIGURE 22–6
Odontoid fractures. Fracture of the odontoid process, the superior projection of the body of C2 that projects into the ring of C1 and orients the two vertebrae, results in instability at this level. Stabilization is required, with the method being determined by the exact type of fracture. (From Barker, E. [1994]. *Neuroscience nursing* [p. 357]. St. Louis, Mosby–Year Book.)

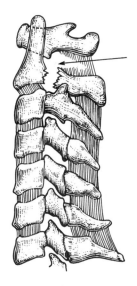

FIGURE 22–5
Hangman's fracture. A fracture through the pedicles of the second cervical vertebra, separating the posterior neural arch from the body of the axis, resulting in an anterior dislocation with angulation of C1 and the body of C2. These fractures usually heal spontaneously with prolonged traction or immobilization with a halo brace. (From Barker, E. [1994]. *Neuroscience nursing* [p. 357]. St. Louis, Mosby–Year Book.)

but most injuries of this type do not result in death or neurological deficits.

Dislocation of a vertebra occurs when one vertebra overrides another and there is unilateral or bilateral dislocation of the facets. This injury usually results from tearing or stretching of ligaments that allows excessive movement of the vertebra. A *subluxation* is a partial or incomplete dislocation of one vertebra over another.

Fractures may be stable or unstable. Stability is maintained if all of the anterior and posterior ligaments, plus one additional structure such as the lamina or spinous process, remain intact (Walleck, 1994).

Nontraumatic Spinal Cord Disorders

The pathophysiology of nontraumatic SCI is due more to changes caused by compression and ischemia than to actual injury and destruction of the spinal cord.

Common pathophysiological changes occurring in nontraumatic SCI are as follows (Hinkle, 1994):

- Compression, irritation, and traction on the spinal cord nerve roots or blood supply
- Mechanical displacement of the spinal cord from forces other than direct trauma

- Ischemia caused by interference with spinal cord blood supply
- Obstruction of cerebrospinal fluid circulation
- Invasion and destruction of spinal cord tracts

Spinal cord tumors, either primary or metastatic, constitute a major source of nontraumatic spinal cord disorders. Infections in the spinal cord, although rare, may be (1) pyogenic, usually abscesses or osteomyelitis; (2) fungal; or (3) parasitic. Spinal tuberculosis also occurs. Arteriovenous malformations consist of abnormalities of one or many arteriovenous channels that cause ischemic necrosis of the spinal cord. "Degenerative disc disorders of the spine have risen dramatically and account for as much as 92.7% of spinal disorders" (Hinkle, 1994).

Syringomyelia is the most common name for abnormal fluid-filled cavities in the central canal of the spinal cord. Another name often used is *syrinx* (cavity). Syringomyelia occurs more commonly in men in their 30s and 40s. The conditions most commonly associated with syringomyelia are the Chiari I congenital brain malformation and severe spinal cord trauma (Michals & Ramsey, 1996). "Disassociated sensory findings of impaired pain and temperature with preservation of light touch sensation are the classic presentation" (Michals & Ramsey, 1996). Syringomyelia can destroy any portion of the spinal cord but tends to attack anterior and lateral structures while preserving posterior structures. Successful decompression of the syrinx cavity involves surgical correction of the underlying abnormality that led to its formation. After surgery, most people experience a decrease in syrinx cavity size; the functional results are less encouraging. The majority of patients show little improvement.

Vascular disease of the spinal cord can result in an infarction and subsequent compromise of blood supply to the spinal cord. The infarction is generally abrupt and disabling. Causes of infarction include trauma, clamping of the aorta during surgery, stenosis, emboli, and hypotension.

Treatment of nontraumatic spinal cord disorders may be medical, surgical, or a combination of both.

PATHOPHYSIOLOGY

Levels of Injury

Cervical and lumbar injuries are the most common because these areas have the greatest flexibility. A cervical injury may result in paralysis of all extremities, traditionally called *quadriplegia*. The term *tetraplegia*, which has replaced quadriplegia, refers to an injury to the cervical region of the spinal cord.

From C3 to C7, there is a relationship between the mechanism of injury, the type of fracture, and the likelihood of neurological deficit. With pure flexion or extension injuries, there is usually no neurological deficit, and the spine is stable. Rotation combined with flexion is more damaging to the vertebral column because the rotational force disrupts the posterior vertebral elements. The flexion component, thus unrestrained, causes a forward dislocation of one or both facet joints, or a *teardrop fracture*, with displacement of the remainder of the vertebral body into the spinal canal, causing SCI. *Compression burst fractures*, due to axial loading, frequently result in SCI because the burst fragments are pushed into the spinal canal; diving accidents are a common cause of this type of injury (Stass et al., 1993).

Injuries of the thoracic, lumbar, or sacral regions of the spine result in paralysis of the lower extremities, called *paraplegia*. Spinal cord injuries are classified according to the International Standards for Neurological and Functional Classification of Spinal Cord Injury. This classification requires a systematic neurological examination of sensory and motor function (Yarkony & Chen, 1996).

The level of injury is determined by the physician's examination of the 28 dermatomes for sensitivity to pinprick and light touch (Fig. 22–7). Motor levels are tested in the 10 pairs of myotomes. The sensory and motor levels are evaluated for right and left sides of the body. It is not unusual to have a discrepancy between the lowest motor and lowest normal sensory levels. The neurological level is the most caudal segment that tests as normal for both sensory and motor function on either side of the body. Muscle responses are graded from 0 (total paralysis) to 5 (normal). Each dermatome has a key sensory point. Light touch and pinprick are used to determine the sensory score, and the motor score is determined by adding the results of the muscle tests of the 10 groups on each side.

The ASIA Impairment Scale (Table 22–3) is a modified version of the Frankel Scale developed by the American Spinal Injury Association. It is the most commonly used scale for the classification of SCI and is the standard used for national data entry. The ASIA scale has five levels, from A through E, that define the extent of the injury. *A* is a complete

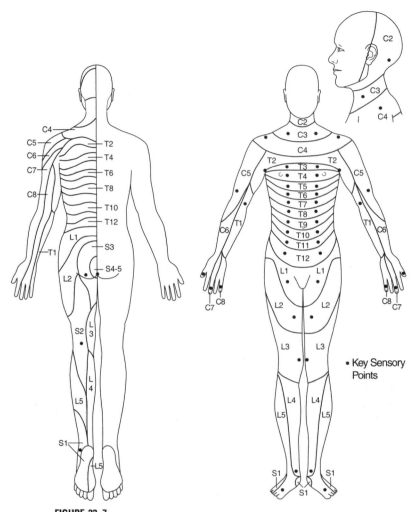

FIGURE 22–7
Posterior and anterior views of dermatomes and key sensory points.

spinal cord lesion with no motor or sensory function in the S4–S5 segment. *B* is an incomplete lesion in which sensation is preserved but not motor function below the neurological level. *C* is an incomplete lesion in which motor function is preserved below the neurological level but the key muscle responses below the neurological level are graded below 3. *D* is an incomplete lesion in which motor function is preserved below the neurological level and the key muscles below the neurological level have a muscle grade equal to or greater than 3. *E* is a normal motor and sensory examination with normal function.

Degree of Involvement

Complete Injury

The degree of involvement may be complete or incomplete. *Complete injury* is used when

both sensory and motor functions below the level of injury are absent. People with complete spinal cord injuries show no evidence of motor or sensory nerve fiber function across the immediate zone of injury into the caudal segment. In *incomplete injury,* partial preservation of sensory or motor function or both is found below the level of injury (see later discussion).

Sacral sparing is sensation at the anal mucocutaneous junction as well as deep anal sensation. The test of motor function is the presence of voluntary contraction of the external anal sphincter upon digital examination. Some patients may present with injuries that appear initially to be at a higher level and that decrease one or two levels with improved neurological function. Spinal cord edema may cause the injury to appear complete until the edema subsides. Patients who present in spinal shock may initially appear

TABLE 22–3 ■ ASIA IMPAIRMENT SCALE

A = **Complete:** No motor or sensory function is preserved in the sacral segments S4-S5.

B = **Incomplete:** Sensory but not motor function is preserved below the neurological level and extends through the sacral segments S4-S5.

C = **Incomplete:** Motor function is preserved below the neurological level, and the majority of key muscles below a neurological level have a muscle grade less than 3.

D = **Incomplete:** Motor function is preserved below the neurological level, and the majority of key muscles below the neurological level have a muscle grade greater than or equal to 3.

E = **Normal:** Motor and sensory function is normal.

From American Spinal Injury Association (1992). International standards for neurological classification of spinal cord injury, Chicago, 1992.

to have complete injuries; however, as spinal shock resolves, the neurological injury may be found to be incomplete.

Overall, slightly more than half of all spinal cord injuries result in quadriplegia. Statistics collected by the NSCISC (National Spinal Cord Injury Statistical Center) (1995) show that the most common neurological category of injury following traumatic spinal cord injury is incomplete tetraplegia at 31.2%, followed by complete paraplegia at 28.2%, incomplete paraplegia at 23.1%, and complete quadriplegia at 17.5%. This organization also has found the proportion of injuries resulting in tetraplegia to increase with age, accounting for two thirds of all injuries in people older than 60 years, and for 87% in people older than 75 years (NSCISC 1995). "It is evident that likelihood of improvement from a complete injury is poor while the prognosis for those with incomplete injury is less bleak. Recovery of an additional root level is expected to occur in approximately 60% of patients, including those with complete lesions" (Frost, 1993). Predictions regarding neurological prognosis should not be made earlier than 72 hours after injury.

Incomplete Injury

Incomplete injuries are categorized according to the area damaged (Fig. 22–8).

Central cord syndrome is a lesion occurring almost exclusively in the cervical region that produces greater motor weakness in the upper extremities than in the lower extremities. Sensory deficits occur to varying degrees but are less severe than motor deficits. The syndrome commonly occurs from hyperextension of the neck, usually caused by a fall. It is most commonly seen in older people with vertebral osteophytes. Bowel and bladder dysfunction is common with this syndrome. *Brown-Séquard syndrome* is a hemisection of the cord that results in (1) ipsilateral (same-side) loss of proprioceptive, motor function, vibration, and deep touch sensations and (2) contralateral (opposite-side) loss of pain, light touch, and temperature sensations.

Anterior cord syndrome results from a lesion that produces loss of motor function and sensitivity to pain and temperature while preserving position, vibration, and touch sensations. It is characterized by acute compression of the anterior portion of the spinal cord. This syndrome commonly results from a flexion injury but is also associated with herniation of an intervertebral disc or thrombosis of the anterior spinal artery. *Posterior cord syndrome* is a rare disorder caused by injury to the posterior cord. It is characterized by loss of proprioception and sensation below the level of lesion with preservation of motor function, sense of pain, and light touch. *Conus medullaris syndrome* results from injury of the sacral cord (conus) and lumbar nerve roots within the neural canal. It usually results in an areflexic bladder, bowel, and lower limbs. Sacral segments may occasionally show preserved reflexes—that is, bulbocavernosus and micturition reflexes.

Cauda equina syndrome affects the lower end of the spinal cord at the first lumbar vertebra. It is a result of injury to the lumbosacral nerve roots within the neural canal, which causes areflexic bladder, bowel, and lower limbs. Such a lesion is often incomplete owing to the great number of nerve roots involved and the large surface area they encompass. The loss of motor or sensory function or both with cauda equina injuries varies. There is often some recovery of function with regeneration of the peripheral nerves, but full return of innervation is not common (Table 22–4).

ACUTE PHASE

Prevention of Additional Cord Injury

"Spinal stabilization and ensuring a patent airway begin at the scene of the accident with traumatic SCI" (Waters, Apple, Meyer, Cotler, & Adkins, 1995). Immobilization of the neck is critical to prevent further injury to the spine. Emergency medical technicians (EMTs) are trained in the use of immobilization and stabilization techniques as well as extrication and transportation of an SCI victim. The com-

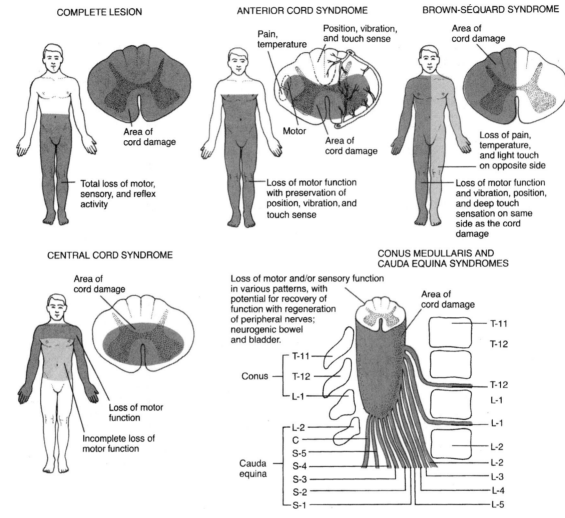

FIGURE 22–8

Common spinal cord syndromes. (From Ignatavicius, D. D., Workman, M. L., and Mishler, M. A. [Eds.]. [1999]. *Medical-surgical nursing across the health care continuum* [3rd ed., p. 1067]. Philadelphia: W. B. Saunders.)

bined use of sandbags, tape across the forehead, and a hard cervical collar has been found to restrict flexion, extension, lateral bending, and rotation of the spine. Studies indicate that 3 to 25% of the injury to the spinal cord occurs after the initial injury, either during transport or early in the course of treatment. Optimal cervical spinal positioning and effective immobilization are necessary to protect neurological function. It is important that EMTs directly transport victims of SCI to identified hospitals in all areas of the country that have a full range of diagnostic and treatment facilities available for spinal cord–injured patients.

Damage to the spinal cord results from several factors, including (1) morphological damage to the spinal cord, (2) hemorrhage, (3) vascular damage, (4) ischemia, (5) structural changes in the gray and white matter, and (6) other biochemical responses to the trauma. The systemic hemodynamic changes that occur after the SCI are a major factor in the resulting damage to the spinal cord. As blood flow to the cord is decreased, ischemia results, causing changes in the tissue oxygen tension that affect all the metabolic functions of the cells. The optimal time for intervention to limit or reverse this destructive process is within 4 hours of injury. The necrotic process consumes approximately 40% of the cross-sectional cord at the level of injury within 4 hours of trauma, and 70% within 24 hours (Walleck, 1994).

TABLE 22–4 ■ LEVELS OF INJURY AND EXPECTED FUNCTIONAL OUTCOMES

Spinal Cord Level	Muscle Function	Functional Goals
C1–C3	Limited head control Talking, chewing, sipping, blowing	Relies on mechanical ventilation Uses computer and environmental control unit Electric wheelchair with sip-and-puff control
C4	Normal head control Diaphragmatic breathing Scapular elevation	Controls electric wheelchair with mouth stick or chin control Mobile arm support for limited self-feeding
C5	Shoulder external rotation Shoulder abduction to 90 degrees Limited shoulder flexion Normal elbow flexion	Dresses upper body Feeds self with adapted utensils Turns self in bed with side rails Pushes wheelchair with handrim projections Operates electric wheelchair Drives with hand controls
C6	Shoulder control Forearm supination Wrist extension (tenodesis grasp)	Dresses lower body Feeds self with hand or tenodesis splints Able to do bowel and bladder program with equipment Independent in transfer to bed, wheelchair, or car with sliding board
C7	Has triceps control Elbow extension, wrist flexion Finger extension	Independent in dressing, feeding, bathing, and transfer to bed, wheelchair, or car Propels wheelchair without handrim projections Able to drive with hand controls
C8–T4	Normal upper extremity function except for fine finger control	Independent in all transfers, including floor Pushes wheelchair up and down curbs Independent with homemaking Independent with bowel and bladder program
T5–T12	Good trunk stability	Independent with wheelchair Able to do all activities more easily T12: walks with walker and long-leg braces with difficulty
L1–L5	Full hip motion Knee flexion and knee quadriceps extension Limited ankle control	Walks with short-leg braces and Lofstrand crutches with some difficulty Uses wheelchair for convenience and energy conservation
S1–S5	Full knee and ankle motion	Functional ambulation Locomotion Partial or complete bowel and bladder control

From Schmidtz, T. (1994). *Physical rehabilitation: assessment and treatment* (pp 554–556). Philadelphia. Copyright 1994 by F.A. Davis Company. Adapted by permission

The use of methylprednisolone, 30 mg/kg body weight) IV within 8 hours of injury, followed by 5.4 mg/kg per hour for 23 hours, has been advocated to lessen neurological deficits, specifically motor function and sensation to pinprick and light touch, since Bracken et al. published results of their clinical trials in 1990. George et al. (1995) conducted a study at two Level I trauma centers from 1989 to 1992 to evaluate the use of methylprednisolone within 8 hours of injury in patients with SCI. Using mobility upon discharge from the hospital and FIM (functional independence measure) scores as outcome measures, this group found no difference. The concern is that the apparent benefit of achieving additional segments of motor and sensory function may not translate to achieving a greater level of function. More research is needed, but meanwhile, the standard of care is the use of methylprednisolone after injury.

Spinal shock is a physiological disruption of the function of the spinal cord that accompanies SCI. It is a temporary suspension of function and reflexes below the level of injury. Symptoms are as follows:

■ Flaccid paralysis of all skeletal muscles and loss of all spinal reflexes
■ Loss of pain, proprioception, and other sensations
■ Bladder and bowel dysfunction with paralytic ileus
■ Loss of thermoregulation

Spinal shock usually occurs immediately after injury but may occur up to 1 week later. It usually lasts 7 to 10 days after injury, although it may be prolonged by infection or other medical complications. The end of spinal shock is indicated by the return of reflexes. Flaccidity gives way to spasticity in the affected muscle groups.

Prognosis for neurological recovery in patients with complete motor and sensory lesions (ASIA level A) tends to be poor, whereas that for those with incomplete lesions is more favorable.

Initial Management

The acute management of SCI care involves spinal stabilization and ventilatory support. The goal of initial care is to provide and maintain optimal oxygenation and perfusion of all vital organs, including the spinal cord.

Assessment begins at the time of injury and focuses on motor and sensory function, including voluntary motor ability and light touch, pinprick, and pain sensations. Patients with injury at T6 and above, especially those with a cervical injury, are at risk for development of spinal shock. Hypotension, bradycardia, and hypersecretion of mucus are a common result.

Nursing interventions include close monitoring of vital signs and respiratory status. Respiratory insufficiency is one of the most serious complications and remains a major cause of death during the acute phase. Subsequent development of atelectasis and pneumonia is an unfortunate complication. Nursing staff must be prepared to perform frequent suctioning, abdominal compression, and cough assistance while collaborating with respiratory and physical therapy to provide chest therapy, bronchodilators, and secretion-altering drugs.

Patients with injury above the C4 level require intubation and ventilation because of the loss of phrenic innervation to the diaphragm. Injuries at C4 and below may involve respiratory compromise and temporary ventilation, so patients with such injuries require frequent respiratory assessment as well.

Neurodiagnostic studies generally consist of cervical spine radiographs as well as thoracic and lumbar views. If a lower level of injury is suspected or there is evidence of multiple trauma, myelogram, tomograms, computed tomography scans, and magnetic resonance imaging will facilitate therapeutic decisions. Radiographs must be taken with the patient in a neutral position to prevent further injury.

Spinal stabilization is further achieved through surgical intervention. Surgery may be performed to restore bony anatomical alignment, to prevent further cord damage, and to stabilize the site (Fig. 22–9). A small percentage of patients require surgery for progressive loss of neurological function occurring after injury. Surgical intervention for cervical injuries involves (1) decompression (anteriorly, posteriorly, or both) and (2) fusion, the use of a bone graft (placed anteriorly, posteriorly, or both), and (3) instrumentation to provide a framework for bony fusion. Surgery for thoracic and lumbar fractures requires use of instrumentation, often with a bone graft. "Harrington rods are the standard of treatment for an unstable spine fracture in the thoracic spine. For injuries caudal to the 9th thoracic vertebra and those with injuries in the lumbar spine, internal fixators transpedicular screws are used" (Alho, 1994).

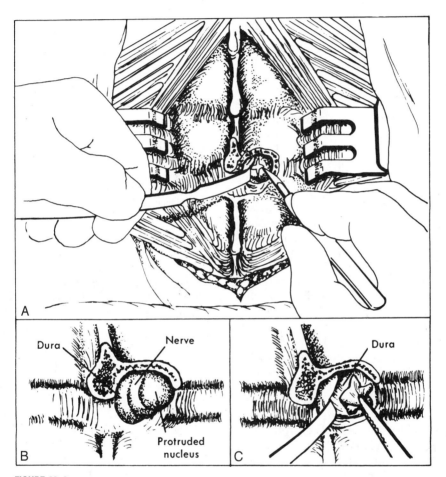

FIGURE 22–9
Laminectomy procedure. *A,* Window has been made in lamina, and ligament has been incised to expose underlying dura mater and nerve root. *B,* Relationship of dura mater, nerve root, and protruded nucleus pulposus (disc). *C,* Retraction of nerve root over dura mater and removal of disc. (From Meeker, J. H., Rothrock, J. C. [1991]. *Alexander's care of the patient in surgery* St. Louis: Mosby–Year Book.)

Immediate surgical intervention is necessary only if the patient demonstrates neurological decline or for treatment of other medical conditions. Surgical stabilization is usually performed after the patient is hemodynamically stable, although associated injuries may preclude stabilization even then. "Studies indicate that patients with incomplete lesions gain more function if decompression and stabilization are done as a single procedure within the first 2 weeks after injury or if stabilization is initially performed" (Rimoldi, Zigler, Capen, Hu, 1992). Campagnolo, Esquieres, and Kopacz (1997) reported a study of 64 patients with cervical, thoracolumbar, or cauda equina injuries who underwent spinal stabilization. For the subjects who had surgery less than 24 hours after injury, the average length of hospital stay was 37.5 days; for those who underwent surgery more than 24 hours after injury, the average length was 54.7 days. There was no reported difference in the two groups as regards medical complications. This study replicates the trend in treatment by the 1980s toward use of early surgical reduction and stabilization of spinal column fractures so patients could start rehabilitation.

The importance of instrumenting as few spinal segments as necessary and of maintaining the normal contour of the spine has been well recognized in recent years. Surgical stabilization is usually supplemented with external stabilization for about 3 months. External stabilization is achieved with traction through tongs inserted into the skull (Fig. 22–10) or with the use of a halo fixation device with body jacket for high cervical injuries (Fig. 22–11). A custom-molded thoracolumbosacral flexion-extension–lateral control, a lumbosacral flexion-extension–lateral control, or a clamshell thoracolumbosacral orthosis is used for thoracic and lumbar spine instability.

Neurological recovery has not been improved by early reduction and stabilization of the spine in severe fractures. The goal of spinal surgery is to reduce or remove displaced fragments and obtain stable healing of the skeletal injury. The advantage of operative fixation is to improve early mobilization. Early mobilization prevents many complications, such as skin problems, deep vein thrombosis, and respiratory difficulties. Patients who undergo early reduction and stabilization often experience less chronic back pain. Also, the patient's social and psychological well-being are enhanced by the ability to be out of bed as early as possible after injury.

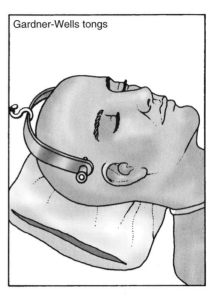

FIGURE 22–10
Gardner-Wells tongs. (From Ignatavicius, D. D., Workman, M. L., and Mishler, M. A. [Eds.]. [1999]. *Medical-surgical nursing across the health care continuum* [3rd ed., p. 1070]. Philadelphia: W. B. Saunders.)

High-Risk Nursing Diagnosis: Alteration in Respiratory Function Related to Ineffective Airway Clearance, Muscle Paralysis, and Ineffective Breathing Patterns

The respiratory system depends on the following four groups of muscles innervated by spinal nerves:

- "Accessory muscles" in the neck, which expand the upper chest and rib cage and are innervated at C2–C8
- Muscles of the diaphragm, which are innervated at C3–C5 via the phrenic nerve
- The intercostal muscles, innervated at T1–T8, which facilitate coughing
- The abdominal muscles, innervated at T6–T12, which are used in expiration and coughing

The patient with an injury *above* C4 requires mechanical ventilation because of loss of innervation of the intercostal muscles and diaphragm at the phrenic nerve. The patient with a neurological injury at C1 to C2 needs permanent ventilator support, phrenic nerve pacemaker support, or both, whereas the patient injured at C3 to C4 may need only supplemental ventilator assistance.

Patients with injuries above C4 have shallow respirations, a vital capacity of 800 to 1500 mL maximum, and no voluntary cough,

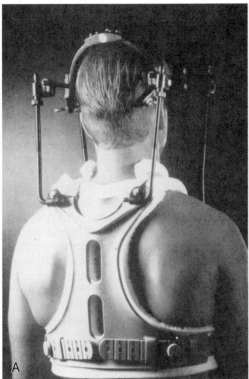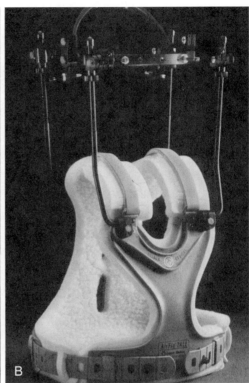

FIGURE 22–11
A and *B*, Halo fixation device.

and they need help to eliminate secretions. They require extensive pulmonary hygiene, including chest percussion with vibration, assisted cough, suctioning, and frequent turning.

The use of an assistive cough, also called *quad coughing*, augments the abdominal muscles during the expiratory phase of a cough and helps loosen pulmonary secretions and force them into the upper respiratory tract, where they can be expectorated or suctioned. This technique is performed as follows:

1. The patient is either lying on the back or sitting in an upright position.
2. The nurse places the heel of one hand cupped under the xiphoid process and instructs the patient to take several deep breaths and then try to hold the breath for a few seconds.
3. The patient is then asked to cough. As he or she coughs, the nurse pushes inward and upward with the heel of the hand against the diaphragm with a quick thrust.
4. This sequence may be repeated until secretions are cleared.

This technique may also be performed two-handed, with the hands on the rib cage and the thumbs meeting at the xiphoid process, or with the patient in the side-lying position and one of the nurse's hands along the upper rib cage.

With an injury *at the C5 level*, patients may have weakness of the diaphragm but generally have adequate voluntary respirations and a vital capacity of 1000 to 1800 mL maximum. These patients also require assistance for elimination of secretions, including aggressive suctioning, incentive spirometry, percussion and drainage, and assisted coughing.

In patients with a *C6 to C7* injury, the diaphragm movement remains normal but the intercostal and abdominal muscles are paralyzed. Preventive respiratory management is needed for such patients, which consists of assistance for coughing and the elimination of secretions.

Those injured at *T1 to T7* incur partial paralysis of the intercostal muscles so generally have an impaired cough and ultimately compensate with diaphragmatic breathing. They require assistance with secretion removal by means of the quad coughing maneuver. Patients with injuries at the *T7 to T12* level have only weakness of the abdominal muscles with some impairment of cough. After injury, compensatory diaphragmatic breathing develops in those with T1 to T7 injuries.

Respiratory failure is divided into problems of ventilation and problems of oxygenation. The most immediate problem is ventilatory failure due to muscle paralysis. Pneumonia and atelectasis, especially of the left lung, develop frequently during the acute phase of tetraplegia. Pulmonary embolism is always of concern. Ventilation is adequate in the patient with (1) normal arterial blood gas values, (2) adequate vital capacity and tidal volume, (3) absence of respiratory distress, (4) absence of pulmonary complications, (4) absence of fever, and (5) demonstration by auscultation and radiographs that lungs are clear.

The nurse must perform physical assessment of the chest, including observation, inspection, palpation, percussion, and auscultation along with vital signs. Changes from baseline respiratory status should be reported. Serial vital capacity measurements should be made frequently to determine decline in mechanical pulmonary failure. Arterial blood gas concentrations and pulse oximetry are monitored to detect impaired oxygenation and guide the type of ventilatory support needed. Initially, the PaO_2 (arterial partial pressure of oxygen) is maintained at 90 mm Hg because systemic hypoxemia can exacerbate the SCI. Supplemental oxygen should be used for the first 24 hours and then as needed to maintain an O_2 saturation value above 90%. Chest radiographs are obtained frequently to rule out pulmonary complications and allow for early treatment if they arise. Assessment of the abdomen is important because abdominal distention interferes with respiratory excursion.

A patient who is ventilator dependent either is intubated or has a tracheostomy tube in place and so is unable to communicate verbally. Patients who are ventilated for any length of time have a tracheostomy tube. In the initial stages, a cuffed tracheostomy tube is used. The cuff is inflated to hold the tracheostomy tube in place and prevent air flow around the outside of the cannula, allowing for more effective ventilation of the patient and preventing aspiration. The lack of air flow across the vocal cords from the fully inflated cuff prevents patients from speaking. A communication system should be initiated at this time to establish a method of communication, such as (1) blinking for "yes" or "no," (2) use of an alphabet board with a mouth pointer, or (3) use of an external device placed on the neck or larynx to facilitate some speech.

When the patient is medically stable, a protocol for deflating the cuff is begun. The speech therapist then can evaluate the patient for the possible use of a "talking trach" or Passey-Muir valve to allow some form of oral communication. The Passey-Muir valve is a one-way valve that allows air to be taken in through the trachea. When the patient exhales, air is forced over the vocal cords, allowing speech. The tracheostomy tube must be deflated when the Passey-Muir valve is used; this is critical because the patient would be unable to exhale otherwise.

In this acute phase, the speech therapist can also help the patient learn to swallow his or her saliva. Positioning is important to aid in mobilizing secretions. If spinal stability has been achieved, elevation of the patient's head serves the dual purpose of assisting with secretion expectoration and allowing some contact with the outside environment. Such contact is important for the patient with an SCI, who is psychologically very fragile at this point in the recovery.

Ventilator-dependent patients with high SCI may also experience dysphagia, which can lead to aspiration and pneumonia. Often, oral feedings are discontinued, and nutrition is provided through a nasogastric or gastrostomy tube. The speech therapist often recommends swallowing studies to identify any dysfunction. The therapist works on swallowing retraining with the patient and reintroduces oral feedings when appropriate. Tracheobronchial suctioning by nursing or speech therapy staff after oral feedings is recommended to prevent aspiration.

Airway clearance is often impaired in the person with a high SCI because of flaccid paralysis of the abdominal and intercostal muscles. The paralysis reduces the strength and quality of the patient's cough. Aggressive chest physical therapy is needed to mobilize and clear secretions to prevent atelectasis and pneumonia. The use of hourly incentive spirometry should be encouraged. The patient with a tracheostomy requires frequent suctioning and good pulmonary hygiene, consisting of chest percussion, vibration and drainage, and assisted coughing, to mobilize secretions and prevent pneumonia.

The ability to cough is also reduced in a patient with a high-level injury. Family members and friends can be taught to manually assist coughing with the quad cough technique. Patients can be taught to perform this procedure independently by putting their wrists one on top of the other under the xiphoid process. Because respiratory complications are a long-term risk for patients with high SCI, this technique should be taught to all patients and caregivers.

Routine nursing interventions consist of turning the patient every 2 to 3 hours and ensuring adequate hydration, which aids in liquefying and mobilizing secretions. Family members can be encouraged to participate by reminding the patient to drink fluids, turning the patient, and performing frequent pulmonary hygiene measures. Mobility and an upright position are critical to reducing respiratory complications.

For the patient with an injury at C4 level or below, a ventilator weaning program is usually instituted during the rehabilitation phase. The objective of such a program is to remove the individual from dependency on the ventilator by (1) gradually increasing the time "off," or disconnected from, the ventilator as tolerated and (2) progressive strengthening of the muscles used in respiration. The success of weaning depends on the patient's physiological stability and psychological readiness. Often, the patient with an SCI better tolerates a weaning program in which periods off the ventilator on a T-piece are alternated with rest periods on the ventilator, which is set to assist-control, than a program in which the rate of intermittent mandatory ventilation is reduced. T-piece trials, beginning with 5 to 15 minutes three or four times a day, provide periods of rest and exercise for the muscles that need strengthening. The weaning program must ultimately be tailored to the individual patient.

Removal of the tracheostomy tube begins after success of the ventilator weaning program, as the need for frequent suctioning diminishes. Weaning from the tracheostomy tube is performed with the Passey-Muir valve initially; as the patient tolerates, the tracheostomy tube is capped with a closed valve. The nurse, speech therapist, or respiratory therapist must closely monitor the patient for any signs of respiratory distress when the tube is capped. Periods of tracheostomy tube capping are increased until the patient tolerates it at all times. The tracheostomy tube is generally changed to a smaller size at this point. It is finally removed when the patient tolerates the smallest size. Some patients with SCI cannot tolerate removal of the tracheostomy tube and incur less respiratory dysfunction with the tube left in place.

For those patients who cannot be weaned from a ventilator, consideration should be given to *diaphragm pacing* or *phrenic nerve stimulation*. Lesions above C3 usually leave the anterior horn cells to the phrenic nerve viable, with the potential to be stimulated electrically. A prosthetic device or "pacer" is surgically implanted bilaterally over the diaphragm. External activation of the pacer results in movement of the diaphragm and thus in "breathing." It is recommended that consideration for surgical implants be delayed 6 to 12 months after an SCI. Chawla (1993) reports that phrenic nerve conduction studies conducted in the early days following injury may yield a false-negative response to stimulation. Of patients in whom phrenic nerve stimulation is successful, many still require the presence of a tracheostomy tube and ventilator as a backup, in case of respiratory complications or malfunction of the pacer (p.89).

Nurses must also consider the emotional stressors associated with ventilator dependence. The process of mechanical ventilation necessitates the loss of independence and control over the most basic function— breathing. Tracheostomy tubes impair not only the ability to speak but also the ability to sigh, gasp, sneeze, or produce any emotional expression. Patients often find the experience of suctioning unpleasant and feel as if they are "suffocating" during the procedure. Noises of the ventilator and the alarms contribute to feelings of apprehension and anxiety. The nurse should provide an environment that minimizes isolation and maximizes interaction and communication. Caregivers must remember that although the patient cannot speak, he or she is very aware of the environment. Every effort should be made to establish a method of communication with the patient.

High-Risk Nursing Diagnosis: Impaired Physical Mobility Related to Muscle Paralysis

Following surgical spinal stabilization, immobilization is maintained by means of external stabilization for up to 3 months (see Figs. 22–10 and 22–11). As already described, halo fixation devices with body jackets are most often used to maintain cervical stability, whereas lumbosacral orthoses (most commonly the LSFEL or Knight spinal orthosis) and thoracolumbosacral orthoses (the TLSFE or thoracolumbar standing orthosis brace) are used for injuries in the thoracic and lumbar areas.

Nursing interventions in the acute phase after SCI require repositioning every 2 to 3 hours to prevent skin breakdown and further respiratory difficulties. Nurses should "log-roll" patients in bed to maintain spinal alignment. For patients who have significant spinal instability or thoracic and lumbar fractures, immobilization is further achieved by the use of special beds that allow movement to prevent pressure ulcers and decrease the risk of pulmonary complications while keeping the spine rigid. Roto-Rest beds and Stryker or Foster frames are often used (Fig. 22–12). It should be stressed that special flotation beds or mattresses do not negate the need for regular turning of the patient.

Nursing care includes management of the halo vest (body jacket) device. It should be checked daily for loosening of the pins, and the patient's skin should be checked for signs of infection. Indications of infection are (1) pain at the site of the pins, (2) wrinkling of the skin at the pin sites, (3) drainage at the pin sites, and (4) an open area. The physician should be notified immediately if pin loosening is suspected.

Pin care should be performed once or twice daily with a cotton-tipped swab dipped in normal saline. Use of solution of half-strength peroxide followed by a rinse with normal saline is indicated if there is crusting around the pin sites. Bacitracin ointment may be applied if drainage or redness is present or an infection is suspected. Care of the vest consists of opening it daily to check the skin and washing it with a mild soap, rinsing with water and drying well. Alcohol can be used under the vest to toughen the skin. No lotion or powder should be used under the vest because it may irritate the skin. Many patients prefer to wear a cotton undershirt under the vest to prevent irritation.

Care must be taken to ensure that staff do not use the halo to turn the patient in bed or during a transfer. Pressure should not be applied to the frame because it may loosen the pins. The nurse should check daily to be sure the wrench (used to tighten the frame) is taped to the front of the halo vest. Presence of the wrench ensures that the vest can be released quickly in an emergency situation, for example, to allow for cardiopulmonary resuscitation.

Monitoring the skin is of utmost importance for patients who have any type of orthotic device. The nurse should use a flashlight to look under the brace if it cannot be removed. Daily skin assessment is critical, and assessment should be performed more often if redness appears. Lotions should be avoided because they may soften skin, leading to maceration and breakdown; powders, which often irritate, should also be avoided. When the patient is wearing a removable orthosis, the skin should be checked carefully each time the device is removed.

Therapy interventions include assessment of the sensory and motor levels, muscle tone,

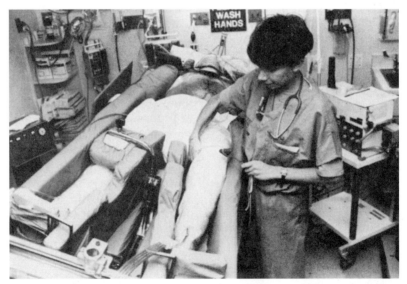

FIGURE 22–12
Neuroscience nurse performing neurological assessment on a patient with spine injuries on a Roto-Rest bed. (From Barker, E. [1994]. *Neuroscience nursing* [p. 366]. St. Louis: Mosby–Year Book.)

deep tendon reflexes (especially biceps, triceps, quadriceps, and gastrocnemius), range of motion, and overall level of function. Treatment plans are individualized for each patient and the level of injury, but they generally comprise the following types of treatments:

1. Respiratory care, including pulmonary hygiene, assisted coughing, and deep breathing techniques.
2. Range-of-motion exercises and positioning. Physical and occupational therapy services will collaborate with nursing to establish a turning schedule, appropriate turning techniques, and the use of positioning splints. Positioning splints for the wrists, hands, and fingers are an early consideration for occupational therapy. "Alignment of the fingers, thumb and wrist must be maintained for functional activities or future dynamic splinting. For high-level lesions the wrist is positioned in neutral, the web space is maintained, and the fingers are flexed" (Schmitz, 1994). Physical therapists will order ankle boots or splints to maintain alignment and prevent heel cord tightness and pressure sores.
3. Mobilization. Once spinal stabilization is ensured and there are no medical contraindications, mobilization is encouraged. The patient should be started on a schedule designed to increase tolerance to sitting. The patient with a high SCI should be able to tolerate sitting at 90 degrees for 15 to 20 minutes in bed without significant blood pressure changes before transferring activities are initiated. The use of an abdominal binder or elastic stockings retards venous pooling and helps eliminate severe postural hypotension. Once the patient is able to leave the bed, a reclining wheelchair with elevating leg rests is optimal for this patient population.

High-Risk Nursing Diagnosis: Alteration in Nutrition: Less Than Body Requirements Related to Inability to Access Nutrients and Increased Metabolism

Gastric emptying is delayed in patients with quadriplegia secondary to alterations in autonomic function. In the acute phase of recovery from the injury, such patients are at risk for gastric atony, paralytic ileus, and gastrointestinal bleeding. Patients at greatest risk are those with injury above the level of T5. Following spinal cord trauma, smooth muscle function ceases, resulting in an accumulation of fluid in the stomach and intestine. This fluid puts the patient at risk for aspiration and hypoventilation. Treatment consists of stomach decompression with a nasogastric tube and elimination of oral intake to prevent respiratory and cardiac compromise due to gastric distention. An abnormal release of catecholamines in response to stress and the use of steroids contribute to gastrointestinal ulceration, perforation, and hemorrhage. Complaints of shoulder pain should be regarded as pain from the gastrointestinal tract and require immediate attention.

Although patients with SCI have larger nutritional requirements during the acute phase, their energy expenditures over the long term are below those of able-bodied people, most likely as a result of loss of muscle mass. Because of the decreases in metabolic rate and physical activity, patients with SCI have a tendency to gain weight. It is important to minimize weight gain both because of its association with medical problems and because of the additional burden on caregivers. It has been suggested that the ideal body weight for persons with paraplegia is 5 to 10% below that of their able-bodied counterparts, and for those with tetraplegia, 10 to 15%.

The nursing intervention related to this diagnosis consists of teaching the benefits of a well-balanced diet that is high in protein, vitamins, and minerals to promote and maintain health and that supplies sufficient calories to maintain an appropriate weight. Iron should be maintained at adequate levels to deliver essential oxygen to the cells. Obviously, the presence of a pressure sore requires special attention to nutritional management.

Potential Complications in the Acute Phase

Prevention of Deep Vein Thrombosis

Deep vein thrombosis is a cause of early mortality and morbidity after SCI. The period of greatest risk is 7 to 10 days after injury. Nursing interventions include the measurement of bilateral calf and thigh circumferences upon admission and on a regular basis. Doppler ultrasound studies or a venogram is often performed as a baseline study. When the patient is sitting up in a chair, the nurse should avoid putting the legs in a dependent position (i.e., the legs should be elevated). Another prophylactic intervention is the use of thigh-high compression stockings or external pneumatic calf-compression boots. The role of pneumatic compression boots is still being evaluated, with initial studies recommending their use 23 hours a day but many rehabilitation centers using them for only 8 hours at night. The use of heparin as prophylaxis has also been a standard of practice; enoxaparin, a low-molecular-weight heparin, has been shown to produce effective prophylaxis but with fewer side effects than with unfractionated heparin.

Many surgeons prophylactically place a filter into the inferior vena cava (Greenfield filter) in the patient with high quadriplegia considered at highest risk for deep vein thrombosis. The nurse must be careful not to dislodge the filter when assisting with quad coughing. Some SCI centers have continued to use manual assisted cough but others have discontinued the technique in patients with Greenfield filters.

If deep vein thrombosis is confirmed, treatment is bed rest with intravenous heparin for 7 to 10 days followed by 3 months of oral warfarin (Coumadin). The presence of deep vein thrombosis puts the patient at risk for a pulmonary embolus. The nurse must carefully watch for signs and symptoms in the patient who is ventilator dependent or has high quadriplegia. Signs and symptoms of pulmonary embolus include the following:

- Heavy feeling in the chest
- Fever
- Irritability or feeling of anxiety
- Increased pulse
- Referred shoulder or scapula pain
- Hemoptysis

Diagnosis of pulmonary embolus is made with a ventilation-perfusion ratio scan or pulmonary angiography. Treatment consists of bed rest with intravenous heparin followed by 6 months of oral warfarin.

Heterotopic Ossification

Heterotopic ossification, the abnormal formation of new bone between layers of connective tissue, occurs in 16 to 53% of patients with SCI. The etiology is unknown. This disorder occurs only below the level of injury although not in the limbs below the knees or elbows. The hips are most commonly affected, followed by the knees, shoulders, and elbows. Heterotopic ossification is typically noted 1 to 4 months after injury. It is also known as ectopic bone formation; if pieces of bone form between the muscles, the condition is known as myositis ossificans (Colachis, Clinchot, & Venesy, 1993).

Onset of heterotopic ossification occurs in one of the following ways:

- Sudden or acute onset, characterized by swelling, pain, and localized temperature at the affected joint
- Insidious onset, with the nurse or therapist noting a decrease in range of motion
- Sudden occurrence of knee effusion without a history of trauma

Nursing assessment for possible development of heterotopic ossification includes early identification of

- Swelling at the affected area
- Warmth
- Pain
- Stiffness
- Limited motion
- Redness

After 4 to 10 weeks, new bone formation can be seen on radiographs or bone scans. Over 3 to 6 months, new bone will continue to form and grow. This process can result in (1) permanent restriction of range of motion in the affected joint, (2) peripheral nerve entrapment, and (3) pressure sores.

Nursing interventions related to heterotopic ossification are as follows:

1. Teach the patient that he or she is at risk for this complication.
2. Mobilize the patient as early as possible.
3. Perform range-of-motion exercises for all joints.
4. Ensure proper patient positioning in bed and in the wheelchair.

Banovac, Gonzalez, and Renfree (1997) reported on a new protocol consisting of the intravenous administration of disodium etidronate (Didronel) in 46 patients after SCI. The dosage, which was higher than previously recommended, was 300 mg given intravenously for 3 days followed by 20 mg per kg body weight daily for 6 months. The data from this study suggested that etidronate may prevent heterotopic ossification in the majority of patients when administered during the early stages of the disease and in higher doses than routinely recommended. The drug does not affect the mature stage of heterotopic ossification.

Cardiovascular Problems

With the onset of spinal shock and the subsequent loss of sympathetic input, the cardiovascular system may lose its ability to effectively regulate blood pressure and heart rate. Patients with injuries above T5 exhibit the most profound symptoms because of interruption of the sympathetic nervous system and loss of vasoconstrictor response below the level of injury. Hypotension occurs as a result of peripheral vasodilation, venous pooling, and decreased cardiac filling pressures. Patients with SCI can usually tolerate a systolic blood pressure of 90 mm Hg in a supine position. If the pressure is too low to maintain adequate tissue perfusion, however, fluid replacement may be necessary. With the absence of normal blood pressure and heart rate reflexes, fluid overload may develop easily in the patient with SCI. Careful monitoring of the patient's fluid volume is necessary to maintain a homeostatic balance.

Because of the inability to regulate internal temperature, the body of the patient with a high SCI assumes the temperature of the environment. Hypothermia and hyperthermia can contribute to cardiac dysrhythmias. Nursing efforts should be directed at maintaining a constant temperature by adding or removing blankets or adjusting the room's thermostat controls.

One result of SCI is the reduced ability to perform aerobic exercise and thus stimulate the cardiovascular system. Long-term effects potentially include decreased muscle tone, a rise in cardiac risk factors, increases in serum cholesterol and low density lipoprotein levels, obesity, and early degenerative changes associated with aging. People with functional levels of C5 to T1 can perform arm exercises and ergometry. It is questionable, however, whether the sympathetic nervous system in such cases is sufficiently activated to provide central circulatory support for voluntary arm exercise. When a patient with an SCI exercises, the heart rate and oxygen levels increase but reach lower levels than in healthy people who exercise.

Peripheral vascular insufficiency and inactivity of the skeletal muscle venous pump may induce excessive venous pooling in the legs and abdomen, reduce the circulating blood volume, and diminish venous return, thus limiting blood flow to exercising arm muscles. People with quadriplegia or high paraplegia are frequently hypotensive during upright arm exercise because of vasodilation in exercising muscles, for which peripheral vasoconstriction in the legs and viscera does not adequately compensate. This dysfunctional syndrome of inadequate acute hemodynamic responses to increased metabolic demands has been called *circulatory hypokinesis* (Figoni, 1990).

The physiological response to exercise in people with paraplegia may be more consistent with that in able-bodied people because of more variable innervation of the peripheral sympathetic system. People with paraplegia may be able to use voluntary upright arm exercise to recruit a muscle mass sufficient to induce adequate volume and pressure levels in the heart and thereby improve cardiovascular fitness.

The voluntary use of the upper extremities facilitates independence in wheelchair mobility and other activities of daily living. To promote cardiovascular fitness, however, rehabilitation of the patient with an SCI must also encompass activities that emphasize upper body fitness, such as weight training, wheelchair-accessible exercises, and wheelchair sports. Membership in a fitness club should be considered as part of the rehabilitation continuum.

REHABILITATION PHASE

The rehabilitation nurse has the opportunity to be an integral part of the transition of the patient with an SCI from disability to return to community. Professional health care workers need to shift their emphasis from "rehabilitation in the hospital" to "rehabilitation in the home, community and at work." Rehabilitation of people with SCI occurs along the continuum, with the goal being "the development of a satisfying and productive lifestyle after discharge" (Brown, 1992).

Alteration in Autonomic Regulation

Altered Temperature Regulation Related to Disruption in Hypothalamic Control

Injuries above T6 often cause problems associated with disruption in the autonomic regulation of body functions. Temperature regulation involves ascending and descending pathways in the spinal cord and integrative structures in the brain. After a complete spinal cord lesion, information from the temperature receptors below the level of the lesion does not reach the brain. Autonomic responses to regulate temperature, such as sweating and shivering, do not occur below the level of the lesion. Although some of the capacity for temperature regulation remains

TABLE 22–5 ■ NURSING INTERVENTIONS FOR ALTERED TEMPERATURE REGULATION

Environment	Patient Response	Nursing Action(s)
Cool	Very cold Shivering Goosebumps above level of injury Skin cool to touch	Dress patient in warm clothing Apply warm blankets Give warm fluids Do not use electric blanket, heating pad, or hot water bottle on areas without sensation
Hot	Headache Flushing of skin Nausea or vomiting Dizziness Sweating above level of injury	Keep patient out of sun Give cool fluids Use fan or air conditioning Have patient wear hat Avoid hot tubs Monitor for decreased urine output

after a high SCI, autonomic temperature regulation is impaired in patients with tetraplegia. As already mentioned, the body often adopts the temperature of the environment. Nursing assessment includes identification of the temperature of the environment and the patient's response to it (Table 22–5).

Autonomic Response: Potential or Actual Hypotension

Postural or orthostatic hypotension tends to be a problem for people with lesions above T6 as a result of interruption of splanchnic control. Movement from a horizontal to a vertical position in people with high lesions is followed by rapid, uninhibited accumulation of blood in the viscera and lower extremities because of disruption in control of the splanchnic nerve roots. The results are decreases in blood supply to the central veins, return of venous blood, and cardiac output. Blood pressure drops, and pulse rises. Patients complain of dizziness, lightheadedness, and even loss of consciousness.

Nursing actions are as follows:

1. Elevate the head of the bed gradually and leave patient in the upright position in bed for 10 to 15 minutes before transfers.
2. Apply elastic stockings before the patient gets out of bed.
3. Use an abdominal binder.
4. Use a recliner wheelchair with elevating leg rests so patient can be gradually moved to a 90-degree position.
5. Consider liberal salt and fluid intake if the problem is persistent.
6. Avoid or correct dehydration.
7. Monitor blood pressure.

If hypotension occurs when the patient has been moved to the wheelchair, the nurse should

1. Tip the wheelchair back carefully; if symptoms do not resolve, return the patient to bed.
2. Monitor blood pressure.
3. Not leave the patient alone.

Autonomic Dysreflexia

Autonomic dysreflexia, also known as *hyperreflexia*, is the most dangerous of all the potential complications of SCI because it can be life-threatening. Autonomic dysreflexia is the result of the body's inability to restore autonomic equilibrium when presented with a noxious stimulus from below the level of injury. "Autonomic dysreflexia occurs in patients with injury at T6 level and above, although episodes have been reported in people with injuries as low as T10" (American Association of Spinal Cord Injury Nurses, 1996). This condition is considered a medical emergency requiring immediate intervention.

SCI not only causes motor and sensory loss but also impairs autonomic nervous system functioning. The autonomic nervous system functions at an unconscious level to regulate and coordinate vital visceral functions. The two branches of the autonomic nervous system, the sympathetic and parasympathetic, balance each other by providing antagonistic innervation to most effector organs of the body (Fig. 22–13). The sympathetic branch evokes a maximum energy response, while the parasympathetic branch is responsible for energy conservation functions. Individuals with high SCI are subject to autonomic dys-

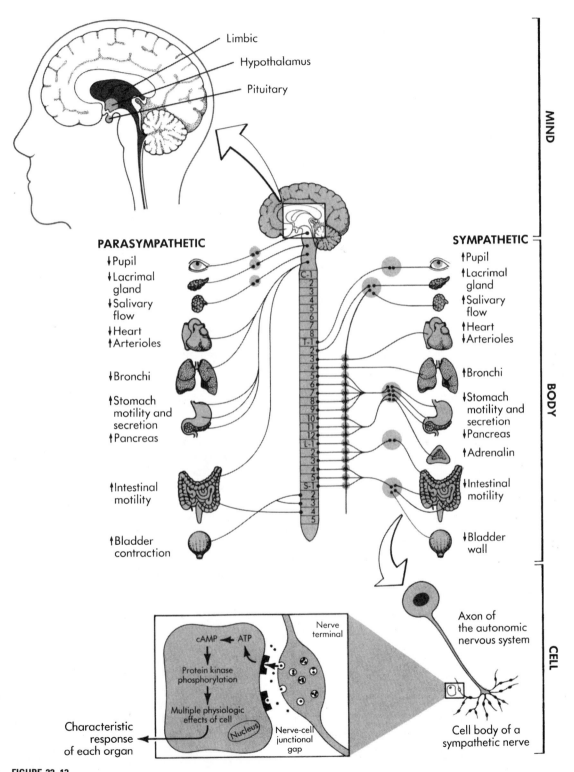

FIGURE 22–13

Diagramatic representation of the autonomic nervous system and its two divisions, sympathetic and parasympathetic. (From Guzzetta, C. E., Dossey, B. M. [1992]. *Cardiovascular nursing: Holistic practice*. St. Louis: Mosby–Year Book.)

function because the injury separates the parasympathetic branch from the sympathetic branch, thus affecting the negative feedback loop. Parasympathetic fibers exiting the brain stem continue to stimulate effector organs as before the injury, but the sympathetic outflow is severely diminished. Stimulation of an intact parasympathetic system in the presence of a diminished sympathetic system results in symptoms of autonomic dysfunction. An example of such stimulation is the abnormal vasovagal response that occurs during tracheal suctioning of an individual with a high spinal cord lesion.

Among the processes affected by autonomic dysreflexia are regulation of blood pressure, bladder and bowel function, sweating, and regulation of body temperature. Any noxious stimulation to the body below the level of cord injury causes elevation of blood pressure and bradycardia as a result of stimulation of cranial nerve X (vagus nerve) below the level of injury. Common noxious stimuli are an overdistended bladder, fecal impaction, and skin breakdown. The body's attempt to reduce blood pressure causes vasodilation above the level of injury.

Patients may experience one, several, or all of the following signs and symptoms related to autonomic dysreflexia:

- Elevation of blood pressure to more than 20 mm Hg above baseline
- Pounding headache
- Bradycardia
- Goose bumps above the level of injury
- Bronchospasm
- Chills without fever
- Flushing and sweating above level of injury
- Nasal congestion
- Changes in vision—blurring, tunnel vision
- Anxiety or apprehension

Nursing Management

The following outline, from the U.S. Department of Health and Human Services AHCPR guidelines, summarizes the components of nursing management for patients at risk for autonomic dysreflexia.

I. Initial assessment—identification of risk factors
   A. Level of injury at T6 or above
   B. Any recent episodes of autonomic dysreflexia
   C. Episodes of headache
   D. Blood pressure elevations to more than 20 mm Hg above baseline
   E. Altered bowel or bladder management
   F. Altered skin integrity
   G. Pain or pressure
   H. Current medications
II. Plan of care—prevention of episodes
   A. Monitor urinary output, and make necessary changes to the bladder management program to prevent overdistention.
   B. Assess for urinary tract infection, ensure appropriate treatment, and evaluate effectiveness.
   C. Monitor bowel program, and make necessary changes to the program to prevent constipation or fecal impaction.
   D. Provide appropriate skin and wound care to prevent noxious stimuli.
   E. Provide other treatment measures as appropriate to alleviate the causes of noxious stimuli.
   F. Provide the patient's family and/or caregiver with educational information about the causes, signs and symptoms, prevention, and management of autonomic dysreflexia.
   G. Assess the ability of the patient's family and/or caregiver to recognize and carry out management techniques designed to avoid autonomic dysreflexia.
   H. Provide information concerning autonomic dysreflexia on a medical alert bracelet or necklace, or have the patient carry such information on a card kept in the wallet.
   I. When planning invasive diagnostic procedures, especially those involving the genitourinary or gastrointestinal system, collaborate with the physician regarding administration of nifedipine, 10 mg orally, prior to the procedure.
III. Interventions for treatment of episodes of autonomic dysreflexia
   A. Sit patient at a 90-degree angle to decrease blood pressure elevation; place the legs in a dependent position, if practical.
   B. Loosen constrictive clothing and/or appliances; remove all vascular support (bandage wraps, abdominal binder, elastic stockings).
   C. Monitor blood pressure and pulse every 2 to 3 minutes throughout the episode.
   D. Assess and remove noxious stimuli below the level of injury until the cause is found and eliminated.

E. For the patient with an indwelling bladder catheter
   1. Check patient for bladder distention.
   2. Remove any mechanical tubing kinks, mucus plugs, urethral constrictions, or gravitational obstructions to urine flow.
   3. Check for blockage by gently irrigating with sterile fluid (total volume not to exceed 30 mL).
   4. If the catheter remains clogged, replace it; if available, use an anesthetic jelly when inserting the new catheter.
F. For the patient with an external urine collection device
   1. Remove the external collecting device.
   2. Catheterize the patient using anesthetic jelly; to prevent a rebound hypotensive effect, empty the bladder by draining 500 mL of urine, clamping the catheter for 5 minutes, and repeating until the bladder is emptied.
G. If systolic blood pressure is greater than 140 mm Hg, apply 1 inch of Nitropaste (15 mg) to the skin, per physician's order, to control blood pressure as a temporary measure until the cause of autonomic dysreflexia can be found.
H. Reassess blood pressure every 2 to 3 minutes, and remove Nitropaste if blood pressure falls below 100 mm Hg.
I. Remove stool gently from the rectal vault; insert anesthetic ointment or jelly into the rectal vault and allow 3 to 5 minutes for the anesthetic effect, then remove fecal impaction from the rectum.
J. Check the wheelchair seat for hard or sharp objects.
K. Observe the patient for pressure sores, ingrown nails, and burns.
L. In a male patient, check to see that genitalia are not pinched and that patient is not having a reflexogenic erection.
M. In a female patient, check for menstrual cramps and vaginal infections.
N. Observe for sensitivity to wrinkled sheets.
O. Administer nifedipine, 10 mg sublingually every 20 to 30 minutes, if systolic blood pressure is greater than 160 mm Hg, per physician order (capsule must be pierced or punctured before administering). *Note:* Administer a maximum of three doses before seeking emergency treatment.
P. Seek further emergency medical treatment if these measures do not resolve the episode; autonomic dysreflexia can lead to seizures, stroke, or death and therefore must be treated immediately.
Q. After the episode resolves, continue to monitor blood pressure and pulse every 2 to 3 minutes until they return to baseline; continue to observe patient over the next 2 to 3 hours, and monitor for any return of symptoms.

Impaired Physical Mobility Related to Muscle Paralysis

Mobilization is an integral component of the SCI patient's rehabilitation, both physical and emotional. Initial sitting begins gradually because of the tendency for orthostatic hypotension in most patients after injury and a period of bed rest. Once the patient is up in a wheelchair, if orthostatic hypotension occurs, the patient can be tilted backward for a few moments until the symptoms subside. Although the experience of orthostatic hypotension is frightening, the patient should be reassured that the body will compensate over time.

The physical and occupational therapy programs (1) continue to emphasize respiratory management, range of joint motion, and positioning and (2) progress to include resistive exercises for the muscles that remain innervated. "Emphasis in physical therapy is on the development of motor control and muscle reeducation techniques for appropriate muscles, regaining postural control and balance by substituting upper body control and vision for lost proprioception, and improved cardiovascular response to exercise" (Schmidtz, 1994).

Activities conducted on an exercise mat constitute a major component of treatment. The sequence of activities begins with achievement of stability within a posture and advances through controlled mobility to skill in functional use. Mat activities begin with rolling, which is of functional significance for bed mobility, independent positional changes in bed for pressure relief, and lower extremity dressing. Ultimately, a level of sitting balance is achieved. Both long and short sitting positions are essential for many activities of daily living, such as dressing, independent performance of range-of-motion exercises, transfers, and wheelchair mobility. "The sitting position varies greatly with the level of injury. Patients with low thoracic lesions will sit with an erect trunk; those with low cervical and high thoracic lesions will maintain sitting balance by forward head displacement and trunk flexion. Patients with high cervical lesions will demonstrate poor sitting posture" (Schmidtz, 1994).

Transfer training is initiated once the patient has gained adequate sitting balance. Training begins on a firm mat and progresses to surfaces such as a bed, toilet, or car seat. The level of a patient's independence in the transfer depends on the level of injury. The technique used most often by patients with SCI is a sliding transfer using a transfer (sliding) board. Stand-pivot transfers are also used commonly for patients needing maximal assist. Nurses and therapists need to communicate about the type of transfer and the patient's ability to participate, so that the same transfer is performed by practitioners in all disciplines and teaching is consistent. As most patients with spinal cord injuries require a wheelchair for the primary mode of mobility, a custom-made wheelchair and appropriate cushions are ordered. The specific adaptations necessary depend on the level of injury.

Patients with low-level injuries who possess good muscle strength, good postural alignment, good range of motion, and sufficient cardiovascular endurance progress to ambulation activities. The orthotic prescription, type of gait pattern, use of functional electrical stimulation, and type of assistive device vary according to the level of injury.

Occupational therapy works on functional activities of daily living. Therapists recommend adaptive dressing modifications and equipment (Fig. 22–14), such as elastic shoelaces and hook-and-loop tape (Velcro) replacements for buttons. The utensil cuff, a palmar strap with a slot at the palm where small items such as a fork or toothbrush can be placed and stabilized, may be used (Fig. 22–15). Nurses must be diligent about incorporating adaptive equipment into patient care to encourage as much functional independence as possible.

Splints are modified as the patient gains strength and range of motion. Nurses and therapists set up splinting schedules that often continue after discharge to achieve and

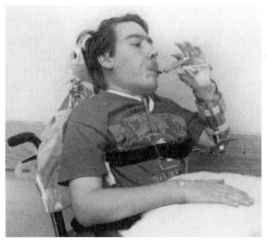

FIGURE 22–14
Mobile arm support used with long opponens splint and vertical holder to aid in feeding: Mobile arm supports upper extremity function when shoulder or forearm strength is weak. The subject also has a long opponens splint with a utensil and vertical holder for a spoon for feeding. (From Braddom R. L. [1996]. *Physical medicine and rehabilitation.* [p. 516]. Philadelphia: W. B. Saunders.)

maintain functional range of motion. Therapists and nurses work closely to encourage functional independence in such activities as the use of a labia spreader by a female patient for self-catheterization and the use of a suppository inserter for a bowel program. Rehabilitation nurses are in a key position to continue the therapy program throughout all shifts.

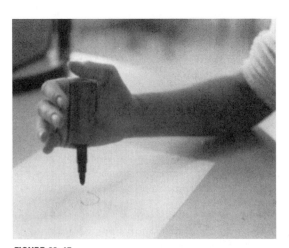

FIGURE 22–15
Utensil cuff holding a writing tool fits over the hand. It can also hold other tools, such as feeding utensils and grooming tools. (From Braddom R. L. [1996]. *Physical medicine and rehabilitation.* [p. 524]. Philadelphia: W. B. Saunders.)

Alteration in Elimination: Bladder and Bowel Function

Patients with SCI have some impairment of bowel and bladder function. Bowel and bladder management is important for physical and psychological well-being. The goal is to establish a program of management that is safe, effective, economical, and minimally disruptive of the patient's lifestyle. Avoidance of medical complications and establishment of control into the patient's lifestyle are critical elements in success.

Bladder Management

Classification of Bladder Dysfunction
The classification of bladder dysfunction depends on the level of injury. Following traumatic injury and during the phase of spinal shock, the bladder is *flaccid*, with the absence of reflex voiding even when the bladder is distended. This can result in urinary retention, requiring continuous or intermittent catheter drainage. In the acute phase of hospitalization, use of an indwelling catheter is often the method of choice. A program of intermittent catheterization is generally initiated when the patient is admitted to the rehabilitation setting.

The patient with a spinal cord lesion above T12 to L1 (upper motor neuron lesion), in whom the reflex arc is still intact, has a *spastic bladder* following the phase of spinal shock; this condition may also be referred to as *automatic* or *reflex bladder*. Disruption of both the sensory and motor nerve tracts above segments S2, S3, and S4 results in uninhibited, involuntary detrusor contractions and uncontrolled, sometimes incomplete voiding. There is decreased bladder capacity with high volumes of residual urine. The inability of the external sphincter to relax in coordination with the detrusor contraction may result in detrusor–external sphincter dyssynergia. The external sphincter contracts as the detrusor muscle contracts in the bladder rather than relaxing; serious consequences, such as bladder hypertrophy, reflux, and upper urinary tract disease, can result.

Patients with spinal cord lesions at or below T12 to L1 (lower motor neuron lesion) have autonomous neurogenic bladder, also called *areflexic* or *flaccid bladder* (see Fig. 11–3). This condition occurs as a result of damage to the cauda equina, which disrupts pathways carrying sensory impulses from the bladder to the cord, motor impulses from the cord to the detrusor muscle, and motor impulses from the spinal cord to the external sphincter. Patients experience decreased sensation of fullness, weakness or absence of detrusor contractions, and increased bladder capacity with high volumes of residual urine. There is complete loss of voluntary voiding, and overflow incontinence is common. The bladder in such a patient functions like the bladder does during spinal shock.

Urinary Tract Infection
One of the most common complications of SCI is urinary tract infection. Although more progress has been made in reducing the incidence of renal failure than in any of the other serious complications of SCI, urinary tract infections and complications continue to be of serious concern and to account for significant morbidity. "Several factors seem to be responsible for an increased risk of infection in the patient with a neurogenic bladder. Repeated bladder instrumentation, placement of an indwelling catheter, impaired emptying with residual urine in the bladder between voids, vesicoureteral or intrarenal reflux, and mucosal ischemia associated with obstructed high-pressure voiding or poor bladder wall compliance may all facilitate bacterial invasion" (Stover, Lloyd, Waites, & Jackson, 1989).

Diagnosis of urinary tract infection in the patient with an SCI may be difficult because the usual signs and symptoms, such as frequency, urgency, nocturia, and dysuria, depend on the level of injury and may be unreliable as diagnostic criteria. The rehabilitation nurse should be aware that the signs may be subtle and may include malaise ("just not feeling well") or only a slight fever (100°F). Cloudy, malodorous urine and changes in urine pH may be signs of urinary tract infection but may also represent colonization or changes of bacterial organisms. Greater spasticity is often a sign of urinary tract complications. Increased spontaneous voiding or larger residual urine volume, including acute urinary retention, may indicate acute infection, demonstrating that the neurogenic bladder does not always respond like the normal bladder. Assessment of the patient and early reporting of signs and symptoms to the physician are immediate nursing interventions for urinary tract infection in the patient with an SCI.

Management of Neurogenic Bladder
Management of the neurogenic bladder involves a variety of options, discussed here.

The level of injury, hand function, lifestyle, or recurrent urinary tract infections may necessitate a combination of these options. Compliance and financial resources also need to be considered.

Intermittent Catheterization. The bladder is emptied periodically through catheterizations, usually every 6 hours. Timing of catheterizations can be adjusted, with the goal of maintaining volumes below 400 to 500 mL. Men with lesions at C7 and below can usually manage self-catheterization.

Indwelling Catheter. Catheters that remain in the bladder provide continuous drainage. They may either be placed through the urethra (urethral catheter) or enter through a stoma in the suprapubic area (suprapubic catheter).

External Collection System (Condom Catheter). An external collection system may be used to collect urine and allow the bladder to empty spontaneously by the reflex action at S2 to S4. The patient may need to perform periodic postvoid residuals to ensure that the bladder is completely emptying.

Often, the condom catheter approach is used in conjunction with a sphincterotomy because many patients with high SCI experience sphincter detrusor dyssnergia. High bladder pressures necessitate the use of medications or surgical intervention to complement the use of an external device. The goal of the condom catheter is to achieve a "balanced bladder" or low-pressure approach, and this device is used most often by men with tetraplegia who are unable to catheterize themselves and do not want to rely on family or caregivers. About a third of men with SCI use condom catheters for long-term urinary drainage. Stelling and Hale (1996) reported a study of 113 patients with SCI who were observed for 5 years to determine the appropriate frequency for routine changing of condom catheters. Eighty of the subjects changed condom catheters daily, whereas 33 changed them every other day. The results showed no significant differences in incidence of skin or urinary complications between the two groups.

Transurethral Resection External Sphincterotomy (TURES). The TURES is a surgical procedure that diminishes bladder neck and sphincter resistance, resulting in continuous emptying. Patients must always wear an external collecting device and leg bag. Any patient for whom this choice is considered must understand that the procedure is irreversible.

Augmentation. Augmentation is a surgical procedure in which a segment of bowel, usually ileum, is sewn into the bladder to create a 600-mL reservoir. The patient continues on a program of intermittent catheterization. No medications are needed, and long-term consequences of this procedure are unknown.

Medications. Medications are also used as part of the bladder management program. The medications used depend on the voiding dysfunction. "Wein has used a classification based on bladder dysfunction: incontinence due to the bladder, incontinence due to the outlet (sphincter), retention due to the bladder, or retention due to the outlet" (Linsenmeyer & Stone, 1993, p. 743). Medications can be prescribed on the basis of this functional classification (Table 22–6).

For instance, a man with tetraplegia, who is unable to perform self-catheterization, may opt for use of a condom catheter for bladder management. Because of detrusor sphincter dyssynergia, however, he has high outlet pressures with the risk of long-term complications. The physician, before suggesting a surgical alternative, may try a medication such as terazosin (Hytrin). This agent relaxes the spastic sphincter, allowing for decreased resistance at the time of bladder emptying and lower pressures.

Long-term management of the neurogenic bladder is often difficult in the patient with SCI. A catheter-free status poses the lowest risk for significant long-term urinary tract complications. Only a minority of patients with SCI can manage with no form of collecting device or catheter.

Indwelling urethral and suprapubic catheters, when used for long-term management of the neurogenic bladder, are associated with a bladder bacterial colonization rate of virtually 100%. Infection rates in patients who develop reflex voiding but require an external collecting device for control of incontinence have been variously reported. Approximately 80% of such patients have either chronic or recurrent bacteriuria.

Formation of bladder calculi is another common complication, related both to infection and to the presence of foreign bodies (urethral or suprapubic catheters). Bladder stones are not a serious complication. Renal calculi are perhaps the most serious complica-

TABLE 22–6 ■ MEDICATIONS USED FOR BLADDER MANAGEMENT IN SPINAL CORD INJURY

Problem	Medications Used	Action	Example(s)
Incontinence			
Due to the bladder	Anticholinergic agents	Smooth muscle relaxants; diminish bladder spasms and increase bladder capacity	Dicyclomine Oxybutynin Propantheline Imipramine
Due to the outlet	α-Adrenergic agonists	Increase bladder neck resistance to decrease leaking around indwelling catheter	Ephedrine Phenylpropanolamine
Retention			
Due to the bladder	Cholinergic agents	Increase detrusor activity and thus increase contractions to improve bladder emptying	Bethanechol chloride
Due to the outlet	α-Adrenergic blockers	Relax smooth muscle at the bladder neck (external or internal sphincters) to improve bladder emptying	Prazosin Phenoxybenzamine Terazocin

Data from Linsenmeyer, T. A., & Stone, J. M. (1993). Neurogenic bladder and bowel dysfunction. In J. DeLisa (ed.), *Rehabilitation medicine: Principles and Practice*. Philadelphia: J. B. Lippincott.

tion in the upper urinary tract. About 8% of patients with SCI have renal calculi, and 98% of the stones are found to have developed from urease-producing infections. Untreated calculi generally progress to obstruction of the kidney (Stover et al., 1989).

Nursing Interventions for Bladder Management

Nursing interventions for bladder management in the patient with SCI are as follows:

1. Reduce or eliminate factors leading to incontinence, such as presence of urinary tract infection, medications that exacerbate incontinence, and environmental barriers.
2. Maintain adequate hydration.
3. Instruct the patient in the amount and type of fluids appropriate for his or her bladder program.
4. Ensure adequate bowel elimination.
5. Prevent overdistention of the bladder.
6. Teach the patient about changes that have occurred in bladder function as a result of SCI.
7. Teach the patient the causes, prevention, and treatment of complications such as urinary tract infections and autonomic dysreflexia.
8. Teach the patient management of a bladder program, which the patient achieves either through independent actions or by directing others.

Bowel Management

The classification of bowel dysfunction or type of *neurogenic bowel*, like bladder dysfunction, is determined at the level of injury. With a spinal cord lesion above T12 to L1, the upper motor neuron damage disrupts voluntary cortical influence on defecation but leaves the reflexes intact. Thus, when the rectum is full, emptying occurs as a reflex response. This condition is called a *reflex* or *spastic bowel*.

A spinal cord lesion at or below T12 to L1 results in *automatic* or *flaccid bowel*. The lesions are at the S2 to S4 neural level, and damage involves the spinal nerves and lower motor neuron segments. A lesion at this level damages the sacral segments necessary for reflex defecation, so the bowel remains relaxed and unresponsive to bowel filling. Fecal incontinence and fecal retention can be problems with this type of injury.

Both types of neurogenic bowel can be managed with bowel training programs. The goal of such a program is to develop a predictable pattern of bowel elimination in which defecation is planned at socially acceptable times and accidents are minimized. The components of a successful bowel program are as follows:

- Eating the proper foods
- Ensuring adequate fluid intake
- Using bowel medications

■ Using techniques to stimulate reflexes and enhance peristalsis

Methods Not Involving Medication

Several nonmedication methods can be used to facilitate defecation in the patient with neurogenic bowel. These techniques are designed to enhance the functioning that remains intact.

Manual disimpaction: physical removal of stool from the lower rectum; can be combined with the Valsalva maneuver for individuals with lower motor neuron lesions.

Abdominal massage: massaging the abdomen from right to left in a circular downward motion that follows the direction of peristalsis in the colon.

Valsalva maneuver: increases intrathoracic pressure by forcible exhalation against a closed glottis; is helpful for those with intact abdominal musculature.

Digital stimulation: manual stimulation of the anal sphincter, which increases peristalsis and relaxes the sphincter muscle; used to "speed up" results and ensure complete emptying of the bowel.

Many people with SCI are able to eventually perform a bowel program using only digital stimulation, thus eliminating oral medications and suppositories.

The procedure for digital stimulation is as follows:

1. The patient may be in bed or on the commode or toilet. Digital stimulation is best performed with the patient in a sitting position to obtain the benefit of gravity. If the procedure must be performed with the patient in bed, have the patient lie on the left side, and use a protective pad underneath. *Never* use a bedpan.
2. Glove a hand and lubricate one finger.
3. Check the rectum for any stool that may block the anal opening, and remove it gently.
4. Gently reinsert the lubricated, gloved finger into the rectum about ½ to 1 inch, and rotate the finger, using a circular motion against the sphincter wall, for about 30 seconds.
5. Remove the finger and allow 15 to 20 minutes for a bowel movement.
6. After the bowel movement is completed, reinsert a lubricated, gloved finger to check for any remaining stool. If stool is present, remove it manually.

If the patient experiences discomfort during the procedure, deep breathing may help. Plenty of lubrication should be used on the gloved finger. Also, the use of an anesthetic lubricant should be considered, especially if the patient is prone to episodes of autonomic dysreflexia.

Enemas are to be avoided in the patient with neurogenic bowel, for two reasons. First, they are too irritating to the bowel to be used on a regular basis. Second, the bowel will become dependent on enemas, and the bowel program will eventually require more and more use of enemas.

The bowel program should be performed at the same time of day, and that time should be chosen to fit in with the patient's lifestyle (Table 22–7).

Methods Involving Use of Medications

The program usually begins with the insertion of a suppository or mini-enema. Many patients, especially initially, need the addition of an oral laxative the evening before. Other assistive bowel medications may also be needed, such as milk of magnesia as a laxative; docusate sodium (Colace) as a stool softener; senna concentrate (Senokot) or casanthranol with docusate sodium (PeriColace) to increase peristalsis; and psyllium hydrophilic mucilloid (Metamucil) if bulk is

TABLE 22–7 ■ LEVEL OF INJURY AND PARTICIPATION IN BLADDER AND BOWEL PROGRAM

Level	Participation
C4 and above	Program may be done in bed or on commode or toilet
	Dependent; can direct program
C5	Able to sit on commode or toilet with safety straps and trunk support
	Dependent; can direct program
C6 and C7	May be able to perform bowel program with adaptive equipment, such as a suppository inserter and digital stimulator
	May be able to perform bladder program with adaptive equipment, depending on particular program
C8 and below	Need for assessment as to whether easier to perform program in bed or in chair
	Independent with program

needed. These medications can often be stopped after the patient is home and the bowel program is successful. There is a waiting period of 15 to 20 minutes after insertion of the suppository to allow it to work.

Initially, this part of the program is performed with the patient lying on the left side on a protective incontinence pad. When stable, the patient should be on the commode or toilet, which must have a padded seat. After the waiting period, digital stimulation (or one of the other maneuvers) is performed to ensure complete emptying of the bowel. The bowel program should be completed within 30 to 60 minutes.

Actual or Potential Alteration in Skin Integrity

"The annual incidence of pressure ulcers among individuals with a spinal cord injury is 23–30% but up to 85% of individuals with spinal cord injury develop a pressure ulcer at some time in their life. Among those with pressure ulcers, 7–8% will die of complications from them" (Byrne & Salzberg, 1996). Pressure ulcers account for one fourth of the cost of caring for a patient with an SCI. The Agency for Health Care Policy and Research (AHCPR) convened a panel of experts to develop clinical guidelines for pressure ulcers. The National Pressure Ulcer Advisory Panel (NPUAP) defines *pressure ulcer* as "any lesion caused by unrelieved pressure resulting in damage of underlying tissue" (Bergstrom, Bennett, Carlson, et al., 1994).

During hospitalization, one responsibility of the nursing staff is to prevent pressure ulcers. Prior to discharge, the patient with an SCI should have been taught how to prevent pressure ulcers, either through his or her own actions or by directing others providing care. The patient with an SCI is at high risk for pressure sores because of (1) immobility and (2) the loss of sensation and autonomic function, which control the reaction of blood vessels to pressure. With poor blood flow, any prolonged pressure puts the skin at risk for breakdown (Fig. 22–16).

A management program for pressure ulcers consists of the following three elements (Kirk, 1996):

- Identifying the factors that contribute to pressure ulcer development and minimizing the risks for them
- Assessing the patient's condition, nutritional status, and pressure ulcer characteristics

- Treating pressure ulcers, which consists of management of the tissue load, débridement, wound care, and prevention or management of infection

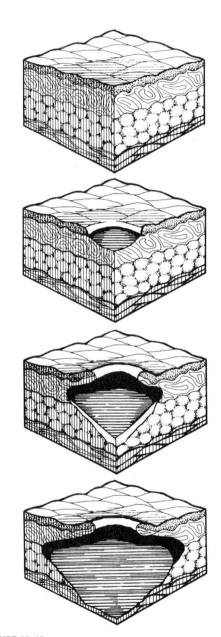

FIGURE 22–16
National Pressure Ulcer Advisory Panel (NPUAP) classification: Identification and staging of pressure ulcers. *Stage 1:* Nonblanchable erythema not resolved in 30 minutes; epidermis intact; reversible intervention. *Stage 2:* Partial-thickness loss of skin involving epidermis, possibly into dermis; may appear as blisters with erythema. *Stage 3:* Full-thickness destruction through dermis into subcutaneous tissue. *Stage 4:* Deep tissue destruction through subcutaneous tissue to fascia, muscle, bone, or joint. (Used with permission from the National Pressure Ulcer Advisory Panel.)

Byrne and Salzberg (1996) critically evaluated the medical-nursing and nutritional research literature pertaining to risk factors for development of pressure ulcers. They found that numerous risk assessment tools are available. The Norton, Gosnell, and Braden scales have been used and tested most extensively. The Norton scale, developed in 1962 and based on geriatric patients, has been evaluated since then in diverse settings, such as medical-surgical units, intensive care units, and nursing homes. The Gosnell scale was developed in 1973, also with geriatric patients. The Braden scale, developed in 1987, has been tested on numerous elderly subjects in hospital settings. Byrne and Salzberg (1996) found little information, however, on pressure ulcers in the SCI population. These researchers then studied 219 patients with SCI for 6 years and developed a pressure risk assessment tool specifically for people with SCI (Fig. 22–17).

The key element is that the nurse perform a systematic skin inspection of the patient at least daily, paying close attention to the bony prominences.

The most common cause of pressure ulcers is prolonged or intense pressure, which results in ischemia of the underlying tissue. The normal capillary pressure is 17 mm Hg; higher pressure impairs blood circulation and produces ischemia. Pressure lasting longer than 30 minutes causes redness. Higher pressure lasting longer than 2 hours causes irreversible damage of fat, fiber, and muscle cells, leading to tissue death. Along with pressure, shearing is an important contributor to pressure ulcer development. Shearing occurs when tissue is forced to move in opposite but parallel sliding directions, making it vulnerable to pressure. Placing the patient in a supine position when the head of the bed is elevated above 30 degrees can result in skin tears. Sacral slits are a very common result of shearing.

Friction, the force of two surfaces moving across each other, is also a factor. Pulling the patient across a sheet, for example, combined with moisture from incontinence or insensible loss can lead to pressure ulcer formation. Immobility is a major factor associated with risk for pressure ulcers. Other pressure factors that may occur when the patient is farther along in the rehabilitation process, when immobility is not as great as factor, are damage or deterioration of support surfaces, new orthoses or shoes, and increased participation in activities that cause pressure, shear, or friction to a bony prominence. The nurse must be vigilant in skin inspection, particularly after any new activity or equipment is introduced.

After pressure itself, malnutrition is a major contributing factor. A patient with the following characteristics is considered to be malnourished:

- Serum albumin value less than 3.5 mg/dL
- Total lymphocyte count less than 1800/mm
- Decrease in body weight of more than 15%
- Presence of vitamin and mineral deficiencies

Adequate protein, calories, vitamins, and minerals are essential components of healing. The recommendation is 30 to 35 calories per kg per day and 1.25 to 1.5 g of protein kg per day (Kirk, 1996, p. 11).

Pressure ulcer assessment should be performed consistently, and a uniform assessment system should be used throughout the practice setting. Using the same system allows for all caregivers to describe the progress of healing and the effectiveness of interventions.

Classification systems have been developed to more accurately describe the extent of tissue damage. The Panel for the Prediction and Prevention of Pressure Ulcers in Adults (1992) recommends using the staging system recommended by the NPUAP in 1989, as follows:

Stage I: Nonblanchable erythema of intact skin (limited to epidermis); the heralding lesion of skin ulceration.

Stage II: Partial-thickness skin loss involving epidermis, dermis, or both; ulcer is superficial, clinically presenting as an abrasion, blister, or shallow crater.

Stage III: Full-thickness skin loss involving damage to or necrosis of subcutaneous tissue that may extend superficial to but not through deep fascia; manifests as a deep crater with or without undermining of the adjacent tissue.

Stage IV: Full-thickness skin loss with extensive destruction of tissues deep to the muscle, bone, and support structures; undermining and sinus tracts may be associated with stage IV pressure ulcers.

Pressure ulcers should be measured and photographed weekly.

The guidelines provided by the U.S. Department of Health and Human Services AHCPR Reference Guide for Clinicians (pp. 15–22) for skin care and the early treatment of pressure ulcers are as follows:

1. All individuals at risk should have a systematic skin inspection at least once a day, paying particular attention to the bony

Pressure Ulcer Risk Assessment Scale

Name _____

Date _____

RISK FACTOR	CODED VALUE	SCORE
1. Level of Activity	0 ( ) ambulatory	_____
	1 ( ) wheelchair	
	4 ( ) bed	
2. Mobility	0 ( ) full	_____
	1 ( ) limited	
	3 ( ) immobile	
3. Complete SCI	0 ( ) no 1 ( ) yes	_____
4. Urine incontinence or constantly moist	0 ( ) no 1 ( ) yes	
5. Autonomic dysreflexia or severe spasticity	0 ( ) no 1 ( ) yes	
6. Age (years)	0 ( ) <34	_____
	1 ( ) 35–64	
	2 ( ) >65	
7. Tobacco use/smoking	0 ( ) never	_____
	1 ( ) former	
	3 ( ) current	
8. Pulmonary disease	0 ( ) no 1 ( ) yes	_____
9. Cardiac disease or ABN.EKG	0 ( ) no 1 ( ) yes	_____
10. Diabetes or glucose > 110 mg/dL	0 ( ) no 1 ( ) yes	_____
11. Renal disease	0 ( ) no 1 ( ) yes	_____
12. Impaired cognitive function	0 ( ) no 1 ( ) yes	_____
13. In a nursing home or hospital	0 ( ) no 1 ( ) yes	_____
14. Albumin < 3.4 or total protein < 6.4	0 ( ) no 1 ( ) yes	_____
15. Hematocrit < 36.0% (hemoglobin < 12.0)	0 ( ) no 1 ( ) yes	_____

Total Score (0–25): _____

RISK: LOW 0–2   MODERATE 3–5   HIGH 6–8   VERY HIGH 9–25

NURSE ASSESSOR'S SIGNATURE: _____

FIGURE 22–17
Pressure ulcer risk assessment scale for individuals with spinal cord injury (version 1.16, revised 10/25/99). (From Salzberg, C., Byrne, D., Cayten, G., Van Niewerburgh, P., Murphy, J., & Vehbeck, M. [1996]. A new pressure ulcer risk assessment scale for individuals with spinal cord injury. *American Journal of Physical Medicine & Rehabilitation, 75*(2), 96–104. Copyright 1996, The Williams & Wilkins Company.)

prominences. Results of skin inspection should be documented.

2. Skin cleansing should occur at the time of soiling and at routine intervals. The frequency of skin cleansing should be individualized according to need and/or patient preference. Avoid hot water, and use a mild cleansing agent that minimizes irritation and dryness of the skin. During the cleansing process, care should be taken to minimize the force and friction applied to the skin.

3. Minimize environmental factors leading to skin drying, such as low humidity (less than 40%) and exposure to cold. Dry skin should be treated with moisturizers.

4. Avoid massage over bony prominences.

5. Minimize skin exposure to moisture due to incontinence, perspiration, or wound drainage. When these sources of moisture cannot be controlled, underpads or briefs made of materials that absorb moisture and present a quick-drying surface to the skin can be used. Topical agents that act as barriers to moisture can also be used.

6. Skin injury due to friction and shear forces should be minimized through proper positioning, transferring, and turning techniques. In addition, friction injuries may be reduced by the use of lubricants (such as cornstarch and creams), protective films (such as transparent film dressings and skin sealants), protective dressings (such as hydrocolloids), and protective padding.

7. When apparently well-nourished individuals develop an inadequate dietary intake of protein or calories, caregivers should first attempt to discover the factors compromising intake and offer support with eating. Other nutritional supplements or support may be needed. If dietary intake remains inadequate and if consistent with overall goals of therapy, more aggressive nutritional intervention such as enteral or parenteral feedings should be considered. For nutritionally compromised individuals, a plan of nutritional support and/or supplementation should be implemented that meets individual needs and is consistent with the overall goals of therapy.

8. If potential for improving mobility and activity status exists, rehabilitation efforts should be instituted if consistent with the overall goals of therapy. Maintaining current activity level, mobility, and range of motion is an appropriate goal for most individuals.

9. Interventions and outcomes should be monitored and documented.

The U.S. Department of Health and Human Services AHCPR Guidelines for Mechanical Loading and Support Surfaces (pp. 22–27) are as follows:

1. Any individual in bed who is assessed to be at risk for developing pressure ulcers should be repositioned at least every 2 hours if consistent with overall patient goals. A written schedule for systematically turning and repositioning the individual should be used.

2. For individuals in bed, positioning devices such as pillows or foam wedges should be used to keep bony prominences from direct contact with one another, according to a written plan.

3. Individuals in bed who are completely immobile should have a care plan that includes the use of devices that totally relieve pressure on the heels, most commonly by raising the heels off the bed. Do not use donut-type devices.

4. When the side-lying position is used in bed, avoid positioning directly on the trochanter.

5. Maintain the head of the bed at the lowest degree of elevation consistent with medical conditions and other restrictions. Limit the amount of time the head of the bed is elevated.

6. Use lifting devices such as a trapeze or bed linen to move (rather than drag) individuals in bed who cannot assist during transfers and position changes.

7. Any individual assessed to be at risk for developing pressure ulcers should be placed when lying in bed on a pressure-reducing device, such as foam, static air, alternating air, gel, or water mattresses.

8. Any person at risk for developing a pressure ulcer should avoid uninterrupted sitting in a chair or wheelchair. The individual should be repositioned, shifting the points under pressure at least every hour, or be put back to bed if consistent with overall patient management goals. Individuals who are able should be taught to shift weight every 15 minutes.

9. For wheelchair-bound individuals, the use of a pressure-reducing device such as those made of foam, gel, air, or a combination is indicated. Do not use donut-type devices.

10. Positioning of persons who use wheelchairs should include consideration of

postural alignment, distribution of weight, balance and stability, and pressure relief.

11. A written plan for the use of positioning devices and schedules may be helpful for chair-bound individuals.

Treatment

The goal of the treatment of pressure ulcers is to create an environment that enhances soft tissue viability and promotes healing. This is accomplished by decreasing the duration and intensity of pressure as well as providing the proper temperature and moisture to support tissue growth. The area should be kept free from pressure; if this is not possible, a specialty bed or device that redistributes pressure should be used. It is helpful if the patient can lie prone. The avoidance of shearing is critical. The head of the bed should be kept at the lowest degree possible.

Débridement

Wound healing is promoted by a noninfected and nonnecrotic surface. Wound débridement, which is used to create a nonnecrotic area, can be accomplished surgically, mechanically, or chemically.

Surgical. Surgical wound débridement involves the use of a scalpel or knife to remove the devitalized tissue.

Mechanical. Mechanical wound débridement is the use of wet-to-dry dressings, hydrotherapy, or wound irrigation to remove devitalized tissue.

Wet-to-dry dressings should be administered every 4 to 6 hours, allowing time for the dressing to dry so that when removed, it will remove the devitalized tissue. To be effective, a wet-to-dry dressing must be used properly, as described here:

1. The gauze should not be packed too tightly, or it will create pressure in the wound and cause further deterioration.
2. The gauze should be a loose weave to allow adherence to the tissue.
3. The wet gauze must not be placed on the healthy tissue around the ulcer, as it would cause maceration of the wound margins.

Both *hydrotherapy* and *wound irrigation* apply enough force to remove eschar, bacteria, and other debris. The water must be applied with enough pressure to remove eschar but not enough to cause trauma to newly formed tissue or drive bacteria into the wound. Enough irrigation pressure should be used to enhance wound cleansing without causing trauma to the wound bed. Safe and effective ulcer irrigation pressures range from 4 to 15 pounds per square inch (psi).

Chemical. Chemical enzymatic ointments contain enzymes that aid in severing the collagen fibers that bind the necrotic tissue to the ulcer. This treatment is usually effective and is less painful than wet-to-dry dressings. A variety of these ointments are available (Kirk, 1996).

Wound Care

After the wound is débrided of devitalized tissue, wound care consists of wound cleansing with each dressing change to remove any exudate or other debris. The nurse must be careful not to cause trauma to the wound during cleansing. A variety of cleansing agents are available. Many of the previously accepted agents, such as hydrogen peroxide, Dakin's solution, acetic acid, and povidone-iodine, have been found to be cytotoxic and to actually inhibit healing. The safest solution is normal saline. Use of a soft mesh gauze for cleansing is suggested so as to not cause trauma to the wound. Whirlpool should be considered as a method of wound irrigation. There are many wound care products available.

The U.S. Department of Health and Human Services AHCPR Reference Guide for Clinicians (pp. 13–17) on pressure ulcer management include guidelines for selection of a dressing according to the condition of the ulcer bed and the function of the dressing. These guidelines are as follows:

1. Use a dressing that will keep the wound moist.
2. Use clinical judgment to select a type of moist dressing suitable for the ulcer.
3. Keep the surrounding tissue dry and intact while keeping the ulcer bed moist.
4. Control exudate but do not desiccate the ulcer bed.
5. Consider caregiver time.
6. Eliminate wound dead space by loosely filling all cavity without overfill to prevent abscess formation.
7. Keep dressings intact by taping edges around difficult areas (anus, for example).

Management of Infection

The management of infection is critical because infection is the most common deterrent to wound healing. Stages II, III, and IV pressure ulcers are colonized with bacteria. Generally, scrupulous cleaning and débridement are adequate to prevent bacterial colonization from spreading to the point of clinical infection. Any foreign body, such as threads from the dressing, devitalized tissue, or dead space in the open wound contributes to bacterial growth by acting as a bacterial support. All open wounds are considered to be contaminated and are associated with some degree of chronic inflammation until healed. Infection occurs when the bacterial burden overcomes the local tissue defenses. Bleeding in the absence of trauma, purulent drainage, and/or foul odor suggest infection in a wound.

AHCPR guidelines for managing bacterial colonization and infection are as follows:

1. Minimize pressure ulcer colonization and enhance healing by effective wound cleansing and débridement.
2. Do not use swab cultures to diagnose wound infection as all wounds are colonized. Swab cultures may be used to determine the presence of drug-resistant organisms that require special treatment and handling precautions.
3. Consider a 2-week trial of topical antibiotics for clean pressure ulcers that are not healing or are continuing to produce exudate after 2–4 weeks of optimal patient care. The antibiotic should be effective against gram-negative, gram-positive, and anaerobic organisms.
4. Osteomyelitis is a serious complication that can result from infected full-thickness wounds. Treatment often involves weeks of intravenous antibiotics and amputation of bone and tissue. Early diagnosis of soft tissue infection or osteomyelitis is essential as healing may be impaired when bacterial levels reach 105 organisms per g of tissue or if there is evidence of osteomyelitis present.
5. Use appropriate systemic antibiotic therapy for patients with bacteremia, sepsis, advancing cellulitis, or osteomyelitis.
6. Protect pressure ulcers from any sources of contamination.

Adjunctive Therapy

"There are several adjunctive therapies available for wound healing, many reported to be effective in some situations. There has not been adequate research to recommend any of the therapies for clinical use. At this time, electrotherapy is the only adjunctive therapy with sufficient supporting evidence to warrant recommendation by the panel" (Bergstrom, Bennett, Carlson, et al., 1994).

The mechanism of electrical stimulation is not well understood but does appear to produce some biological effects that enhance wound healing. Salzberg, Cooper-Vastola, Perez, Viehbeck, and Byrne (1995) reported on a randomized, double-blind study of 30 men with SCI, 20 with stage II pressure ulcers and 10 with stage III pressure ulcers, in whom nonthermal, pulsed, high-frequency electromagnetic energy (Diapulse) treatments, 30 minutes twice daily, were used for 12 weeks or until the wound healed. Their results indicated that for spinal cord–injured men with stage II pressure ulcers, active Diapulse treatment significantly improved healing.

Hyperbaric therapy is another adjunctive treatment designed to deliver oxygen to tissue to improve oxygen tension within tissue, encourage collagen synthesis, promote revascularization, retard bacterial growth, and reduce edema. Topical agents and human growth factors have also been used in the management of pressure ulcers. Findings have been promising in some studies. Ultraviolet and laser irradiation and ultrasound are some of the other therapies being used and studied.

Surgical Treatment

Surgical intervention for wound closure is sometimes performed (1) for a stage III or IV wound that is not healing with conservative treatment or (2) when the time required for conservative healing will be very long and will negatively affect the patient. Various surgical techniques are described in the literature, including split-thickness skin grafts, local flaps, myocutaneous flaps, and gluteus maximus island myocutaneous flaps.

The major considerations before any type of surgical intervention apply here; the patient must be medically stable, well nourished, and able to comply with the postoperative restrictions. Smoking cessation, control of spasticity, and elimination of infection all should occur before surgery is attempted. Preoperatively, patients should begin practicing lying prone; a high-protein, low-residue diet should be initiated; and bowel cleansing should be completed.

Postoperatively, a fluid air loss bed is needed for a minimum of 2 to 4 weeks; the low-residue diet is continued; and the patient is kept prone as much as possible. When the surgical site is determined to be ready for weight bearing, the time of weight bearing should be increased very slowly, with diligent inspection of the site after removal of the pressure. If pallor, redness, or both at the operative site do not decrease after 10 minutes of pressure relief, it must be considered that the flap viability has been compromised, and the weight-bearing schedule must be adjusted.

Patient and Family Education

Patient and family education are critical components of the rehabilitation nurse's plan of care in terms of prevention or management of pressure ulcer prevention. Patients must know prevention and management techniques as well as available resources, and they must believe they can succeed.

Nursing teaching interventions for pressure ulcers are as follows:

- Skin inspection
  - The patient or caregiver should visually inspect with a mirror and by palpation of the bony prominences and under orthotic devices.
  - The patient or caregiver should check for redness, warmth, edema, blisters, and rash.
  - The patient or caregiver should lightly massage around erythema but should not rub the reddened area.
- Skin care
  - The patient should be turned every 2 hours while in bed.
  - The caregiver should use draw sheets to lift the patient up in bed to prevent shearing.
  - The patient should lie prone if tolerated to allow better weight distribution, and the patient or caregiver should check the skin after 2 hours; any area that remains red for 20 minutes after pressure has been removed is in danger.
  - The patient or caregiver should protect bony areas from direct contact with skin surfaces by means of pillows or positioning devices.
  - The patient or caregiver should not use donut devices or other rings that compromise circulation
  - The patient should gradually increase sitting time in the wheelchair; begin with 30 minutes three times daily and increase by 15 minutes per day if no skin problems occur.
- Precautions secondary to insensate skin
  - The patient or caregiver should check bath water for temperature.

- The patient should avoid holding hot drinks between the legs or on the lap.
- The patient should keep feet away from heaters or other hot objects.
- The patient should avoid using heating pads.
- Pressure relief in the wheelchair: Shift weight every 15 to 20 minutes for at least 60 seconds of pressure relief by
  - Pushing up using the arms with hands or armrests
  - Leaning sideways or forward
  - Reclining backward (used most commonly for tetraplegics in power wheelchairs)
- Proper positioning
  - The patient should sit straight
  - The patient should distribute weight equally
  - For tetraplegic patients: Using the wheelchair arms for stability, alternate sides frequently
  - The patient should sit in a properly fitting wheelchair
  - The patient should sit on appropriate cushions
- Hygiene
  - The patient or caregiver should avoid excessive use of soap, which is very drying.
  - The patient or caregiver should avoid alcohol and powder because of their drying properties.
  - The patient or caregiver should avoid excess lotion, which may cause maceration.
  - The patient or caregiver should not use plastic or rubber sheets because they retain heat and moisture.
  - The patient or caregiver should avoid the use of bedpans because they cause pressure.
  - The patient should not wear constrictive clothing.
  - The patient or caregiver should remove any wrinkles in clothing.
  - The patient should wear properly fitting shoes to prevent blisters and sores; it is recommended that patients wear shoes one size larger than before the SCI.
  - The patient or caregiver should remove elastic stockings every 8 hours.

Outcomes for such interventions specify that the patient is able to state the skin care program, which consists of

- Turning schedule when in bed
- Sitting tolerance when up
- Wheelchair pressure relief

❑ Skin checks
❑ Resources for medical intervention if skin condition is changing

Alteration in Sexual Functioning

Sexual functioning is often severely impaired following SCI. That disruption often represents the area of greatest concern to patients. Sexuality is viewed by many as the physical act of sexual intercourse. That definition alone causes severe worry to patients with SCI, the majority of whom are young men. This is often the first time they look at sexual functioning in terms other than the physical. Sexuality has been described as the "feelings, attitudes, and behaviors that express being a man or being a woman. It encompasses the way we view and think about ourselves, the way we dress, sensuality, and relationship patterns" (Alexander, Griggs, & Ledwell, 1987). The World Health Organization has defined *sexual health* as "an integration of somatic, emotional, intellectual, and social aspects of sexual being, in ways that are positive, enriching, and that enhance personality, communication, and love" (Greco, 1996).

Culture and society determine what are usual and acceptable sexuality and sexual performance. It is the role of the rehabilitation nurse to (1) explore the issues of sexual functioning with the patient with SCI, (2) be willing to discuss sexual functioning, (3) accept the patient's need to know, (4) be comfortable with alternative sexual orientation, (5) accept not discussing the subject until the patient is ready, and (6) overcome the silence that so often surrounds this issue.

The PLISSIT Model

The PLISSIT model developed by Annon is the most helpful model for a nursing intervention. It matches clinical competence with the presenting sexual problems in patients, thus allowing the nurse to counsel at his or her own level of comfort. The PLISSIT model consists of the following four levels of involvement in discussions about the patient's sexuality (Greco, 1996):

Level I—Permission *(P)*. Permission is given to the patient by the nurse to discuss sexual concerns. This may be done initially during the nursing admission assessment or at any time during the patient's rehabilitation. Permission may be given verbally or nonver-

bally, but the importance is that the patient knows he or she has permission to ask questions and seek information when ready.

Level II—Limited Information *(LI)*. The nurse gives information about general sexual problems, often dispelling myths. The information can be given verbally or in written form. Such an opportunity often occurs as the nurse is catheterizing a man, and he sustains a reflexogenic erection. His response is one of excitement, for this means that "everything is working again!" This interaction provides an opportunity for the nurse to give basic information about the level of injury and its impact on an erection. The information need not be detailed because the patient may not be emotionally ready to hear about the full impact of the disability, but it provides the opening for provision of information about future sexual functioning.

Level III—Specific Suggestions *(SS)*. If knowledgeable and comfortable, the nurse may give specific suggestions about sexual functioning, including new positions to use, new ways of experimenting with the partner, fertility, and treatment options. This type of information necessitates a knowledge of the patient's sexual history and sexual problems.

Level IV—Intensive Therapy *(IT)*. This level is a referral mechanism used to meet the long-term needs of the patient (and sexual partner). This level requires a full sexual history of the patient and offers specialized advanced treatment skills. This level of intervention is not required for all individuals with SCI but is appropriate for those with significant psychosocial sexual dysfunction. It is the role of the nurse to identify the need for this level of intervention and to refer the patient to a sexual counselor. A member of the rehabilitation team may be skillful and knowledgeable at this level of counseling and education.

Effects of SCI on Sexual Functioning

Basic to dealing with sexuality and SCI is a knowledge of the alterations in sexual functioning following SCI. "Erection in the neurologically intact individual is a complex process involving the vasculature, endocrine factors, peripheral nervous system, and central nervous system. In order for erection to occur, intricate vascular changes are necessary which are controlled through intact neurologic pathways" (Smith & Bodner, 1993). SCI can affect either the upper motor neurons, as in tetraplegia, or the lower motor neurons, as in cauda equina syndrome. These lesions involve motor and sensory pathways, causing motor weakness, diminished sensation, and changes in the ability to have and sustain erections.

Erections can be either reflexogenic or psychogenic. "Reflex erections occur in response to neural transmission from the pelvic parasympathetic nerves, which originate in S2–4 and also supply parasympathetic innervation to the urinary bladder, causing bladder emptying when stimulated. Direct tactile stimulation of the penis by rubbing of the glans or shaft results in reflex erections when the sacral reflexes (S2-4) are intact. Reflex erections are poorly maintained without constant tactile stimulation" (Smith & Bodner, 1993). Upper motor neuron injuries, those above the sacral reflex arc, produce spasticity below the level of injury, with reflex contraction of the bladder, hyperactive lower extremity reflexes, and reflexogenic erections. Reflex erections occur most often in patients with lesions above T11 and those with incomplete injuries.

"Psychogenic erections originate from the cerebral impulses mediated by the hypothalamus and limbic system, which travel through the thoracolumbar portion of the spinal cord and the sacral roots to the sacral erection centers" (Smith & Bodner, 1993). Lower motor neuron injuries produce a flaccid bladder, diminution or absence of anal and external urethral sphincter tone, and the ability to have both reflexogenic and psychogenic erections of poor quality and short duration. Men with complete lower motor neuron lesions involving S2 to S4 (cauda equina or conus medullaris) have poor erectile function because the S2 to S4 reflex arc is interrupted. They may have penile tumescence secondary to sympathetic psychogenic activity. Erections tend to be inadequate for intercourse. Psychogenic erections are generally lost with lesions above T10 to T12.

Female sexual functioning has been less well studied. In women, reproductive function is not affected at any level of injury, although amenorrhea generally occurs and lasts for up to 1 year after injury. Pregnancy and normal delivery are quite possible, although not without risks. Women with SCI face complications such as urinary tract infections, pressure ulcers, anemia, spasticity, impaired pulmonary function, leg edema, thrombophlebitis, and autonomic dysreflexia. Because the uterus is innervated at T10 to T12 level, women with lesions above that level will not feel uterine contractions or fetal movement.

Women with lesions above T6 are at risk for autonomic dysreflexia during labor and delivery. The most effective preventive and therapeutic approach for autonomic dysreflexia in labor and delivery is regional anesthesia, with the most common technique being continuous epidural anesthesia. Prenatal care is determined by standard obstetrical practice, with the only strong indication for delivery by cesarean section being intractable autonomic dysreflexia that is unresponsive to anesthetic interventions. The surgical procedure will continue to incite the process of autonomic dysreflexia but may be necessary if the duration of vaginal delivery is prolonged.

The issue of orgasm in women with SCI is less clear. Sipski, Alexander, and Rosen (1995) reported on a study of 25 women with SCI matched with 10 able-bodied control subjects. They used a 75-minute protocol to obtain information about the physiological events accompanying orgasm. The results indicated that 100% of the able-bodied subjects achieved orgasm but only 52% of the subjects with SCI did so. Level of injury and degree of injury did not play a significant role; women with SCI took longer than able-bodied women to reach orgasm, and those with no voluntary movement in their legs required the most time.

Treatment of Erectile Dysfunction

Several treatments for erectile dysfunction are available for men with SCI. Although many men are capable of attaining an erection, the erections achieved are often not suitable for intercourse. Options include the surgical implantation of a penile prosthesis, vacuum erection devices, topical nitroglycerin, and intracorporeal therapy. Several types of penile prostheses are available, but individual patients must be counseled about the potential complications. Penile prostheses range from rigid to a semirigid, hinged type, from those left inflated at all times to those manually inflated prior to intercourse, from those used to keep an external condom catheter on the penis to those used to correct sexual dysfunction.

A variety of vacuum erection devices are available. Vacuum tumescence constrictive therapy (VTCT) is the term for this technique, which functions as follows: A vacuum is created inside a plastic tube placed over the penis, drawing blood into the penis, and tumescence is maintained by placing a constriction band around the base of the penis. Erections can be maintained for up to 30 minutes. Smith and Bodner (1993) reported in one study that all of the patients using a Synergist vacuum device were able to have intercourse and that 88% of the men were satisfied with their erections.

A third treatment for erectile dysfunction is intracorporeal injection of vasoactive medications to cause erection; it can be used when the vasculature is intact. The medication is injected into the base of the penis by the individual or his partner. The dose of medication required for erection in men with SCI is generally much lower than in other impotent men, so the initial injections should be at very low doses to prevent priapism. The dose should then be titrated upward until an erection adequate for intercourse but lasting less than 4 hours is attained. "Papaverine with its direct smooth muscle inhibition and phentolamine with smooth muscle relaxation have been found to be most effective. Recently, prostaglandin E_1 has shown to be effective with less morbidity than papaverine or phentolamine. Reports of less penile discomfort in those with intact sensation, less tunical scarring, and decreased incidence of priapism have added to its popularity" (Watanabe, Chancellor, Rivas, Hirsch, Bennett, Finocchiaro, Razi, Bennett, Green, Foote, Killorian, Juma, Linsenmeyer, & Lloyd, 1996).

Another treatment is "the use of transcutaneous nitroglycerin as topical therapy to produce erections suitable for intercourse in some patients for whom papaverine injections had induced rigid erections. Oral levadopa has also been used with 55–60% of patients reporting rigid erections" (Gilbert, 1996).

Male fertility after SCI is a major problem. Fewer than 10% of men with SCI are able to impregnate their partners spontaneously after injury (Gilbert, 1996). Much of the research and techniques designed to restore ejaculation are aimed at restoring fertility. Penile vibratory stimulation (PVS) and electroejaculation (EEJ) have gained widespread acceptance as methods of semen retrieval. Sonksen, Sommer, Sorenson, Ziebe, Lindhard, Loft, Anderson, and Kristensen (1997) reported that PVS ejaculation rates range from 24 to 91%. The method of PVS can be refined to induce

ejaculation in men with SCI by focusing on the importance of vibratory amplitude. As a consequence, ejaculation may be induced by PVS in more than 80% of all men with spinal cord lesions above T10. These researchers report that EEJ is nearly as effective in obtaining ejaculation in men with SCI but should be reserved for those in whom PVS fails.

Risk of Autonomic Dysreflexia

All people with SCI at T6 level or above are at risk for autonomic dysreflexia during sexual activity. If autonomic dysreflexia occurs, all activity should stop. The individual should sit up and should seek medical attention if the symptoms do not subside.

It is important for the rehabilitation nurse to acknowledge that sexually related problems are part of SCI but also to stress that the individual's sex life is not "over." Body image, self-esteem, roles, and gender identity are all issues surrounding sexuality and SCI that should be dealt with along with the physical changes. Nurses must be comfortable with their own sexual identity and must be prepared to integrate issues of sexuality into care of the patient with an SCI. The nurses not only should discuss knowledge about sexual functioning as an integral part of the rehabilitation process but also should emphasize that a partnership and sexual relationship are still possible for the person with an SCI.

Potential Long-term Complications

Spasticity

Spasticity is not a complication but is the most commonly associated neurological phenomenon in patients with SCI. It is an abnormal increase in muscle tension, often referred to as "spasm," "twitching," "jerking" or "tone." During the early phase of spinal shock, flaccidity occurs in both lower motor neuron and upper motor neuron injuries. In cervical or thoracic injuries, the flaccid state evolves into a state of spasticity over several weeks or months.

The signs of spasticity are (1) increased resistance to passive movement, (2) increased tendon reflexes, and (3) involuntary jerky movements. Spasticity can be helpful when it enables the person to perform functional activities. It can create postural integrity at higher levels of injury. For instance, the increased stability and stiffness of the quadriceps muscle may enable some patients to transfer more easily and independently. Conversely, greater spasticity may limit proper hygiene and raise the potential for skin breakdown. Spasticity may also hasten the development of joint contractures.

Interventions include the use of medications such as baclofen or dantrolene, phenol nerve blocks, or surgical tendon releases. When spasticity is intractable to oral baclofen, the continuous intrathecal administration of baclofen has been a powerful treatment for severe spinal spasticity. Azouri, Mane, Thiebaut, Denys, Remy-Nevis, and Bussel (1996) reported on 18 patients with severe spinal spasticity selected for continuous treatment with intrathecal baclofen using implantable pumps. After 3 years, there was significant decrease in tone and spasms for all patients; tolerance appeared in the first 6 to 9 months. The subjects showed an increase in functional independence measure scores for bathing and lower extremity dressing and transfers, especially subjects with thoracic spinal cord lesions. FIM scores were improved for sitting balance and positioning in those with high-level injury, resulting in greater comfort in the wheelchair and making it easier to provide nursing care.

Nursing actions for spasticity include

- Daily stretching exercises
- Use of resting splints, made by occupational therapy personnel
- Protection of bony prominences
- Daily skin inspection

Chronic Pain

People with SCI experience a range of sensations, including acute pain, usually skeletal or radicular, which is a universal concomitant of acute SCI. Its course parallels that of acute injury and resolves with healing of bone and soft tissue. Nonpainful phantom sensations are almost universally experienced. Somatic pain is experienced by those with mechanical spine instability or chronic infection.

The most common pain following SCI is *neuropathic pain*. This term describes the varieties of chronic pain that arise following injury to the spinal cord, spinal roots, and cauda equina; they include (1) nerve root pain, experienced about the level of injury; (2) central or "phantom" pain, a sharp, burning pain below the level of injury; and (3) pain in the perineal area, lower extremities, or abdominal region.

Pain commonly occurs within 6 months to 1 year of injury. It affects every level but is most common in people with incomplete injuries of the conus medullaris and cauda equina. The actual incidence of pain in those with SCI is unclear. "Reported incidence varies: one study of 471 patients found that over 90% complained of diffuse burning pain. Another study of 102 patients found a figure of 13%" (Stass et al., 1993). The actual cause of the pain is unknown. The primary pathophysiological change after injury of peripheral and spinal nerves is believed to be an increase in electrical excitability owing to abnormal differentiation of the axonal membrane at the site of damage (Segatore, 1994). It has been suggested that the nerve root pain may be caused by incomplete damage to one or more nerve roots. The phantom pain may occur because a damaged nerve fires inappropriately or because nerves may sprout after trauma, causing abnormal and uncontrollable electrical outbursts. The abdominal pain may come from distention or increased reflux activity in the bladder, stomach, uterus, or colon.

There is no specific treatment for this pain because the etiology is unknown. A medical evaluation should be performed first to check for possible underlying complications. Nonmedication interventions include hypnosis, acupuncture, biofeedback, meditation, imagery techniques, and transcutaneous electrical nerve stimulation. Anticonvulsants such as phenytoin (Dilantin) and carbamazepine (Tegretol) have been used to treat phantom and deafferentation pain. Gabapentin (Neurontin), a new anticonvulsant drug, is currently being prescribed for neurogenic pain. Psychotropic medications with antidepressant effects have also been used to treat neurogenic SCI pain. They include imipramine (Tofranil), doxepin (Sinequan), desipramine (Norpramin), and amitriptyline (Elavil). Narcotics are used for severe unremitting pain.

Patient education is important to give reassurance that this pain does not represent an active medical problem. Psychological support should be considered for uncontrollable pain, as well as admission to a pain clinic. One neurosurgical procedure sometimes considered is dorsal root entry zone (DREZ) microcoagulation, a five-level laminectomy that destroys abnormal secondary neurons within the dorsal root entry zone. The procedure has been found to be effective for SCI-related pain at or below the level of injury in 78% of people with segmental pain but to be ineffective (26 to 32%) for people with deafferenta-tion central pain (Ragnarsson, 1997). Patients with such pain should be encouraged to continue mobilization and normal activities of socialization as much as possible.

Lower Extremity Fractures

Incidence of lower extremity fractures after SCI has been reported as 1.5 to 6% (Stass et al., 1993). This statistic does not take into account osteoporosis in lower extremity bones, vigorous physical therapy programs, falls, and other trauma, making the true incidence much higher. Also, some fractures occur in people with SCI and go unnoticed.

The femur is the most common site of fractures in SCI. Fractures are more common in people with paraplegia and in those with complete injuries. The most common cause is a fall during transfer.

Treatment is usually conservative, using a soft, well-padded splint. The patient is often out of bed and in the wheelchair within several days of the fracture. Traction is rarely used. Plaster casts or splints should be avoided because inadequate padding can cause the development of pressure sores. The most problematic fractures are those of the femoral neck and subtrochanteric regions. A femoral neck fracture may develop a nonunion, but this result may be functionally acceptable. A subtrochanteric fracture may develop angulation, which may not be acceptable and may require open reduction and internal fixation.

Overworked Upper Extremity Syndrome

A common complication that occurs after SCI as a result of excessive overwork is shoulder pain. Stass et al. (1993) reported one study in which 51% of subjects with SCI reported shoulder pain and 43% described the pain as severe enough to interfere with sleep. Hand and wrist pain also occurs frequently in people who have used crutches or wheelchairs for many years. A study of subjects with paraplegia found that 68% had complaints of pain somewhere in the upper extremities; 30% complained of shoulder pain during transfers. Upper extremity compressive neuropathies are common in paraplegic patients.

Management of these problems is essentially the same as in other people. Advising rest is problematic in the person with an SCI, whose upper extremities are necessary for transfers. Temporary use of an assistive de-vice for transfers and a power wheelchair for locomotion may be indicated. Surgical decompression in cases of impingement in the weight-bearing shoulder has been reported to have some success (Stass et al., 1993).

COMMUNITY REINTEGRATION

The health care system needs to focus on rehabilitation goals for people with SCI; a plan of care that uses these goals is shown in Figure 22–18. "SCI rehabilitation strives to provide, for persons with an acquired disability, the opportunity to lead a fruitful and satisfying personal and vocational life" (Frost, 1993).

Successful adjustment to SCI includes promoting a separation of the disabled person from the medical model of rehabilitation. As DeVivo and Richards (1992) remark, "The long term goal of SCI rehabilitation is to achieve community reintegration with the maximum possible level of functional independence and a return to pre-injury lifestyle." These researchers report that data from the National Spinal Cord Injury Statistical Center database collected from the model regional SCI care system institutions indicate that people who complete rehabilitation are almost always (94.1%) discharged to a private residence within the community. People who become employed shortly after injury virtually always return to the same job and employer they had prior to injury. Among people treated at model system units after SCI who were not married at the time of injury, 12% marry within the next 5 years. Among people who were married at the time of injury, 80.7% were still married 5 years later. Most people are able to achieve what they define as a satisfactory quality of life after SCI.

During the first year after discharge, there is evidence of a decrease in depression and hostility over time. Beyond the first year, acceptance of disability increases and life satisfaction improves as the time since injury lengthens. People with SCI living in the community consistently report their greatest challenges to be (1) accessibility in the community; (2) vocational opportunities, including the capacity to earn an income; and (3) the length of time it takes to perform self-care activities. Nurses can begin exploring these issues with patients early in the rehabilitation period.

Life expectancy and the quality of life for people with SCI have increased dramatically over the past 20 years. Renal failure is no

PLAN OF CARE

Estimated Length of Stay: _____

ADMISSION

Area of Assessment	**Suggested Interventions**
	Medicine/Nursing
• Skin	Establish appropriate skin care protocol
• Bladder	Establish appropriate bladder program
• Bowel	Establish appropriate bowel program
• Neuromuscular	Establish spine stability and care of stabilizing device
	Evaluate level of spasticity and pain
• Respiratory status	Establish level of pulmonary hygiene
• Cardiovascular status	Assess potential for orthostatic hypotension
	Autonomic dysreflexia and deep vein thrombosis
	Obtain baseline leg measurements
• GI	Evaluate for potential for ileus, GI bleed
• Knowledge of medications	Medication teaching for frequency, usage, and side effects

	Physical/Occupational/Speech Therapy
• Joint and muscle function	Establish ROM, positioning, and splinting schedules
• Activity tolerance	Initiate activity as appropriate to LOI and medical status
• Feeding	Provide with appropriate adaptive devices
• Bathing, grooming, and dressing	Provide with appropriate assistive equipment
• Pt./caregiver training	Provide instruction in all areas (positioning, splinting, ROM, equipment, transfers, mobility, pressure relief).
• Wheelchair/cushions	Evaluate for electric/manual wheelchair with adaptive equipment and appropriate seating cushions for pressure relief
• Mobility	Establish functional patterns of mobility
• Swallowing	Swallowing evaluation
• Communication	Communication board, talking trach

	Nutrition
• Diet and fluid status	Establish diet to meet fluid and protein requirements
• Current weight	Establish IBW and diet to meet 100% of nutritional needs

	Psychosocial/Education
• Understanding of disability and prognosis	Provide information to patient and family through education group and written material
	Provide for individual counseling, support group, and peer visitation through spinal cord chapter
• Understanding of rehab program goals, LOS	Review program, goals, LOS with pt. and family
• Understanding of complications of spinal cord injury	Implement individualized teaching plan
	Provide for group education
• Access to medical care after discharge	Provide information of availability of medical resources
• Discharge to appropriate environment	Equipment needs met, home environment adapted to meet functional needs

	Recreational Therapy/Vocational Rehab
• Preinjury recreational interests	Integrate community reentry into rehab program by introducing pt. to new activities and interests
	Driving evaluation
• Preinjury vocational status	Make vocational referral to appropriate agencies
• Discharge disposition	Identify financial, community, and support resources available after discharge to ensure accessible housing

FIGURE 22–18

See legend on following page

PLAN OF CARE *Continued*

DISCHARGE

Expected outcomes:

- Skin remains intact.
- Pt. demonstrates pressure relief measures, and/or directs others.
- Pt. performs bladder management program with moderate to maximal assist and/or directs others.
- Pt. performs bowel management program with moderate to maximal assist and/or directs others and has less than 1 incontinent episode/week.
- Pt. verbalizes mechanisms to control spasticity and pain.
- Lungs remain clear; pt. and caregiver demonstrate quad cough technique; pt. verbalizes interventions for adequate pulmonary hygiene.
- Pt. verbalizes current medication regime—frequency, usage, and side effects.
- Pt. knowledgeable about S/S of medical complications and how to access medical care.
- Pt. transfers to chair with moderate to maximal assist with sliding board.
- Pt. controls electric/manual wheelchair using appropriate device.
- Pt. knowledgeable in proper seating cushions.
- Pt. bathes, grooms, and dresses with appropriate assist and/or directs others.
- Diet meets 100% of nutritional requirements.
- Pt. displays appropriate interaction with others in environment.
- Pt. verbalizes understanding of Americans with Diabilities Act.
- Pt. aware of assistive technology opportunities.
- Pt. connected with registry of motor vehicles to obtain information on license, plate, and adaptive equipment for motor vehicle or other transportation options.
- Pt. aware of community resources for leisure/recreational pursuits.
- Pt. knowledgeable of vocational opportunities.
- Pt. connected with local chapter of National Spinal Cord Injury Association.

FIGURE 22–18

Suggested plan of care for the patient with high spinal cord injury (quadriplegia) in the rehabilitation setting. GI, gastrointestinal; IBW, ideal body weight; LOI, level of injury; LOS, length of stay; pt., patient; rehab, rehabilitation; ROM, range-of-motion exercises; S/S, signs and symptoms; trach, tracheostomy.

longer a leading cause of death in spinal cord–injured patients. The use of low-dose heparin, external pneumatic compression devices, and electrical stimulation have reduced the incidence of deep vein thrombosis, pulmonary embolism, and death in people with SCI. Intrathecal catheters and pumps have allowed for administration of agents directly into the spinal cord for the treatment of spasticity and pain. People with high tetraplegia successfully live in the community; some, like actor Christopher Reeve, become role models for the disabled.

Rehabilitation needs to focus on goals for return to the community, with nurses and therapists being teachers. The following areas of focus must be included:

- The need for transportation services with access to public areas
- Accessible housing
- Employment and vocational retraining
- Access to continued medical care after discharge from the hospital
- Financial assistance
- The need for services of a personal care attendant

- Assistive technology in the areas of
  - Personal—tools for self-care
  - Activity-specific—eating, reading, writing
  - Environmental—to maximize access to society and its resources

Part of a comprehensive rehabilitation program involves assessment of the person's home environment and ability to function within it. Nursing staff should participate in the home visit; if that is not possible, the nurse should be part of the follow-up discussion of the problems identified and the areas to be addressed before discharge. Areas not sufficiently addressed before discharge should be referred to a home care agency or outpatient care setting for continued intervention.

Driving and being a passenger in an appropriate vehicle must be considered part of community reintegration. Evaluation of the patient for the potential to drive should be considered and is available through driver education programs. The occupational therapist is often the one to complete the predriving screening. Many rehabilitation hospitals have a driving simulator, enabling parts of the driving evaluation to be performed while the patient is still hospitalized. Selection of the proper vehicle with the necessary equipment and modifications is the next step. The state's registry of motor vehicles will validate proper vehicle identification and issue a new license after the patient has completed a driver education program.

Rehabilitation engineering has made gains through the use of computer technology, metallurgy, and the development of new materials. These advances have positively affected the level of independent activity achievable by people with high quadriplegia. Computers, environmental control units, one-handed joystick control drive cams, and voice-controlled wheelchairs all have liberated such people in the areas of banking and money management, word processing, electronic mail, shopping, and pursuing vocational activities. Computer activities should be integrated into the rehabilitation process whenever possible. Recreational therapy can play an active role in setting up computer games for patients to play with other patients and staff.

Improvements in wheelchairs and wheelchair cushions have led to longer sitting times and greater mobility for people with SCI. Wheelchair prescription is a complex task and involves the entire rehabilitation team, patient, family, and insurance provider. The basic components and accessories of a wheelchair can make the difference in an individual's functional independence level for skills, including propulsion, distance, endurance, manipulation of varied environmental factors, transfers, balance, and availability of upper extremities for functional tasks. For the person with high tetraplegia, a power wheelchair may be the only functional mode of mobility. It must have a system for pressure relief as well as appropriate control mechanisms, such as activation by chin, tongue, head, gaze, voice, or pneumatic action (sip-and-puff device). Some environmental control units can be interfaced with a power wheelchair's mechanisms to further increase the individual's independence.

Proper seating and positioning are critical to enhanced independence. The development of improved cushions has led to better pressure relief and the ability to be functional for longer periods in homemaking, community, school, and vocational activities. In evaluating seating and positioning, the rehabilitation team should pay attention to range of motion, tone, respiratory function, skin integrity, ex-

isting deformities, communication, environmental control, cognition, safety, motor function, psychological acceptance, and funding.

Education must include the need for continual reassessment of the seating and positioning program, especially as patients grow older. According to Edwards (1996), one study evaluating postrehabilitation services for SCI patients found that among the services desired but not obtained were an exercise program (43%); testing of muscle function (29%); referral to a fitness center (26%); classes on relaxation techniques (21%); and referral to a physical therapist to prevent contractures. Edwards (1996) suggests that a fitness assessment, an exercise prescription, and a fitness plan registered with a fitness center should be considered for people with SCI, pointing out, "Health care providers need to develop health promotion activities, specifically exercise and physical fitness activities for individuals with SCI; they have the same needs for health promotion services as the general population."

Preparation for community reintegration also includes management of self-care and medical issues. Determination of the method of bladder management, establishment of the proper bowel program, hiring of a personal care attendant if appropriate, an understanding of skin management and pressure relief, and access to health care services should all be accomplished before discharge. Intermittent self-catheterization has become a widely accepted method of bladder management. Percutaneous surgical techniques for removing stones from kidneys have greatly decreased the morbidity from renal operations and have improved kidney function. Advances in electrical stimulation have enabled many people with SCI to become continent. Improved bladder surgery has improved bladder capacity, continence, and bladder emptying. Medications, intrathecal pumps, and nerve blocks have all improved treatment for spasticity.

Exposure to leisure activities and recreational pursuits should also be part of the preparation. People with SCI can participate in activities such as camping, hunting, and fishing. Sporting pursuits include water skiing, downhill skiing, basketball, and rugby (Fig. 22–19). There are organized groups for wheelchair sports and other athletic pursuits.

Taking trips out into the community while still a patient in the rehabilitation unit is important for adjustment to the community (Fig. 22–20). Nurses should work with recreational

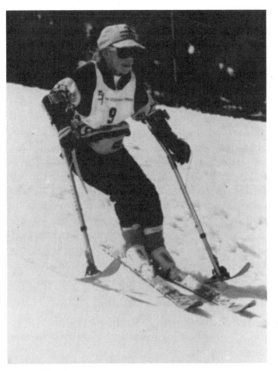

FIGURE 22–19
Outrigger skis used while skiing by a person who has difficulty shifting weight, maintaining upright stance, and maintaining balance. To ski with outriggers, a person must be able to stand independently but may have difficulty with coordination. (From Braddom R. L. [1996]. *Physical medicine and rehabilitation.* [p. 527]. Philadelphia: W. B. Saunders.)

of fatigue and pain, and decreases in activity level; bladder infections, stomach problems, pressure ulcers, respiratory and bowel problems" (Pentland, McColl, & Rosenthal, 1995). There has been a lack of information about long-term survival of people with SCI and the services needed to meet these long-term problems.

Alexander, Parker, and Stauffer (1997) reported on 41 patients who were 50 years or older at the time of SCI. Thirteen had complete injuries and the remaining 28 had incomplete injuries. None of the subjects with complete injuries improved, and all went to nursing homes after rehabilitation. Of the 28 with incomplete injuries, 20 went home, six went to nursing homes, and two died. The mortality of those with complete injuries was 77% after 1 year; the leading cause of death was respiratory failure. For those with incomplete injuries, the mortality was 50% after 5 years; respiratory failure was again the leading cause of death. The investigators concluded that the components of aging appear to be accelerated in people with spinal injur-

therapists to let them know when patients have the endurance and knowledge of important issues such as pressure relief and bladder management to be able to go on an outing to the local mall, a restaurant, or a movie theater. The patient can learn much about social readjustment, accessibility, and management from such short outings with staff. The "debriefing" with staff members afterwards is a vital component of the rehabilitation process. If the insurance company allows, overnight visits home provide valuable insight about the patient's eventual transition to the community. If that is not possible, an overnight stay in the hospital's transitional living apartment must be a prerequisite to discharge.

As people with SCI age, they face secondary and tertiary disabilities, many of which are preventable. "Studies which interviewed 34 persons with an average duration of SCI of 22 years and a relatively young mean age of 45 years, noted that this group had already begun to have problems with increased levels

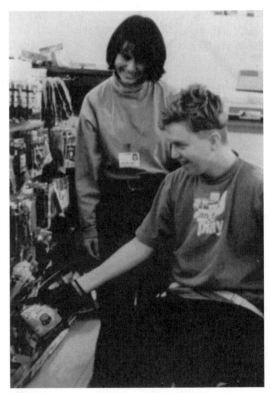

FIGURE 22–20
Therapist facilitating independence in the community. Person is solving problem of how to take items off the shelf in a grocery store. (From Braddom R. L. [1996]. *Physical medicine and rehabilitation.* [p. 526]. Philadelphia: W. B. Saunders.)

ies, compounding the difficulties of independence, home help, mobility, and independent living.

Information about insurance coverage and benefits is integral to rehabilitation, growing in importance as hospital lengths of stay are shortened. Patients and families need to be well informed about what services and equipment third-party payers will cover, in both inpatient and outpatient settings. Technology has made so much more available for people with SCI, but many of the new devices are extremely expensive. An improved health care system should address

- Better education for people with disabilities
- Better-trained community of health care practitioners
- Greater availability of personal assistance and technological services focused on the needs of people with disabilities
- More accessible environment
- More accommodation to the unique needs of the disabled in the workplace
- Revision of social and health policies affecting people with disabilities
- A pervasive societal effort to enhance the

self-esteem of disabled people in order that they use the proposed improvements in the health care system

Professionals in rehabilitation should not emphasize ill health but rather stress that the patient is healthy but disabled. The rehabilitation program needs to have physical skills training but should focus on the redevelopment of life skills as well. There is a need for the early involvement of the psychosocial disciplines of psychiatry, psychology, neuropsychology, family therapy, social service, and chaplaincy in rehabilitation for people with SCI. Nurses should identify interpersonal techniques they can use to help patients develop strategies to gain more control of their lives. The rehabilitation nurse is in the ideal position to provide information to patients with SCI about their new lifestyle.

Peer support is important—a system linking former patients and their families with new patients is extremely helpful as the person with an SCI reenters the community. Resources are available for patients and families to take advantage of early in the rehabilitation process; a partial list of resources is given in Table 22–8.

TABLE 22–8 ■ COMMUNITY RESOURCES FOR PEOPLE WITH SPINAL CORD INJURIES

The following national organizations can be contacted by telephone:

American Association of SCI Nurses	718-803-3782
American Paralysis Association	800-225-0292
American Paraplegic Society	718-803-3782
American Spinal Cord Injury Association	312-908-6207
Eastern Paralyzed Veterans Association	718-803-3782
Miami Project to Cure Paralysis	800-782-6387
National Spinal Cord Injury Association (NSCIA@aol.com)*	800-962-9629
National Spinal Cord Injury (PVA) Hotline	800-526-3456
Information Center for Individuals with Disabilities	800-727-5540
National Spinal Cord Injury Statistical Center	205-934-5359
Paralyzed Veterans of America (PVA)	800-424-8200
Internet Information Services	800-642-0249
Disability Resources Affiliate and Groups Network	612-338-2535
New Mobility Magazine: Lifestyle, Culture & Resources	800-543-4116
National Audiovisual Database of Educational Materials on SCI	713-797-5945

Written information is available on a variety of topics through periodicals, publications, and books. A sampling follows:

The Wheelchair Traveler (Ball Hill Road, Melford, NH 03055)—information on 4,000 airports, hotels, and tourist attractions in the United States, Canada, and Mexico

A Guide to Recreation, Leisure and Travel for the Handicapped (Resource Directories, 3103 Executive Parkway, Toledo, OH 43606)

Diasabled Outdoors (National Wheelchair Athletic Association, 2107 Templeton Gap Road, Suite C, Colorado Springs, CO 80907)—information on wilderness sports

Job Hunting for the Disabled (Marks & Lewis, New York: Barton's Educational Series, Inc., 1983)

Working Together—A Key to Jobs for the Handicapped (AFL/CIO Organizations, 815 16th Street NW, Washington, DC 20006)

A Handbook on Sexuality after SCI (J.M. Toggie & S.M. Manley, 4325 S. Clarkson, Englewood, CO 80110)

*Many areas have local chapters of the National Spinal Cord Injury Association. The national office can provide listings of local chapters as well as of resource material available throughout the country.

SPINAL CORD INJURIES IN CHILDREN

Every year, SCIs occur in 230 to 500 people younger than 15 years and in 1500 to 2000 people younger than 20 years (Vogel, 1997). Unlike the sex ratio in adults, males and females are equally represented among young children; the ratio of males with SCI increases in adolescence along with risk-taking behaviors. As in adults, motor vehicle injuries are the most common cause of SCI in children and adolescents, with violence being the next leading cause. "Unique etiologies of pediatric SCI include lap belt injuries, birth injury, child abuse, high cervical lesions related to juvenile rheumatoid arthritis, Down syndrome, and skeletal dysplasias such as achondroplasia, Morquio syndrome and metatropic dwarfism" (Vogel, 1997a and b).

Young children tend to have a lower rate of tetraplegia and a higher rate of complete paraplegia because of motor vehicle accidents' being the leading cause of injury. Survival rate in children increases as severity of injury decreases; the lower the level of injury and degree of impairment (Frankel grade or ASIA level), the longer the survival. The most common causes of death after the acute phase are pneumonia, pulmonary emboli, and septicemia.

Anatomical and physiological characteristics of children are responsible for (1) SCI without radiological abnormalities (SCIWORA), (2) a higher frequency of complete SCI, (3) delayed onset of neurological findings, and (4) consequent neurological levels. Approximately 20 to 40% of children and adolescents with SCI have SCIWORA. The high incidence of SCIWORA in children younger than 10 years relates to the anatomical and biomechanical characteristics of the spine at this stage. Despite the benign radiological picture in SCIWORA, these injuries are more commonly associated with complete neurological lesions and a poor prognosis for neurological return (Vogel, 1997a).

A unique aspect of pediatric SCI is the interaction of growth and development with the manifestations and complications of the injury. Growth is responsible for a number of orthopedic problems. Spine deformity is prevalent in many children as a result of muscle weakness or imbalance, residual deformity of the spinal column following a fracture, or surgery. Other problems can subsequently develop from the spine deformity, including diminished upper extremity function, pressure ulcers, pain, poor fit of lower extremity orthoses, and gastrointestinal or cardiopulmonary dysfunction. Hip instability is another major and common orthopedic problem, resulting most often from muscle imbalance, which pushes the hip out improperly, or poor socket control from flaccid hip muscles. Contractures can result within weeks or months of an injury. Prevention is the key to management of this orthopedic problem. Pathological long bone density fractures occur secondary to loss of bone mineral density. Caregivers must focus on safety during risky activities. Encouraging weight bearing for as long as possible with braces or full extension splints is recommended, as well as good nutrition and adequate sunlight. Spinal cord syrinx is found in children, caused by regions of hemorrhage or ischemia within the spinal cord. Health care providers and caregivers should be aware of these and other orthopedic complications that occur as a result of growth in children with SCI.

Medical complications are also found in the pediatric population with SCI. Prevention of urinary tract infections and renal complications are primary goals of bladder management. Clean, intermittent catheterization is most often utilized, and children are taught intermittent self-catheterization by 5 years of age. In adolescence, the use of an indwelling catheter or suprapubic tube for males or the surgical creation of a catheterizable stoma for females is sometimes considered to allow more freedom and independence. Children with SCI are at high risk for latex allergy and may require the use of nonlatex equipment. "Hypercalcemia occurs in 10–23% of patients with SCI and most commonly affects adolescent and young adult males one to twelve weeks after injury" (Vogel, 1997b).

Pulmonary complications are the most common cause of death during the acute and rehabilitation phases of SCI in children and adolescents. "Initially, the most common pulmonary complications are atelectasis, pneumonia and ventilatory failure. Subsequently, the most common pulmonary complications are pneumonia and ventilatory failure, related to deteriorating pulmonary function as patients grow older, superimposed on ventilatory weakness as a consequence of the neurological deficit" (Vogel, 1997b). Heterotopic ossification also occurs in the pediatric population, although not as frequently as in adults. Deep vein thrombosis and pulmonary embolism are life-threatening complications that develop in the pediatric population early after injury; early detection and management are the same as for the adult population.

Rehabilitation of children with SCI is similar to that of adults, with the focus being on maximizing mobility, muscle strength, range of motion, and accomplishment of the activities of daily living. Standing and ambulation are encouraged for children younger than 18 months to provide physical strengthening and psychological development comparable to that of able-bodied children. Children should be evaluated early on for both upper and lower extremity orthoses. Consideration of the child's desire to stand and ambulate, family support, and ease of use in school and during toileting will all determine the successful use of orthoses. Older children often abandon standing and ambulation and actually gain more independence using a wheelchair. For a young child without effective ambulation, the rehabilitation team must consider a means of mobility that gives the child freedom of movement and exploration. Children can learn to mobilize in a wheelchair as young as 18 to 24 months. As children age, rehabilitation should include wheelchair sports and other activities that mimic those available to able-bodied peers.

Rehabilitation of the child with SCI must incorporate the developmental changes. The interdisciplinary team needs to develop a plan of care that meshes the normal growth and developmental changes with the special needs of the injury. Treatment must be developmentally based, and goals must be relevant to the child's stage of development. To enable the child with SCI to view life as satisfying, the goals must survive the stressful periods of adolescence and young adulthood. Compliance with treatment plans is often compromised during adolescence; complications such as urinary tract infections, respiratory problems, bowel incontinence, pressure ulcers, and substance abuse can all occur as the adolescent struggles with the journey into adulthood carrying the additional burden of a chronic disability.

The child or adolescent's ability to explore the environment physically, sexually, educationally, and vocationally can be impaired by limited function and mobility. Normal behavioral responses are difficult when one is dependent on caregivers. The need to address sexuality is often overlooked in children with SCI. It is critical that this issue be addressed with children and parents because of the significant impact the SCI may have on sexual functioning and fertility. Children and adoles-

cents need to be reassured of their sexuality and their ability to be sexual beings and to have meaningful relationships.

Emotional adjustment to SCI is intertwined with the physical adaptation and is important at all ages of injury. Although adjustment to injury seems easier for infants and young children, the overall impact continues throughout their years of development. Harper has proposed the following model for understanding adjustment to childhood disability, which is relevant to pediatric SCI (Anderson, 1997):

A developmental perspective: The child's developmental level is related to (a) how aware the child will be of the disability, (b) how the child will understand and respond to treatment, (c) how much the family will be involved in caregiving, (d) how the disability may interfere with development.
A life span process: Adaptation will change as the child develops and meets new challenges.
Family focus: The child's disability occurs within the family and (a) the family's attitudes and resources affect the child's adjustment and (b) the child's disability affects the whole family.
Peer feedback and socialization: Disability can limit opportunities for socialization and peer feedback at every developmental level.

Inherent in this model is the assumption that psychological assessment, guidance, and counseling are ongoing processes in the treatment of children with SCI. The goal is normal cognitive, emotional, and social development despite the SCI.

Children with SCI are at risk for a lack of independence and control, social isolation, immature social development, and lower self-esteem. Rehabilitation should focus on not only individual counseling but also peer support groups, wheelchair sports or other recreational group activities, assistance with adapted driving, education, and career planning. Rehabilitation involves the whole family. Parents and siblings need support and guidance as well. A father may feel anger at a son who cannot play sports; a mother may be frustrated that her child's needs keep her at home rather than allowing her to return to the workforce; siblings may feel jealous of the attention the disabled child requires. Counseling should include all members of a family with a disabled child.

Contact with the school system should be made while the child is in the rehabilitation process. Tutoring should be started in the hospital, as soon as the child is medically stable. Reintegration into the mainstream school system should be encouraged early on. The school nurse should be contacted to ensure arrangements for special treatments or medications required during the school day. Attending school with a personal care attendant may be part of the program; any special arrangements for classroom space or seating should be identified so that the child's reentry is as smooth as possible. Preparation for career planning should begin in high school; although playing football may not be realistic, the adolescent needs assistance to envision coaching or sports management as a viable option.

■ CASE STUDY 22–1

Nate is a 23-year-old student injured in a fall from the balcony of an apartment on a college campus. Emergency medical technicians found him unresponsive, lying on his right side, and bleeding from the mouth. Emergency care at the scene consisted of a backboard, neck collar, and immediate transfer to the trauma unit of a nearby medical center. Initial x-rays revealed a fracture subluxation of C3 on C4 with gross displacement and fragments in the spinal canal, as well as C5 body fracture without significant cord compression. The initial impression was C3 on C4 fracture-subluxation with quadriplegia. The patient was placed in Crutchfield tongs for neck stabilization. He was intubated and mechanically ventilated. His past medical history included severe childhood asthma. Initial physical examination found facial abrasions from the fall. He was started on high-dose steroids; chest tubes were inserted into both lungs for bilateral hemopneumothoraces; and a Foley catheter was inserted. Vital signs were closely monitored. Once stabilized, the patient was transferred to the spinal intensive care unit.

Two days later, Nate was taken to the operating room for surgical decompression and spinal stabilization with a halo body vest, insertion of a tracheostomy tube, and placement of a Greenfield filter for prevention of pulmonary embolus.

While in the spinal intensive care unit, he demonstrated temperature spikes secondary to pneumonia and was treated with intravenous antibiotics. A gastrostomy tube was placed for supplemental feedings. Mechanical ventilation was switched from assist-control (AC) to pressure-support mode as weaning was initiated. The patient's O_2 saturation values (sats) remained at 90 to 96%; vital signs were stable; and his appetite improved. A right pneumothorax developed, as did a stage II sacral pressure ulcer. Physical medicine and rehabilitation specialists assessed his injury as C4 sensory incomplete quadriplegia, ASIA impairment level B. Therapists initiated treatment programs.

Nate was admitted to the rehabilitation unit 23 days after initial injury. By that time, he was off the ventilator some of the day and taking food completely by mouth. The chest tubes had been removed and the Foley catheter was in place; there was a quarter-size stage II pressure sore on his sacrum.

Nate's primary rehabilitation nurse established the following nursing diagnoses during the initial assessment:

I. Alteration in respiratory function related to ineffective airway clearance, muscle paralysis, and ineffective breathing pattern.
II. Alteration in elimination: bowel and bladder dysfunction related to paralysis.
III. Impaired skin integrity related to altered circulation, immobility, and mechanical factors.
IV. Impaired physical mobility related to muscle paralysis.
V. Alteration in thermoregulation related to disruption in hypothalamic control.
VI. Altered coping related to psychological effect of catastrophic illness.
VII. Altered self-esteem and feelings of self-worth related to changes in body image, increase in dependency, and change in lifestyle.
VIII. Knowledge deficit related to lack of knowledge about SCI.
IX. Alteration in sexual functioning related to paralysis.

I. Alteration in Respiratory Function Related to Ineffective Airway Clearance, Muscle Paralysis, and Ineffective Breathing Pattern

Interventions

1. Weaning schedule established; ventilator on AC mode when patient on; ventilator checks every 4 hours when patient on.
2. O_2 calibrated to keep sats at 90 to 95% with weaning to room air.

3. Frequent suctioning by nursing and respiratory therapy, and use of quad coughing to encourage mobilization of secretions after suctioning.
4. Incentive spirometry every 4 hours while awake.
5. Trach care every shift.
6. Chest physical therapy twice daily and as needed.
7. Nebulizer treatments every 4 hours and as needed.
8. Speech therapy consult for use of the Passey-Muir valve and swallowing trials.

II. ALTERATION IN ELIMINATION: BOWEL AND BLADDER DYSFUNCTION RELATED TO PARALYSIS

Interventions

1. Remove indwelling catheter and begin intermittent catheter program.
2. Implement bowel program.
3. Education regarding autonomic dysreflexia.

III. IMPAIRED SKIN INTEGRITY RELATED TO ALTERED CIRCULATION, IMMOBILITY, AND MECHANICAL FACTORS

Interventions

1. Initial treatment for stage II pressure ulcer was Dermagram and the use of a fluid air loss mattress.

As the wound worsened, a course of electrical stimulation and a normal saline wet-to-dry dressing twice daily was instituted. Despite these interventions, the wound continued to enlarge and worsen to a stage III wound. Complicating factors in this pressure ulcer included

■ The use of steroids for the chronic asthma.
■ Nate's noncompliance with a turning schedule; he wished to stay on his back.
■ Shearing forces because the head of the bed was often up. Nate had many visitors and liked to be on his back sitting up when they were there.

A surgical consultation was ordered, and Nate was moved from the fluid air loss mattress to a fluid-air-loss bed. The surgeon debrided the wound and ordered strict bedrest with the head of the bed elevated no more than 30 degrees at any time, including for meals. Nursing staff instituted a strict turning schedule of every 2 hours during the day and every 3 hours at night. The wound was measured and photographed every 2 weeks. Nate received a picture of the wound at his request. Upon examining the picture, he

greatly improved his compliance with the turning schedule and keeping the head of the bed at less than 30 degrees. Wound cultures ultimately revealed osteomyelitis. A course of intravenous antibiotics followed, with Nate's admission to the acute care hospital for a myocutaneous flap procedure. He returned to the rehabilitation unit with orders to remain at bed rest and completely flat for 4 weeks.

IV. IMPAIRED PHYSICAL MOBILITY RELATED TO MUSCLE PARALYSIS

Interventions

1. Assess safety level.
2. Halo vest care.
3. Establish range of motion, positioning, and splinting schedules.
4. Mobilization with therapists after wound heals.

Admission examination revealed the following findings:

Motor findings:

	Right	Left
Deltoids	2+ to 3/5	1/5
Biceps	4/5	1/5
Wrist extensors	0/5	0/5
Triceps	0/5	0/5
Hand extensors	0/5	0.5

Sensory findings:
■ Sensation to pinprick intact at C5 bilaterally
■ No voluntary rectal control
■ Patchy sensation to light touch below the level of injury

V. ALTERATION IN THERMOREGULATION RELATED TO DISRUPTION IN HYPOTHALAMIC CONTROL

Interventions

1. Assess issues of thermoregulation versus medical complications.
2. Teach patient and family about the concept of thermoregulation: to know response of SCI to internal temperature regulation.
3. Regulate environment to maintain normal body temperature.

VI. ALTERATION IN COPING RELATED TO PSYCHOLOGICAL EFFECT OF CATASTROPHIC ILLNESS

Interventions

1. Support Nate and his family through the grieving process.
2. Arrange family therapy and psychiatric consultations.

3. Referral to Peer Visitation program through local chapter of National Spinal Cord Injury Association (NSCIA).
4. Obtain referral for recreational therapy.
5. Encourage participation in patient/family education group.
6. Obtain referral for vocational rehabilitation.

VII. ALTERED SELF-ESTEEM AND FEELINGS OF SELF-WORTH RELATED TO CHANGES IN BODY IMAGE, INCREASE IN DEPENDENCY, AND CHANGES IN LIFESTYLE

Interventions

1. Arrange referral to Peer Visitation program through the local chapter of the NSCIA.
2. Arrange for previous patients on the unit to visit.
3. Give Nate the opportunity to vent his feelings.
4. Support Nate with realistic responses without taking all hope away. A response, when he would initially ask about recovery, was, "We don't know yet what your final level of injury will be, but right now, let's work with what you have." We encouraged him to deal with the present rather than think too far into the future.
5. Encourage participation and support from family and friends.
6. Allow the patient as much control and decision making as possible. One of Nate's dreams was to play soccer professionally. One of his roommates arranged for a former Boston Bruins hockey player to visit him. This visit really lifted his spirits and offered him hope for the future.

VIII. KNOWLEDGE DEFICIT RELATED TO LACK OF KNOWLEDGE ABOUT SPINAL CORD INJURY

Interventions

1. Give patient and family the Spinal Cord Injury Education Manual.
2. Introduce family to the local chapter of the NSCIA and their resource information.
3. Encourage attendance at the weekly patient/family SCI education series.
4. Primary nurse to share information while providing care and answer questions matter-of-factly as they arise.
5. Work with recreation therapy to plan outing for reintegration into the community.

IV. ALTERATION IN SEXUAL FUNCTIONING RELATED TO PARALYSIS

Interventions

1. Allow patient to express feelings and concerns.

2. Provide patient with information, both verbal and printed.

OUTCOME

Nate was successfully weaned from the ventilator, the tracheostomy was removed, and his respiratory condition returned to pre-injury status, using as-needed asthma medications only. The halo vest was removed after 3 months. He wore a soft collar only when up.

He was discharged with an intermittent catheterization program of 4/day catheterizations. The local visiting nurse agency and family members planned to perform catheterizations until a personal care attendant could be hired and trained. A decision was not made on long-term bladder management program at the time of discharge. Because Nate's neurological status was still improving, the hope was that eventually he could perform self-catheterization. If not, his physician was considering use of an external device and medication for a "balanced bladder" approach. Nate did not want to be dependent on others over the long term for his bladder management. He was using a successful bowel program every other day, which the visiting nurse continued after discharge, also until a personal care attendant could be hired.

Nate hoped he could eventually be independent with the use of adaptive equipment. His sacral wound had healed; he knew how to perform pressure relief measures while in the wheelchair and how to monitor his skin for potential breakdown. He was independent in his power wheelchair using hand controls. He had a manual wheelchair with handrim projections, which he used on level surfaces for short periods to help regain strength and function. At the time of discharge, he was transferring with a sliding board and a moderate assist from one person.

Nate was knowledgeable about controlling his environment for thermoregulation problems. He continued to be sensitive to environmental temperature and became easily chilled. Nate found it comfortable to keep his external environment at close to 80°F.

Nate showed steady improvement in upper extremity strength, with some trace movements extending down to the C8 level on the right side. He had trace finger flexion on the right side without clear intrinsic hand function. Sensation was intact on the right side through C6, and on the left side to C5 with partial preservation at C6 level. Light touch was grossly intact on the right side with some patchy decreases in the lower extremities; and grossly intact on the left side to C7–C8 with some patchy decreases in the lower extremities as well. No voluntary rectal contraction was ever noted. The possibility of his gaining function in the triceps and right wrist extensors over the next 6 to 12 months was anticipated by the physiatrist and therapists. He was determined to be classified as having C5 incomplete SCI with ASIA impairment level B at the time of discharge.

Nate was coping better with the effects of his disability. He found a great deal of support from the peer visitors and was able to share many thoughts and feelings with them. The college waived the three remaining courses he needed, so he graduated that year. He was working with the vocational counselor, exploring employment opportunities or a return to school for a degree in sports management. Although his dream to play professional soccer after college had been dashed by his injury, he realized he could still pursue a career in the world of sports. Nate was able to acknowledge that his drinking while at college had been a mechanism to help him deal with women. He was aware that he had to deal with dating relationships on a different, more appropriate level now.

Nate was discharged from the rehabilitation hospital and returned home to live with his father. He had services of the Visiting Nurses' Association initially; eventually, he hired a personal care attendant and traveled for outpatient services. His father set up his computer at home. Using a utensil cuff and wrist splint for support, with a pencil in the cuff, Nate gained a great deal of independence in his environment. With this adaptation, he could turn the computer on and off, press the mouse as well as the keyboard, turn pages in a book, push the buttons on the television remote, and dial numbers on the touch-tone telephone. He could cradle the phone on his shoulder and talk to his friends independently.

One month after returning home, Nate was functioning at a semi-independent level and continuing with return of neurological function. He had regained slight triceps function in his left arm, although his right arm continued to be more functional. He had sensation on his left side down to his hand, and could "wiggle" his toes in conjunction with a spasm when positioned in bed at 90 degrees. He had a sense of independence returning and hope for the future.

REFERENCES

Alexander, D. H., Parker, J., & Stauffer, E. S. (1997). *Spine,* 22 (11); 1189–1192.

Alexander, T., Griggs, W., & Ledwell, K. (1987). Sexuality. In C. Carlson (Ed.), *Spinal cord injury: A guide to rehabilitation nursing* (pp. 57–66). Rockville, MD: Aspen Publishers.

Alho, A. (1994). Operative treatment as a part of the comprehensive care for patients with injuries of the thoracolumbar spine: A review. *Paraplegia, 32,* 509–516.

American Association of Spinal Cord Injury Nurses: (1996). *Clinical practice guideline: Autonomic dysreflexia,* (pp. 1–18). New York: Author.

Anderson, C. (1997). Unique management needs of pediatric spinal cord injury patients: Psychosocial issues. *Journal of Spinal Cord Medicine, 20* (1), 21–23.

Banovac, K., Gonzalez, P. A., & Renfree, K. (1997). Treatment of heterotopic ossificans after spinal cord injury. *Journal of Spinal Cord Medicine 20* (1), 60–65.

Bergstrom, N., Bennett, M. A., Carlson, C. E., et al. (1994). *Pressure ulcer treatment.* (Clinical Practice Guideline: Quick Reference Guide for Clinicians, No. 15.) (AHCPR Pub. No. 95–0653.) Rockville, MD: Agency for Health Care Policy and Research.

Bracken, M. B., Shephard, M. J., Collins, W. F., et al. (1990). A randomized, controlled trial of methylprednisolone or naloxone in the treatment of acute spinal cord injury: Results of the Second National Acute Spinal Cord Injury Study. *New England Journal of Medicine, 332,* 1406–1411.

Brown, D. J. (1992). Spinal cord injuries: The last decade and the next. *Paraplegia, 30,* 77–82.

Byrne, D. W., Salzberg, C. A. (1996). Major risk factors for pressure ulcers in the spinal cord disabled: A literature review. *Spinal Cord, 34* (5), 255–263.

Campagnolo, D., Esquieres, R., & Kopacz, K. (1997). Effect of timing of stabilization on length of stay and medical complications following spinal cord injury. *Journal of Spinal Cord Medicine 20* (3), 331–334.

Chawla, J. C. (1993). Rehabilitation of spinal cord injured patients on long term ventilation. *Paraplegia, 31,* 88–92.

Colachis, S., Clinchot, D., & Venesy, D. (1993). Neurovascular complications of heterotopic ossification following spinal cord injury. *Paraplegia, 31,* 51–57.

DePace, D. (1994). Anatomy and physiology of the nervous system. In E. Barker (Ed.), (President), *Neuroscience nursing* (pp. 3–47). St. Louis: Mosby–Year Book.

DeVivo, M., & Richards, J. (1992). Community reintegration and quality of life following spinal cord injury. *Paraplegia, 30,* 108–112.

Edwards, P. (1996). Health promotion through fitness for adolescents and young adults following spinal cord injury. *SCI Nursing, 13* (3), 69–73.

Emick-Herring, B. (1993). Normal motor control and neurophysiological approaches to care. In A. McCourt (Ed.), *The specialty practice of rehabilitation nursing: A core curriculum* (pp. 28–34). Skokie, IL: Rehabilitation Nursing Foundation.

Figoni, S. (1990). Perspectives on cardiovascular fitness and SCI. *Journal of the American Paraplegic Society, 13* (4), 63–71.

Fletcher, D., Taddonio, R., Byrne, D., Wexler, L., Cayten, C., Nealon, S., & Carson, W. (1995). Incidence of acute care complications in vertebral column fracture patients with and without spinal cord injury. *Spine, 20* (10), 1136–1146.

Frost, F. (1993). Role of rehabilitation after spinal cord injury. *Spinal Cord Injury, 20* (3), 549–559.

George, E., Scholten, D., Buechler M., Jordan-Tibbs, J., Mattice, C., & Albrecht, R. (1995). Failure of methylprednisolone to improve the outcome of spinal cord injuries. *American Surgeon, 61,* 659–663.

Gilbert, D. M. L. (1996). Sexuality issues in persons with disabilities. In R. Braddom (Ed.), *Physical medicine and rehabilitation* (pp. 605–629). Philadelphia. W. B. Saunders.

Greco, S. (1996). Sexuality, education and counseling. In S. Hoeman (Ed.), *Rehabilitation nursing: Process and application* (2nd ed, pp. 594–627). St. Louis: Mosby–Year Book.

Hinkle, J. (1994). Nontraumatic spinal cord disorders. In E. Barker (Ed.), *Neuroscience nursing* (pp. 391–420). St. Louis: Mosby–Year Book.

Kirk, P. (1996). Pressure ulcer management following spinal cord injury. *Topics in Spinal Cord Injury Rehabilitation, 2* (1),9–20.

Linsenmeyer, T. A., & Stone, J. M. (1993). Neurogenic bladder and bowel dysfunction. In J. DeLisa (Ed.), *Rehabilitation medicine: Principles and practice,* (pp. 733–762). Philadelphia: J. B. Lippincott.

Kirk, P. (1996). Pressure ulcer management following spinal cord injury. *Topics in Spinal Cord Injury Rehabilitation, 2* (1), 9–20.

Michals, E. & Ramsey, R. (1996). Syringomyelia. *Orthopaedic Nursing, 15* (5), 33–39.

Panel for the Prediction and Prevention of Pressure Ulcers in Adults. (1992). *Pressure ulcers in adults: Prediction and prevention* (Clinical Practice Guideline No. 3. AHCPR Pub. No. 92–0047.) Rockville, MD: Agency for Health Care Policy and Research.

Pentland, W., McColl, M. A., & Rosenthal, C. (1995). The effect of aging and duration of disability on long term health outcomes following spinal cord injury. *Paraplegia, 33,* 367–373.

Pires, M. (1996). Bladder Elimination and Continence. In S. Hoeman (Ed.) 2nd edition. Rehabilitation Nursing Process and Application (pp. 417–451). St. Louis, Mosby-Year Book.

Pires, M., & Adkins, R. (1996). Pressure ulcers and spinal cord injury: Scope of the problem. *Topics in Spinal Cord Injury Rehabilitation, 2* (1); 1–8.

Ragnarsson, K. (1997). Management of pain in persons with spinal cord injury. *Journal of Spinal Cord Medicine, 20* (2); 186–197.

Rimoldi, R., Zigler, J., Capen, D., & Hu, S. (1992). The effect of surgical intervention on rehabilitation time in patients with thoracolumbar and lumbar spinal cord injuries. *Spine, 17* (12); 1443–1449.

Salzberg, C., Cooper-Vastola, S., Perez, F., Viehbeck, M., & Byrne, D. (1995). The effects of non-thermal pulsed electromagnetic energy (Diapulse) on wound healing of pressure ulcers in spinal cord–injured patients: A randomized double-blind study. *Wounds, 7* (1); 11–16.

Schmidtz, T. (1994). Traumatic spinal cord injury. In S. B. O'Sullivan & T. J. Schmitz (Eds.), *Physical rehabilitation: Assessment and treatment* (3rd ed. pp. 533–575). Philadelphia: F. A. Davis.

Segatore, M. (1994). Understanding chronic pain after spinal cord injury. *Journal of Neuroscience Nursing, 26* (4), 230–236.

Sipski, M., Alexander, C., & Rosen, R. (1995). Orgasm in women with spinal cord injuries: A laboratory-based assessment. *Archives of Physical Medicine and Rehabilitation, 76,* 1097–1102.

Smith, E., & Bodner, D. (1993). Sexual dysfunction after spinal cord injury. *Urologic Clinics of North America, 20* (3); 535–542.

Sonksen, J., Sommer, P., Sorenson, F., Ziebe, S., Lindhard, A., Loft, A., Anderson, A. N., & Kristensen, J. K. (1997). Fertility treatment in men with spinal cord injury. *Archives of Physical Medicine and Rehabilitation, 78* (10); 1059–1061.

Stass W., Formal, C., Gershkoff, A., Hirschwald, J., Schmidt, M., Schultz, A., & Smith, J. (1993). Rehabilitation of the spinal cord–injured patient. In J. DeLisa (Ed.), *Rehabilitation medicine: Principles and practice* (2nd ed., pp. 886–915). Philadelphia: J. B. Lippincott.

Stelling, J., & Hale, A. M. (1996). Protocol for changing condom catheters in males with spinal cord injury. *SCI Nursing, 13* (2); 28–31.

Stover, S., Lloyd, L., Waites, K., & Jackson, A. (1989). Urinary tract infection in spinal cord injury *Archives of Physical Medicine and Rehabilitation, 70,* 47–54.

Thomas, J. P. (1995). The model spinal cord injury concept: Development and implementation. In S. Stover, J. DeLisa, & G. Whiteneck (Eds.); *Spinal cord injury: Clinical outcomes from the model systems.* Gaithersburg, MD: Aspen Publishers.

U.S. Department of Health and Human Services (Dec. 1994). AHCPR Reference Guide for Clinicians. #15. Pressure Ulcer Treatment. Publication No. 95–0653. Rockville, MD: Author.

U.S. Department of Health and Human Services. AHCPR Clinical Practice Guidelines. #3. Pressure Ulcers in Adults: Prediction and Prevention. Publication No. 92–0047. Rockville, MD: Author.

Vogel, L. (1997a). Unique management needs of pediatric spinal cord injury patients: Etiology and pathophysiology. *Journal of Spinal Cord Medicine, 20* (1); 10–12.

Vogel, L. (1997b). Unique management needs of pediatric spinal cord injury patients: Medical issues. *Journal of Spinal Cord Medicine, 20* (1); 17–19.

Walleck, C. (1994). Neurotrauma: Spinal cord injury. In E. Barker (Ed.), *Neuroscience nursing* (pp. 352–375). St. Louis: Mosby-Year Book.

Watanabe, T., Chancellor, M., Rivas, D., Hirsch, I., Bennett, C., Finocchiaro, M., Razi, S., Bennett, J., Green, B., Foote, J., Killorian, R. W., Juma, S., Linsenmeyer, T., & Lloyd, K. (1996). Epidemiology of current treatment for sexual dysfunction in spinal cord injured men in USA Model SCI centers. *Journal of Spinal Cord Medicine, 19* (3); 186–189.

Waters, R., Apple, D., Meyer, P., et al. (1995). Emergency and acute management of spine trauma. In S. Stover, J., DeLisa, & G. Whiteneck (Eds), *Spinal cord injury. Clinical outcomes from the model systems.* Gaithersburg, MD: Aspen Publishers.

Yarkony, G. M., & Chen, D. (1996). Rehabilitation of atients with spinal cord injuries. In R. Braddom (Ed.), *Physical medicine and rehabilitation* (pp 1149–1179). Philadelphia: W. B. Saunders.

BIBLIOGRAPHY

Aggarwal, A., Sangwan, SS., & Siwach, R. C. (1996). Gluteus maximus island flap for the repair of sacral pressure sores. *Spinal Cord, 34* (6); 346–350.

Azouri, P., Mane, M., Thiebaut, J. B., Denys, P., Remy-Nevis, O. & Bussel, B. (1996). Intrathecal baclofen administration for control of severe spinal spasticity: Functional improvement and long-term follow-up. *Archives of Physical Medicine and Rehabilitation, 77* (1), 35–39.

Betz, R. (1997). Unique management needs of pediatric spinal cord injury patients: Orthopedic problems in the child with SCI. *Journal of Spinal Cord Medicine, 20* (1), 14–16.

Carola, R., Harley, J., & Noback, C. (1992). *Human anatomy & physiology* (2nd ed.). New York: McGraw-Hill.

DeLisa, J. A. (1992) Clinical rehabilitation research advances in spinal cord injury. *Paraplegia, 30,* 73–74.

DiLima, S. N., Hildebrand, U., & Schust, C. (Eds.). (1996). *Spinal cord injury: Patient education manual.* Rockville, MD: Aspen Publishers.

Formal, C., & Smith, J. (1996). Upper extremity function in spinal cord injury. *Topics in Spinal Cord Injury Rehabilitation, 1* (4), 1–14.

Hughes, M. (1990). Critical care nursing for the patient with a spinal cord injury. *Critical Care Nursing Clinics of North America, 2* (1), 33–40.

Ignatavicius, D., & Varner Bayne, M. (1991). Implications for clients with central nervous system disorders. In *Medical-surgical nursing: A process approach* (pp 865–959). Philadelphia: W. B. Saunders Company.

LaFavor, K., & Ang, R. (1997). Managing autonomic dysreflexia through use of the clinical practice guidelines. *SCI Nursing, 14* (3); 83–86.

Marino, J., & Stineman, M. (1996). Functional assessment in spinal cord injury. *Topics in Spinal Cord Injury Rehabilitation, 1* (4); 32–45.

Matthews, P. (1987). Elimination. In C. Carlson (Ed.), *Spinal cord injury: A guide to rehabilitation nursing* (pp 97–120). Rockville, MD: Aspen Publishers.

Mix, C., & Pieper Specht, D. (1996). Achieving functional independence. In R. Braddom (Ed.), *Physical medicine and rehabilitation* (pp 514–530). Philadelphia: W. B. Saunders.

Mulcahey, M. (1997). Unique management needs of pediatric spinal cord injury patients: Rehabilitation. *Journal of Spinal Cord Medicine, 20* (1); 25–29.

National Spinal Cord Injury Statistical Center (2000, January). *Factsheet: Facts and figures at a glance.* Birmingham, AL: University of Birmingham.

Nolan, S. (1994). Current trends in the management of acute spinal cord injury. *Critical Care Nursing Quarterly, 17* (1); 64–78.

Patterson, T. (1994). Rehabilitation. In E. Barker (Ed.), *Neuroscience nursing* (pp 376–390). St. Louis: Mosby–Year Book.

Peterson, W., Charlifue, M. A., Gerhart, A., & Whiteneck, G. (1994). Two methods of weaning persons from mechanical ventilators. *Paraplegia, 32,* 98–103.

Platts, R., & Fraser, M. (1993). Assistive technology in the rehabilitation of patients with high spinal cord lesions. *Paraplegia, 31,* 280–287.

Salcido, R., Hart, D., & Smith A. M. (1996). The prevention and management of pressure ulcers. In R. Braddom (Ed.), *Physical medicine and rehabilitation* (pp 630–648). Philadelphia: W. B. Saunders.

Salzberg, C., Byrne, D., Cayten, G., Van Niewerburgh, P., Murphy, J., & Viehbeck, M. (1996). A new pressure ulcer risk assessment scale for individuals with spinal cord injury. *American Journal of Physical Medicine and Rehabilitation, 75* (2); 96–104.

Waldon, M. (1996). From head to toe. *Paraplegia News,* February, 15–18.

Hammell, K. R. Whalley (1994). Psychosocial outcomes following spinal cord injury. *Paraplegia, 32,* 771–779.

CHAPTER 23

Nursing Management of the Patient with an Orthopedic Disorder

Mary Jean Kotch

Orthopedic rehabilitation nursing encompasses a variety of conditions and disabilities. This chapter focuses on two chronic orthopedic diseases, osteoarthritis and osteoporosis. Osteoarthritis affects 16 million Americans (Arthritis Foundation, 1997b). Clients with osteoarthritis are seen in rehabilitation settings as a result of functional decline and as a result of pain, either in association with the disease or after arthroplasty. Osteoporosis affects approximately 10 million Americans (Osteoporosis and Related Bone Diseases–National Resource Center [ORBD-NRC], 1998). Clients with vertebral and hip fractures resulting from osteoporosis are often seen in rehabilitation.

The chapter begins with an overview of the etiology, risk factors, and pathophysiology of osteoarthritis. Pharmacological multidisciplinary treatment modalities and surgical interventions are described. Potential complications, and collaborative problems, which are physiologic complications that nurses manage using both nursing and physician-prescribed interventions (Carpenito, 1997), are reviewed. Key nursing diagnoses and interventions are presented. The same approach is used for the presentation of osteoporosis. The reader should understand that some potential complications and collaborative problems as well as nursing diagnoses and interventions can apply to both diseases. The diagnoses and interventions highlight information essential to the practice of rehabilitation nursing. An overview of cultural care in relation to clients' teaching needs, pain, and the therapeutic regimen follows. Finally, discharge planning, home care considerations, and community reintegration issues are presented.

OSTEOARTHRITIS

Overview, Definition, Etiology, Incidence, Risk Factors, and Pathophysiology

Arthritis is a term meaning inflammation of the joint. More than 100 diseases included in the category arthritis affect an estimated 40 million Americans (Arthritis Foundation, 1997b). Arthritis was the leading cause of disability in people older than 15 years in the United States in 1991 to 1992 (U.S. Department of Health and Human Services [USDHHS], 1998).

Osteoarthritis is the most common type of arthritis, accounting for 40% of cases. It is often referred to as *degenerative joint disease* or "wear and tear" arthritis. Osteoarthritis is a condition of synovial joints that causes both breakdown of the cartilage and bony changes, which result in pain and loss of motion. It may be primary or secondary. *Primary* osteoarthritis has no known cause and is referred to as *idiopathic*. The *secondary* type has predisposing factors or causes. It includes generalized, posttraumatic, congenital, neuropathic, and types associated with metabolic or crystal disease (Loeser & Kammer, 1997).

Osteoarthritis commonly affects older adults in the fifth and sixth decades of life, but it should not be considered a normal part of aging. In contrast to rheumatoid arthritis, osteoarthritis is noninflammatory, develops slowly, and affects joints asymmetrically without systemic symptoms. In people younger than 45 years, osteoarthritis is more common in men. After this age, it is more prevalent in women. Risk factors for development of secondary osteoarthritis are as follows:

- Aging
- Obesity
- Joint trauma
- Crystal deposits in cartilage of joint fluid
- Congenital or developmental disorders
- Repetitive joint overuse
- Enhanced bone mineral density
- Prolonged immobility
- Joint hypermobility
- Peripheral neuropathy

The joints most often affected are (1) the cervical and lumbosacral spine, (2) the hip, and (3) the knee. Other common sites are the joints at the bases of the great toe and thumb (Loeser & Kammer, 1997). Osteoarthritis of the hands is more common in women, whereas osteoarthritis in weight-bearing joints and the spine is more common in men (Clyman, 1996). The incidence of osteoarthritis will rise as the elderly population in the United States grows. In addition, rates of disability and of subsequent treatments such as surgery will increase (Lozada & Altman, 1997).

Cartilage acts as a shock absorber between the surfaces of bones. The breakdown of cartilage in osteoarthritis starts with softening and a loss of elasticity (Fig. 23–1). As larger sections wear away, friction on the bones increases. The ends of the bones form growths called *spurs*. *Heberden's nodes* are spurs that develop at the distal finger joints, and *Bouchard's nodes* develop in the middle finger

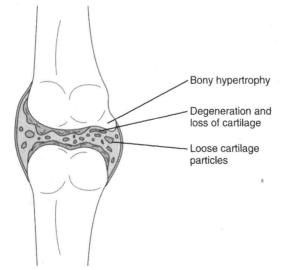

Bony hypertrophy

Degeneration and loss of cartilage

Loose cartilage particles

FIGURE 23–1
Degenerative joint changes. (From Hansen, M. [1998]. *Pathophysiology: Foundations of disease and clinical intervention* [p. 1007]. Philadelphia: W. B. Saunders.)

joints (Arthritis Foundation, 1997b). Synovial fluid can be forced into bone defects and cause cysts.

Deformity, localized pain that worsens with activity, morning stiffness, and loss of joint motion are some of the common symptoms of osteoarthritis. Diagnosis is made from the history, physical findings, and radiographs. Complications of this disease include pain, decreased range of motion, joint contractures, and loss of abilities necessary to remain independent in the activities of daily living (ADLs).

Treatment Modalities

Pharmacological Measures

Medications can control the symptoms of osteoarthritis. They may be administered around the clock or on an "as needed" (prn) basis. A 24-hour, around-the-clock dosing schedule may be more effective in the initial rehabilitation program. Medication provided in this manner can reduce anxiety, pain, and suffering (McCaffrey & Beebe, 1989). The goal of treatment is to prescribe a medication at the lowest possible dose to relieve the symptoms while causing no adverse effects.

Acetaminophen is considered the first choice of treatment. Gastrointestinal side effects are rare. Renal or hepatic toxicity can occur in clients with impaired kidney or liver function. Topical ointments containing capsaicin, an extract from the chili pepper plant, can provide relief.

The most commonly prescribed drugs for osteoarthritis are of the nonsteroidal anti-inflammatory drug (NSAID) category. Lower doses of NSAIDs can be prescribed for treating osteoarthritis than for treating rheumatoid arthritis because inflammation is not usually present in osteoarthritis. Gastritis, peptic ulcers, and bleeding are potential side effects. Misoprostol (Cytotec) may be prescribed to prevent gastrointestinal problems. This synthetic prostaglandin has been shown to be effective in protecting the stomach from the ulcerating effects of NSAIDs and aspirin.

Narcotic analgesics are prescribed for significant pain that has not been relieved by other agents. Tramadol (Ultram), a dual-acting analgesic affecting both opioid and serotonin pathways, is useful in relieving moderate to severe pain. Intraarticular corticosteroids may be used for osteoarthritis, but should be limited to three to four injections per year. Repeated use can cause further cartilage damage. Systemic steroids are not indicated in osteoarthritis. Antispasmodic agents and tricyclic antidepressants are useful to enhance sleep, which is often impaired by pain in the client with arthritis (Lozada & Altman, 1997). The tricyclic antidepressant amitriptyline hydrochloride (Elavil) should not be combined with tramadol; the combination can increase seizure risk in epileptics (Medical Economics, 1997). In addition, amitriptyline hydrochloride should be used with caution in elderly clients (Lozada & Altman, 1997).

Multidisciplinary Measures

Various modalities are used to treat the symptoms of osteoarthritis. Physical therapists, occupational therapists, and nurses are involved in nonpharmacological adjunctive treatments. Although analgesics play a major role in osteoarthritis treatment, a team approach with multiple modalities is most beneficial and is the approach most commonly implemented in the rehabilitation setting.

Thermal modalities are used alone or as part of a medication regimen. The application of heat to affected joints promotes circulation, relaxes muscles, and relieves pain. Hot water bottles, moist or dry heating pads, paraffin treatments, and warm showers or baths can improve symptoms. Ice packs are preferred by some clients to provide pain relief and to decrease inflammation and swelling. Both heat and cold can interrupt the cycle of muscle spasm–pain–muscle spasm. Ultrasound treatments, which can deliver deep heat, may be used by physical and occupational therapists (Lozada & Altman, 1997).

Exercise can assist in maintaining mobility and independence in ADLs. Muscles that are in good condition are less likely to spasm, thereby breaking the spasm-pain cycle. Range-of-motion exercises reduce stiffness and improve flexibility. Both isometric and isotonic exercises strengthen muscles. *Isometric* exercises involve muscle tightening but do not involve movement of the joints. In *isotonic* exercises, joints are moved, and light weights can be added to enhance strengthening. Finally, *endurance (aerobic)* exercises strengthen the cardiovascular and pulmonary systems. Walking, bicycling, and water exercises are forms of endurance exercise. Swimming in warm water cannot only increase strength and endurance but also relieve pain and stiffness (Arthritis Foundation, 1997a). Exercise, performed under the guidance of a physical

therapist and a physiatrist, should be a comprehensive part of the treatment plan.

Transcutaneous electrical nerve stimulation (TENS) may block pain messages as they travel from peripheral sites to the brain. The three components of a TENS unit are the pulse generator, skin electrodes, and cable wires. The small, portable unit sends electrical impulses to nerve endings under the skin. The correct amount of current is ordered by the physician. Physical therapists usually initiate application of the modality and supply the rehabilitation nurse with instructions for electrode placement and electric current settings. The electrodes should be applied only over intact skin. Clients with pacemakers should not use a TENS unit. A week-long trial period of TENS is considered essential to assess the client's response (Shealy, Liss, Kornhauser, and Cannizzaro, 1997). Rehabilitation nurses reapply the unit as directed and monitor the client's response to the TENS unit being used as an intervention to relieve pain.

Relaxation methods, such as guided imagery, prayer, and audio or video tapes, may assist in relieving arthritic pain. The psychologist, utilizing biofeedback, can help the client master the relaxation technique. A biofeedback machine sends out external auditory or visual signals to validate that relaxation is occurring. This serves to familiarize the client with cues that he or she is beginning to relax (Tan, 1998). Psychologists, who are part of the interdisciplinary team, may also be consulted for the client with osteoarthritis who is experiencing chronic pain. Depression is often a component of prolonged pain. Support groups may also play a role in helping clients feel good about themselves. Sharing experiences and information about their disease can assist with coping.

Assistive devices for ADLs, mobility aids, and joint stabilizers are interventions initiated by the physical or occupational therapist. Maintaining proper joint alignment and decreasing stress on painful joints can provide both protection and stability to the joint, thereby decreasing pain (Block & Schnitzer, 1997). Energy conservation techniques can prevent fatigue. The importance of pacing and of planning activities and chores is stressed.

Body weight has been shown to be a factor in the development of osteoarthritis, particularly in the knee. Studies show that weight gain during middle and later years of life can contribute to osteoarthritis (Arthritis Foundation, 1997b). Weight gain and its connection with the development of osteoarthritis in the hip has also been noted, but this association is not as prevalent as that in the knee (Felson, 1996). Weight loss in an overweight client with osteoarthritis will decrease both the pain and the progression of the disease to other joints (National Institute of Arthritis and Musculoskeletal and Skin Diseases [NIAMS], 1998). Counseling with a dietitian is indicated for overweight clients, particularly those planning to undergo arthroplasty in the near future.

Arthroplasty

Description

Arthroplasty is the replacement of a worn or injured joint with a prosthesis made of metal and plastic (Fig. 23–2). Recent advances in alternative surface materials for joint replacement now include ceramic as an option. More than 900,000 hip joint replacements have been performed since this type of surgery began in 1970 (National Institutes of Health [NIH], 1994b). The main indication for arthroplasty is to decrease both pain and disability that have not responded to pharmacological or multidisciplinary treatment modalities. Although joint replacement is a therapeutic intervention for rheumatoid arthritis, more than 70% of knee and hip replacements are performed for osteoarthritis (Felson, 1996). Contraindications to arthroplasty are (1) infection, (2) severe osteoporosis, and (3) uncontrolled medical problems. Clients with obesity and neuropathic joints need to be carefully considered and evaluated because they have higher surgical risks and may not have a satisfactory outcome (Goldberg, 1994). Revision procedures are more difficult to perform and have less successful outcomes (NIH, 1994b).

Three methods of prosthesis fixation used in arthroplasty are (1) cemented, (2) noncemented, and (3) hybrid. The major benefit of a cemented prosthesis is the ability to bear weight as tolerated on the surgical leg immediately after surgery. Also, recovery is quicker for cemented fixation, which is usually the method chosen for older, less active clients. In uncemented fixation, the prosthesis is porous coated. Time is required for bone to grow into the prosthesis. Partial weight bearing is maintained for several weeks if the uncemented method is chosen. Uncemented prostheses have a slightly longer life span, a benefit to younger clients, who may eventually need a revision surgery after the joint surface wears away. Hybrid fixation consists of both cemented fixation and noncemented fixation. In hip replacement with hybrid fixation, the femoral component is cemented and the acetabular component is noncemented; in knee replacement, the tibial component is cemented and the femoral component is noncemented (NIAMS, 1997b).

It is essential for the rehabilitation nurse to understand the weight-bearing status for a client who has undergone arthroplasty. Weight-bearing status is defined in terms of how much of the client's body weight the prosthesis is allowed to bear, as follows (Mont, Tankersley, Mont, & Hungerford, 1997):

> *Non–weight bearing (NWB):* 0% (none) of body weight
> *Toe-touch weight bearing (TTWB):* 20% of body weight
> *Partial weight bearing (PWB):* 20 to 50% of body weight
> *Weight bearing as tolerated (WBAT):* 50 to 100% of body weight
> *Full weight bearing (FWB):* 100% of body weight

Rehabilitation for postarthroplasty clients accounts for a large number of admissions to inpatient rehabilitation settings in the United

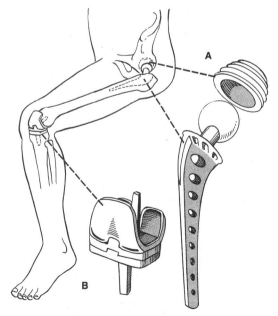

FIGURE 23–2
Total hip and knee replacement. (From Black, J., & Matassarin-Jacobs, E. [Eds.]. [1993]. *Luckmann and Sorensen's medical-surgical nursing* [4th ed., p. 603]. Philadelphia: W. B. Saunders.)

States. In the past, private insurance companies' clients have been noted to receive rehabilitation services less frequently than Medicare and Medicaid recipients (Munin, Kwoh, Glynn, Crosset, & Rubash, 1995). However, changes in Medicare laws may affect the program's reimbursement for rehabilitation services. The growing influence of managed care will also have an impact on inpatient rehabilitation after arthroplasty, in terms of both earlier admission to and earlier discharge from rehabilitation. Community-based rehabilitation in the home or outpatient setting is a new trend.

Research has been conducted to identify the benefits of participation in inpatient rehabilitation programs. Subjects in a study by Munin, Rudy, Glynn, Crossett, and Rubash (1998) consisted of high-risk clients who underwent total hip or knee arthroplasty. Their risks included being elderly, living alone, having comorbid conditions, or having multiple risk factors. The objective of the study was to determine whether admission to rehabilitation at postoperative day 3 versus postoperative day 7 provided a more rapid functional improvement at a lower cost. The data showed that clients who were able to tolerate the early intensive rehabilitation benefited from it. In this and a previous study (Munin et al., 1995), the importance of aggressive pain management in early inpatient rehabilitation was noted. Rehabilitation nurses play an important independent and collaborative role in ensuring that clients' level of comfort is adequate to facilitate positive rehabilitation outcomes.

Procedures

Total Knee Replacement. In 1995 in the United States, 216,000 total knee replacements were performed. The average age of the clients was 68.3 years, and 65.1% of the procedures were performed in women (American Academy of Orthopaedic Surgeons [AAOS], 1998a). Outcomes indicated that 95 to 97% had good to excellent clinical results and 90% continued with success at 10 years. Joint strength and range of motion are usually achieved by 3 months, and full benefit of the knee replacement surgery is realized at about 1 year postoperatively. Outcomes of total knee replacement can be influenced by both the condition of the knee before surgery and the motivation of the client to participate in rehabilitation (Tankersley et al., 1997).

Hip Replacement. Hip replacement surgery is one of the most successful orthopedic procedures. Total hip replacement resurfaces both the acetabulum and the femoral head with prostheses, whereas a hemiarthroplasty replaces only the femoral head. In 1995, 134,000 hip arthroplasties were performed in the United States. The average age of the client was 67 years, and 59.9% of the procedures were performed in women (AAOS, 1998a). Outcomes indicated that 95% of clients had excellent clinical results at 1 year and that the success rate was 90% at 10 years. Joint strength and range of movement are usually regained by 3 months, and full benefit of the procedure is realized at 1 year postoperatively (Mont et al., 1997). Poorer outcomes are clearly related to comorbid diseases rather than age (NIH, 1994b).

Potential Complications and Collaborative Problems

Deep Vein Thrombosis. Development of deep vein thrombosis is a risk of surgery. Clients undergoing hip surgery and knee reconstruction have a 45 to 70% risk of this complication (NIH, 1986). Venous thromboembolism occurs in at least 50% of hip surgery clients who are not protected by anticoagulation (Spiegel, 1997). Hereditary risk factors contributing to the development of deep vein thrombosis constitute problems and deficiencies related to coagulation. Acquired risk factors are (1) increased age, (2) immobilization, (3) obesity, (4) prior thromboembolism, (5) cancer, (6) heart failure, (7) myocardial infarction, (8) sepsis, and (9) oral contraception.

Clients at high risk for deep vein thrombosis should receive low-dose warfarin (Coumadin), dextran, or adjusted-dose heparin for 7 days. If the client is immobile, anticoagulant therapy should continue for longer (NIH, 1986). With warfarin use, the International Normalized Ratio (INR) must be closely monitored and kept in the 2.0 to 3.0 range. INR is the standard reporting of prothrombin time. Hematoma formation from anticoagulation treatment carries a higher risk of infection. The American College of Chest Physicians (cited in Clagett, Anderson, & Heit, 1995) recommends a minimum of 7 to 10 days of anticoagulant prophylaxis for patients undergoing elective total hip or knee replacement. Low-molecular-weight heparin (enoxaparin, Lovenox) in a dose of 30 mg subcutaneously twice daily can be used in high-risk patients for 7 to 14 days. Aspirin has not been shown to be effective compared with other treatments. Regardless of the length of hospitalization, the risk for development of deep vein thrombosis can persist for at least 2 months after total hip or knee replacement (Tan, 1998).

An admission nursing assessment should include identification of risk factors to alert health care professionals to a client's predisposition to deep vein thrombosis. Symptoms of a lower extremity deep vein thrombosis include (1) edema of the leg and foot, (2) tenderness of the calf, (3) pain in the posterior thigh or popliteal area, (4) low-grade fever, and (5) cramping pain on ambulation. A positive Homans' sign is pain associated with dorsiflexion of the foot; some sources discourage the performance of the check for Homans' sign because it could dislodge a thrombus. Fifty to 90% of cases of deep vein thrombosis are undetected by physical examination (Tan, 1998).

Interventions that can reduce the incidence of deep vein thrombosis are elevation of the foot of the bed and use of pneumatic compression (NIH, 1986). Intermittent pneumatic leg compression can be used in high-risk clients in the rehabilitation setting for whom anticoagulation is contraindicated. Early ambulation, active and passive range-of-motion exercises, adequate hydration, and avoiding the use of the knee gatch on hospital beds are other nursing interventions (Carroll, 1993). The effectiveness of thromboembolitic disease stockings (TED) is controversial; however, they are reportedly more effective than elastic bandage (Ace) wraps (Tan, 1998). TED stocking may be of use in low-risk patients. Proper size, fit, and application are essential. The stockings should be applied in the morning before the client gets out of bed. Stockings should be routinely removed to check skin integrity. Elastic bandage wraps are an alternative, but their proper application is critical to provide the correct amount of compression.

Baseline measurements of the calf and ankle circumference are important to the detection of deep vein thrombosis. Clients and family members should be instructed about both the signs and symtoms of this complication and the need to promptly report them. If signs or symptoms occur, the physician must evaluate the situation. The rehabilitation nurse should monitor the size and temperature of the calf. If a deep vein thrombosis is suspected, it is important to limit self-care activities; apply warm, moist compresses; and monitor the INR values (Tucker, Cannobbio, Paquette, & Wells, 1996).

Clients started on anticoagulant therapy must be instructed about precautions, food and drug interactions, and the need for routine blood tests. Outcomes of interventions should be the prevention of the development of both deep vein thrombosis and pulmonary embolism (see later).

Because deep vein thrombosis and pulmonary embolism are serious medical complications for inpatient rehabilitation clients, studies have been conducted to identify the usefulness of screening procedures in asymptomatic clients. A noninvasive test that has been used in the rehabilitation setting is impedance plethysmography (IPG). It is considered to be cost-effective and safe. Katz and McCulla (1995) conducted a study of this test in 483 rehabilitation clients with varying diagnoses. IPG was conducted within several days after admission in each client. Routine use of this test, however, showed that it had poor value as a screening tool for deep vein thrombosis in asymptomatic clients undergoing inpatient rehabilitation. Additional conclusions were that anticoagulant prophylaxis is a better prevention method and that duplex ultrasonography is a better assessment tool.

Anticoagulation treatment for confirmed deep vein thrombosis should continue for 3 months or more. The most serious result of this complication is pulmonary embolism (see later). A delayed complication of deep vein thrombosis is postphlebitic syndrome. Persistent leg swelling, pain associated with exercise, and skin ulcerations are problems associated with this syndrome.

Pulmonary Embolism. A *pulmonary embolus* is a clot that travels to and obstructs the pulmonary artery or its branches. The incidence of pulmonary embolism is 20% in patients undergoing hip surgery and lower in those receiving knee replacement (NIH, 1986). The period of highest risk for pulmonary embolism after hip replacement is the 2 to 3 weeks after surgery, during which time 70% of cases occur (Spiegel, 1997). When it occurs it is usually 24 to 72 hours postoperatively.

Risk factors for the development of this complication are the same as for deep vein thrombosis. As with deep vein thrombosis, almost 50% of cases of pulmonary embolism are asymptomatic. Clients with submassive pulmonary embolism may have symptoms such as tachycardia, tachypnea, hemoptysis, dyspnea, rales, cough, pleuritic chest pain, fever, and malaise. Massive pulmonary embolism has a sudden onset of the preceding symptoms along with cyanosis, restlessness, agitation, apprehension, and jugular vein distention. Arterial blood gas levels may show a decrease in oxygen, but this measurement can be used only as a screening test. A ventilation-perfusion ($\dot{V}/\dot{Q}$) scan is more sensitive than a chest radiograph in detecting pulmonary embolism. In any setting, pulmonary embolism is an emergency; 20% of the cases that cause clinical symptoms are fatal. Death can occur within 30 minutes of a massive pulmonary embolism (Tan, 1998).

Thrombolytic agents (streptokinase, tissue plasminogen activator, and urokinase) can be used when the diagnosis is definite. Inferior vena cava filters, such as the Greenfield filter, can be inserted percutaneously to trap emboli before they enter the pulmonary circulation. Such filters do not, however, prevent deep vein thrombosis. Anticoagulant treatment for confirmed pulmonary embolism should continue for 3 months or more (Tan, 1998).

In the event of symptoms of pulmonary embolism, the nurse must remain with the client and monitor vital signs, level of consciousness, pain, dyspnea, tachypnea, neck vein distention, and hemoptysis. A semi-Fowler's position and oxygen therapy ensure adequate oxygenation. Emotional support and pain management are appropriate interventions until the patient can be transferred to an acute care setting. The outcome of nursing interventions performed for the collaborative problem of pulmonary embolism should be to manage and minimize the complications of embolism (Carpenito, 1997).

Infection. The most serious complication of arthroplasty is infection. Incidence of infection after hip replacement is estimated to be 1% (Apley & Solomon, 1993). Prevention is the best approach to this potential problem, which can progress to systemic infection, removal of the prosthetic hip, or amputation (Nasser, 1992).

Classification. Stages of infection have been classified on the basis of the interval since arthroplasty and the cause.

Stage I infection occurs postoperatively. The cause can be a superficial wound infection or hematoma formation. Signs are fever, increased pain, incisional drainage, inflammation, and elevations in white blood cell count and erythrocyte sedimentation rate.

Stage II infection can occur 6 to 24 months postoperatively and is more difficult to diagnose. Return of pain to the operative site may be the only symptom; however, this symptom may also represent loosening of the prosthesis.

Stage III infection occurs 2 years or more postoperatively. Diagnosis at this stage is easier because symptoms are usually associated with dental procedures, surgical procedures, or infection of the urinary, respiratory, or gastrointestinal tract (Fitzgerald, 1992; Fitzgerald, Nolan, & Ilstrup, 1977).

Causes. Infection can begin at the time of surgery as a result of contamination either by airborne bacteria in the operating room or by skin flora. Hematoma formation, secondary to anticoagulant therapy, can contribute to infection. The urinary and gastrointestinal tracts, oral cavity, and skin can be sources of infection that spreads to the arthroplasty site via the blood or lymphatic system (Hanssen, Osmon, & Nelson, 1996).

Risk factors. Clients with a history of type 1 diabetes, previous prosthetic joint infection, poor nutrition, or hemophilia are at higher risk for infection. The development of hematogenous total joint infection is increased when risk factors of an immune system compromised by inflammatory arthropathies, rheumatoid arthritis, systemic lupus erythematosus, or radiation treatments are present. The critical period for development of infection is the first 2 years after arthroplasty (American Dental Association & American Academy of Orthopaedic Surgeons, 1997). Revision of total joint replacement imposes a higher risk of infection because of both the longer operating time and the larger surgical exposure (Nasser, 1992).

Prevention. Prior to arthroplasty, a preoperative physical examination should be performed, with special attention paid to the general skin condition. A dental examination and any necessary treatment should be completed before arthroplasty. In addition, clients in whom urinalysis revealed presence of infection should be treated with the appropriate antibiotic. Routine parenteral administration of antibiotics immediately preoperatively and for 48 hours postoperatively is advised. Indwelling Foley catheters should be removed as soon as possible to avoid infection. If either the Foley catheter remains in place for more than a few days or wound drainage continues, appropriate antibiotics should be prescribed (Nasser, 1992).

A joint advisory statement issued by the American Dental Association and the American Academy of Orthopaedic Surgeons (1997) provides guidelines for practitioners treating clients who have had arthroplasty and now require dental treatment or dental surgical procedures. Routine antibiotic therapy is not indicated for most such clients. For high-risk clients, identified earlier, administration of antibiotics 1 hour before dental procedures is recommended. Stratification of dental procedures with high and low incidence of bacteremia is included in the advisory statement to guide decision making regarding antibiotic prophylaxis.

Routine antibiotic prophylaxis is controversial and may contribute to bacterial resistance. Infection with vancomycin-resistant enterococci has occurred in orthopedic clients with prosthetic joints (Morris, Shay, Hebden, McCarter, Perdue, Jarvis, Johnson, Dowling, Polish, & Schwalbe, 1995). The Centers for Disease Control and Prevention reports increases in the occurrence of these organisms. The American Academy of Orthopaedic Surgeons (1998b) issued an advisory statement related to the use of prophylactic antibiotics in orthopedic medicine for vancomycin-resistant organisms, including enterococci, *Staphylococcus epidermidis*, and *Staphylococcus aureus*. Recommendations include reducing both the use of vancomycin and the spread of staphylococci and enterococci. Hand washing with antibacterial soaps and contact isolation of clients infected with vancomycin-resistant organisms are two key interventions recommended. *Contact isolation* involves (1) the use of sterile gowns and gloves, (2) placement of the client in a private room, and (3) limited movement of the client out of the room. The latter component of contact isolation raises issues in the rehabilitation setting because the environmental design is open and interactive.

Nursing interventions related to infection include monitoring joint temperature and checking for swelling, pain, and drainage at the surgical site. Sterile technique with dressing changes should be maintained until healing is complete. If a Foley catheter remains in place for several days, monitoring the character of urinary output and encouraging adequate fluid intake are essential. Collaboration with the physician is essential if signs and symptoms of infection either at the surgical site or elsewhere are noted.

Because of the controversy that exists regarding antibiotic prophylaxis and treatment of potential or actual infections, signs and symptoms of infections need to be reviewed with the client so they can be reported to the physician. All clients also should be taught that they must alert dentists and physicians caring for them that they have a joint prosthesis.

Dislocation. Hip dislocation is the most common early complication of hip replacement. The incidence of hip dislocation is about 2% after arthroplasty, with the greatest possibility of occurrence in the first 8 weeks postoperatively (Altizer, 1998). It occurs when the articular surfaces are completely separated. The components of a prosthesis are slightly smaller than the client's bones, and this difference contributes to the risk (NIAMS, 1997b). Treatment involves either a manual closed reduction or, possibly, surgical reduction (Morrey, 1992). After surgical correction, the client may wear an abduction brace for a period of time specified by the physician to limit hip movement.

Two surgical approaches are used in hip arthroplasty, anterior and posterior. Positioning precautions to prevent dislocation differ for the type of approach used. After an *anterior* approach, the client's operated leg should be turned slightly inward to decrease pressure on the head of the femur against the anterior joint capsule. An abductor wedge (Fig. 23–3) or pillow is placed between the legs, and a trochanter roll is positioned along the outside of the affected femur (Dunajcik, 1989). After a *posterior* approach, the legs should be kept spread, and the operated leg should be turned slightly outward. An abductor wedge or pillow is used between the legs, but a trochanter roll is not used (Dunajcik, 1989).

The client may lie on the unoperated side, but this positioning requires the use of an abductor wedge. Lying on the operated hip is allowed when the surgeon approves. Clients should continue to use the abductor wedge or pillow when in bed for 6 to 12 weeks postoperatively. After this time, a pseudocapsule surrounds the hip joint, and improved muscle strength provides stability (Mont et al., 1997).

Hip flexion greater than 90 degrees is not permitted because it exerts pressure on the posterior capsule. Also, the operated leg should not cross the midline or roll inward (Fig. 23–4) (Altizer, 1998). Total hip precautions should be followed for at least 12 weeks

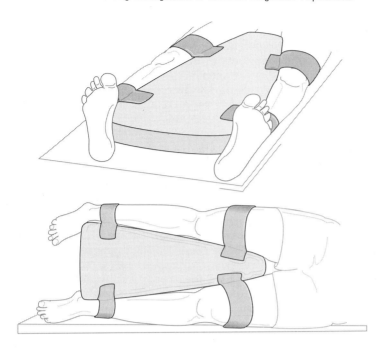

FIGURE 23–3
Abductor pillow/wedge with positioning. (Redrawn from illustration provided courtesy of A. Kotch, copyright 1998.)

or longer, according to the recommendation of the orthopedic surgeon. After that time, the incidence of dislocation of the hip is reduced by 95% (Mont et al., 1997).

Symptoms of a hip dislocation are (1) pain, (2) change in the position or length of the leg, (3) neurovascular impairments, (4) a popping sound, (5) acute groin pain, (6) bulge at the hip, and (7) inability to move the leg (Carpenito, 1997). Figure 23–5 shows the differences in the signs and symptoms of anterior and posterior dislocations. In anterior dislocations, which are rare, the knee is flexed and the leg turns outward. In the more common posterior dislocation, the leg turns inward and appears shorter than the other leg, and the femoral head is prominent (Dunajcik, 1989). Anterior dislocation may cause femoral nerve injury, whereas posterior dislocation may cause sciatic nerve injury (Spiegel, 1997).

Knee Dislocation. Little information is available on dislocation after total knee replacement, but shifts in position of the prosthesis are more common in the uncemented type of fixation (Dood, Hungerford, & Krackow, 1990). The knee should be kept in a neutral position, with the degree of flexion as ordered by the physician.

Nursing interventions for dislocation are preventive. Proper positioning and assessment for signs of dislocation are key (Carpenito, 1997). Clients must be educated about proper positioning, and interdisciplinary

team members should reinforce precautions through pictures, demonstrations, and reminders. Crossing the legs, having the knees higher than the hips, rolling the operated leg inward, bending at the waist, and positioning the ankles and knees too close together are to be avoided in total hip replacement.

Kneeling and deep knee bends should be avoided after total knee replacement (Altizer, 1998).

Signs of dislocation and the importance of seeking prompt medical attention should be included in client and family teaching. If signs of a dislocation are noted in the rehabilitation setting, the patient should be kept immobile until he or she is seen by the physician and the dislocation is either confirmed or ruled out by a radiograph.

Loosening. Loosening of the prosthesis is the most common cause of failure after total hip replacement. Young, active, or obese patients are at higher risk for its development (Mont et al., 1997). Loosening can occur at either the cement-to-bone location or the cement-to-prosthesis location. Small pieces of cement wear off the joint surfaces, beginning an inflammatory response. Osteolysis and loosening of the implant follow. New thigh or groin pain that is worse with transfers is a sign of loosening (Spiegel, 1997).

Loosening is usually a later problem and may be the reason for eventual failure of the prosthesis. Treatments include anti-inflam-

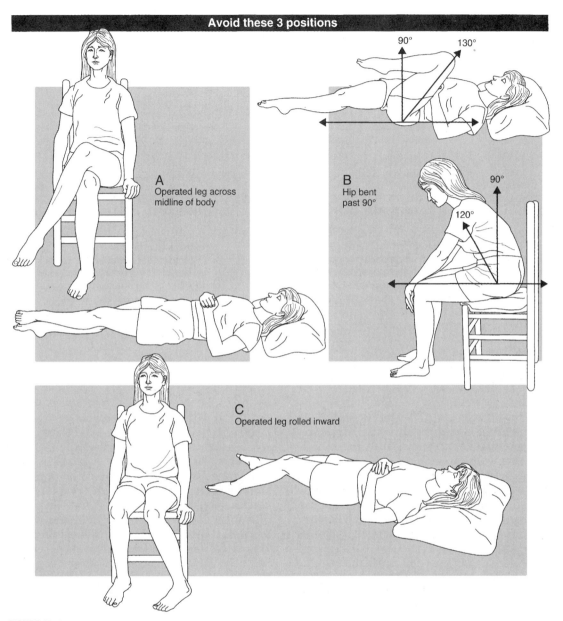

Avoid these 3 positions

A
Operated leg across
midline of body

B
Hip bent
past 90°

C
Operated leg rolled inward

FIGURE 23–4
Rules to follow after total hip arthroplasty. (From Altizer, L. [1998]. Degenerative disorders. In A. Maher, S. Salmond, & T. Pellino [Eds.], *Orthopaedic nursing* [2nd ed., p. 500]. Philadelphia: W. B. Saunders.)

matory medications, revision surgery, and replacement surgery (NIAMS, 1997b). Polyethylene prosthetic material may be the source of the wear particle. Use of alternative surface materials of prostheses such as ceramics may decrease the incidence of loosening of joint prostheses (Goldberg, 1994).

Nursing interventions for loosening of the prosthesis include provision of comfort measures and pain management. The client should be instructed to report to the physi-

cian any increase or change in pain after arthroplasty.

Neurovascular Impairment. Nerves and blood vessels can be damaged by fractures or orthopedic surgery. Clients who have undergone orthopedic surgery require neurovascular monitoring. Neurovascular assessment should be performed by the rehabilitation nurse during admission assessment and then daily.

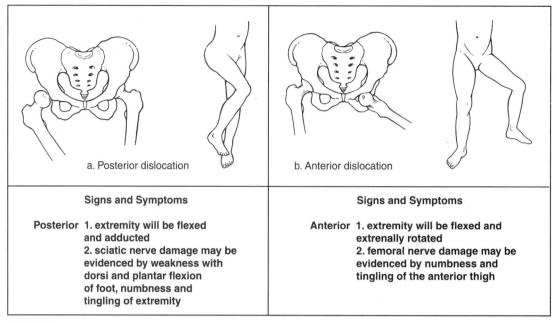

a. Posterior dislocation	b. Anterior dislocation
Signs and Symptoms	**Signs and Symptoms**
Posterior 1. extremity will be flexed and adducted 2. sciatic nerve damage may be evidenced by weakness with dorsi and plantar flexion of foot, numbness and tingling of extremity	**Anterior 1. extremity will be flexed and extrenally rotated 2. femoral nerve damage may be evidenced by numbness and tingling of the anterior thigh**

FIGURE 23–5
Signs and symptoms of posterior *(A)* and anterior *(B)* hip dislocation. (Reprinted with permission from Slye, Debra Anne, and Theis, Luann M. [1981]. p. 61. *An introduction to orthopaedic nursing: an orientation module.* Pitman, N. J.: National Association of Orthopaedic Nurses.)

Vascular Assessment. Peripheral vascular assessment involves observing the extremity for color, temperature, capillary refill, edema, and pulses. A normal inspection shows a pink color, warm temperature, 1- to 2-second capillary refill time, and full turgor. A pale appearance indicates poor arterial supply, whereas a dusky, mottled, or blue appearance signifies poor venous return.

Temperature is best felt with the back of the hand or fingertips placed on the operated leg and compared with the unoperated leg. Cool temperature indicates poor arterial supply, and heat may signify venous congestion. Capillary refill should occur in less than 2 to 3 seconds. It is tested by squeezing a nail bed for 2 to 3 seconds, at which time it should blanch, and then monitoring the time it takes for the color to return. Less than normal time to refill indicates poor venous return, and longer time indicates poor arterial supply (Kunkler, 1991).

Peripheral pulse checks should be monitored in clients who have undergone total knee or hip replacement. The best position for the femoral pulse check is with the client lying in bed. Femoral pulses, located in the groin, should be checked simultaneously. Popliteal pulses, located on the backs of the knees, are more difficult to check. Slight flexion of the client's knee and the use of both of the examiner's hands to feel the pulse is helpful; each limb is checked separately, with firm pressure. Injury to femoral or popliteal blood vessels can occur during total knee replacement but is rare (Rand, 1993). The posterior tibial pulse is located behind and above the ankle (Fig. 23–6). The dorsalis pedis pulse is near the top of the foot, above the second and third digits; however, it is absent in about 10% of people (Schoen, 1986). Use of a standard key for grading pulse amplitude is essential. One such key rates pulse amplitude from 0 through 4 as follows (Swartz, 1994):

0 = Absent
1 = Diminished
2 = Normal
3 = Increased
4 = Bounding

Some edema in the operated leg and foot is common after surgery, but it must be monitored, and the skin integrity must be checked. Antiembolism stockings and exercises such as ankle pumps can help decrease edema. Scheduling periodic rest periods with the legs elevated or raising the leg rests slightly on the wheelchair can also minimize edema.

Neurological Assessment. Peripheral neuro-

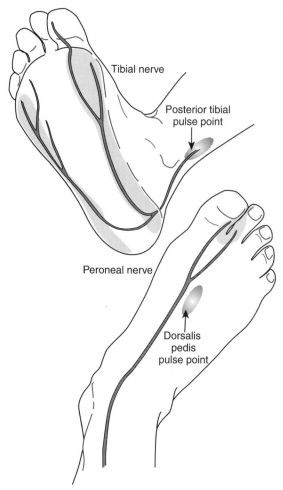

FIGURE 23–6
Peripheral vascular and sensory assessment. (Redrawn from illustration provided courtesy of A. Kotch, copyright 1998.)

logical assessment involves sensation, motor function, and pain. For tests of sensation, the client closes the eyes; then the examiner lightly touches the extremity and asks the client where he or she feels pressure. Neural injury can occur after hip arthroplasty but is not common. It is caused by compression from retractors or from a hematoma. The peripheral nerves most commonly damaged after total hip replacement are the sciatic and peroneal nerves. Damage to both nerves is more common during revision surgery, after dislocation, and with hematoma formation (Wasilewski, Crossett, & Rubash, 1992).

Peroneal palsy is infrequent but can be associated with total knee replacement; its frequency is increased in revision procedures (Rand, 1993). It can occur when the use of a

continuous passive motion (CPM) machine causes pressure on the peroneal nerve at the fibular neck (James & Wade, 1991). Motor function of the peroneal and tibial nerves should be tested. Because injury to the peroneal nerve can cause footdrop, assessment of dorsiflexion of the foot can be used to check for nerve damage. Tibial nerve damage is evident by the inability to plantar flex or to flex and extend the toes.

Femoral compressive neuropathy can be caused by either hemorrhage from anticoagulant therapy or heat produced by cement during total hip replacement. A rehabilitation client who experiences sudden pain in the groin or thigh may have bleeding into the retroperitoneal space because of anticoagulant therapy. Femoral neuropathy can occur in this situation (Spiegel, 1997).

Finally, the presence of pain should be assessed by all interdisciplinary team members using a standard pain scale. Pain that either resumes after being controlled or increases with ambulation or passive stretching should be reported to the physician.

Nursing Diagnoses and Interventions

Alteration in Comfort

Alteration in comfort is a common nursing diagnosis in rehabilitation. It can be related to a chronic musculoskeletal disorder such as osteoarthritis or to an acute event such as arthroplasty or fracture. In arthritis, pain and discomfort can be due to inflammation of tendons and ligaments or to fatigue and muscle strain. The pain experience is variable and individual (NIAMS, 1998).

The first step in successful nursing interventions is to assess the pain and discomfort, including its characteristics and source. Factors that decrease pain tolerance, such as fatigue, should be identified and addressed. Depression, which is common in clients with chronic pain and arthritis, can increase the perception of pain. Energy conservation and pacing of activities are helpful interventions to prevent fatigue and should be taught to the client and incorporated into the rehabilitation program.

Collaboration between the client and the interdisciplinary team members is essential to identify methods of improving comfort. The use of heat or ice may be of benefit. If the source of discomfort is exercise in physical therapy, administering pain medication about

1 hour before therapy may be an effective intervention. Prevention of pain is the best approach. Educating the client regarding his or her role in both requesting "as needed" pain medication and taking it before the pain becomes severe is an important part of this process.

Clients with arthritis have chronic pain. The desired outcome of interventions for such clients is to manage their pain and increase their functional mobility and independence in ADLs. Discussion with both the client and the family is essential, because the client's chronic pain has effects on all of them. The chronic pain cycle can begin because of ineffective pain management. Depression, fatigue, inactivity, increased pain, spasm, and more pain can ensue. The inactivity will decrease strength and endurance. Spasm due to anxiety will increase pain.

Chronic pain syndrome, which is persistent pain that has an organic cause but also has a host of psychological, social, and behavior problems, can occur (Patil, 1997). It is essential to discuss with the client the methods suggested to relieve the pain, because issues such as cost, complexity, and convenience affect the client's compliance with the pain management program after discharge.

Pain after arthroplasty is most severe during the first 2 days. The arthritic component of the pain is almost completely relieved soon after surgery. The surgical component of the pain lasts about 2 to 3 weeks (Mont et al., 1997). Acute pain management in the orthopedic patient involves several principles; they are (1) establishing a therapeutic relationship with the client, (2) realizing that unrelieved pain can have negative physical and psychological consequences, and (3) understanding that prevention of pain is better than treatment. Around-the-clock dosing is preferred to maintain adequate blood levels of analgesics. Opioid analgesics are usually recommended for severe postoperative pain. NSAIDs have an opioid dose–sparing effect and have a role in pain management after surgery (USDHHS, 1992). Multidisciplinary measures, as discussed earlier, can be used for acute and chronic pain.

Ongoing assessment of the success of the modality chosen for pain relief is critical to effective pain management. It is important to remember that pain is a subjective experience—pain is what the client says it is. A standard pain scale, used by all involved disciplines in the rehabilitation setting, is necessary to accurately assess both the pain and

the effectiveness of the interventions. A standard pain diary may be useful to the client and rehabilitation nurse in identifying pain patterns and allowing the client to be an active participant in the plan. Involving clients in the pain management plan will empower them to take an active role.

Pain assessment in the elderly presents a challenge, for several reasons. Health care professionals often believe that aging increases tolerance to pain. Older clients may think that pain cannot be relieved and therefore underreport it. Also, cognitive and sensory impairments can interfere with the use of pain scales (USDHHS, 1992). Pain cues, such as behaviors, sounds, and appearance, may help the nurse determine whether the client is uncomfortable. Aggressiveness, restlessness, moaning, screaming, wincing, tenseness, insomnia, and resistance to care and eating are some ways that pain can be expressed. In addition, knowing a client's usual pattern of response to pain is beneficial (Parke, 1998). This information is easier for a nurse or caregiver who truly knows the client to recognize.

Because many patients with arthritis and joint replacements are elderly, proper medication choices and dosing are essential. The decline in renal and liver function with age may cause medications to have a stronger, longer-acting effect in the elderly patient. Careful monitoring for both therapeutic and side effects is important (Novy & Jagmin, 1997). The prevalence of polypharmacy in the elderly needs to be addressed.

In the rehabilitation setting, a variety of modalities can be used for pain. Because pain is multidimensional, it is best approached with various modalities according to the nature of the pain and the client's preferences. Outcomes of effective pain management are that the client (1) verbalizes comfort and relief of pain and (2) participates in the rehabilitation program.

Impaired Physical Mobility

Impaired physical mobility can be related to fatigue, pain, motivation, and musculoskeletal problems as well as poor strength, endurance, balance, and muscle tone. An assessment of the impairment determines the severity of the functional mobility problems.

Four aspects of mobility significant to rehabilitation nursing are bed mobility, transfers, wheelchair mobility, and ambulation, which can be regarded as occurring in four stages.

Stage I is bed mobility. It is the most basic form of mobility, involving activities such as turning from side to side, lifting the hips, and moving up in bed. It may be accomplished independently or with aids such as a trapeze. *Stage II*, transfers, involves the ability to move from the wheelchair to the bed, toilet, chair, bathing bench, and motor vehicle seat. The transfers can be accomplished independently or with partial assistance from either a helper or a sliding board. *Stage III*, wheelchair mobility, can be manually or electrically managed. *Stage IV*, ambulation, can be accomplished with devices such as crutches, canes, walkers, prostheses, and orthoses (McCourt, 1993).

Another way to describe problems with mobility in the rehabilitation setting is the level of assistance required. *Level I* mobility is accomplished with the use of a device or equipment only. *Level II* mobility is achieved with help from a person in the form of hands-on assistance, supervision, or teaching. *Level III* mobility requires the assistance of both a person and equipment. *Level IV* is dependent and the client does not participate in movement (Mumma, 1987).

The Functional Independence Measure (FIM) is the most widely used functional assessment tool. Eighteen items are assessed in the FIM scale, including the motor areas of transfers and locomotion. A seven-level number scale describes the type and amount of assistance required by subject. The assistance can be in the form of a person or assistive device. Levels of function and score are as follows:

1 = Total assistance (subject = 0%)
2 = Maximal assistance (subject = 25% +)
3 = Moderate assistance (subject = 50% +)
4 = Minimal assistance (subject = 75% +)
5 = Supervision or setup (no assist from person)
6 = Modified independence (assistive device used)
7 = Complete independence (timely, safe)

The FIM scale is frequently used to measure outcomes of rehabilitation (Deutsch, Braun, & Granger, 1997).

The client who has undergone hip or knee arthroplasty with a cemented prosthesis is usually allowed immediate weight bearing as tolerated, with the use of a walker for at least 6 weeks, beginning on postoperative day 1. Clients who have undergone noncemented (ingrowth) or hybrid-fixation arthroplasty are usually held to toe-touch weight-bearing status with use of a walker for 6 to 8 weeks

postoperatively. Progression to crutch or cane walking is permitted after 6 weeks, when the client's status is weight bearing as tolerated (Cameron, Brotzman, & Boolos, 1996). By 3 months after arthroplasty, 70% of clients are ambulating without an assistive device (Tankersley et al., 1997; Mont et al., 1997).

Traveling up and down stairs is possible with the use of a crutch or cane. Use of the saying "Up with the good, and down with the bad" or "The good go to heaven and the bad go to hell" often helps clients remember the correct sequences for ascending and descending stairs after surgery (Cameron et al., 1996). The correct procedure for ascending stairs is as follows:

1. Take the first step up with the unoperated ("good") leg.
2. Keeping the crutches on the level below, bring the operated ("bad") leg up onto the step.
3. Bring both crutches up onto the step.
4. Repeat the process for the next step.

Going down the stairs, the client proceeds as follows:

1. Place the crutches down on the step below.
2. Step down to that step with the operated ("bad") leg.
3. Bring down the unoperated leg.
4. Repeat the process for the next step.

Although controversy exists regarding its use after total knee replacement, the CPM machine (Fig. 23–7) is often used in the acute care, rehabilitation, and home settings for clients who have undergone total knee arthroplasty (Cameron et al., 1996). The goal for range of motion after knee arthroplasty is 105 to 110 degrees. The inpatient rehabilitation goal at 2 weeks after surgery is that the client is achieving 90 degrees of range of motion in the knee. Some studies, including one reported by Pope, Corcoran, McCaul, and Howie (1997), indicate that range of motion is initially achieved more rapidly with the use of CPM but that there are no significant differences 1 year later between clients who did and did not use a CPM. Table 23–1 outlines benefits and disadvantages of the use of CPM. Its use is contraindicated in clients who have diabetes or are taking steroids, because they are at higher risk for poor wound healing (Cameron et al., 1996). In addition, a CPM machine should not be used in clients with unstable fractures and wound dehiscence (Addamo & Abba Clough, 1998).

CPM is an adjunct to an exercise program

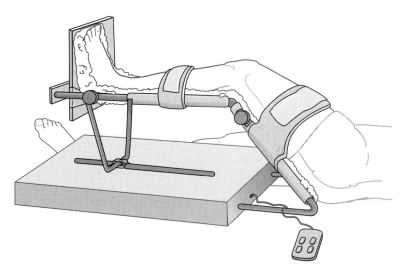

FIGURE 23–7
Continuous passive motion machine. (Redrawn from illustration provided courtesy of A. Kotch, copyright 1998.)

(Tan, 1998). It is generally believed to increase flexion and decrease the necessity of manipulation. If, at 2 weeks after knee arthroplasty, the client has not achieved at least 70 degrees of flexion, manipulation by the orthopedic surgeon is usually attempted (Tankersley et al., 1997).

TABLE 23–1 ▪ **POTENTIAL ADVANTAGES AND DISADVANTAGES OF CONTINUOUS PASSIVE MOTION (CPM)**

Advantages	Disadvantages
Decrease in disuse atrophy	Cost: health care provider and purchase or rental of the device
Decrease in capsular contractures	
Maintenance of articular cartilage	Increased postoperative drainage of total knee arthroplasty suture line
Aids in nutrition of involved tissues	Patient's activity is restricted during CPM use
Early, continuous mobilization to enhance healing and tissue remodeling	
Decrease in joint effusions and associated pain	
Decrease in joint hemarthrosis	
Reduction in the amount of time required to attain range-of-motion goals	
Decreases total knee arthroplasty postoperative hospitalization	
Reduction in the incidence of postoperative knee manipulation	

From Addamo, S., & Abba Clough, J. (1998). Modalities for mobilization. In A. Maher, S. Salmond, & T. Pellino T (Eds.), *Orthopaedic nursing* (2nd ed., pp. 323–350). Philadelphia: W. B. Saunders.

Before use of the CPM machine can be initiated, a physician's order that indicates specifics as to the degree of flexion, degree progressions, and the number of hours of therapy is required. Rehabilitation nurses are often responsible for initially setting up the machine, instructing client's about its operation, and assessing the client's ability to use the hand control. Additionally, the nurse monitors a client's response to the CPM exercise and keeps the physician informed of any difficulties with tolerance or poor progress in increasing the degree of flexion.

Proper positioning in the CPM machine is important. The knee should be in the center of the CPM frame, with the foot against the plate. Sheepskin padding lines the machine. Hook-and-loop material (Velcro) straps secure the leg in the machine, and they should not interfere with the gears. It is essential that there be no external rotation of the lower leg or undue pressure from the strap while the leg is in the machine; either condition could cause peroneal nerve damage.

Clients who have undergone total hip replacement have additional precautions related to mobility, as discussed earlier along with the potential complication of dislocation. Weight-bearing status, along with the total hip precautions shown in Figure 23–4, needs to be emphasized. Selection of an assistive mobility device depends on the weight-bearing status. The angle of movement of the operated leg should be no greater than 90 degrees.

Selection of chairs is also critical. A helpful way to explain the selection of a chair to a client is to say that the seat of the chair should be at the level of the back of the knees or higher, so that the angle of the operated leg remains within the hip precautions when the client is seated. Getting out of the chair is easier if it has arms to push down on. Use of a wheelchair cushion or pillow in a chair may be necessary for added seat height. Twisting movements, common in vacuuming and filling a dishwasher, for instance, are prohibited. Seat height and avoidance of twisting movements are essential to remember during car transfers. The client's mobility in bed will be limited because of the use of the abductor wedge or "pillow" for several weeks postoperatively. Positioning on the unoperated side is possible, but the client will need help assuming this position while the abductor wedge is being used.

Nursing interventions include promoting optimal mobility and movement through active or passive range-of-motion exercises. Active range of motion is achieved by the client independently, whereas passive range-of-motion exercises are performed by a helper (Carpenito, 1997). Other interventions related to impaired mobility involve monitoring for deep vein thrombosis, pneumonia, skin, and elimination problems. Gradually increasing activities and providing a balance of rest and exercise are two principles to reinforce. Outcomes of nursing interventions for the client with impaired mobility are for the client to (1) regain an optimal level of mobility, (2) participate in the rehabilitation program, (3) verbalize restrictions, and (4) seek assistance when needed (Tucker et al., 1996).

Self-Care Deficit

Self-care deficits related to activity intolerance, pain, and musculoskeletal impairment are seen in the rehabilitation client. Difficulties with ADLs, such as dressing, grooming, toileting, and bathing, are included in this deficit. In the inpatient rehabilitation setting, addressing self-care skills is largely the responsibility of both occupational therapists and nurses. The areas to assess include the client's abilities, energy, and safety, all of which are related to accomplishing the tasks. Adaptive devices are issued as needed. Pacing, planning, and protection are techniques taught in occupational therapy and reinforced by rehabilitation nurses. *Pacing* involves resting frequently and spreading out the tasks of the day. *Planning* consists of limiting the number of strenuous activities, such as shopping trips and visits to the doctor, to one per day. Protection involves doing certain tasks

differently to avoid putting excess stress on joints.

Instrumental ADLs (IADLs) include preparing food, driving, shopping, using the phone, and doing laundry. These are also areas addressed by occupational therapists. An important area for the rehabilitation nurse in this category of higher-level activities is the self-management of medications. This task is ideally introduced in the rehabilitation setting when a self-medication program is in place. Formal and informal teaching about medications should begin on admission to give the client adequate time to gain knowledge and competence with managing what is often a complex regimen.

The rehabilitation nurse is responsible for reinforcing teaching related to adaptive equipment issued and techniques taught by other disciplines. Verbal cues and demonstration of equipment are essential. Outcomes of the interventions for clients with self-care deficit should include that they: (1) can identify preferences, (2) achieve maximal independence, and (3) participate in the rehabilitation program (Carpenito, 1997).

Constipation

Constipation, which is related to an irregular bowel evacuation pattern, lack of privacy, change in diet, and decreased activity, is a common problem in rehabilitation. Pain and iron medications can be contributory. Prophylactic treatment of constipation, such as the routine use of a stool softener, may be initiated with a physician's order. The dietitian can increase fruits, vegetables, and whole grains in the client's diet. Adequate fluid intake is essential. It is important to increase fluid intake prior to the introduction of fiber. Client education about constipation includes stressing the need for the client to report difficulties so that a satisfactory routine can be established. Constipation is often an embarrassing problem for the client. Rehabilitation nurses need to address the issue during the assessment and reinforce the importance of reporting any difficulties with bowel movements. It should be understood that prevention is the best strategy.

Nursing interventions begin with assessing the client to identify both previous normal habits and the cause of the constipation. Providing privacy and natural stimulants such as coffee or prunes may help. Replicating the client's home routine can improve bowel regularity. Taking the client to the toilet after meals takes advantage of the gastrocolic reflex, which stimulates peristalsis. Use of the commode rather than the bedpan is preferred (McCourt, 1993). Reassuring the client that activity, diet, fluids, and medications will help with the difficulties is important. Cultural background can also determine how the client prefers to treat the problem; some cultures have some folk medicine for elimination problems. Complications of constipation are abdominal pain, nausea, decreased appetite, anxiety, impaction, intestinal obstruction, and perforation.

Outcomes of interventions for constipation should be (1) regular or improved bowel evacuation, (2) client verbalization of the factors contributing to and improving the problem, and (3) client reporting of difficulties (Carpenito, 1997).

Sleep Pattern Disturbance

Sleep pattern disturbances can occur with both arthritis and osteoporosis. Other contributing factors are surgery, psychological stress, and change in the environment. Six to 8 hours of sleep daily is preferred. The inpatient rehabilitation program may be a challenge for clients, and it is critical that they have adequate, restful sleep in order to fully participate in their rehabilitation schedule. Sleep deprivation can enhance pain perception. In addition to their use in pain management, tricyclic antidepressants may be beneficial to clients with arthritis who have sleep disturbances. Amitriptyline (Elavil) has been used as an effective bedtime medication, but it must be used cautiously in the elderly (Lozada & Altman, 1997).

Tips suggested by the Arthritis Foundation to improve sleep patterns (1997b) include keeping a regular sleeping schedule and avoiding exercise, alcohol, and caffeinated beverages before bedtime. Soothing music and reading can help. Finally, warm milk and high-protein snacks at bedtime may be of benefit. Clients should understand that persistent sleep problems need to be discussed with a health care professional.

A quiet environment promotes sleep. Other nursing interventions include coordinating nursing care activities to limit nighttime interruptions. Therapists and nurses should incorporate rest periods into the client's rehabilitation program, but daytime sleep should be kept to a minimum. If medications are used to promote sleep, their effectiveness should be monitored.

Outcomes of nursing interventions for sleep disturbance are that the client identifies both the factors contributing to sleep difficulties and the techniques to induce sleep (Carpenito, 1997).

Alteration in Sexual Activity Patterns

Alteration in sexual patterns related to arthritis or arthroplasty may be identified in the rehabilitation setting. Arthritis and joint replacement may impose constraints on the client's sexual role functioning. Health care professionals often overlook the issues of sexuality and intercourse for the client. Positioning constraints, fatigue, pain, and fear can impose physical and emotional strain. Sexual functioning can improve quality of life and self-concept, so it is essential to be addressed.

Clients with total arthroplasty have position restrictions initially. Hip precautions should be maintained for at least 6 weeks. Positions used for sexual activity should not violate any of the hip precautions described earlier. Clients with knee replacements should avoid kneeling until the incision is healed. Clients who have undergone arthroplasty should consult their physicians regarding limitations. If the joint replacement is due to arthritis, sexual activity after healing may be more enjoyable and easier than in the recent past.

Arthritis imposes constraints on sexual relations through pain, stiffness, and decreased range of motion. Experimentation with different positions is important. Partners with joint pain and limitations should assume the position that requires the least movement (Houtchens, 1998).

Client communication with partners and health care professionals is critical. Rehabilitation nurses are in an excellent position to address intimacy and sexuality issues with the client. Respect, confidentiality, and empathy are essential to a discussion of this topic (Drench & Losee, 1996). Being nonjudgmental and being a good listener are important. Culture and religion may affect the client's willingness to discuss issues related to sexuality.

Client and partner education is an essential nursing intervention. The PLISSIT (permission, limited information, specific suggestions, and intensive therapy) model can guide the rehabilitation nurse in addressing this topic. Permission, as the initial level of counseling, consists of engendering an atmosphere that allows the client to feel free and comfortable in addressing sexual questions. Including questions related to sexuality in a nursing assessment may open the door to such a discussion. *Limited information* can be provided by the rehabilitation nurse through verbal or written material. Statements such as "Patients with hip replacements often have concerns about resuming sex after surgery," "Many clients who have had hip replacements for arthritis report that their sexual relations improve after surgery," and "Arthritis has no effect on the physical aspects of sex" are examples of limited information. *Specific suggestions* involve recommendations for problems and dysfunction. Such suggestions include use of certain positions, taking pain medications prior to sexual relations, and recommending that the client discuss problems and difficulties with the physician. *Intensive therapy* should be handled only by individuals with special training in this field (Tan, 1998).

Outcomes of nursing interventions for altered sexual activity patterns should be that the client (1) identifies factors causing limitations in sexuality, (2) understands suggested modifications, and (3) reports satisfying sexual activity (Carpenito, 1997).

Knowledge Deficit

Knowledge deficit can be related to a new diagnosis or treatment. A previous lack of interest in learning may also be contributory. Inadequate following of instructions, verbalization of poor understanding, and requests for information may be defining characteristics of a client's knowledge deficit (Tucker et al., 1996).

Management of arthritis, particularly in the initial stages, includes client education. This is an important role of a rehabilitation nurse. Issues such as pain management, disease process, exercise, nutrition, and joint protection are important. A client's knowledge can be measured through the use of tests and questionnaires. Edworthy, Devins, and Watson (1995) describe the development of the Arthritis Knowledge Questionnaire. Behavior, self-management, arthritis in general, and rheumatoid arthritis are topics of the subtests in this questionnaire. This psychometrically sound instrument can facilitate client education by identifying learning needs and measuring the success of education interventions. Although these investigators developed and evaluated the Arthritis Knowledge Questionnaire for patients with rheumatoid arthritis, it and other available tests can be adapted with permission for use in clients with osteoarthritis and arthroplasty.

Clients with total joint replacements need to know what signs and symptoms to report to their physician, such as those of infection, deep vein thrombosis, pulmonary embolism, and dislocation. Weight-bearing status, positioning precautions, medications, anticoagulation precautions, food and drug interactions, antibiotic prophylaxis, and the importance of making and keeping follow-up appointments should be included in client teaching.

Principles of client education for the rehabilitation nurse are as follows:

- Initiate teaching on admission.
- Provide verbal and written information appropriate to the client's ability to understand.
- Present information in small segments.
- Allow time for questions.
- Prioritize the information according to the client's rehabilitation goals.

Readiness to learn, preferred learning style, client and family priorities, and cultural influences need to all be taken into consideration (Tucker et al., 1997). Rehabilitation nurses have many roles, but client and family education, being essential to community reintegration and self-care, is one of the most important.

Table 23–2 lists the titles and sources of materials on various subjects related to osteoarthritis and arthroplasty that can complement the nurse's education efforts. Use of the client's preferred learning style and use of several teaching methods both enhance retention.

Outcomes of teaching include the client's verbalization or demonstration of understanding. In addition, the client or family who asks questions shows the need for reinforcement and readiness to accept information; this is a positive outcome.

OSTEOARTHRITIS

Overview, Definition, Etiology, Incidence, Risk Factors, and Pathophysiology

Osteoporosis simply means "porous bone." It refers to a metabolic disease in which there is low bone mass and alteration in bone cell functioning, which decrease skeletal strength (Levy, 1997). Former U.S. Surgeon General Dr. C. Everett Koop called osteoporosis a pediat-

TABLE 23–2 ■ **CLIENT AND FAMILY EDUCATION RESOURCES FOR ARTHRITIS AND ARTHROPLASTY**

Topic	Source	Available Information
Arthritis in general	Arthritis Foundation (AF) 1330 West Peachtree Street Atlanta, GA 3309 (800) 283-7800 http://www.arthritis.org	*Arthritis Answers: Basic Information About Arthritis* *Bone Up on Arthritis: Self-Care Program*
	National Institute of Arthritis and Musculoskeletal and Skin Diseases (NIAMS) U.S. Dept. of Health and Human Services Bethesda, MD 20892-3675 (301) 495-4484 http://www.nih.go/niams	*Arthritis Fact Sheet* (No. AR-27) *Arthritis in General: Key Words* (No. AR-27)
	National Institute on Aging (NIA) 31 Center Drive, Bldg. 31 Room 5C-27 Bethesda, MD 20892-2292 (301) 496-1752 http://www.nih.gov/nia	*Age Page: Arthritis Advice*
Arthroplasty	American Academy of Orthopaedic Surgeons (AAOS) 6300 North River Road Rosemont, IL 60018 (800) 346-AAOS http://www.aaos.org	*Total Joint Replacement*
	AF	*Surgery: Information to Consider*
	NIAMS http://www.nih.gov/niams/healthinfo/	*Questions and Answers About Hip Replacement* (No. AR-149QA) *Knee Replacement: Fact Sheet* *Knee Replacement: Keywords* (No. AR-102)
	National Association of Orthopaedic Nurses (NAON) East Holly Avenue, Box 56 Pitman, NJ 08071-0056 (609) 256-2310 http://naon.inurse.com/	*Patient Education for Total Hip Replacement* [Video] *Patient Education for Total Knee Replacement* [Video]
Exercise	NIAMS	*Questions and Answers About Arthritis and Exercise* (No. AR-103 QA)
	AF	*Exercise and Your Arthritis* *PEP: Pool Exercise Program* [Video]
Medications	AF	*Aspirin and Other NSAID's* *Medications: Using Them Wisely*
	NIA	*Age Page: Arthritis Medicines*
Osteoarthritis	AF	*Osteoarthritis*
	NIAMS	*Osteoarthritis: Key Words* (No. AR-73)
Pain	AF	*Managing Your Pain*
	NIAMS	*Questions and Answers About Arthritis Pain* (No. AR188QA)
Public Policy	AF	*Americans With Disabilities Act Resource Guide*
Sexuality	AF	*A Guide to Intimacy with Arthritis*

ric disease because half of the adolescents in this country consume less than 500 mg of calcium per day, far short of the recommended amount they should take (Deal, 1997). Symptoms of osteoporosis are relatively absent until a fracture occurs, explaining why it is often called the "silent disease."

Two types of osteoporosis have been identified, primary and secondary. *Primary* osteoporosis is related to aging and decreased hormonal activity. Within the primary category are senile osteoporosis and postmenopausal osteoporosis. Senile osteoporosis typically occurs in the seventh and eighth decades of life and has more serious symptoms than the postmenopausal type. A classic event of senile osteoporosis is a fracture of the femoral neck, often with very little trauma involved. Postmenopausal osteoporosis can manifest as increased back pain or kyphosis.

Secondary osteoporosis can be caused by various factors, such as endocrine, metabolic, and neoplastic conditions. Hypercortisolism from corticosteroid use can contribute to its development. Gonadal hormone insufficiency in younger women with amenorrhea or surgical menopause and decreased testosterone levels in men contribute to secondary osteoporosis. Hyperthyroidism, multiple myeloma, alcohol abuse, and immobilization facilitate the development of osteoporosis (Apley & Solomon, 1993).

It is estimated that 10 million Americans have osteoporosis. It can strike at any age, but certainly, advancing age increases the incidence. Eighty percent of those affected are women. Osteoporosis is a major public health problem, with large numbers of existing cases. It is estimated that 18 million more people have low bone mass and are at risk for developing osteoporosis (ORBD-NRC, 1998). Although more is heard about women with osteoporosis, the disease can occur in men. Because men have more bone mass, die at an earlier age, and do not experience a rapid decline in sex hormone production, as do females, the incidence of osteoporosis is lower than in women (National Institute of Arthritis and Musculoskeletal and Skin Disease [1995], Osteoporosis in Men: Fact Sheet No. AR-167 rev. ed. Bethesda, US Department of Health and Human Services).

Risk factors for the development of osteoporosis can be separated into modifiable and nonmodifiable categories. *Modifiable* risk factors include low testosterone in men (NIAMS, 1994). If testosterone deficiency is identified, testosterone replacement should be considered. Sharp decreases in estrogen during menopause cause the most rapid rate of bone loss in the first 6 to 8 years after menopause (NIH, 1994). Estrogen replacement in menopausal women should be weighed carefully as a prevention strategy. The risks and benefits of that treatment should be considered in a conversation between the client and physician.

Other modifiable risk factors are amenorrhea due to excessive exercise and anorexia. Diet-related factors are low intake of calcium and vitamin D and excess consumption of caffeine and alcohol. Cigarette smoking causes less calcium to be absorbed, and smokers have been shown to also have decreased estrogen levels. An inactive lifestyle, standing for less than 4 hours per day, and being immobile also contribute to the development of osteoporosis. Medications such as glucocorticoids and certain anticonvulsants (phenytoin, divalproex sodium) are additional risk factors for osteoporosis.

Nonmodifiable risk factors include being of female gender, advanced age, small build, and white or Asian descent. A family history of fractures, rheumatoid arthritis, multiple myeloma, or type 1 diabetes increases the risk of osteoporosis. Previous bone loss from conditions such as malabsorption and immobility are also risk factors (ORBD-NRC, 1998).

A new population of clients with osteoporosis is appearing among women who have survived breast cancer. History of that disease prohibits the use of estrogen therapy, which is known to prevent osteoporosis. In addition, long-term survivors of breast cancer may have decreased bone mass because of cyclophosphamide, methotrexate, or glucocorticoid therapy (Mahon, 1998).

Bone tissue is continually remodeling. New bone is replacing old bone. Peak bone mass is achieved at about age 30. After this age, bone mass or density can decrease or remain steady. Osteoblasts are involved in bone formation, whereas osteoclasts are the prime mediators of bone reabsorption. When the rate of bone reabsorption is greater than the rate of bone formation, osteoporosis occurs (Apley & Solomon, 1993).

Regular radiographs are poor at detecting osteoporosis until 25 to 40% of the bone is depleted (ORBD-NRC, 1995). Bone density measurement can detect osteoporosis before fractures occur and can even predict the chance of its development. Dual-energy x-ray absorptiometry (DXA or DEXA) is the best method of measuring bone density (Deal, 1997). The Balanced Budget Act, passed by the U.S. Congress in 1997, established national criteria enabling the cost of bone density diagnostic testing in high-risk people to be covered under the Medicare program (National Osteoporosis Foundation [NOF], 1997).

In the rehabilitation setting, clients with osteoporosis are seen with postural abnormalities, decreased mobility and functioning, and pain due to an acute rib or vertebral fracture (Kanner & Roth, 1997).

Treatment Modalities

Pharmacological Measures

Medications are used in osteoporosis to control pain and to slow or reverse the disease process. Several new medications have been developed, and research continues. A summary of drugs used to treat osteoporosis is given in Table 23–3.

Estrogen replacement therapy after menopause can limit bone loss and decrease the risk of osteoporotic fracture by almost 50%. Risks of estrogen replacement therapy include the possibility of endometrial cancer. Cyclical or continuous regimens may be prescribed (Levy, 1997). Oral or transdermal forms of estrogen can be used.

Pain associated with osteoporosis can be managed with NSAIDs. Calcitonin (Calcimar) inhibits osteoclasts and impairs bone reabsorption. Initially, this drug was given by the intramuscular and subcutaneous routes. It is now available in a nasal spray (Miacalcin) which is associated with fewer side effects than the previously used routes. Calcitonin also has an analgesic effect, which is helpful in clients with acute fractures (Levy, 1997).

Alendronate (Fosamax) has been proven to increase bone mineral density in the femoral head, greater trochanter, and lumbar spine. It is 1000 times more potent than etidronate (Didronel) (Deal, 1997). Once-a-day dosing with alendronate is guided by a strict protocol to prevent esophageal irritation and to ensure maximum absorption. It must be taken immediately after the client gets up in the morning, on an empty stomach, and with a full glass of water. No other medications, foods, or liquids can be taken for a half-hour afterward; during that period, the client must sit upright (Medical Economics, 1997).

Raloxifene hydrochloride (Evista) is the newest drug for osteoporosis. It is used only to prevent osteoporosis in postmenopausal women. Clients with a history of blood clots should not take this drug because clots are a rare side effect. Women taking any form of estrogen or cholestyramine should not take raloxifene. Women who are expected to be on prolonged bed rest should stop taking the medication. It is recommended that raloxifene therapy be stopped 72 hours prior to elective surgery because of the chance that postoperative immobility will contribute to clot development (Lilly, 1997).

Sodium fluoride increases bone formation; however, it can also increase bone fragility. Its use remains controversial, and it is considered an investigational drug. Research is being conducted to develop a slow-release preparation of this drug (Levy, 1997).

Multidisciplinary Measures

Inactivity contributes to the development of osteoporosis. However, there is controversy about the effect of exercise on both bone mass density and decrease of the risk in premenopausal and postmenopausal women. The American College of Sports Medicine (1995) position statement declares that exercise cannot replace estrogen hormone replacement for menopausal women. Sedentary women may have a slight increase in bone mass with activity, but the main benefit will be to prevent further loss. The American Medical Association (1994) reported in a news release that high-intensity strength training for 45 minutes twice weekly achieves gains not only in bone mass but also in muscle mass. Additional benefits of exercise are improvements in strength and balance.

The role of exercise in decreasing fracture rates is not known. A general summary of studies on osteoporosis and exercise compiled by Vargo (1995) found that exercise helps achieve peak bone mass, which will offer protection in later years. Exercise should start at an early age. High-impact exercises such as running and aerobic dancing are best. Low-impact aerobic exercises such as walking and bicycling are beneficial. Home exercise programs should fit the lifestyle of the individual in order to ensure compliance. The main benefit of exercise in the elderly is to prevent bone loss from disuse. It will also improve mobility, agility, strength, coordination, and balance (Christansen, 1993). Being in better physical condition can help reduce the chances of falling.

TABLE 23–3 ■ COMMON MEDICATIONS USED IN THE MANAGEMENT OF OSTEOPOROSIS

Agent	Dose and Route	Nursing Considerations and Patient Instructions
Estrogen	0.3–0.625 mg/d PO or 0.05–0.1 mg via transdermal patch, applied twice weekly	Instruct patient regarding progesterone (e.g., 10 mg medroxyprogesterone on days 15–25) as prescribed by physician Instruct patient regarding monthly breast self-examination, yearly mammography, reporting of any abnormal vaginal bleeding, and annual gynecological examinations Instruct patient to take missed dose as soon as remembered but not to "double up" doses to make up for a missed dose Review anticipated benefits and possible drug side effects with patient Caution patients who are taking estrogens to stop smoking
Calcitonin	50–100 IU SC or IM daily or 3 times/wk of salmon calcitonin or 0.5 mg SC or IM daily or 2–3 times/wk of human calcitonin	Perform skin test before initial dose Review anticipated benefits and possible side effects with patients and family; side effects include nausea and vomiting, anorexia, mild transient flushing of palms of hands and soles of feet, and urinary frequency Recommend that patient take medication at bedtime, because this practice tends to minimize side effects Teach patient and family how to administer drug subcutaneously, including injection technique, aseptic technique, accurate dosage preparation, recording of injection sites, and rotation of sites Ensure proper nutrition and intake of calcium and vitamin D
Calcitonin nasal spray (Miacalcin)	200–400 IU given in daily dose Alternate nares daily; i.e., use right nostril one day and left nostril next day	Perform skin test before initial dose Side effects include mild nasal discomfort and rhinitis Is contraindicated in people who were previously allergic to injectable forms of salmon calcitonin Ensure proper nutrition and intake of dietary calcium and vitamin D
Alendronate sodium (Fosamax)	10 mg/d PO (treatment) 5 mg/d PO (prevention)	To ensure adequate absorption, pill must be taken on an empty stomach and with 6–8 of plain water 30–90 minutes before first food or beverage of the day Patient must remain in upright position for 1 hour after taking medication Side effects include gastric distress, esophagitis, and headache Must not be taken by anyone taking aminoglycoside antibiotics
Fluoride (slow fluoride)	25 mg bid PO Investigational drug	Review anticipated benefits and potential side effects with patient, which include gastrointestinal upset (*must* be taken with food) and painful joints Monitor serum fluoride levels every 3 months Give with calcium citrate (Pak et al., 1995) Perform bone mineral density studies at 6-month intervals to document progress of bone density Reinforce importance of adequate calcium intake while taking fluoride

Table continued on following page

TABLE 23–3 ▪ COMMON MEDICATIONS USED IN THE MANAGEMENT OF OSTEOPOROSIS *Continued*

Agent	Dose and Route	Nursing Considerations and Patient Instructions
Calcium	1000–1500 mg PO in divided doses	Gastrointestinal distress may occur Free hydrochloric acid is needed for calcium absorption; calcium should be taken with meals Should be taken in divided doses Monitor for history and ongoing presence of hypercalcemia or hypercalciuria
Raloxifene hydrochloride (Evista)	60 mg/d PO	Used in women after menopause to prevent osteoporosis Immobility from prolonged bed rest, as after surgery, can increase risk of blood clots When travelling, client should get up and move around periodically Client should report signs of blood clots as pain in leg or calves, chest pain, shortness of breath, coughing of blood, or change in vision; other side effects are swelling of hands and feet

bid, twice a day; d, day; IM, intramuscularly; PO, by mouth; SC, subcutaneously.
Modified from Hunt, A. (1998). Metabolic conditions. In A. Maher, S. Salmond, & T. Pellino (Eds.). *Orthopaedic nursing* (2nd ed., pp. 431–479). Philadelphia: W. B. Saunders.

Clients with established osteoporosis must be cautious about the types of activities they engage in. Something as simple as picking up a toddler or grocery bag can cause a fracture. Spinal flexion exercises can predispose women with osteoporosis to vertebral fractures (Levy, 1997). Back extension exercises, however, can prevent kyphosis. Skiing, skating, and activities that put torque on the spine, such as golf and racquet sports, should be avoided (Vargo, 1995).

Calcium is essential to building and maintaining the strength of bones. Guidelines for amounts of calcium intake are as follows (NIH, 1994a):

1200 to 1500 mg per day for everyone aged 11 to 24 years

1000 mg per day for women aged 25 to 50 years, men aged 25 to 65 years, and postmenopausal women who are taking estrogen

1500 mg per day for women during initial menopause, women aged 50 to 65 years who are not taking estrogen, and men and women older than 65 years

Foods high in calcium include milk, other dairy products, and green vegetables. A simple comparison of foods containing 300 mg of calcium is (1) 1 oz of Swiss cheese, (2) 1 cup of milk, and (3) 1 cup of yogurt (Levy, 1997). A diet high in caffeine-containing foods increases bone loss. Additionally, high levels of protein and sodium can increase calcium excretion. In 1997, the National Academy of Science made recommendations for daily calcium intake that are higher than the previously listed amounts (OBRD-NRC, 1998).

Hip Fractures

Osteoporosis causes approximately 300,000 hip fractures per year, 90% of which occur as the result of a fall. Of clients with hip fractures, 25% fully recover, 40% are placed in nursing homes, 50% ambulate with a cane or walker, and 20% die within a year (AAOS, 1997). As populations age, the number of hip fractures is anticipated to double in less than 50 years (European Foundation for Osteoporosis & National Osteoporosis Foundation, 1997).

White postmenopausal women are at greatest risk for hip fractures (Levy, 1997). Physiological contributing factors are stroke, parkinsonism, neurological deficits, decreased orientation, and osteoporosis. Predisposing home factors are problems with the environment, such as poor lighting. Medications, such as sleeping pills, pain medications, and diuretics, can also increase the risk for a fall (Theis, 1991).

Hip fractures can occur in the intracapsular or extracapsular area (Fig. 23–8). The *intracap-*

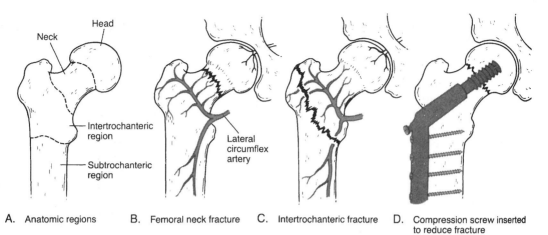

A. Anatomic regions   B. Femoral neck fracture   C. Intertrochanteric fracture   D. Compression screw inserted to reduce fracture

FIGURE 23–8

Hip fractures. *A*, Normal proximal end of the femur. *B*, Intracapsular fracture of the proximal end of the femur. Note the blood supply. *C*, Extracapsular intertrochanteric fracture. Note the effect of the fracture on the blood supply. *D*, Femoral neck fracture with compression screw inserted for reduction. (From Black, J., & Matassarin-Jacobs, E. [Eds.]. [1993]. *Luckmann and Sorensen's Medical-surgical nursing* [4th ed., p. 1924]. Philadelphia: W. B. Saunders.)

sular fracture occurs within the joint capsule and is often caused by minor trauma in a person with osteoporosis. Femoral neck fractures are an example of intracapsular fractures. They occur between the two trochanter bones. The fracture can be displaced, with pieces of broken bone either not aligned and impacted or comminuted with the bone fragments scattered. A comminuted fracture has a higher risk of avascular necrosis because the fragments may interrupt the blood supply. Intracapsular fractures can be repaired by open reduction and internal fixation with pins, nails, plates, and screws. Such a repair involves a postoperative period of toe-touch weight bearing.

Extracapsular hip fractures occur below the joint capsule and are always comminuted. They are often seen in clients with metastatic disease. Fixation is often by open reduction and internal fixation with a nail, pins, or a compression hip screw. Subtrochanteric fractures occur below the trochanter (Black & Matassarin-Jacobs, 1993; Resnick, 1994).

Vertebral Compression Fractures

In the United States yearly, 700,000 vertebral compression fractures occur. Forty percent of women have at least one spinal fracture by the age of 80 years (NOF, 1998b).

A vertical compression fracture can be one of three types—anterior wedge, biconcave, or crush deformity (Fig. 23–9). The fractures commonly occur when the client puts a load on the outstretched arms, such as when picking up a child or raising a window. In a client with severe osteoporosis, a simple cough, sneeze, or turn in bed can cause a fracture.

Pain is severe for a few days but can persist and remain intense for 2 to 3 months. Changes in posture such as kyphosis (dowager's hump) can cause chronic pain and sleep problems. Shortening and loss of height due to fractures, reduction in the size of the abdominal and thoracic cavities, and the development of a protuberant abdomen can occur with vertebral fractures (Lukert, 1994).

Some vertebral fractures are asymptomatic. With each new fracture, functional limitation increases. A study by Nevitt, Ottinger, Black, Stone, Jamal, Ensrud, Segal, Genant, and Cummings (1998) of 7223 women older than 65 years demonstrated that both women and their doctors may not recognize vertebral fractures, even when they are causing pain. Women who had vertebral fractures were at a fourfold greater risk to have a second fracture. Clients with vertebral fractures are seen in the rehabilitation setting because of either the functional decline related to the chronic condition or an acute fracture associated with pain.

Physical therapy for osteoporosis may include weight-bearing activities and low-impact exercises such as walking. Swimming provides chest expansion, spinal extension, and cardiopulmonary fitness. Spinal flexion exercises are contraindicated in clients with vertebral compression fractures (Levy, 1997).

Potential Complications and Collaborative Problems

Fat Embolism

Fat embolism is an acute respiratory insufficiency. The occurrence of fat embolism is most prevalent in fractures of the long bones, bones of the pelvis, and bones with marrow. Both a delay in treatment by open reduction with internal fixation and nonsurgical treatment of fractures increase the incidence of fat embolism. Other risk factors are sickle cell disease, diabetes, and alcoholism. Fat embolism is also a serious complication that can occur after joint replacement, from reaming of the medullary canal, or with fractures of bones that contain marrow fat (Johnson, 1986).

Fat globules released from the marrow of long bones can enter into the peripheral circulation and deposit in the lung capillaries. Subclinical, overt, and fulminating forms of fat embolism can occur. The *subclinical* form of fat embolism appears about 3 days after surgery or injury. Signs are decreases in oxygen level and hematocrit along with thrombocytopenia. Bleeding into the lungs causes the drop in hematocrit. The *overt* form occurs within 24 to 72 hours of a fracture. Cerebral and respiratory symptoms are common signs. The *fulminant* form of fat embolism occurs within hours after an injury or surgery (Pellino, Polacek, Preston, Bell, & Evans, 1998). Fat embolism does not usually occur more than 1 week after injury.

Respiratory arrest can occur in this syndrome. Symptoms can be similar to those of pulmonary embolism, such as chest pain, shortness of breath, rales, tachypnea, tachycardia, and fever. An early sign is alteration in the level of consciousness, which may appear as anxiety, agitation, restlessness, or disorientation. One difference between fat embolism and pulmonary embolism is the frequent presence of a petechial rash on the chest, axilla, and neck, as well as on the conjunctiva and retina with fat embolism. Diagnosis is made from changes in arterial blood gas levels, the fall in hematocrit, and associated signs and symptoms. The key to treatment of fat embolism is prevention by the early stabilization of fractures. Treatment consists of corticosteroids and oxygen therapy (Pellino et al., 1998).

Nursing interventions are supportive. They include (1) keeping the client in a high Fowler's position to promote easier breathing, (2) administering oxygen as ordered, and (3) providing emotional support. In addition, monitoring breath sounds, vital signs, and

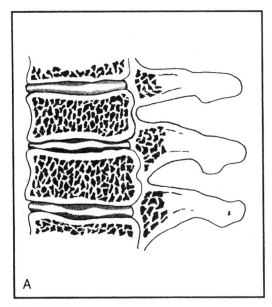
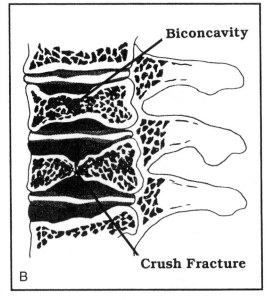

FIGURE 23–9

Effects of osteoporosis on the vertebrae. The normal vertebrae *(A)* differ substantially from the osteoporotic vertebrae *(B)*. Note the compression of crush fracture in the middle vertebra pictured *(B)*. These various abnormalities lead to shortened stature of the patient with osteoporosis and can cause both pain and structural changes, such as thoracic kyphosis. (From Hunt, A. [1998]. Metabolic conditions. In A. Maher, S. Salmond, & T. Pellino [Eds.], *Orthopaedic nursing* [2nd ed., p. 438]. Philadelphia: W. B. Saunders.)

blood gas levels is integral (Carpenito, 1997). Prompt recognition of symptoms is critical to ensure a satisfactory outcome.

Avascular Necrosis

Avascular necrosis, also known as septic necrosis or osteonecrosis, is death of bone due to ischemia. It can occur following a hip fracture or dislocation. Long bones, such as the femur, are commonly affected. Each year, 10,000 to 20,000 people are diagnosed with avascular necrosis (NIAMS, 1997b). The disorder is seen often in clients older than 60 years with fractures of the femoral neck, which impair blood supply to the femoral head. Almost 20% of clients with fractures of the femoral neck experience avascular necrosis (Hunt, 1998). The disorder accounts for 10% of total hip replacement procedures performed in the United States (Mont et al., 1997). Posterior hip dislocations have a 10 to 20% higher risk for the development of avascular necrosis (Spiegel, 1997).

The femoral head is the most common site of symptomatic avascular necrosis. Its peculiar blood supply makes it vulnerable to any cutoff of the arterial supply. This process may begin soon after a severe hip injury, but it may take months for signs and symptoms to appear. If the femoral head deteriorates enough, it can collapse; the only treatment for collapse is total hip replacement (Apley & Solomon, 1993).

Risk factors for development of avascular necrosis include corticosteroid therapy and excessive alcohol use. Other factors are Gaucher's disease, radiation treatments, and chemotherapy (NIAMS, 1997b). Magnetic resonance imaging is a very sensitive means of diagnosing the condition in early stages.

In the client with total joint replacement, mild to severe pain and progressive loss of function may signal avascular necrosis (Apley & Solomon, 1993). There may be no symptoms in the initial stages, but about 85% of clients experience joint pain (NIAMS, 1992). Continued pain after a fracture or decreased range of motion may be evident. The pain can be associated with motion, but complaints of pain at night are common. Treatment involves prolonged weight-bearing restrictions and anti-inflammatory medication. Total hip replacement or joint fusion may be necessary (Hunt, 1998).

Rehabilitation nurses may see this complication in a client with a hip fracture, dislocation, or arthroplasty. A rehabilitation program for a client with avascular necrosis includes pain management, joint protection, and exercises. Pool therapy and isometric exercises are used to increase range of motion (Mont et al., 1997). Nursing interventions include pain management with the use of NSAIDs and multidisciplinary measures. Reinforcement of weight-bearing status is critical. Client education after fracture or total hip replacement should stress the importance of reporting new or increased hip or leg pain.

Nursing Diagnoses and Interventions

Alteration in Body Image

An alteration in body image may occur in clients with osteoporosis. The realization of vulnerability to fractures can affect how clients feel about themselves. Other problems related to self-esteem and body image are pain and disfigurement from kyphosis. Decrease in functional ability and mobility can affect self-esteem. Height loss, abdominal protrusion, dowager's hump, and poorly fitting clothes are also factors contributing to an alteration in body image (Hunt, 1998). Because of the poor self-esteem and body image, the client may not continue with social events outside the home. Psychosocial issues associated with osteoporosis include poor quality of life, anxiety, depression, and low self-esteem (Ross, 1997).

Nursing interventions include allowing the client to express these feelings and promoting self-care. Suggestions can be made about clothing that may be helpful, such as using scarves as a way to camouflage kyphosis. Encouraging the client to communicate with their significant other may be helpful. Osteoporosis support groups may assist with coping. Outcomes of interventions should be the client's ability to (1) share feelings, (2) use adaptive equipment, (3) dress to enhance appearance, and (4) participate in social activities (Tucker et al., 1996).

Alteration in Mobility

Clients with fractures and osteoporosis may experience an alteration in mobility. Approximately one fourth of clients who were ambulatory before a hip fracture are placed in long-term care facilities afterward. Ambulation may eventually be achieved in the home but not in the community (NOF, 1998b). Of women who sustain a hip fracture, 15 to 25%

lose independence within the first year, 50% require nursing home placement, and 50% of those in nursing homes remain there after 1 year (Kanner & Roth, 1997). Of clients surviving, 25 to 50% regain their premorbid level of function (Spiegel, 1997). Negative predictors of ambulation after hip fracture are (1) lack of social support, (2) age more than 85 years, (3) lower limb contractures, and (4) poor prefracture functional status (Mont et al., 1997).

Vertebral deformity contributes to decreased spinal mobility in clients with osteoporosis. With this change comes difficulties with ADLs, ambulation, standing, rising from chairs, bending, and bathing. Fear of falls and fractures may lead clients to decrease their activity (Ross, 1997).

Client education related to mobility includes the importance of participation in an exercise program under the guidance of a physical therapist and physiatrist. Certain exercises are contraindicated in clients with osteoporosis. In cooperation with occupational therapists, rehabilitation nurses can reinforce the use of adaptive equipment to foster independence (Hunt, 1998). Safety with mobility is critical, and it is important to stress the use of the ambulation device, if one was recommended, to improve stability and prevent falls. In the client with severely impaired mobility, it is essential to monitor skin integrity. Outcomes of interventions should be the client's demonstration or use of adaptive devices and walking aids and improved mobility.

Alteration in Comfort

Osteoporosis can cause either acute or chronic pain. Pain from vertebral fractures causes discomfort, sleeping difficulties, functional decline, and social isolation. Clients recuperating from vertebral fractures are seen in the rehabilitation setting.

The duration of the acute pain varies from weeks to months. Pain from a fracture is initially due to periosteal irritation from local bleeding and muscle spasm. Discomfort can occur from other clinical consequences, such as constipation and organ compression due to vertebral collapse from fractures causing kyphosis (Ross, 1997). The client with a hip fracture may also experience acute pain. Chronic pain results from vertebral deformities, kyphosis, or nerve root compression. It is important to stress to the client that the pain is not permanent (Lukert, 1994).

Bracing stabilizes the spine but is often underutilized as a comfort measure for verte-

bral fractures (Lukert, 1994). The type of brace depends on the location of the fracture. The simplest brace is an elastic binder, which reminds the client to be careful with movement and increases intraabdominal pressure. The Jewett brace and the thoracolumbosacral orthosis (TLSO) offer greater control. A Taylor brace is used to decrease kyphosis. Short-term use of braces for 7 to 10 days after thoracic fracture is recommended (Levy, 1997).

Nursing interventions for alteration in comfort include pain management through either administration of medications or adjutant nonpharmacological measures presented earlier. NSAIDs can control pain and decrease the need for narcotics. The latter may be needed for short periods. After an acute fracture, calcitonin (Miacalcin, Calcimar) provides an analgesic effect (Levy, 1997). Because the average client with osteoporosis is elderly, drug side effects should be closely monitored.

Bed rest is recommended initially, but sleeping can be difficult because of trouble finding a comfortable position. The principles related to improving sleep discussed earlier may be necessary. Ice massage for 7 to 10 minutes may help with acute pain, and heat can relieve a spasm (Lukert, 1994). Education should include reinforcing the fact that pain from vertebral fractures is not permanent, and that bracing can be of benefit. The rehabilitation nurse should show the client how to apply and remove the brace as well as how to check skin integrity. It is important to emphasize that braces should be used only for the limited time they are prescribed because their prolonged use actually causes back muscles to weaken (ORBD-NRC, 1997).

Outcomes of interventions are that the client (1) verbalizes an increased level of comfort, (2) demonstrates increased activity and self-care, and (3) participates in the rehabilitation program (Carpenito, 1997).

Acute Confusion

Many clients with osteoporosis are elderly. Hospitalization can contribute to their confusion, in relation to a change in environment, medications, or electrolyte imbalance. Other risk factors for the development of confusion are pain, infection, sleep deprivation, blood loss, and anesthesia after-effect. The altered level of consciousness has a negative effect on recovery, including rehabilitation (Currie, 1990).

Confusion, which is common in clients after hip surgery, is evidenced by disorientation, getting out of bed, removing dressings, or having hallucinations. O'Brien, Grisso, Maislin, Chiu, and Evans (1993) describe a study of 202 elderly patients with hip fracture. Key points of the study's results are that (1) confusion is often underdiagnosed, (2) severely confused clients experience more medical complications and higher rate of discharge to a nursing home, and (3) the risk of being physically restrained increases in the severely confused client. This study, as well as others, showed that more than half of clients with hip fractures are admitted with confusion or experience it during hospitalization.

Initial nursing interventions include identifying the cause of the confusion and ensuring client safety. In addition, accurately assessing cognition, monitoring responses to medications, and ensuring adequate nutrition and fluid intake must be addressed. The environment should have calendars and clocks to assist with orientation. Providing a client with a copy of the rehabilitation schedule and the names of nurses and therapists for the day is beneficial. In the instance of sensory impairment that can contribute to confusion, clients must wear and use their hearing aids and eyeglasses.

Nurses should explain procedures and keep the client's routine consistent. Encouraging family members to spend time with clients and accompany them to therapy sessions may be therapeutic and may ultimately be an alternative to restraining a confused client to prevent injury. If confusion increases with excessive visitors or noise, the overstimulation should be limited (Tucker et al., 1996). Family support and education are essential for the severely confused client.

Outcomes of nursing interventions for confusion should be that (1) the confusion resolves, (2) the client remains oriented and safe, and (3) the client interacts in the rehabilitation setting.

Knowledge Deficit

Knowledge deficit in the client with osteoporosis and fracture may be related to the diagnosis or treatment. Key topics that need to be addressed are safety, diet, recommended exercises, risk factors, lifting limitations, weight-bearing status, and medications. Themes of client education are (1) managing continued care, (2) limiting the use of alcohol and drugs affecting balance, and (3) reducing environmental hazards that contribute to falls (Hunt, 1998).

Table 23–4 outlines titles and sources of materials related to osteoporosis and fractures that can reinforce teaching. Outcomes of client education should be verbalization or demonstration of understanding.

CULTURALLY SENSITIVE CARE

Our nation's changing demographics were reflected in the 1990 census. The U.S. Census Bureau anticipates that when the 2000 census is completed, groups previously classified as minorities will become national majorities. It is important to understand that culture has an effect on issues such as complying with a therapeutic regimen, seeking medical care, and responding positively to client teaching. Leininger (1991) defines culture as the learned, shared, and transmitted values, beliefs, norms, and lifeways of a certain group that guides their thinking, decisions, and actions. The goal of culturally congruent care is to provide health care or well-being services that are meaningful, satisfying, and beneficial (Leininger, 1991). Other components of a client's background, such as socioeconomic status, sexual orientation, disability, and religion, also affect values and beliefs.

The American Nurses Association's Position Statement on Cultural Diversity in Nursing Practice emphasizes the importance of having knowledge and skills related to cultural diversity. The nurse's culture and the environment are part of the nurse-client interaction. *Ethnocentrism*, or the belief that one's own culture is superior, is evident in health care and must be avoided to provide effective nursing interventions (American Nurses Association, 1996). Nurses need to first explore their own attitudes, beliefs, and biases. Being an active and reflective learner about the clients who are being served is an important element in providing culturally appropriate care (Leininger & Cummings, 1996).

Table 23–5 summarizes some key aspects of culture in the largest ethnic population groups in the United States as they relate to nursing care. Lipson, Dibble, and Minarik (1996) compiled the information to assist nurses in providing culturally congruent nursing care. It is important to note that cultures have certain characteristics but they should not be used to stereotype all clients within a group. Table 23–5 summarizes cultural values and beliefs related to pain, client teaching, and management of a therapeutic regimen. Rehabilitation nurses caring for clients with osteoarthritis and osteoporosis need to understand cultural values and beliefs as they relate to these three aspects of care.

TABLE 23–4 ■ CLIENT AND FAMILY EDUCATION RESOURCES FOR OSTEOPOROSIS

Topic	Source	Available Information
Osteoporosis in general	Osteoporosis and Related Bone Diseases–National Resource Center (ORBD-NRC) 1150 17th Street NW, Suite 500 Washington, DC 20036-4603 (800)624-BONE http://www.osteo.org	*Osteoporosis Overview* *Strategies for People With Osteoporosis: The Diagnosis*
	National Osteoporosis Foundation (NOF) 1150 17th Street NW Washington, DC 20036 http://www.nof.org	*Fast Facts on Osteoporosis* *Living With Osteoporosis* *How Strong Are Your Bones?* *Talking With Your Doctor About Osteoporosis* *The Older Person's Guide to Osteoporosis*
	National Institute on Aging (NIA) 31 Center Drive, Bldg. 31 Room 5C-27 Bethesda, MD 20892-2292 (301)496-1752 http://www.nih.gov/nia/	*Age Page: Osteoporosis, The Silent Bone Thinner*
Diet	ORBD-NRC	*Calcium: Important at Every Age*
Fall prevention	NIA	*Age Page: Preventing Falls and Fractures*
	American Academy of Orthopaedic Surgeons (AAOS) 6300 North River Road Rosemont, IL 60018 (800)346-AAOS http://www.aaos.org	*Don't Let a Fall Be Your Last Trip* [On-Line]
Hip fracture	ORBD-NRC	*Strategies for People With Osteoporosis: Recovery From Hip Fracture*
Medications	NOF	*Medications and Bone Loss*
	Eli Lilly and Co Indianapolis, IN 46285 http://www.evista.com/pi/htm1#patient http://www.evista.com/safety.htm1	*Information for the Patient: EVISTA* *Additional Safety Information Regarding EVISTA* *How to Take Fosamax* *A Woman's Guide to Bone Health* *Osteoporosis and Bone Loss: What You Should Know and What You Should Do*
	Sandoz Pharmaceutical Corporation, East Hanover, NJ 07936	*Facts About Miacalcin Spray* *Bone Matters* *Bone Matters Educational Program*, a 12-month educational mailing, 1-800-347-2663
Men	National Institute of Arthritis and Musculoskeletal and Skin Diseases (NIAMS) U.S. Dept. of Health and Human Services Bethesda, MD 20892-3675 (301) 495-4484	*Osteoporosis in Men: Fact Sheet* (No. AR-169, Rev. ed.)
	NOF	*Men With Osteoporosis: In Their Own Words*
Menopause	NOF	*Menopause and Osteoporosis*
Vertebral fracture	ORBD-NRC	*Strategies for People With Osteoporosis: After the Vertebral Fracture*

TABLE 23–5 ■ CULTURAL CARE ISSUES FOR ORTHOPEDIC CLIENTS

Culture or Ethnic Group	Pain	Patient Teaching	Compliance with Therapeutic Regimen
American Indian	Generally undertreated Complain in general terms If initial complaint to health care professional (HCP) provides no relief, may complain to trusted person to relay fact to HCP	Keep respectful distance from client Place value on personal autonomy Communicate respect by avoiding eye contact Literacy assessment advised	Traditional medicine may be used initially or in combination with Western medicine Holistic and wellness oriented Traditional medicine view does not recognize "silent disease" Self-care valued Physical stamina, relaxation; and harmonious living along with religion and prayer believed to promote health
Black or African American	Generally open about pain Avoid medications, fearing addiction	Silence may indicate lack of trust Respect privacy—will provide personal information if trust and respect present Literacy assessment advised	Home remedies used initially Open to and accepting of health information Diet, proper behavior, and exercise maintain health Illness caused by poor diet, exposure to cold, God's punishment Use both folk medicine and biomedical systems
Chinese Americans	May not complain HCP must be aware of nonverbal cues	Avoid eye contact with authority figures Keep respectful distance from client Shy, especially in unfamiliar environment Extremely modest Allow family involvement and participation Literacy assessment advised	May use herbal preparations and special soups Treat minor symptom with food remedies Some fearful of having blood drawn Many avoid surgery Major illness ignored until advanced Seek advice of relatives before that of HCPs Maintain health by balance between "Yin" and "Yang" influences Balanced diet and harmony with family and friends believed to maintain health
Cuban	Express pain, men seem hypersensitive, women more tolerant Fear addiction and prefer not to take medications	Typically outgoing and confronting Expect direct eye contact Silence signifies awkwardness Only the family selected by the patient should be included in conversation High degree of literacy	Understand modern germ theory Also believe stress and nervousness cause disease Use medical facilities and religious assistance concurrently Poor diet habits–view overweight as healthy Do not accept concept of self-care

Table continued on following page

TABLE 23–5 ■ CULTURAL CARE ISSUES FOR ORTHOPEDIC CLIENTS *Continued*

Culture or Ethnic Group	Pain	Patient Teaching	Compliance with Therapeutic Regimen
Filipino	Can be stoic; should be offered pain medications Fearful of addition Prefer medications by mouth or intravenous route; dislike intramuscular route	Sensitive to tone and manner of speaker Speak slowly to client and use simple medical terms Typically shy Make little direct eye contact with authority figures Literacy assessment advised	Do not respond to illness until advanced Believe that illness is a result of an imbalance or bad behavior, or a punishment Believe concurrently in modern and folk medicine Regard being overweight as indication of good socioeconomic standing Associate health with good food Exercise not a part of daily living
Mexican Americans	Tend not to complain; HCP should assess for nonverbal cues Stoicism common Men may believe that expression of pain shows weakness	Frequently avoid direct eye contact with authority figures Silence sometimes shows lack of agreement with care plan Regard touch as disrespectful Literacy assessment advised—great diversity in abilities	Believe that health is controlled by environment, fate, and God Rely on health care providers and family for care Believe self-care can adversely affect recovery Self-medication common Believe that disease is a result of imbalance between individual and environment May use folk medicine for chronic symptoms Many believe illness is not being treated unless medicine is prescribed Define health as feeling well and functioning in role Diet generally nutritious and low in fat
Puerto Ricans	Speak loudly and openly Do not censure pain expression as exaggeration Use herbal teas, heat, and prayer to manage pain	Information should be provided slowly Expect a respectful environment Option should be provided for language preference for oral and written information Respect personal space	Most prefer independence in care Use herbal teas for signs and symptoms of illness Consult family and friends before an HCP Believe that illness is a result of heredity, punishment, sin, or lack of personal attention to health Do not regard exercise as essential and discourage it in illness Believe that "happy and oversized" is healthy Prefer female physicians

TABLE 23–5 ▪ CULTURAL CARE ISSUES FOR ORTHOPEDIC CLIENTS *Continued*

Culture or Ethnic Group	Pain	Patient Teaching	Compliance with Therapeutic Regimen
Russian	High pain threshold Stoic—may not ask for medications Pain Medication should be encouraged	Make direct eye contact Nodding is a gesture of approval Often mistake registered nurses for medical doctors Many are very highly educated	Illness caused by poor nutrition, cold, or stress Will self-treat before seeking medical advice as a last resort Believe that drugs can poison and that excessive drug use is harmful Define health as absence of symptoms and regularity of bowel movements Selective about choosing health care facility
West Indian	Try various home remedies before seeking medical advice Use herbal and bush teas and ointments Fear that prescription medications may cause harm or addiction	Audiovisual method with direct patient teaching should be used Unlikely to ask question or admit to poor understanding Avoid direct eye contact with HCPs	May discontinue drugs as soon as symptoms disappear Believe that illness is caused by germs, cold air, and not eating properly Seek medical attention when physically ill and at an advanced stage of disease Define health as absence of pain, weight gain, and ability to perform usual activities Exercise and healthy eating are not cultural values

Data from Lipson, J., Dibble, SI, & Minarik, P. (eds.): *Culture and nursing care: A pocket guide.* San Francisco, UCSF Nursing Press, 1996.

A cultural assessment is the starting point for providing culturally appropriate care. A conversational approach to obtaining the information is preferred over a rigid question-and-answer period. The following key areas should be covered in a cultural assessment (Bozeman, 1996):

- Social structure and family
- Views on health care
- Attitudes and beliefs about pain, illness, and suffering
- Communication methods and building of relationships
- Diet and food preferences

Pain

A client's cultural background has an effect on his or her *pain perception threshold*—the smallest stimulus that causes the client to report feeling pain. *Pain threshold* is the point at which the client can no longer tolerate pain. Cultures have different ways of expressing pain. Some manifest pain by moaning, whereas others are stoically silent. The meaning of pain also varies with cultures. Pain may be viewed as either a punishment or a means to salvation (Jeans & Melzak, 1992). These differences affect whether clients will accept or comply with recommended therapeutic regimens.

Correct assessment of pain requires a cultural pain assessment. A respectful and non-threatening approach is essential. Questions should address not only the characteristics of the pain but also how the client usually deals with pain. Some cultures prefer folk remedies over medications (Bozeman, 1996).

Client Teaching

Culturally sensitive client teaching can be guided by a four-step approach, which consists of (1) examination of personal culture, (2) familiarity with the client's culture, (3) identification of the client's adaptation for living in the American culture, and (4) modification of client teaching based on the previous three steps (Kittler & Sucher, 1990).

Assessment is the starting point in the teaching-learning process. Language, verbal and nonverbal cues, and understanding of health care are explored. Verbal and nonverbal communication can differ with ethnicity. Some groups do not make eye contact with the health care professional as a sign of respect. An interpreter may be necessary.

Next, a teaching plan is prepared on the basis of mutual goals. Culturally appropriate tools, such as handouts and videos prepared in the client's language, may reinforce the teaching. The combination of visual, auditory, and psychomotor teaching methods improves retention of the information. The plan should be implemented when the client is well rested and free of pain. The decision to include a family member in teaching varies according to the client's preference and cultural background.

Finally, evaluation of learning can be accomplished through return demonstrations of techniques and observation of changes in behavior and attitudes (Price & Cordell, 1994).

Therapeutic Regimen

It is essential that aspects of the therapeutic regimen be integrated into a client's daily living routine. Ineffective management of the regimen can occur as a result of a treatment's cost and complexity. Situational issues contributing to difficulties can be barriers to comprehension, including fatigue and language. Mistrust of health care professionals and weak understanding of the seriousness of the medical situation can also contribute to poor compliance (Carpenito, 1997).

A trusting relationship is essential to ensure compliance. Clients must not be pressured into adherence to the program. Mutual goal setting, which is so important in rehabilitation, is also significant in the choice of the therapeutic regimen. Cultural imposition, which is imposing one's personal beliefs, values, and behavior patterns on a client of another culture, does not ensure compliance (Cooper, 1996). Outcomes of adherence to the therapeutic regimen include maintenance of symptoms within a normal range of expectation and verbalization of the desire to manage the therapeutic regimen.

DISCHARGE PLANNING

Discharge planning begins on admission. It requires interdisciplinary teamwork and communication. Issues such as financial considerations and community resources need to be explored. The rehabilitation nurse has a role in assessing the physical and psychological status of the client and family. The level of self-care expected at the time of discharge and the abilities of the client and family must be assessed. Both ADLs and IADLs need to be addressed (Hester, 1996). Adjuncts to interdisciplinary discharge planning are home visits, therapeutic passes, and family conferences (Mumma, 1987). Issues such as equipment, medication, and assistive devices are integral to discharge planning.

Discharge planning goals for the rehabilitation nurse are to (1) maintain the client's optimal health and functional abilities, (2) complete client and family education, and (3) to provide referrals to the appropriate community resources (Mumma, 1987).

Community Reintegration

The ultimate goal of rehabilitation is to reintegrate the client into family and community settings. The rehabilitation nurse, as a generalist or case manager, should be involved in the client's discharge planning and community reentry. Referrals to community agencies and services are necessary to ensure reintegration.

Figure 23–10 lists some services that receive state or federal funding. They can be used to facilitate community reintegration. As the client moves from acute care to rehabilitation and then to home or alternative placement, access to services is essential. Case management, Visiting Nurse Association, proprietary (for-profit) agencies, public health services, elderly and adult services, Alpha I (member of the National Council on Independent Living), and general services may be necessary. Communication with agencies that will offer support services is critical during the transition phase to home (McCourt, 1993).

Five aspects of independent home recovery are (1) physical activity, (2) health care monitoring, (3) medications, (4) self-care measures, and (5) reasons to call a health care professional. Formal and informal teaching throughout the rehabilitation stay, not just at discharge, is critical (Wells, 1996). Collaboration with all disciplines is essential to achieving the best discharge plan.

Accessibility

The Americans with Disability Act (ADA) of 1990 is a civil rights law intended to prohibit discrimination against employment, public

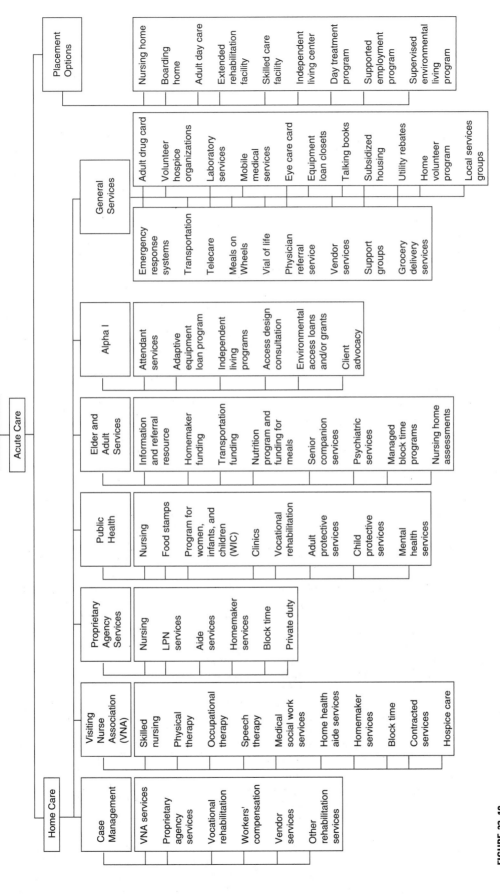

FIGURE 23-10

Gaining access to community resources. (Reprinted from *The Specialty Practice of Rehabilitation Nursing: A Core Curriculum* [3rd ed.], 1993, with permission of the Rehabilitation Nursing Foundation, 5700 Old Orchard Road, Skokie, IL 60077–1057. Copyright 1993.)

services, public accommodation, and communications for disabled people. A goal of the ADA is to integrate disabled people into community life. A person is *disabled* if he or she (1) has a physical or mental impairment that significantly limits one or more major life activities, (2) has a record of such impairment, or (3) is regarded as having such an impairment. Walking, caring for oneself, and working are included in major life activities (U.S. Equal Employment Opportunity Commission, 1992).

Clients with arthritis or osteoporosis may be considered disabled. It is not just those traumatically injured or born with disabilities who can benefit from the ADA. The elderly often lack knowledge about the law and its privileges, but they can benefit from it. They may not realize that their chronic disease or functional disability will permit them to use some of the privileges of the ADA. Rehabilitation professionals need to educate clients about the ADA and advocate for them to ensure that necessary services are provided and rights are upheld (Bachelder & Hilton, 1994).

Accessibility involves housing, transportation, work, education, recreation, health care services, and supportive services. Public transportation and accommodations are required by the ADA to be accessible. Buses, trains, restaurants, hotels, stores, banks, pharmacies, hospitals, senior centers, and museums are included in these categories.

Housing transitions may be necessary for the client to live independently. Home accessibility adaptations, such as ramps, mechanical lifts, and wide doorways, are necessary for some clients to return home. Bathroom accessibility is a common problem, and bathrooms are often in need of modification. Barriers to accessibility are not only physical but also economic; examples are poverty, perceived inability to afford services, and inability to meet eligibility criteria for special programs (Woodruff, 1995). Cultural barriers to health services in the community include the client's inability to speak English, distrust of health care professionals, lack of familiarity with bureaucracy, and stigma associated with using a service (Woodruff, 1995). Rehabilitation nurses, in cooperation with practitioners of other disciplines, can help clients gain access to health care and other community resources.

Recreation

Traveling with a disability is possible, but good planning is critical. Clients should choose a location, climate, accommodations, and mode of travel on the basis of their limitations. Rest periods are critical, and the length of the trip is best determined by the client. Group tours need to be investigated to learn the pace and timing. Room location near elevators and bathroom equipment is another concern. An aisle seat in the bus, airplane, car, or train provides easier access (American Society of Travel Agents and UpJohn). Clients with artificial joint replacements need to be reminded that the metal components of their prostheses may trigger the metal detectors in airports. The orthopedic surgeon can issue a card attesting to the presence of the prosthesis.

Clients with total hip replacement should not drive for 6 weeks after surgery. Total hip precautions must be maintained in the initial postoperative period. Clients who have total knee replacements should refrain from driving for 4 to 6 weeks. A consideration in deciding when driving can resume is which side the hip or knee surgery was performed on (Cameron et al., 1996). Handicapped stickers, licenses, and special parking privileges are beneficial to the client recovering from joint replacement surgery.

Work

Chronic health conditions are the most common cause of work limitation. Osteoarthritis and allied disorders account for 1.3 million conditions reported to cause work limitations (Kraus, Stoddard, & Gilmartin, 1996). Many people with osteoarthritis and osteoporosis are older; however, they may still desire to work on a part-time basis. They may believe that their age and disability force them to early retirement.

Reasonable accommodations for employees with disabilities must be made by employers. Example are modifying schedules or equipment and reassigning the client to a new position. People with adult-onset chronic disorders often do not realize their ability to benefit from the ADA (Freeman, Blalock, Holman, Liang, & Meenam, 1996).

Health Care Considerations

Support Services

Discharge to home often requires support services. Obstacles to receiving services have a variety of causes, which should be identified and addressed in the rehabilitation setting.

Support services and their delivery are affected by many factors, including the type and number of public services, geographic location, insurance and personal funding, and community commitment to assisting the disabled (McCourt, 1993). In the discharge planning for the client with osteoporosis or osteoarthritis, support services such as home health nurses may be necessary to monitor wound status and anticoagulant treatment. Transportation to follow-up doctor's appointments may be required. Meals on Wheels delivery of a hot meal once a day may be indicated for clients living alone.

Support groups can provide counseling, peer support, and education. They can also help the client with coping strategies. The National Osteoporosis Foundation recognizes the importance of support groups in helping cope with the disease. Building Strength Together, a National Osteoporosis Foundation affiliated support group, assists clients with osteoporosis. The leader's manual for the program contains suggestions for meetings. Linking-Up is another NOF-sponsored support activity in which clients with osteoporosis can make contact with a confidential telephone network. There are also groups for women younger than 50 years and for men (NOF, 1998a). Many local communities have Arthritis Support Groups.

Caregiver Training

Assessment of a caregiver's abilities is important to discharge planning. People responsible for the client's care after discharge must have the knowledge and practical experience to confidently and safely provide care. They must be able to learn and to provide care, which involves physical, emotional, and financial resources (Mumma, 1987). Caregiver training sessions with either the primary rehabilitation nurse or a clinical nurse specialist with advanced knowledge in coaching and teaching are essential throughout the rehabilitation process. Responses to assuming the caregiver role vary according to (1) the relationship between the client and caregiver, (2) the support system, and (3) the caregiver's knowledge about the client's disability (Williams, Oberst, Bjorklund, & Hughes, 1996).

Williams et al. (1996) studied 57 family caregivers of clients with hip fractures. Information about caregiving demands, expectations, and mood was presented. Tasks included in caregiving were providing medical and nursing treatments, providing personal care, assisting with mobility, providing emotional support, monitoring, transporting, managing finances, performing household tasks, structuring activities, and managing behavior. This abbreviated list of identified tasks points to the fact that training in the rehabilitation setting in a small way prepares the caregiver for all the responsibilities. The demands of caregiving can go far beyond the mobility assistance and personal care that might have been the focus of the training. Advice from the study's caregiver subjects include (1) having a network of support people to provide some relief, (2) adjusting the home to maximize the client's independence, and (3) speaking with a caregiver in a similar situation. The study concluded that caregiving for the elderly client after a hip fracture is often a difficult and lengthy process.

Slauenwhite and Simpson (1998) conducted a qualitative research study to determine the effect of early discharge on the families of older adults with repaired hip fracture. It is important to note that transition from hospital to home and the interaction with the health care system were reported as often being problematic for caregivers. Pain management was an area, both in the hospital and at home, in which the expectations of both clients and families were not met by the health care providers.

Equipment

Mobility devices may be necessary for clients with osteoporosis or osteoarthritis. It has been estimated that 7.4 million persons in the U.S. population use assistive devices for mobility. Of that number, almost 5 million use canes (National Center for Health Statistics, 1997).

Gait aids include walkers, crutches, canes, wheelchairs, and scooters. Proper height adjustment is essential. The client must have upper extremity strength and balance to use a walker safely. The gait patterns vary with the weight-bearing status. Crutches provide more stability than a cane, but upper extremity strength must be adequate to raise the body 1 to 2 inches off the floor. Canes can be single- or several-point. The cane is to be held in the hand on the side of the unaffected lower extremity to widen the base of support and to reduce the workload on the affected joint (Tan, 1998). Wheelchairs and scooters may be necessary for community mobility, such as for shopping.

Self-care tasks, such as eating, dressing, grooming, bathing, and toileting, may require assistive devices. Equipment for ADLs may be necessary. The client with osteoarthritis may require built-up handles on forks and spoons to improve grip or a rocker knife to facilitate cutting. Button hooks, zipper pulls, elastic shoelaces, and reachers can simplify dressing. Clients who have undergone arthroplasty will need a sock aid to help with donning stockings. Elastic shoelaces or Velcro tabs, a long-handled shoehorn, and a reacher facilitate independence with lower extremity dressing. Long-handled brushes or sponges and shower or tub chairs facilitate bathing. A raised toilet seat or commode chair with armrests is necessary for clients with total hip replacement to maintain their hip precautions.

Home activities such as meal preparation and household maintenance may require equipment for functional independence and safety. Wheeled utility carts to push items and baskets on walkers are easier ways to transport items. Household cleaning is easier with a self-propelled vacuum and long-handled dust pan and duster.

Community living skills include shopping and medication management. Motorized carts, bags with handles, and shopping at nonpeak hours are helpful. Medication management is a critical issue to be identified by nurses. Use of a calcitonin nasal spray may be new for the client with osteoporosis, and the nurse must assess whether the client can assemble the vial and sufficiently squeeze it to administer the full dose. Clients with arthritis may need non-childproof containers for their medications. An automatic insulin injector may make administration easier if fine motor movement is difficult because of arthritis. Special schedules or pill organizers can serve as reminders of doses and times.

Safety

Safety instruction is essential for a successful discharge plan. Falls are the major cause of both fatal and nonfatal injuries in people 65 and older in the United States. The most common serious injuries are wrist, spine, and hip fractures. Sixty percent of fractures occur in the home. The falls are generally incurred during everyday activities (AAOS, 1997). Contributing factors in falls are poor vision, poor mobility, orthostatic hypotension, loss of muscle strength and balance, medications, alcohol, and chronic diseases such as Parkinson's disease and dementia.

If ambulation devices are recommended, their use should be reinforced to provide added stability and safety. Rising slowly when getting up, having a lamp at bedside, using night-lights in hallways, and wearing properly fitting slippers, clothes, and shoes are all important. Throw rugs, electrical cords, and phone wires should not be in the path of walking. Grab bars and nonskid mats are beneficial in the bathroom. Clients should be advised not to lock the bathroom door, so that in case of injury, someone can enter easily to help (AAOS, 1997).

For clients who will be discharged alone with little or no support services or family supervision, it is essential that issues related to medications be addressed. Prior to discharge, rehabilitation nurses must assess the client's knowledge regarding medications. In addition, the ability to open containers, self-administer medication, and identify symptoms to report to a health care professional are essential to the safe management of medications. For clients taking anticoagulant medications, a fall can be especially serious, and clients need to know the importance of safety and when to report and seek medical attention if this occurs.

SUMMARY

This chapter provides a comprehensive overview of information essential to the nursing care of clients with osteoporosis and osteoarthritis and their families. As the trend toward shorter hospitalizations continues, rehabilitation nurses need to have knowledge and skills in orthopedic nursing to be prepared for caring for clients with complications that in the past may have been seen only in the acute care facility. In addition, rates of the orthopedic conditions described in this chapter are expected to increase as the U.S. population ages. As integral members of interdisciplinary teams, rehabilitation nurses need to be ready for future challenges and changes and prepared to assist practitioners of other disciplines in caring for orthopedic rehabilitation clients with complex needs.

REFERENCES

Addamo, S., & Abba Clough, J. (1998). Modalities for mobilization. In A. Maher, S. Salmond, & T. Pellino (Eds.), *Orthopaedic nursing* (2nd ed., pp. 323–350). Philadelphia: W. B. Saunders.

Altizer, J. (1998). Degenerative disorders. In A. Maher, S. Salmond, & T. Pellino (Eds.), *Orthopaedic nursing* (2nd ed., pp. 480–544). Philadelphia: W. B. Saunders.

American Academy of Orthopaedic Surgeons. (1997). *Don't let a fall be your last trip* [On-line]. Available: http://www.aaos.org/wordhtml/pateduc/falls bro.htm.

American Academy of Orthopaedic Surgeons. (1998a). *Facts about total hip and total knee replacement* [On-line]. Available: http://www.aaos.org/wordhtml/press/hipknee.htm.

American Academy of Orthpaedic Surgeons. (1998b). *The use of prophylactic antibiotics in orthopaedic medicine and the emergence of vancomycin-resistant bacteria: Advisory statement* [On-line]. Available: http://www.aaos.org.

American College of Sports Medicine. (1995). Position stand on osteoporosis and exercise. *Medical Science Sports Exercise,* (27), 1–7.

American Dental Association & American Academy of Orthopaedic Surgeons. (1997). Advisory statement: Antibiotic prophylaxis for dental patients with total joint replacement. *Journal of the American Dental Association, 128,* 1004–1008.

American Medical Association. (1994, Dec.). *News release: High intensity exercise can help prevent osteoporosis.* Chicago: Author.

American Nurses Association. (1996). Cultural diversity in nursing practice. In *Compendium of ANA Position Statements.* Washington, DC: Author.

American Society of Travel Agents & Upjohn. (n.d.). *Ansaid tablets: Guide to travelling with arthritis* [Brochure]. Author.

Apley, A., & Solomon, L. (1993). *Apley's system of orthopaedics and fractures* (7th ed.). Great Britain: Batte Press.

Arthritis Foundation. (1997a). *Exercise and your joints* [Brochure]. Atlanta: Author.

Arthritis Foundation. (1997b). *Osteoarthritis* [Brochure]. Atlanta: Author.

Bachelder, J., & Hilton, C. (1994). Implication of the Americans with Disabilities act of 1990 for the elderly person. *The American Journal of Occupational Therapy, 48* (1), 73–81.

Black, J., & Matassarin-Jacobs, E. (Eds.). (1993). *Luckman & Sorensen's medical-surgical nursing: A psychophysiologic approach* (4th ed.). Philadelphia: W. B. Saunders.

Block, J., & Schnitzer, T. (1997). Therapeutic approaches to osteoarthritis. *Hospital Practice, 32,* 159–164.

Bozeman, M. (1996). Cultural aspects of pain management. In E. Salerno & J. Willens (Eds.), *Pain management handbook: An interdisciplinary approach* (pp. 67–87). St. Louis: Mosby–Year Book.

Cameron, H., Brotzman, S., & Boolos, M. (1996). Rehabilitation after total joint arthroplasty. In S. Brotzman (Ed.), *Clinical orthopaedic rehabilitation* (pp. 283–311). St. Louis: Mosby–Year Book.

Carpenito, L. (1997). *Nursing diagnosis: Application to clinical practice* (7th ed.). Philadelphia: Lippincott-Raven.

Carroll, P. (1993). Deep vein thrombosis: Implications for orthopaedic nursing. *Orthopaedic Nursing, 12* (3), 33–42.

Christiansen, C. (1993). Consensus development conference: Diagnosis, prophylaxis & treatment of osteoporosis. *American Journal of Medicine, 94,* 646–650.

Clagett, A., Anderson, F., & Heit, J. (1995). Prevention of venous thromboembolism. *Chest, 108* (Suppl.), 312S–334S.

Clyman, B. (1996). Osteoarthritis: What to look for and when to treat it. *Geriatrics, 51,* 36–41.

Cooper, T. (1996). Culturally appropriate care: Optional or imperative. *Advanced Practice Nursing Quarterly, 2* (2), 1–6.

Currie, C. (1990). Rehabilitation in the elderly with fracture neck of the femur. *Seminars in Orthopaedics, 5* (2), 61–67.

Deal, C. (1997). Osteoporosis: Prevention, diagnosis, and management. *American Journal of Medicine, 102* (Suppl. 1A), 35S–39S.

Deutsch, A., Braun, S., & Granger, C. (1997). The functional independence measure (FIM instrument). *Journal of Rehabilitation Outcomes Measurement, 1,* 67–71.

Dood, C., Hungerford, D., & Krackow, K. (1990). Total knee arthroplasty fixation: Comparison of early results in cemented versus uncemented porous coated anatomic knee prosthesis. *Clinical Orthopaedics and Related Research, 260,* 66–70.

Drench, M., & Losee, R. (1996). Sexuality and sexual capacities of elderly people. *Rehabilitation Nursing, 21,* 118–123.

Dunajcik, L. (1989). The hip: When the joint must be replaced. *RN, 52* (4), 62–71.

Edworthy, S., Devins, G., & Watson, M. (1995). The arthritis knowledge questionnaire: A test for measuring patient knowledge of arthritis and self-management. *Arthritis and Rheumatism, 38,* 590–595.

Eli Lilly & Co. (1997). *Evista: Important information for patients using Evista for the prevention of osteoporosis after menopause* [On-line]. Available: http://www.evista.com/pi.html patient.

European Foundation for Osteoporosis & National Osteoporosis Foundation. (1997). Consensus development statement: Who are candidates for prevention and treatment of osteoporosis. *Osteoporosis International, 7,* 1–6.

Felson, D. (1996). Weight and osteoarthritis. *American Journal of Clinical Nutrition, 63* (Suppl.), 430S–432S.

Fitzgerald, R. (1992). Total hip arthroplasty sepsis: Prevention and diagnosis. *Orthopedic Clinics of North America, 23,* 259–264.

Fitzgerald, R., Nolan, D., & Ilstrup, D. (1977). Deep wound sepsis following total hip arthroplasty. *Journal of Bone and Joint Surgery, 59(A),* 847.

Freeman, J., Blalock, S., Holman, H., Liang, M., & Meenam, R. (1996). Advances brought by health services research to patients with arthritis: Summary of the Workshop on Health Services Research in Arthritis: From research to practice. *Arthritis Care and Research, 19,* 142–50.

Goldberg, V. (1994). Surgical treatment of osteoarthritis. *Journal of Musculoskeletal Medicine, 11* (12), 13–24.

Hanssen, A., Osmon, D., & Nelson, C. (1996). Prevention of deep periprosthetic joint infection. *Journal of Bone and Joint Surgery [Am], 78,* 458–471.

Hester, L. (1996). Coordinating a successful discharge plan. *American Journal of Nursing, 96,* 35–37.

Hitch, M. (1991). Complications. In D. Slye and L. Theis (Eds.), *An introduction to orthopaedic nursing: An orientation module* (pp. 105–118). Pitman, NJ: Jannetti.

Houtchens, C. (1998). *A guide to intimacy with arthritis: Answers to the most commonly asked questions* [Brochure]. Atlanta: Arthritis Foundation.

Hunt, A. (1998). Metabolic conditions. In A. Maher, S., Salmond, & T. Pellino (Eds.), *Orthopaedic nursing* (2nd ed., pp. 431–479). Philadelphia: W. B. Saunders.

Iacono, J., & Campbell, A. (1997). *Patient and family education: The compliance guide to the JCAHO standards.* Marblehead, MA: Opus Communications.

Jeans, M., & Melzack, R. (1992). Conceptual basis of nursing practice: Theoretical foundations of pain. In J. Watt-Watson & M. Donovan (Eds.), *Pain management: Nursing perspective* (pp. 11–35). St. Louis: Mosby–Year Book.

James, S., & Wade, P. (1991). Total knee arthroplasty: Postoperative care and rehabilitation. In *Total Joint Replacement* (pp. 533–539). Philadelphia: W. B. Saunders.

Johnson, J. (1986). Respiratory complications of orthopaedic injuries. *Orthopaedic Nursing, 5* (1), 24–28.

Kanner, M., & Roth, M. (1997). Women's issues in rehabilitation. In B. O'Young, M. Young, & S. Stiens (Eds.), *PM&R secrets* (pp. 435–439). Philadelphia: Hanley & Belfus.

Katz, R., & McCulla, M. (1995). Impedance plethysmography as a screening procedure for asymptomatic deep vein thrombosis in a rehabilitation hospital. *Archives of Physical Medicine and Rehabilitation, 76,* 833–839.

Kittler, P., & Sucher, C. (1990). Diet counseling in a multicultural society. *Diabetes Educator, 16,* 127–131.

Kraus, L., Stoddard, S., & Gilmartin, D. (1996). Causes and medical cost of disabilities. In *Chartbook on disability in the United States* (pp. 25–28). Washington, DC: U.S. National Institute on Disability and Rehabilitation Research.

Kunkler, C. (1991). Neurovascular assessment. In D. Slye & L. Theis (Eds.), *An introduction to orthopaedic nursing: An orientation module* (pp. 17–23). Pitman, NJ: Jannetti.

Leininger, M. (1991). *Culture care diversity and universality: A theory of nursing.* New York: National League for Nursing.

Leininger, M., & Cummings, S. (1996). Nursing's new paradigm is transcultural nursing: An interview with Madeline Leininger. *Advanced Practice Nursing Quarterly, 2* (2), 62–69.

Levy, C. (1997). Metabolic bone disease. In B. O'Young, M. Young, & S. Stiens (Eds.), *PM & R secrets* (pp. 501–508). Philadelphia: Hanley & Belfus.

Lozada, C., & Altman, R. (1997). Osteoarthritis: A comprehensive approach to management. *Journal of Musculoskeletal Medicine, 14,* 26–38.

Loeser, R., & Kammer, G. (1997). Osteoarthritis: Following the clinical clues to diagnosis. *Journal of Musculoskeletal Medicine, 14,* 25–34.

Lukert, B. (1994). Vertebral compression fractures: How to manage pain and avoid disability. *Geriatrics, 49,* 22–26.

Mahon, S. (1998). Osteoporosis: A concern for cancer survivors. *Oncology Nursing Forum, 25,* 843–851.

McCaffrey, M., & Beebe, A. (1989). *Pain: Clinical manual for nursing practice.* St. Louis: Mosby–Year Book.

McCourt, A. (Ed.). (1993). *The specialty practice of rehabilitation nursing: A core curriculum.* (3rd ed.) Skokie, IL: Rehabilitation Nursing Foundation of the Association of Rehabilitation Nurses.

Medical Economics. (1997). *Physicians desk reference* (51st ed.). Montvale, NJ: Author.

Mont, M., Tankersley, W., & Hungerford, D. (1997). Hip rehabilitation after surgery. In B. O'Young, M. Young, & S. Stiens (Eds.), *PM & R secrets* (pp. 330–337). Philadelphia: Hanley & Belfus.

Morrey, B. (1992). Instability after total hip arthroplasty. *Orthopedic Clinics of North America, 23,* 237–248.

Morris, J., Shay, D., Hebden, J., McCarter, R., Perdue, E., Jarvis, W., Johnson, J., Dowling, T., Polish, L., & Schwalbe, R. (1995). Enterococci resistant to multiple antimicrobial agents, including vancomycin: Establishment of endemicity in a university medical center. *Annals of Internal Medicine, 123,* 250–259.

Mumma, C. (Ed.). (1987). *Rehabilitation nursing: Concepts and practice—a core curriculum* (2nd ed.). Skokie, IL: Rehabilitation Nursing Foundation.

Munin, M., Kwoh, K., Glynn, N., Crossett, L., & Rubash, H. (1995). Predicting discharge outcome after elective hip and knee arthroplasty. *American Journal of Physical Medicine and Rehabilitation, 74,* 294–301.

Munin, M., Ruddy, T., Glynn, N., Crossett, L., & Rubash, H. (1998). Early inpatient rehabilitation after elective hip and knee arthroplasty. *JAMA, 279,* 847–852.

Nasser, S. (1992). Prevention and treatment of sepsis in total hip replacement surgery. *Orthopedic Clinics of North America, 23,* 265–277.

National Institute of Arthritis and Musculoskeletal and Skin Diseases. (1995) *Osteoporosis in men: factsheet* (No. AR-169, Rev. ed.). Bethesda, MD: U.S. Department of Health & Human Services.

National Institute of Arthritis and Musculoskeletal and Skin Diseases. (1997a). *Questions and answers about avascular necrosis* (No. AR-150QA). Bethesda, MD: U.S. Department of Health & Human Services.

National Institute of Arthritis and Musculoskeletal and Skin Diseases. (1997b). *Questions and answers about hip replacement* (No. AR-149QA). Bethesda, MD: U.S. Department of Health & Human Services.

National Institute of Arthritis and Musculoskeletal and Skin Diseases. (1998). *Questions and answers about arthritis pain* (No. AR-188QA). Bethesda, MD: U.S. Department of Health & Human Services.

National Center for Health Statistics. (1997). *New report on disability from NCHS.* [On-line]. Available: http://www.cdc.gov/nchswww/releases/97facts/97sheets/astecdev.htm.

National Institutes of Health. (1986, March). *Consensus development conference statement: Prevention of venous thrombosis and pulmonary embolism* [On-line]. Available: http://texc.nlm.nih.gov./nih/cdc/www/98txt/html.

National Institutes of Health. (1994a, June). *A summary of NIH consensus: Optimal calcium intake.* Bethesda, MD: Author.

National Institutes of Health. (1994b, Sept.). *Summary of the NIH consensus: Total hip replacement.* Bethesda, MD: Author.

National Osteoporosis Foundation. (1998b). *Fast facts on osteoporosis* [On-line]. Available: http://www.nof.org/stats.html.

National Osteoporosis Foundation. (1997, August). *Cutting edge reports: National Osteoporosis Foundation applauds inclusion of osteoporosis test in Balanced Budget Act* [On-line]. Available: http://www.nof.org/budgtact.html.

National Osteoporosis Foundation. (1998a). *Building strength together: A National Osteoporosis Foundation affiliated support group program* [On-line]. Available: http://www.nog.org/support/html.

Nevitt, M., Ottinger, B., Black, D., Stone, K., Jamal, S., Ensrud, K., Segal, M., Genant, H., & Cummings, S. (1998). The association of radiographically detected vertebral fractures with back pain and function: A prospective study. *Annals of Internal Medicine, 128,* 793–800.

Novy, C., & Jagmin, M. (1997). Pain management in the elderly orthopaedic patient. *Orthopaedic Nursing, 16* (1), 51–57.

O'Brien, L., Grisso, J., Maislin, G., Chiu, G., & Evans, F. (1993). Hospitalized elders' risk of confusion with hip fracture. *Journal of Gerontological Nursing, 19*(2), 25–31.

Osteoporosis and Bone Related Diseases–National Resource Center. (1995). Strategies for People with Osteoporosis: The Diagnosis. Washington, D.C.: National Osteoporosis Foundation.

Osteoporosis and Bone Related Diseases–National Resource Center. (1997). *Strategies for people with osteoporosis: After the vertebral fracture.* Washington, DC: National Osteoporosis Foundation.

Osteoporosis and Bone Related Diseases–National Resource Center. (1998). *Osteoporosis overview.* Washington, DC: Author.

Pak, C., Sakhall, K., Adams-Huet, B., et al. (1995). Treatment of postmenopausal osteoporosis with slow-release fluoride. *Ann Int Med 123,* 401–408.

Parke, B. (1998). Gerontological nurses' ways of knowing. *Journal of Gerontological Nursing, 24*(6), 21–28.

Patil, J. (1997). Chronic pain syndromes. In B. O'Young, M. Young, & S. Stiens (Eds.), *PM & R secrets* (pp. 351–355). Philadelphia: Hanley & Belfus.

Pellino, T., Polacek, L., Preston, M., Bell, N., & Evans, R. (1998). Complications of orthopaedic surgery. In A. Maher, S. Salmond, & T. Pellino (Eds.), *Orthopaedic nursing* (2nd ed., pp. 212–260). Philadelphia: W. B. Saunders.

Pope, R., Corcoran, S., McCaul, K., & Howie, D. (1997). Continuous passive motion after primary total knee arthroplasty: Does it offer any benefits? *Journal of Bone and Joint Surgery [Br], 79*(6), 914–917.

Price, J., & Cordell, B. (1994). Cultural diversity and patient teaching. *Journal of Continuing Education in Nursing, 25*, 163–167.

Rand, J. (1993). Neurovascular complications of total knee arthroplasty. In J. Rand (Ed.), *Total knee arthroplasty* (pp. 417–422). New York: Raven Press.

Resnick, B. (1994). Die from a broken hip? *RN, 57*(7), 22–26.

Ross, P. (1997). Clinical consequences of vertebral fractures. *American Journal of Medicine, 103*(2A), 30S–43S.

Schoen, D. (1986). *The nursing process in orthopaedics.* Norwalk, CT: Appleton-Century-Crofts.

Shealy, N., Liss, S., Kornhausen, S., & Cannizzaro, C. (1997). Transcutaneous electrical nerve stimulation. In B. O'Young, M. Young, & S. Stiens (Eds.), *PM & R secrets* (pp. 542–544). Philadelphia: Hanley & Belfus.

Slauenwhite, C., & Simpson, P. (1998). Patient and family perspectives on early discharge and care of the older adult undergoing fractured hip rehabilitation. *Orthopaedic Nursing, 17*(1), 30–36.

Snyder, P. (1998). Fractures. In A. Maher, S. Salmond, & T. Pellino (Eds.), *Orthopaedic nursing* (2nd ed., pp. 663–717). Philadelphia: W. B. Saunders.

Spiegel, N. (1997). The hip. In B. O'Young, M. Young, & S. Steins (Eds.), *PM & R secrets* (pp. 287–290). Philadelphia: Hanley & Belfus.

Swartz, M. (1994). *Textbook of physical diagnosis: History and examination* (2nd ed.). Philadelphia: W. B. Saunders.

Tan, J. (1998). *Practical manual of physical medicine and rehabilitation.* St. Louis: Mosby–Year Book.

Tankersley, W., Mont, M., & Hungerford, D. (1997). Knee rehabilitation after surgery. In B. O'Young, M. Young, & S. Stiens (Eds.), *PM & R secrets* (pp. 337–340). Philadelphia: Hanley & Belfus.

Theis, F. (1991). Caring for the elderly hip fracture patient. In D. Slye & L. Theis (Eds.), *An introduction to orthopaedic nursing: An orientation module* (pp. 90–101). Pitman, NJ: Jannetti.

Tucker, S., Canobbio, M., Paquette, E., & Wells, M. (1996). *Patient care standards: Collaborative practice planning guides* (6th ed.). St. Louis: Mosby–Year Book.

U.S. Department of Health and Human Services. (1992). *Quick reference guide for clinicians: Acute pain management in adult-operative procedures.* Rockville, MD: Author.

U.S. Department of Health and Human Services. (1998). *Targeting arthritis: The nation's leading cause of disability–at a glance.* Atlanta: Centers for Disease Control.

U.S. Equal Employment Opportunity Commission and U.S. Department of Justice Civil Rights Division. (1992, Sept.). *The Americans with disabilities act: Questions and Answers.* [Brochure]. Washington, DC: Author.

Vargo, M. (1995). Osteoporosis: Strategies for prevention and treatment. *Journal of Musculoskeletal Medicine, 12*(5), 19–30.

Wasilewski, R., Crossett, L., & Rubash, H. (1992). Neural and vascular injury in total hip arthroplasty. *Orthopedic Clinics of North America, 23*, 219–235.

Wells, S. (1996). Adding an at home path to your discharge plan. *American Journal of Nursing, 96*(10), 73–74.

Williams, M., Oberst, M., Bjorklund, B., & Hughes, S. (1996). Family caregiving in cases of hip fracture. *Rehabilitation Nursing, 21*, 124–131, 138.

Woodruff, L. (1995). Growing diversity in the aging population. *Caring, 4*, 7–10.

CHAPTER 24

Nursing Management of the Patient with Amputation

Michelle Young-Stevenson

The person with an amputation must face life with a profound change in body image. Whether it results from trauma or is caused by a complication of diabetes or peripheral vascular disease, and regardless of the age of the person, an amputation is physically challenging. Children, however, accept amputation, whether congenital or due to trauma, more easily than adults.

In children, congenital deformities are generally the cause of amputations in the first decade. After 10 years of age, trauma is the leading cause of amputation, followed by tumors (Jan, 1996). This chapter focuses on the care of adults with amputation.

The geriatric adult sustains an amputation of the lower extremity from complications of diabetes mellitus and peripheral vascular disease. The rate of lower extremity amputation is 15 times greater in diabetic people (Williamson, 1992). According to the American Diabetes Association, there are more than 50,000 lower extremity amputations performed each year on diabetic patients (Sanders, 2000). The young adult may undergo amputation of the upper extremities to a work-related, motor vehicle, or violence-related injury. There are more than 100,000 upper extremity amputations in the United States; the right hand and forearm are the most commonly affected.

The average cost of a nontraumatic amputation—from the initial onset of the problem involving diagnostic testing; through pharmaceutical intervention and surgical procedures to save the limb; to postoperative care, rehabilitation (physical, occupational, and psychological), nursing care, and the fitting of first a temporary, then a definitive prosthetic device—is very difficult to determine. The chronicity of the problem adds to the final cost, which would be greater than that for a traumatic amputation.

LEVEL OF AMPUTATION

The level of the amputation is determined by the severity of soft tissue damage, vascularity, and best level of functioning for the patient (Fig. 24–1). The lowest level of amputation is always the goal of any surgical procedure. The goal is to preserve the function of the extremity, thereby enabling the patient to function at the optimal level after surgery.

An amputation performed after many vascular bypass procedures should be viewed as the best outcome for returning the person to an optimal level of functioning. The person will be free of chronic pain, stress, and immobility. The vascularity of the affected limb after amputation should not compromise the healing. The goal is to make sure the wound, once closed, will heal. Factors that affect the healing process are (1) adequate nutrition, (2) resolution of local infection, and (3) overall medical stability of the patient.

The levels of amputations are as follows:

Syme amputation: Ankle disarticulation with the heel pad preserved

Below-the-knee amputation: Spares the knee joint

Knee disarticulation: Does not spare the knee joint

Above-the-knee amputation: Spares the hip joint

Hip disarticulation: Does not spare the hip joint

PREVENTIVE CONSIDERATIONS FOR KNOWN DISEASE FACTORS

Preventing complications of known disease processes can be difficult to accomplish. The impaired person may deny the disease process. Awareness of disease progression can lead to implementation of strategies to slow or stop the process. Numerous pamphlets

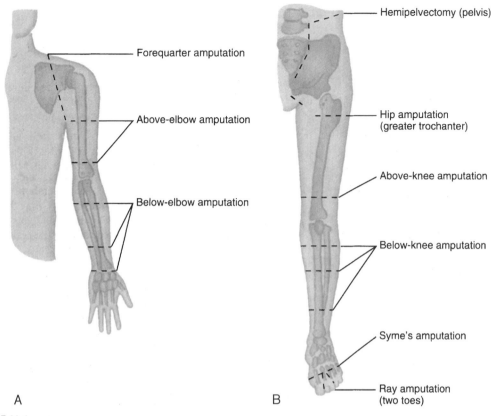

FIGURE 24–1
Common sites of amputation: *A*, Upper extremity. *B*, Lower extremity. (From Black, J., & Matassarin-Jacobs, E. [Eds.]. [1997]. *Medical-surgical nursing* [5th ed., p. 1419]. Philadelphia: W. B. Saunders.)

available from the American Heart Association and the American Diabetes Association provide basic information about the diseases (cardiovascular disease and diabetes) and how to decrease complications.

The knowledge needed to assist clients with their care is available through pamphlets, slides, didactic workshops, and seminars. Small-group sessions in clinics and doctors' offices may enhance self-care knowledge. Patients, families, and significant others must be recipients of such education. Knowledge is power. Through teaching, rehabilitation nurses give individuals, families, and communities the power to take control of the preventive measures needed to stop the advancement of disease. Once a disease or condition is detected, it must be treated to prevent further progression and complications.

Peripheral Vascular Disease

Peripheral vascular disease, also known as arteriosclerosis, is a major cause of amputations. This is a hereditary disease; the impaired person has the genes carrying the tendency to develop the disease. Arteriosclerosis progresses over time by leaving deposits of lipids, calcium, and fibrin, producing calcified plaques in the arterial walls, especially along the bifurcations of the large arteries (Guyton & Hall, 1997). Over time, the arteries narrow and blood flow is restricted.

As a result, pain develops, in the form of either intermittent claudication or ischemic rest pain. *Claudication* is pain that occurs after exercise or walking and is relieved by rest. *Ischemic rest pain* occurs at night, when the legs may be elevated and the circulation is decreased by the cardiac output while sleeping. This pain may awaken the patient. The patient rubs the leg, walks around, or takes medication to relieve the pain.

Early detection of the symptoms can prevent further complications such as occlusion, which can require bypass surgery and amputation. Various assessments, such as detection of a pulse by Doppler and calculation of the ankle-brachial index, can be made to identify vascular occlusions of the circulatory system. The goal is to relieve the pain and prevent an amputation.

Rehabilitation nurses employ many strategies to reduce risk factors, such as

- Diet counseling to modify diets—decrease saturated fats and cholesterol
- Counseling for weight loss—decrease obesity
- Monitoring and control of blood pressure
- Stress management education
- Counseling for smoking cessation

Patients with peripheral vascular disease must avoid trauma to the skin in the form of bruising or laceration. The delayed healing caused by the disease predisposes the person to infection. Safety education is an essential nursing intervention.

Diabetes Mellitus

Diabetes mellitus is also a hereditary disease that affects all systems of the body. Diabetes is a disorder of the metabolism of carbohydrate, fat, and protein. Abnormal secretion of insulin is its hallmark.

Insulin is produced by the beta cells in the islets of Langerhans in the pancreas. The insulin is released into the bloodstream when food is ingested. In diabetes, a decreased amount of insulin is released. Insulin, along with the other hormones that counterregulate glycogen, helps maintain blood glucose levels within normal ranges. Any abnormalities of insulin production or of these counterregulatory hormones cause diabetes.

The goal of management of diabetes mellitus should be to achieve a balance among diet, activity, medication, and monitoring, as well as patient and family education. Monitoring activities help maintain control of the disease process and ultimately prevent complications such as amputations (Ruda, 1996). The goals of diabetes management are as follows:

1. Maintain blood glucose as near normal as possible by balancing food intake, insulin daily dose, activity, and regular exercise.
2. Attain and maintain reasonable body weight by providing sufficient calories for energy expenditure.
3. Achieve and maintain optimal blood lipid levels.
4. Prevent and treat hypoglycemia and hyperglycemia.
5. Improve or maintain overall health through optimal nutrition.

PHYSICAL CARE OF THE LOWER EXTREMITIES

Patients with the hereditary diseases diabetes mellitus and arteriosclerosis must give special care to their lower extremities. Foot ulcers are the cause of 85% of all lower extremity amputations (Reiker, Lipsky, & Gibbons, 1998).

Foot Care

Because sensation may be diminished in diabetic neuropathy, patients may not feel pain until necrosis and/or severe infection is discovered. The Bureau of Primary Health Care (2000) has initiated the Lower Extremity Amputation Prevention Program to determine patient risk. The diabetic foot screen is available through the Division of Programs for Special Populations website (BPHC, 2000). Patient education regarding physical care should include the following points:

1. Inspect the feet daily, especially between the toes, for blisters, cuts, and scratches. The use of a mirror can improve visualization of the bottoms of the feet.
2. Wash the feet daily and dry carefully, especially between the toes.
3. Avoid extreme temperatures. Test the water with a thermometer before bathing.
4. If feet feel cold at night, wear socks. Do not apply hot water bottles or heating pads.
5. Do not use chemical agents for the removal of corns and calluses.
6. Inspect the insides of shoes daily for foreign objects, nails, and torn linings.
7. Wear properly fitted stockings, do not wear mended stockings, avoid stockings with seams, and change stockings daily.
8. Do not wear garters.
9. Shoes should be comfortable at the time of purchase. Do not assume that they will stretch.
10. Do not wear shoes without stockings.
11. Do not wear sandals with thongs between the toes.
12. Do not walk barefooted, especially on hot surfaces such as sandy beaches and swimming pool decks.
13. Cut toenails straight across if you have good eyesight. Visit a podiatrist on a regular basis, at least every 3 months, or more frequently if nails grow fast.
14. Do not cut corns and calluses. Follow special instructions from your physician or podiatrist.
15. See your physician regularly, and be sure your feet are examined at each visit.
16. If your vision is impaired, have a family member inspect your feet daily and trim your toenails.

Skin Care and Daily Maintenance of the Amputated Limb

Daily care of the skin of an amputated limb is just as important as that of the remaining limb. Once the staples or sutures are removed, the stump should be bathed daily with warm water. Mild soap and a soft washcloth must be used to prevent trauma to the skin. Rinsing of the skin thoroughly to remove all the soap will decrease the incidence of irritation. The skin should be dried thoroughly with a soft towel and then allowed to air dry before application of stump socks and the prosthesis.

After the wearing of a pylon or prosthesis, it is important to inspect the skin. Areas of redness and abrasion can occur from improper fit or prolonged use. The areas of concern are as follows:

■ Groin area
■ End of the stump
■ Front of the stump, where the bones end
■ Behind the stump, where there is pressure from the prosthesis

Even with the frequent skin checks, problems may still arise. Table 24–1 lists the problems associated with impaired skin integrity and their possible causes.

In patients who are of African-American descent or have darker skin, the problem of redness is difficult to detect by vision alone. The nurse may need to touch the extremity to determine whether irritation has caused any change in the temperature. Color changes in such patients may appear blue, green, or purple.

There may also be signs and symptoms of more serious problems. Signs and symptoms of potential or actual infection in the ampu-

tated limb are (1) drainage from openings in the stump, (2) low-grade fever, (3) increased pain in the stump area, and (4) elevated blood glucose level in a diabetic patient. The emphasis on impeccable physical care will prevent or identify such problems as early as possible.

Stump Wrapping

Stump wrapping is another important aspect of physical care. Shaping the residual limb, controlling edema, and minimizing pain are the goals of stump wrapping.

The bandages must be clean and dry. The patient must have two sets of bandages so that one can be washed while the other is being worn. Various products can be used for stump wrapping, such as (1) elastic bandage (Ace) wraps and (2) a stump shrinker, an elastic one-piece stocking that fits over the stump. These bandages or stockings need to be washed by hand, not in the washing machine, which would cause them to stretch and lose their elasticity. Members of the client's family should be taught how to wrap the stump and wash the bandages, in the event that the client becomes sick and is unable to provide self-care.

The patient should be taught to always keep the knee extended when wrapping the stump and to wrap using diagonal turns. He or she must also make that sure that there are no puckers or bulges in the skin and that all the skin below the knee is covered. The limb should be rewrapped every 24 hours or whenever the bandage starts to slip or feel loose.

The following procedure should be used for stump wrapping (Fig. 24–2):

1. Hold the bandage in one hand with the roll facing up and toward the head. With the other hand, hold the end of the bandage against the front of the limb, just below the knee. Slowly unroll the bandage diagonally (in figure-of-eight fashion) down the front leg to the inside corner of the limb.
2. Wrap the bandage over the inside corner of the limb. Give it a slight tug so that it will stay firmly against the skin. Bring the bandage around the posterior limb to the outside of the lower leg. Wrap diagonally up the lower leg toward the knee. Cross over the end of the bandage to hold it in place.
3. Go around the back of the lower leg, and bring the bandage to the front, just below

TABLE 24–1 ■ PROBLEMS ASSOCIATED WITH IMPAIRED SKIN INTEGRITY, WITH POSSIBLE CAUSES

Problem	Cause(s)
Abrasion	Scrapes, rough washcloth, rubbing from prosthesis
Reddened area (or warm skin area in people of color)	Pressure from prosthesis
Blister	Improper fitting or not wearing a stump sock
Hair root infection	Ingrown hair
Rash	Perspiration, inadequate drying skin, friction from prosthesis, reaction to sock material

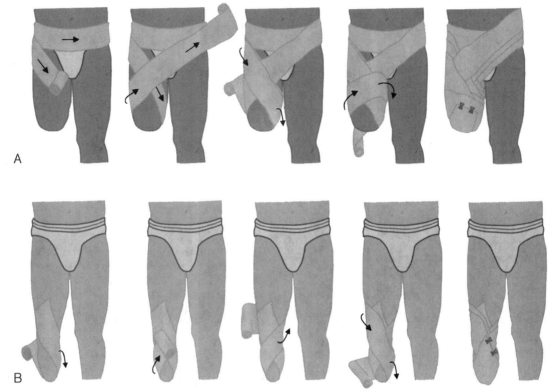

FIGURE 24–2
Common method of stump wrapping. *A,* For an above-knee stump, two bandages are required. *B,* For a below-knee stump, one bandage is usually sufficient. (From Black, J., & Matassarin-Jacobs, E. [Eds.]. [1997]. *Medical-surgical nursing* [5th ed., p. 1421]. Philadelphia: W. B. Saunders.)

the knee. Wrap diagonally down the front of the lower leg to the inside of the limb.

4. Bring the bandage around the back of the limb and forward over the outside corner. Give the bandage another gentle tug to keep it firmly against the skin. Wrap diagonally up the front of the lower leg.

5. Go around to the back of the limb, and come to the front again below the knee. Wrap diagonally down the front of the lower leg toward the inside corner of the limb.

6. To keep the bandage from slipping, bring it up one side of the knee, around the back of the thigh, and down the other side of the knee. Then wrap diagonally down and around the lower leg, to reach the end of the bandage. Attach the end of the bandage to the layer below it with paper tape. Avoid using pins or metal clips.

7. Tingling or throbbing anywhere in the limb may be a sign that the tension is too tight. If it occurs, rewrap the bandage using less tension.

POSITIONING AND EXERCISE

To enable the client to regain and maintain body alignment and to prevent contracture and pain after an amputation, exercise and positioning are a part of the daily routine.

Positioning

Limbs must be flexible, so frequent change of position is needed. Sitting or lying in one position for long periods can cause hip and knee stiffness or contractures. Contracture, which will interfere with the fitting of a prosthesis and ultimately with ambulation, should be prevented. The various positions for comfort and alignment are prone, supine, and sitting. These positions should be used alternately. The physical therapist will instruct the patient in these procedures during the therapy sessions.

The prone position stretches out the hip muscles. Lying prone for 30 minutes twice during the day and sleeping prone at night on a firm bed are recommended. The legs should be together, with both hips flat on the mattress. Supine lying can be used as a change of position. No pillows should be used under hips or knees. The limb should be kept flat so the hip and knee joints are straight. Sitting for long periods can cause muscles in the hip to tighten. The patient should change the position by standing or lying down to stretch out the muscles in the hip.

The person with an above-the-knee amputation should sit straight in a firm chair so that the weight is distributed evenly on the buttocks. The legs should be close together and oriented frontward. The person with a below-the-knee amputation should not cross the legs or let the amputated limb hang dependent. He or she needs to use a stump board to support the limb and keep the knee straight. If a prosthesis is being worn, standing and walking to change position will help straighten the knee joint.

Exercises

Exercise and strengthening of muscles are need to achieve ambulation. The leg muscles after surgery are weak in the amputated limb as well as in the nonamputated limb. The exercises described here focus on the major muscle groups of the lower extremity, which are (1) hip extensors, (2) hip flexors, (3) knee extensors, (4) hip abductors, (5) hip adductors, and (6) knee flexors.

Hip extension exercises strengthen the hip and buttock. They are performed as follows:

1. Lie supine on a firm mattress with a pillow under the head.
2. Bend the nonamputated leg at the knee, and press the amputated leg down into the mattress.
3. Hold, then relax.
4. Switch to a prone position with the hands under the chin.
5. Keeping both hips flat against the mattress, raise the amputated leg to the ceiling.
6. Hold, slowly lower the leg back to the mattress, and then relax.

Hip flexion–knee extension exercises strengthen the hip and the knee. They are performed as follows:

1. Lie supine.
2. Bend the nonamputated leg at the knee. Then raise the amputated leg straight up to be parallel with the other thigh, and hold.
3. Slowly lower the amputated leg, press it into the mattress, and hold.
4. Relax.

Hip abduction-adduction exercises strengthen the hip and buttocks. They are performed as follows:

1. Lie supine on a firm mattress.
2. Keeping both legs straight, slide the amputated leg out to the side as far as possible.
3. Slide the leg back, then relax.
4. Squeeze the legs together, hold, then relax. This exercise can be enhanced by putting a pillow or towel between the thighs.
5. Turn onto the nonamputated side, and bend the knee of the nonamputated leg slightly.
6. Raise the amputated leg toward the ceiling. Push it back slightly to keep it in line with your body, and hold.
7. Lower the leg, and relax.

Knee flexion exercises strengthen the muscles in the knee. They are performed as follows:

1. Lie prone with a pillow under the chest and the hands under your chin or forehead.
2. Keeping both hips flat against the mattress, bend the leg at the knee, and hold.
3. Slowly lower the leg back to the mattress, straighten it out, then relax.

The series of exercises just described will help to prepare the client with an amputation for walking with assistive devices, such as walkers, crutches, and prostheses. Greater energy is required to walk with an assistive device. Balance is also crucial in the success of the rehabilitation process. The client who is going to walk with a walker or crutches must be able to balance on one leg. Exercise and positioning go hand in hand to maintain the proper alignment and functioning for assistive ambulation.

NUTRITIONAL CONSIDERATIONS

Proper nutrition is a major component of treating disease and illness. Conditions such as stroke, heart disease, diabetes, and arteriosclerosis have a direct correlation with dietary intake and metabolism. The U.S. Department of Agriculture developed a food guide to promote health, called the Food Pyramid (ARAMARK Services. Nutrition care manual, 1992). It contains five major food groups. Each group provides nutrients needed for good health. Eating a variety of foods from each group is the foundation of a well-balanced diet.

The selection of foods from each group

should be based on individual needs, such as calories. People with specialized diets, such as diabetic, cardiac, renal, and low cholesterol, should receive counseling from a registered dietitian or nurse. Nutrition-related factors that affect wound healing are as follows:

- Obesity
- Protein deficiency
- Anemia
- Hyperglycemia
- Dehydration
- Atherosclerosis
- Inadequate food intake

An emphasis on good nutrition during the rehabilitation of a patient with an amputation is paramount to the healing of the site. Because many such patients are diabetic and may also have heart disease, the nutritional component must be individualized. Patients with diabetes must also incorporate exercise, lifestyle, and diabetes management into their lives. The goals of diabetes management should include but are not limited to these goals:

- Maintain blood glucose level as near normal as possible by balancing food intake, insulin, and activity.
- Attain and maintain reasonable body weight by providing sufficient calories for energy expenditure.
- Achieve and maintain optimal blood lipid levels.
- Prevent and treat hypoglycemia and hyperglycemia.
- Improve or maintain overall health through optimal nutrition.

Many studies have been done on dietary practices of individuals with diabetes. Approximately 3% of the U.S. population have been diagnosed with diabetes. There are probably an equal number of people with non–insulin-dependent diabetes (NIDDM). The prevalence of NIDDM in the United States is highest in minorities, such as Hispanic, Native American, and African American (Monk, 1995). People with NIDDM are perhaps more at risk for developing complications of diabetes because they may not be aware that they have the disease. Blood glucose control is important for people with both forms of disease.

Coronary heart disease, the leading cause of mortality in the United States, accounts for one third of all deaths annually. Evidence linking dietary intake of saturated fats and cholesterol to the development of coronary heart disease has been mounting. Govern-

ment and private healthcare organizations have led a movement to change dietary habits of all Americans (U.S. Department of Agriculture & Department of Health and Human Services [USDA & DHHS], 1995). Diet should include plenty of vegetables, fruits, and grain products. To maintain health and prevent disease, sugar, salt, and alcohol should be used only in moderation. Fat intake should be no greater than 30% of total daily calories and total carbohydrate intake no more than 50%.

The National Cholesterol Education Step 1 and Step 2 Diets include recommendations that total fat intake be 30% of the total daily calories and total carbohydrate intake be 55%. In more stringent programs, such as the Pritikin diet, total fat intake is 10% of total calories, and total carbohydrate intake is 75 to 80%. The Dean Ornish diet requires that only 10% of total calories come from fat, and 70 to 75% from carbohydrates (Institute for Natural Resources, 1996).

Any severe dietary restrictions should always be made under the supervision of a physician, especially if there are medical problems such as diabetes and heart disease. The primary concern is that the modification of potential and actual risk factors is monitored. The nurse is the primary link in the use of health care services by the patients through education. A complete understanding and adaptation of prudent eating habits can decrease the incidence of heart disease and control the complications of diabetes (Monk, 1995).

Cultural Adjustments

At all age levels, members of minority groups are more likely than whites to consider their health fair or poor. This belief will have a great impact on their nutritional status, because diet and health are so closely linked. Any restrictions of dietary intakes, as described for specialized diets designed for use in specific diseases, need to take in the cultural differences of minority clients. A culturally traditional preparation of foods needs to be modified to comply with the dietary restrictions. This modification will be a monumental task, especially if a client's literacy is an issue. Someone who cannot read above the third-grade level will be unable to read labels or recipes.

PSYCHOSOCIAL SUPPORT

The patient who has lost a body part as a result of trauma or a disease process requires psychosocial support. Such support may ultimately need to come from a professional psychologist to help the patient deal with personal coping patterns. The nurse can initiate some interventions for the most commonly used nursing diagnoses in this situation. These diagnosis are (Williamson, 1992)

- Grieving related to actual loss
- Alterations in comfort
- Disturbances in self-concept, which include body image disturbances, impaired social interaction, and alteration in family process

The nurse must encourage patients to express anxiety and fears openly. Participation in the care as early as possible helps patients recognize that the body image change is real.

The phenomenon of *phantom limb sensation* elicits various reactions. Reports of being able to feel toes moving and pins-and-needles sensations in the absent limb are examples. In phantom limb sensation, the remaining nerves continue to generate impulses that flow through the spinal cord and the thalamus to the somatosensory areas of the cerebral cortex. Most patients with amputation experience the sensation that amputated limb is still present. This sensation is stronger for upper limb amputations than for lower.

Patients with amputation who experience pain for more than 6 months are said to have *phantom pain*. Someone who perceives the (amputated) foot to be in a twisted position may have lost the foot in a traumatic crushing injury. Depression may contribute to the pain in the phantom limb.

Nonpharmaceutical pain management to help control the pain should be tried first. Treatment modalities such as biofeedback, transcutaneous electrical nerve stimulation (TENS), ultrasound, acupuncture, relaxation, and surgical management should also be used. If all else fails, the use of analgesics is acceptable. The nurse should reassure the patient that the pain will diminish over time. The use of alternative treatments decreases the focus on the amputation by centering on an activity in which the person can be a participant (Rounseville, 1992).

EDUCATIONAL PLAN FOR PREVENTION OF COMPLICATIONS

In rehabilitation, the patient is expected to gain the requisite knowledge to achieve self-care. The rehabilitation team members talk to the patient at different times about various aspects of recovery and the road to independence. Teaching begins at the bedside, is reinforced in the therapy areas, and is revisited upon the patient's return to the nursing unit. The goal of teaching is to maintain the optimal level of wellness through the understanding of the disease process.

Education of the patient is a major component of the rehabilitation process. Teaching can be conducted individually, with another patient, or in a group setting. When the setting is selected for the individual patient, the environment is more conducive for that patient's learning.

Before initiation of any educational program, a needs assessment must be performed to determine the patient's level of cognitive function and desire to learn. A simple tool that can address the educational needs and assess the limitations of patients and significant others should be used. The form should be multidisciplinary so that educational contributions made by practitioners of all disciplines in the rehabilitation unit can be recorded in one place. Such a form allows anyone to see at a glance what has been taught or needs to be reviewed.

When educational needs or limitations are assessed, the areas of physical, cognitive, language, psychosocial, and emotional needs; desire to learn; and socialization should be included in the criteria. These areas should direct the plan of care developed for each patient. Figure 24–3 is an example of a form that can be used to record the plan of care and keep track of educational activities. The procedure for using it is as follows:

1. Identify interventions.
2. List topics and procedures, and identify the learner if other than the patient.
3. Evaluate how the person responded to the information by using the codes in the top right corner.
4. Make recommendations for further teaching as listed in the top right corner.
5. Add general comments.

Whatever patient education tool is used, it must be clear and easy to use so the information will be consistently documented. The form in Figure 24–3 is an example of a tool that can be used to monitor teaching.

After assessing the needs and establishing who will be taught, the nurse can decide which setting is most appropriate. Private one-to-one sessions or group sessions can be chosen based on the learner's needs. Handouts, slides, and any type of visual aids

Date & Initials	Educational Needs Assessment Limitations	Yes	No
	Physical		
	Cognitive		
	Language		
	Psych/emotional		
	Desire to learn		

Codes	
Evaluation	Recommendation
1 = No evidence of learning	5 = Reteach
2 = Recalls content	6 = Review
3 = Returns demonstration	7 = Practice
4 = Applies knowledge	8 = Home care follow-up

Date/Initials	Intervention (Topic/procedure taught; identify the learner if other than the patient)	Evaluation (Enter code above)	Recommendation (Enter code above)	Comments

Initials	Signature and Title	Initials	Signature and Title	Initials	Signature and Title

FIGURE 24–3
Patient/family teaching record.

I. Causes of amputation:
   A. Peripheral vascular disease
   B. Diabetes mellitus
   C. Trauma
   D. Tumors
II. Levels of amputation:
   A. Transmetatarsal
   B. Syme
   C. Below-the-knee
   D. Above-the-knee
   E. Hip disarticulation
III. Skin care:
   A. General
   B. Care of the amputated limb
   C. Signs and symptoms of infection
IV. Phantom limb sensation
V. Stump wrapping
VI. Positioning and exercise
VII. Mobility
   A. Transfers
   B. Ambulation:
      1. Walkers, crutches
      2. Devices—temporary/definitive
   C. Nonambulators
VIII. Equipment
IX. Discharge planning

FIGURE 24–4
An example of an outline for the care of the patient with an amputation.

should be used to assist in the teaching process. A time should be allotted for questions and answers after each teaching session.

A course outline should be given to the patient and family (Fig. 24–4). Each area of the outline of care should have objectives, and handouts should be developed to complement its content. The objective should be stated in behavioral terms, with measurable outcomes.

Teaching is only one part of the care of the person with an amputation. Teaching can lead to the prevention of further complications and progression of the condition that necessitated the amputation, which can save the person from future problems.

AVAILABILITY OF HEALTH CARE FOR DISADVANTAGED CLIENTS

Heart disease, diabetes, and their sequelae—peripheral vascular disease and amputations—are major health care concerns. The Health Resources and Services Administration (HRSA), an agency of the U.S. Public Health Service, is responsible for developing national resources and supporting the delivery of health services to disadvantaged populations. The HRSA has compiled data in the *Health Status of the Disadvantaged Chartbook*, which was published in 1990 and reflects the data from the late 1980s (USDHHS, 1990). It shows that the status of health care in minority populations is improving slightly but that the trends in death rates and risk categories for these groups continue to remain high.

The data also found that one of every four Americans is classified as minority, and one of every three minority persons is of Hispanic origin or descent. Minorities have shared in the general improvement in health but lag behind in the health status indicators, such as death rates for chronic diseases and the presence of elevated blood pressure. In 1986, death rates from heart disease were higher in black males and females than in their white counterparts. Also, blacks were more likely to have high-risk serum cholesterol levels and to have borderline or elevated blood pressure. This tendency may be due, in part, to diet, lack of exercise, and income level. Of families with income levels of less than $10,000, 37% had no health care coverage (USDHHS, 1990).

Health care services are underutilized by minority groups. Minorities and low-income families experience the greatest difficulty in acquiring and regularly using medical care. The trend has been to visit hospital emergency rooms for immediate attention to a problem rather than to seek preventive care and ongoing treatment of a condition from a physician or clinic. Two groups, however, utilize health care services better—African Americans who are older than 65 years, and persons who are disabled; members of both these groups are covered by Medicare or Medicaid services (USDA & DHHS, 1990).

SUMMARY

Amputations are often related to peripheral vascular disease and diabetes. Whether an amputation is due to chronic illness or is of a traumatic origin, it represents an insult to the body image and a physical challenge to the person. With proper physical care, including skin care and daily maintenance of the amputated limb, positioning, exercise, nutrition, psychosocial support, and patient education, the person with an amputation can live a fulfilling life. The rehabilitation nurse is in a key position to ensure high-quality care for patients with amputations.

REFERENCES

Bureau of Primary Health Care (BPHC), Division of Special Populations. Lower Extremity Amputation Prevention Program. Available at http://www. hphc. hrsa.gov/leap/screening.htm

Esquenazi, A. (1993). Geriatric amputee rehabilitation. *Clinics in Geriatric Medicine, 9,* 731–743.

Guyton, A. C., & Hall, J. E. (1997). *Human physiology and mechanism of disease* (6th ed.). Philadelphia: W. B. Saunders.

Jan, S. (1996). Rehabilitation in limb deficiency: 3. The pediatric amputee. *Archives in Physical Medicine and Rehabilitation, 77,* 14–17.

Monk, A., Barry & McClain, K. (1995). Practice guidelines for medical nutrition: Therapy provided by dietitians for persons with non-insulin dependent diabetes mellitus. *Journal of the American Dietetic Association,* 999–1006.

Reiber, G E., Lipsky, B. A., Gibbons, G. W. (1998). The burden of diabetic foot ulcers. *American Journal of Surgery, 176,* 58–108.

Rounseville, C. (1992). Phantom limb pain: The ghost that haunts the amputee. *Orthopedic Nursing, 11,* 67–71.

Ruda, S. (1996). Nursing role in management of musculoskeletal problems. In S. Lewis, I. Collier, & M. Heit-kemper (Eds.), *Medical surgical nursing* (pp. 1839–1895). St. Louis: Mosby.

Sanders, C. S. (2000). Caring for diverse populations: Preventing amputation in patients with diabetes. *Patient Care for the Nurse Practitioners* 17–38.

U.S. Department of Health and Human Services, Human Resources and Services Administration, Division of Disadvantaged Assistance. (1990). *Health status of the disadvantaged chartbook* (Publication No. HRS-P-DV 90-1). Rockville, MD: Author.

U.S. Department of Agriculture and Department of Health and Human Services. (1995). *Nutrition and Your Health: Dietary guidelines for Americans* (4th ed.). Washington, DC: Author.

Williamson, V. (1992). Amputation of the lower extremity: An overview. *Orthopedic Nursing, 11,* 55–65.

BIBLIOGRAPHY

ARAMARK Services. (1992). *Nutrition care manual* (pp. 1D–4D). Philadelphia: ARAMARK.

CHAPTER 25

Nursing Management of the Patient with Rheumatoid Arthritis

Mary P. Brassell

The rehabilitation nurse is in a key position to facilitate the patient coping with the daily challenges of arthritis. When the client is newly diagnosed, the focus is on prevention of loss of function, prevention of deformities, and compliance with therapeutic and drug regimens. When and if the client exhibits pain and disability that are associated with arthritis, the nurse's goal is to help the client adapt to functional compromise.

The term arthritis encompasses over 150 diseases, syndromes, and conditions. Some conditions, such as tendinitis or bursitis, are short-term and/or self-limiting. Some types of arthritis, such as osteoarthritis, affect only the joints. However, multisystem or systemic arthritis affects the joints and body systems. These disorders include rheumatoid arthritis (RA), systemic lupus erythematosus, and progressive systemic sclerosis, previously referred to as scleroderma. The etiology of these diseases is unknown. There are no cures and many are life-threatening. These diseases impact adversely on activities of daily living (ADLs), sexuality, economic status, and psychosocial issues. Insufficient arthritis education in both medical and nursing schools impacts negatively on diagnosis, prognosis, and treatment. Rheumatologists are specially trained in the management of these diseases; however, many physicians lack the expertise to diagnose and treat multisystem arthritis.

In 1992, arthritis costs ranged over $50 billion, which accounted for over 3% of the gross national product (Klippel, 1997). Osteoarthritis is the second most common disability in the United States.

This chapter delineates the differences between nonsystemic arthritis and multisystem arthritis. Osteoarthritis is used as the prototype for nonsystemic, joint-related arthritis and is covered in Chapter 23. RA is used as

the prototype for multisystem arthritis and pain. A general view of signs, symptoms, diagnosis, prognosis, and treatment is presented. The major goals according to priority are pain management and arthritis drug therapy, prevention of deformities, and management of ADLs to maintain or prevent loss of function.

RHEUMATOID ARTHRITIS

RA is a chronic inflammatory disease that affects the peripheral joints of the body and is accompanied by extraarticular manifestations that affect other body systems, that is, the eyes, skin, heart, and respiratory, renal, nervous, and gastrointestinal systems. In addition, many people with RA are sensitive to colder temperatures. One of the most devastating aspects of RA is its unpredictable periods of remission and exacerbation of varied intensities. RA is found throughout the world in all ethnic groups. It can occur at any age, but the peak incidence is between the fourth and fifth decades. RA is 2.5 times more prevalent in women. Both the cause and the cure for RA remain a mystery; however, current research seems directed toward genetic, molecular, and cellular factors related to the inflammatory response. There is no laboratory tool that identifies RA; rather, clinical findings establish the diagnosis. The American College of Rheumatology revised the criteria for the classification of RA in 1987, and these criteria serve as a guide for care providers to aid in establishing the diagnosis.

Although a positive rheumatoid factor, present in 90% of the RA population, is a major immunological abnormality in RA, it is not specific for RA. Rheumatoid factor is detected in patients with chronic bacterial infections, organ transplants, and other chronic inflammatory diseases. The presence of rheumatoid factor also increases with age.

The abnormality of RA stems from the two-cell synovial membrane that lines all synovial joints, tendons, and ligaments. Some unknown trigger causes the synovium to become inflamed, and if the inflammation is unchecked, the synovium proliferates, forming a pannus, which destroys the cartilage, and secondary osteoarthritis may occur. The classic signs and symptoms of RA are found in Table 25–1.

Morning Stiffness Related to Rheumatoid Arthritis

Morning stiffness that lasts an hour or longer is one of the hallmarks of RA. It differs from the "gel" syndrome associated with osteoarthritis, which is relieved within 10 to 15 minutes of resumption of movement. The stiffness of RA can last from 1 to 24 hours. A mother with RA who may need help in sending her children off to school in the early morning but is able to play bridge in the afternoon may be chided by her family for

pretending to be incapacitated to avoid maternal duties. Because of extreme sensitivity to cold temperatures, a father may be unable to attend his son's hockey games. RA in one member of the family affects other family members and creates interrelationship difficulties when remissions and exacerabations are unpredictable.

Atlantoaxial Subluxation

Studies have revealed that atlantoaxial subluxation, another hallmark of RA, has been found in 75% of the RA population. Atlantoaxial subluxation occurs in the cervical spine at the C1, C2, and C3 levels. Tenosynovitis of the transverse ligament (which supports C1 and stabilizes the odontoid process of C2) produces significant instability of both C1 and C2. Cervical myelopathy can develop if the ligament becomes lax or ruptures. A neurological examination and radiograph of the cervical spine should be part of the evaluation of the client. The presence of neuropathy may require a cervical fusion of C1 and C2. The manifestation of signs and symptoms of neurological deficits are inconsistent and

TABLE 25–1 ■ SIGNS AND SYMPTOMS OF RHEUMATOID ARTHRITIS

Signs and Symptoms	Explanation
Morning stiffness lasting up to 1 h	This differs from the stiffness of osteoarthritis, which is resolved in 10–15 min on resuming activity. Stiffness in RA is not related to activity and may persist for hours.
Pain and swelling of peripheral joints	Intensity varies according to inflammation.
Alantoaxial subluxation	This occurs from tenosynovitis of the transverse ligament, which produces laxity of C1 and C2, which can cause a step-off subluxation of C3, C4, C5, and C6. It is visualized on radiographs. MRI aids in locating spinal cord compression and the need for cervical fusion.
Hand deformities, including ulnar drift, boutonnière, and swan-neck deformities	This is related to an inflammatory process of metacarpals, phalanges, and wrists; joint immobilization; destruction of cartilage and bone; and alterations in muscles and tendons.
Foot deformities, including MTP, cock-up toes, and subluxation of MTP heads on the sole.	This is related to an inflammatory process of ankles, joint immobilization, destruction of cartilage and bone, and alterations in muscles and tendons.
Neuropathy of the hand and wrist: carpal tunnel syndrome	Synovial swelling causes nerve entrapment, producing parasthesias. If untreated, it causes functional deficits.
Neuropathy of the ankle and foot: tarsal tunnel syndrome	Synovitis results in nerve entrapment of the posterior tibial nerve, which causes radiation of burning paresthesias on the sole.
Dermal vasculitic lesions	Lesions do not usually indicate vasculitis.
Petechiae, ecchymosis	This is related to NSAID and/or steroid therapy.
Respiratory manifestations	This is caused by synovitis of the cricoarytenoid joint.
Cricoarytenoid inflammation	This causes episodic laryngeal pain, dysphonia, and pain on swallowing.
Ocular problems, dryness	Sjögren's syndrome produces episcleritis, which if untreated can result in scleritis.

MRI, magnetic resonance imaging; MTP, metatarsophalangeal; NSAID, nonsteroidal anti-inflammatory drug; RA, rheumatoid arthritis.

can mimic stroke, carpal tunnel syndrome, or other conditions. Since atlantoaxial subluxation is usually asymptomatic, the patient is at risk in the hospital, at home, or while riding any type of transportation such as an automobile, train, or even an elevator that stops suddenly. A sudden stop may project the neck forward and cause spinal cord injury or death. Visits to the beauty salon or dentist can precipitate serious injury because of the possibility of flexion or extension of the neck. Cardiopulmonary resuscitation should be performed in patients with RA with the jaw thrust forward rather than with the head tilted back. The presence of atlantoaxial subluxation should be documented by the nurse, and all team members should be notified of its presence. Caution should be used when writing orders for mobility and ADLs. A sign should be placed over the patient's bed. When a collar is prescribed, compliance by the client should be carefully monitored and documented.

Swelling and Joint Deformity

Swelling of the peripheral joints of the upper and lower extremities varies according to the degree of synovitis, the state of exacerbation or remission, and the inflammatory process. The joint may vary in appearance from normalcy to sausage-type puffiness in early RA and/or may be accompanied by deformities in the later stages of RA that may include ulnar drift and ulnar deviation at the metacarpal joints. This is often associated with radial deviation at the wrists, and the fingers drift toward the ulna. The normal hand can direct the metacarpals (knuckles) toward the ulna and return the metacarpals to normal positioning. In ulnar drift of RA, the metacarpals remain fixed. Swan neck deformity occurs when a flexion deformity occurs at the proximal interphalangeal joint and there is hyperextension of the distal phalangeal joint.

Joint deformities are directly related to the ravages produced by uncontrolled synovitis. The nurse and the occupational therapist should collaborate to teach the client how to protect the joints in order to prevent damage and prevent pain (Fig. 25–1). These principles include using the largest joint for the largest task, avoiding stressing a painful joint, and performing a task in small steps to avoid fatigue and stress. Often the patient with painful metacarpal hand deformities bears weight directly on the metacarpals. Instead, extending the hand and using the palms and

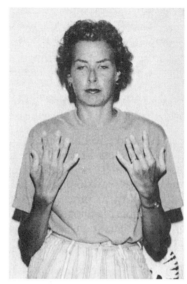

FIGURE 25–1
For people with chronic conditions such as rheumatoid arthritis, daily pain may be a fact of life. (From Ignatavicius, D. D., Workman, M. L., & Mishler, M. A. [1995]. *Medical-surgical nursing: A nursing process* [2nd ed.]. Philadelphia: W. B. Saunders.)

soft tissues accomplishes the task and diminishes joint stress. Some clients hypothesize that one should not baby oneself by not using the joint, and this fallacy adds to joint destruction. Turning a doorknob or ignition key can have destructive effects on wrist tendons, leading to further damage, including rupture. The client must be educated about this. Collaboration with rheumatology colleagues including the occupational therapist "can assist the nurse to educate the client to prevent further damage." Becoming familiar with equipment through observation and catalogs can provide both the nurse and the client with assistive devices that can be incorporated in ADLs and help to prevent joint damage.

The National Arthritis Foundation and its local chapters are an excellent approved source of patient education. The organization provides free literature, which has graphical illustrations of how to avoid and prevent joint injury. Another source of helpful literature is the drug companies that manufacture arthritis drugs.

Pain

A major daily issue for the patient with RA is chronic pain. Pain is subjective. Nociceptors are located throughout the body, and deep somatic nerve receptors can be activated in the bony arthritic joint.

Melzack and Wall (1996) outlined the gate control theory to explain the mechanism of pain (Fig. 25–2). According to the theory, the pain response results from tissue damage and the release of chemicals that stimulate nociceptors. These known substances include prostaglandins, bradykinin, histamines, and serotonin. Once nociceptors are stimulated, neurotransmitters are released. Large-diameter pain, proprioceptor, and touch fibers respond to cutaneous stimulation, massage, cold, vibration, and pain sensation. Small-diameter A-delta fibers and C nociceptor afferent fibers transmit impulses to the substantia gelatinosa in the doral horn of the spinal cord. The substantia gelatinosa has the ability to close the gate to pain transmission and thereby eliminate pain response. If the faster small-diameter A-delta cells are excited, then the C nociceptors can be blocked and the gate is closed to afferent pain transmission. Heat and temperature change, touch, massage, and pressure treatment modalities can therefore close the gate or reduce pain perceptions.

The chronic pain of RA differs from acute pain in physiological and behavioral manifestations (Table 25–2). The degree of chronic

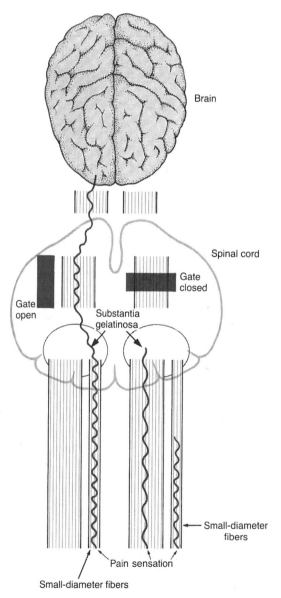

FIGURE 25–2
The gate control theory of pain. (From Ignatavicius, D. D., Workman, M. L., & Mishler, M. A. [1999]. *Medical-surgical nursing: A nursing process approach* [3rd ed.]. Philadelphia: W. B. Saunders.)

TABLE 25–2 ▪ PHYSIOLOGICAL AND BEHAVIORAL RESPONSES TO ACUTE AND CHRONIC PAIN

Pain Type	Physiological Response	Behavioral Response
Acute	Increased blood pressure initially Increased pulse rate Increased respiratory rate Dilated pupils Perspiration	Restlessness Inability to concentrate Apprehension Distress
Chronic	Normal blood pressure Normal pulse rate Normal respiratory rate Normal pupils Dry skin	Immobility or physical inactivity Withdrawal Despair

From Ignatavicius, D. D., Workman, M. L., & Mishler, M. A. (1999). *Medical-surgical nursing across the health care continuum* (3rd ed.). Philadelphia: W. B. Saunders.

pain varies with the progression of the disease process and personal cultural variables that influence sick-role behaviors. Chronic pain can lead to despair and withdrawal. As the pain persists, patients often demonstrate poor self-esteem, learned helplessness, dependency, and sick-role behaviors. Acute or chronic pain interferes with ADLs, including employment, and can cause added financial strain.

NURSING INTERVENTIONS

The primary purpose of management in the newly diagnosed patient is to control inflammation and retard the long-term progression of the disease (O'Sullivan & Schmidt, 1994). Nursing interventions are directed toward preventing loss of function, preventing deformity, reducing pain, and enhancing compliance with therapeutic modalities including physical therapy and occupational therapy. The rehabilitation nurse must perform a careful pain history and physical examination. The McGill-Melzack Pain Questionnaire is an example of an instrument that might be used to support detailed documentation of chronic pain (Fig. 25–3). Plans of care including nursing diagnoses such as (1) chronic pain related to joint inflammation, (2) impaired physical mobility related to fatigue and inflammation, and (3) self-care deficits related to fatigue, pain, and stiffness that must be identified (Table 25–3).

Patient education is critical. The aim of arthritis educational programs is to teach management strategies that increase self-efficacy and self-confidence to meet the physical and emotional challenges posed by the illness (Gonzales, Goeppinger, & Lorig, 1990). With shorter hospital stays and less contact with the nurse, patient education time has been greatly diminished. The nurse must teach in an efficient manner. Patient education must include verbal and written instruction followed by a return demonstration. Patient education materials must be culturally relevant with careful consideration of cultural diversity.

One of the best resources for health care providers is the National Arthritis Foundation. The organization has prepared educational materials for arthritic people of all ages including manuals, coloring books, audiovisuals, and slides. Self-help groups for patients and family members are available. Members of this association work with national and local arthritis chapters to defray the costs of seminars and literature for patients with financial need. Many chapters have equipment loan programs and hotlines to answer questions for patients and health providers.

Patient education should include assessment of the use of nonapproved arthritis remedies. Patients with chronic diseases are often accepting of quick cures. Educating arthritic populations to the dangers of questionable treatments is difficult. During the nursing assessment, the nurse should inquire about the remedies and treatments that have been tried. Consideration of cultural influences is important. Wearing a copper bracelet is not harmful unless the wearer substitutes such a bracelet for essential medical intervention as the disease progresses. Remedies from the 17th and 18th centuries have included herbs, cold and hot baths, massage, application of irritant-producing poultices, and the applica-

McGill-Melzack
PAIN QUESTIONNAIRE

Patient's name _____ Age _____

File No. _____ Date _____

Clinical category (e.g., cardiac, neurologic)

Diagnosis: _____

_____

_____

Analgesic (if already administered):

1. Type _____

2. Dosage _____

3. Time given in relation to this test _____

Patient's intelligence: circle number that represents best estimate.

   1 (low)   2   3   4   5 (high)

****

   This questionnaire has been designed to tell us more about your pain. Four major questions we ask are

1. Where is your pain?
2. What does it feel like?
3. How does it change with time?
4. How strong is it?

   It is important that you tell us how your pain feels now. Please follow the instructions at the beginning of each part.

_____

© R. Melzack, Oct. 1970

Part 1. Where Is Your Pain?

   Please mark, on the drawings below, the areas where you feel pain. Put E if external, or I if internal, near the areas you mark. Put EI if both external and internal.

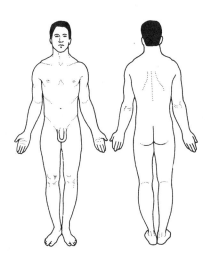

Part 2. What Does Your Pain Feel Like?

   Some of the words below describe your *present* pain. Circle ONLY those words that best describe it. Leave out any category that is not suitable. Use only a single word in each appropriate category — the one that applies best.

1	6	11	16
Flickering	Tugging	Tiring	Annoying
Quivering	Pulling	Exhausting	Troublesome
Pulsing	Wrenching	12	Miserable
Throbbing	7	Sickening	Intense
Beating	Hot	Suffocat-	Unbearable
Pounding	Burning	ing	17
2	Scalding	13	Spreading
Jumping	Searing	Fearful	Radiating
Flashing	8	Frightful	Penetrating
Shooting	Tingling	Terrifying	Piercing
3	Itchy	14	18
Pricking	Smarting	Punishing	Tight
Boring	Stinging	Grueling	Numb
Drilling	9	Cruel	Drawing
Stabbing	Dull	Vicious	Squeezing
Lancinating	Sore	Killing	Tearing
4	Hurting	15	19
Sharp	Aching	Wretched	Cool
Cutting	Heavy	Blinding	Cold
Lacerating	10		Freezing
5	Tender		20
Pinching	Taut		Nagging
Pressing	Rasping		Nauseating
Gnawing	Splitting		Agonizing
Cramping			Dreadful
Crushing			Torturing

Part 3. How Does Your Pain Change With Time?

1. Which word or words would you use to describe the *pattern* of your pain?

1	2	3
Continuous	Rhythmic	Brief
Steady	Periodic	Momentary
Constant	Intermittent	Transient

2. What kind of things *relieve* your pain?

3. What kind of things *increase* your pain?

Part 4. How Strong Is Your Pain?

People agree that the following 5 words represent pain of increasing intensity. They are:

1	2	3	4	5
Mild	Discomforting	Distressing	Horrible	Excruciating

To answer each question below, write the number of the most appropriate word in the space beside the question.

1. Which word describes your pain right now? ____
2. Which word describes it at its worst? ____
3. Which word describes it when it is least? ____
4. Which word describes the worst toothache ____ you ever had?
5. Which word describes the worst headache ____ you ever had?
6. Which word describes the worst stomach ache ____ you ever had?

FIGURE 25–3

McGill-Melzack Pain Questionnaire. (From Melzack, R. [1975]. The McGill Pain Questionnaire: Major Properties and Scoring Methods. *Pain*, 1, 277–299.)

TABLE 25–3 ■ CLIENT CARE PLAN: THE CLIENT WITH RHEUMATOID ARTHRITIS

Expected Outcomes	Nursing Interventions	Rationale
Nursing Diagnosis No. 1: Chronic Pain Related to Joint Inflammation The client will experience a reduction in joint pain.	Give prescribed drugs, as ordered, on time.	Giving drugs on time ensures a consistent blood level (e.g., salicylates).
	Give analgesic drugs as needed, if ordered, and periods of rest, especially after periods of increased activity (e.g., physical therapy).	Supplemental analgesics may be needed to control chronic pain; rest is necessary to prevent the overuse of joints and helps decrease inflammation.
	Provide a warm shower, tub bath, and/or hot compresses after periods of decreased activity or rest.	Heat application increases blood flow to the joints to decrease pain and increase joint mobility.
	Provide nonpharmacological pain-relief measures, such as imagery, massage, and music therapy. (Determine which of these measures are effective for each client.)	Independent nursing interventions help reduce pain and decrease the amount of analgesics needed for pain relief.
	Evaluate the effectiveness of all pain-relief interventions and document/communicate the outcome to the physician and other involved health care team members.	Evaluation of the effectiveness of pain-relief interventions helps the health care team plan care for the client. Changes may be necessary if the plan is not effective in meeting the expected outcome.
Nursing Diagnosis No. 2: Impaired Physical Mobility Related to Fatigue, Inflammation, and Pain The client will ambulate independently, with or without ambulatory aids.	Reinforce the importance of and techniques for therapeutic joint and muscle exercises as taught by the physical therapist.	Therapeutic joint and muscle exercises increase joint mobility, decrease pain, and increase muscle strength.
	Teach the importance of recreational exercises, such as walking and swimming.	Walking and swimming increase muscle tone and enhance psychological well-being.
	Reinforce the importance of and techniques for use of ambulatory aids, such as a cane or walker; allow rest periods during ambulation.	Ambulatory aids help reduce stress on affected joints and, therefore, reduce pain and inflammation.
	Emphasize the client's abilities and strengths in mobility skills.	Focusing on the client's ability rather than deficits builds the client's self-esteem and confidence.

Table continued on following page

TABLE 25-3 ■ CLIENT CARE PLAN: THE CLIENT WITH RHEUMATOID ARTHRITIS *Continued*

Expected Outcomes	Nursing Interventions	Rationale
Nursing Diagnosis No. 3: Self-Care Deficit (Partial) Related to Fatigue, Pain, Stiffness, and Joint Deformity Your client will independently perform activities of daily living with or without the use of adaptive devices.	In collaboration with the occupational therapist, assess the client's abilities in ADLs.	The nurse allows the client to perform all ADLs independently. If the client needs assistance, the nurse plans ways to promote independence in these areas.
	Set up the client's tray, if needed, by opening packages and cartons and cutting food; assess the need for assistive/adaptive devices.	The client may be able to self-feed if the tray is set up and/or if assistive devices, such as plate guards, are obtained.
	For dressing activities, assess the need for long-handled assistive/adaptive devices and other mechanical aids.	The client may be able to dress independently if assistive/adaptive devices are available.
	Encourage the client to use large muscle groups and joints instead of smaller ones, if possible.	Using larger joints helps prevent stress and pain in small joints (joint protection).
	Emphasize the client's abilities in performing ADLs.	Focusing on the client's abilities builds self-esteem and confidence.
	Teach the client to allow rest periods during ADLs.	Rest reduces fatigue that contributes to a decreased ability to perform ADLs.
	Assess the client's pain level, and intervene appropriately (see nursing diagnosis no. 1).	Pain and stiffness contribute to a decreased ability to perform ADLs.

From Ignatavicius, D. D., Workman, M. L., & Mishler, M. A. (1999). *Medical-surgical nursing across the health care continuum* (3rd ed.). Philadelphia: W. B. Saunders.

tion of treacle (Bolander, 1988). Billions of dollars are spent annually by arthritis patients who are lured by the promise of a cure.

PHARMACOLOGICAL MANAGEMENT

Traditionally, medications were prescribed to the patient with RA sequentially, beginning with aspirin and proceeding through the non-steroidal anti-inflammatory agents, antimalarials, and gold salts or penicillamine (Tables 25-4, 25-5 and 25-6). Because pain reduction is often not achieved for 10 to 12 weeks, low doses of corticosteroid therapy may be administered as a bridge therapy until the disease-modifying antirheumatic drugs take effect (O'Sullivan & Schmidt, 1994). Steroids have no direct effect on the disease process but are potent anti-inflammatory agents that inhibit inflammation regardless of mechanical, chemical, immunological, or infective stimuli. It is important to remember that the client on steroids must be informed of the dangers of stopping therapy suddenly because of the adrenal suppression risk. Drug

therapy for arthritis continues to evolve. Currently, etanercept (Enbrel), celecoxib (Celebra), and hylan G-F 20 (Synvisc) are being widely advertised. The reader is advised to check the latest pharmacology references for information on the use and side effects of these and other new medications. It is equally as important for the nurse to remember that pharmacological therapy alone will not have a significant impact on any inflammatory or noninflammatory arthritic disease. Maintenance of proper positioning, adequate nutrition, rest, joint protection, and energy-conservation techniques are equally important to aid in halting the inflammation and joint destruction of RA.

CONCLUSIONS

Arthritis is a constellation of 150 diseases, syndromes, and conditions. This chapter has focused on RA as a prototype to highlight priorities; the prevention of deformities and loss of function; nursing interventions; pain; and pharmacological management. Treatment is continually evolving, and the rehabilitation

TABLE 25–4 ■ ANALGESICS USED IN ARTHRITIS

Generic Name	Trade Name	Side Effects and Patient Cautions
Acetaminophen	Anacin Panadol Tylenol	Patients should avoid excessive use of alcohol and fasting; kidney or liver damage is possible side effect
Acetaminophen with codeine	Fiorcet Phenaphen with codeine Tylenol with codeine	Codeine can produce fatigue, drowsiness, nausea, constipation Contraindicated with drug abuse; asthma; head injury; liver, thyroid, or renal disease
Propoxyphene	Darvon	Side effects include dizziness, lightheadedness, nausea, vomiting
Tramadol	Ultram	Side effects include dizziness, nausea, constipation, headache, sleepiness

TABLE 25–5 ■ NONSTEROIDAL ANTI-INFLAMMATORY DRUGS*

Generic Name	Trade Name	Generic Name	Trade Name
Diclofenac potassium	Cataflam	Ketorolac	Toradol
Diclofenac sodium	Voltaren	Meclofenamate sodium	Meclomen
Etodolac	Lodine	Mefenamic acid	Ponstel
Fenoprofen calcium	Nalfon	Nabumetone	Relafen
Flurbiprofen	Ansaid	Naproxen	Naprosyn
Ibuprofen	Motrin, Motrin IB	Naproxen sodium	Anaprox
	Advil		Aleve
	Nuprin	Oxaprozin	Daypro
Indomethacin	Indocin	Piroxicam	Feldene
Ketoprofen	Orudis, Orudis KT	Sulindac	Clinoril
	Oruvail	Tolmetin sodium	Tolectin
	Actron	Celecoxib	Celebra

*Cautions with nonsteroidal anti-inflammatory drugs (NSAIDs): The purpose of NSAID therapy is to decrease inflammation. The drugs must be taken even if the symptoms disappear, because a certain level is required in the bloodstream to keep the inflammation under control. All NSAIDs must be taken with food to decrease the possibility of gastrointestinal bleeding or ulcers. Side effects include abdominal pain, diarrhea, dizziness, fluid retention, gastric ulcers and bleeding, heartburn, indigestion, nausea, rash, lightheadedness, nightmares, and tinnitus. In persons with heart and kidney disease, side effects may be more pronounced. Elderly persons may exhibit confusion.

TABLE 25–6 ■ DISEASE-MODIFYING ANTIRHEUMATIC DRUGS*

Generic Name	Trade Name	Side Effects
Auranofin	Ridaura	Bloating; abdominal and stomach cramps; loss of appetite; diarrhea; gas; indigestion; nausea and vomiting; skin rash; photosensitivity
Azathioprine	Imuran	Loss of appetite; nausea or vomiting; skin rash; bone marrow suppression; infection; malignancy
Cyclophosphamide	Cytoxan	Infertility in men and women; loss of appetite; bone marrow suppression; hemorrhagic cystitis; malignancy
Cyclosporine	Sandimmune Neoral	Bleeding; enlarged tender gums; fluid retention; hypertension; increased hair growth; loss of renal function; loss of appetite; tremors of hands
Hydroxychloroquine sulfate	Plaquenil†	Diarrhea; loss of appetite; nausea and vomiting; stomach cramps or pain; retinopathy; neuropathy
Methotrexate	Rheumatrex	Cough; diarrhea; loss of hair; loss of appetite; unusual bleeding; bruising; fevers; infection; pneumonitis; stomatitis
Minocycline	Minocin	Dizziness; vaginal secretions; nausea; headache; skin rash; hyperpigmentation
Penicillamine	Cuprimine Depen	Diarrhea; joint pain; decreased or loss of taste; fever; hives; itching; mouth sores; lymphadenopathy; bone marrow suppression; weakness; unusual bleeding
Sulfasalazine	Azulfidine	Stomach pain; diarrhea; achiness; dizziness; headache; photosensitivity; liver problems; lowered complete blood count; nausea and vomiting
Gold sodium thiomalate	Myochrysine‡ (injectable)	Photosensitivity; metallic taste; sore tongue; skin rash; itching; bleeding gums; bruising; oral ulcers; proteinuria; bone marrow suppression
Aurothioglucose (injectable) (gold salt dissolved in oil for slower absorption)	Solganal	Photosensitivity; metallic taste; sore tongue; skin rash; itching; bleeding gums; bruising; oral ulcers; proteinuria; bone marrow suppression

*The disease-modifying rheumatic drugs include both immunosuppressives and remittive drugs. The remittive drugs are primarily gold salts, antimalarials, sulfa drugs, and penicillamine. Azathioprine, cyclophosphamide, methotrexate, and cyclosporine are immunosuppressive drugs. Before either remittive or immunosuppressive drug therapy is begun, baseline laboratory studies are indicated and should be continued throughout the course of the drug therapy. These drugs significantly affect family finances, as they are costly, require additional laboratory fees and physician visits, and may cause time lost from work. Immunosuppressives such as methotrexate are fetotoxic, and cyclosporine affects fertility in both men and women and can also affect the fetus.

†An ophthalmological examination is required before beginning Plaquenil therapy to rule out the presence of hyperpigmentation of the macula lutea, which could lead to blindness. An annual eye examination must be done while patient is on antimalarial therapy. This drug can lead to blindness.

‡Nitrotoid crisis (flushing, tachycardia) can occur with the first dose or subsequent doses. This usually resolves in minutes. There have been no reports of anaphylactic reaction.

nurse maintains a current knowledge base through networking with other professionals, continuing educational development, and research.

REFERENCES

Bolander, V. (1988). Rheumatism remedies of the past. *Orthopedic Nursing, 7,* 71–74.

Gonzales, V., Goeppinger, J., & Lorig, K. (1990). Four psychological theories and their application to patient education and clinical practice. *Arthritis Care Research, 3,* 132–143.

Klippel, J. H. (1997). *Primer on the rheumatic diseases* (11th ed.) Atlanta, GA: The Arthritis Foundation.

Melzack, R., & Wall, P. D. (1966). *The challenge of pain.* London: Penguin.

O'Sullivan, S. B., & Schmidt, T. J. (1994). *Physical rehabilitation: Assessment and treatment* (3rd ed.). Philadelphia: F. A. Davis.

BIBLIOGRAPHY

Brassell, M. P. (1988). Pharmacological management of rheumatic disease. *Orthopedic Nursing, 7,* 29–49.

Chernecky, C. C., Krech, R. L., & Berger, B. J. (1993). *Laboratory diagnostic procedures.* Philadelphia: W. B. Saunders.

McGrory, C., Moore, M. E., & Carroll, E. T. (1997). *An introduction to learning about lupus, a user friendly guide* (2nd ed., pp. 167–172). Ardmore, PA: The Lupus Foundation of Greater Philadelphia.

Moore, M. E., & Caroll, E. T. (1997). *An introduction to learning about lupus, a user friendly guide* (2nd ed., pp. 1–13). Ardmore, PA: The Lupus Foundation of Greater Philadelphia.

Parker, J. C., Frank, R. G., Beck, N. C., Smarr, K. L., Buescher, K. L., Phillips, L. R., Smith, E. I., Anderson, S. K., & Walker, S. E. (1988) Pain management: 1. Rheumatoid arthritis patients: Cognitive-behavioral approach. *Arthritis and Rheumatism, 31,* 593–601.

CHAPTER 26

Cardiopulmonary Rehabilitation

Cynthia Phelan

CARDIAC REHABILITATION

Despite advances in diagnosis, care, and treatment, cardiovascular disease continues to be the leading cause of death in the United States (Figs. 26–1 and 26–2). As the population ages, this disease will continue to have tremendous human and economic impact. Today cardiovascular disease accounts for about 42% of all deaths in the United States, or a total of more than 954,000 deaths per year. The prevalence of cardiovascular disease is staggering. More than one in four Americans have one or more types of cardiovascular disease, including high blood pressure, coronary heart disease (CHD), stroke, and rheumatic heart disease. The American Heart Association (1999) estimates that nearly 50 million people have high blood pressure and 12.2 million have CHD.

Cardiovascular Diseases

Atherosclerosis: A Major Cause of Cardiovascular Disease

Atherosclerosis is an arterial disease most commonly affecting the aorta and the coronary, cerebral, femoral, and other large- or middle-sized arteries. It consists of the proliferation of smooth muscle cells and the accumulation of lipids in the intima of such arteries. The exact pathogenesis of atherosclerosis is unknown. The characteristic lesion of atherosclerosis is the raised fibrous plaque, a yellowish gray elevated area on the surface of the artery. It is characterized by deposits of fatty substances, cholesterol, cellular waste products, calcium, and fibrin. The plaque protrudes to a varying extent into the arterial lumen and may impede arterial blood flow or block it completely.

There are six hypotheses of the pathogenesis of atherosclerosis. According to the *response to injury hypothesis*, a nonspecific injury (mechanical, chemical, hormonal, or immunological) to the endothelial cells of the luminal

arterial surface results in a change in the permeability of the intimal membrane. Supporters of this theory suggest that humans can sustain endothelial injury as a result of hypertension, hydrocarbons from cigarette smoking, plasma cholesterol, and hormones.

The *monoclonal hypothesis* proposes that the atherosclerotic plaque is due to a proliferation of smooth muscle cells that is started by a single smooth muscle cell. The atherosclerotic lesion is the result of clones of that cell.

The *clonal-senescence hypothesis* relates atherosclerosis to age, which is one of the identified risk factors. This hypothesis describes the smooth muscle proliferation in the intima as resulting from an age-dependent decline in replication of stem cells. Stem cells give rise to differentiated, specific cell types.

The *lipid insulation hypothesis* holds that the lipid in the atherosclerotic lesion is derived from lipoproteins in the blood. The *thrombogenic theory* describes the fibrous plaque as a mural thrombus that converts to a mass of connective tissue as fibroblasts and, possibly, smooth muscle cells migrate into the throm-

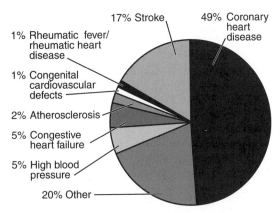

FIGURE 26–1

Percentage breakdown of deaths from cardiovascular diseases in United States, 1997. (Redrawn from American Heart Association [1999]. *2000 Heart and stroke statistical update*. Dallas: Author.)

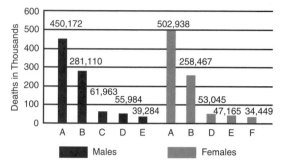

FIGURE 26–2
Leading causes of death for all males and females in United States, 1997. (Redrawn from American Heart Association [1999]. *2000 Heart and stroke statistical update*. Dallas: Author.)

bus from the arterial walls. The *hemodynamic hypothesis* identifies such factors as turbulence and shearing stress as an explanation of why plaques are more often situated in branchings and bends of some arteries or arterial segments than elsewhere.

It is important to note that none of the theories completely describes all aspects of the disease and that they are not mutually exclusive. Each hypothesis might be applicable at a different time during the development of the atherosclerotic lesion. Therefore, much of the research has been focused on the identification of risk factors. Myocardial infarctions and cerebral infarctions are the two major consequences of this disease process (Zierler & Cowan, 1995).

Myocardial Ischemia and Infarction

CHD was responsible for one of every 5 deaths in 1997. In this country, myocardial infarction is the single largest killer of American men and women. This year, as many as 1,100,000 Americans will have a new or recurrent heart attack, and about 40% of the people who experience a heart attack in a given year will die of it. Consider the following statistics about CHD (AHA, 1999):

- 84.9% of the people who die of heart attacks are 65 years or older.
- 80% of CHD mortality in people younger than 65 years occurs during the initial attack.
- In 50% of men and 63% of women who

died suddenly of CHD, there were no previous symptoms of the disease.

Myocardial ischemia and myocardial infarction are two of the most common manifestations of CHD. *Myocardial ischemia* can occur when blood flow through the coronary arteries decreases relative to oxygen demand. If myocardial blood flow is not increased or if myocardial demand is not reduced, ischemia can lead to death of the myocardial cells, resulting in *myocardial infarction.*

Angina pectoris is a symptom used to describe the pain or discomfort associated with CHD. Angina occurs when there is an oxygen deficiency in the myocardium. The most important items to note about the chest pain history are the quality, location, and duration of the pain and any factors that provoke or ameliorate it (Table 26–1).

Myocardial oxygen demands are increased with effort, emotional stress, smoking, eating, and exposure to cold weather. In response to the greater demand, coronary vasodilatation occurs, increasing the blood supply. Coronary atherosclerosis prevents adequate vasodilatation and may result in angina. Advances in the treatment of patients with myocardial ischemia due to CHD have resulted in interventions to improve oxygen supply by reperfusion or revascularization of the myocardium. The goal is to restore perfusion to ischemic or at-risk myocardium. This goal may be accomplished through thrombolysis, angioplasty, atherectomy, placement of an intracoronary stent, or a combination of these interventions (Fig. 26–3) (Osguthorpe & Woods, 1995).

Cardiac Surgery

Coronary artery bypass graft (CABG) surgery is performed primarily to alleviate anginal symptoms as well as improve survival. It may be indicated for patients who have left main coronary artery disease or three-vessel coronary disease or for whom angioplasty or medical management of angina has failed (LeDoux & Shinn, 1995). Caring for patients undergoing cardiac surgery in this era of ever-changing technology is challenging. Today, patients have many options. As of 2000, cardiac surgery may be performed without cardiopulmonary bypass, laser energy may be used to improve myocardial blood flow, and

TABLE 26–1 ■ DIFFERENTIATING CARDIAC FROM NONCARDIAC CHEST PAIN BY SYMPTOMS

Symptom	Cardiac Pain	Noncardiac Pain
Quality of pain	Constricting/squeezing Visceral quality Burning Heaviness	Dull, aching Sharp, stabbing, piercing, knifelike Muscular
Location of pain	Substernal Across precordium Neck One or both shoulders, arms Intracapsular region One or both forearms, hands Epigastrium	Left submammary area, apex of heart Superficial tissues of the left chest Right lower chest Very discrete localization possible
Duration of pain	Angina: 2–10 min Infarction: >20 min–24 hr	<20 sec Persistent without change for >24–48 hr
Precipitating and aggravating factors	Exercise, particularly with hurrying Excitement Cold temperature exposure Stressful stimuli Postprandially, after heavy meal	After completion of exercise With specific body positions, chest wall movement, and respiration With direct palpation of chest wall Spontaneous During fasting, with cold liquids
Relieving factors	Rest Nitroglycerin	Antacids Food Nonsteroidal analgesia

Modified from Braddom, R. L. (1995). *Physical medicine and rehabilitation* (p. 655). Philadelphia: W. B. Saunders.

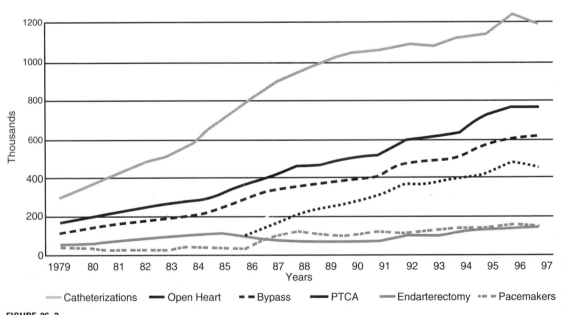

FIGURE 26–3
Trends in cardiovascular operations and procedures. (Redrawn from American Heart Association [1999]. *2000 Heart and stroke statistical update*. Dallas: Author.)

patients may request minimally invasive cardiac surgery rather than standard cardiac surgery. Rehabilitation nurses are challenged to provide comprehensive care for our patients, which consists of blending the latest technology with the nursing and rehabilitation needs of the patient.

Prevention of Coronary Heart Disease

Continued efforts in primary prevention are critical to reducing the incidence of CHD. Most of the principles of risk factor reduction, an essential component of cardiac rehabilitation, can be applied to many populations, throughout the continuum of health care, regardless of the setting. One approach to describing prevention strategies divides them into distinct categories.

A *primary prevention* strategy precludes the initiation of a disease process. A regular program of exercise is an example of primary prevention in a healthy person. Programs designed to intervene before the clinical onset of CHD provide the greatest opportunity to alter the natural history of the disease.

A *secondary prevention* strategy arrests a developing disease while the affected person is still asymptomatic. Examples of secondary prevention are blood pressure screening and cholesterol measurement.

Tertiary prevention is aimed at minimizing disability, morbidity, and mortality associated with a known disease. Certain elements of cardiac rehabilitation, diabetes management, and hypertension control can be classified as tertiary prevention. In working with many patient populations, whether in formal rehabilitation programs or at home, rehabilitation nurses have an opportunity to implement many elements of cardiac rehabilitation in the form of risk factor reduction and prevention strategies (Zimmerman & Horton-La Forge, 1996).

Cardiac Rehabilitation

Continued advances in medical and surgical techniques, combined with comprehensive and focused programs in cardiac rehabilitation, are needed to manage the manifestations and consequences of CHD. *Cardiac rehabilitation* is the process that restores optimal medical, physiological, psychological, social, and vocational performance following recovery from an acute cardiac event. Most commonly, cardiac rehabilitation is initiated after acute myocardial infarction, coronary artery bypass surgery (CABS), and percutaneous transluminal coronary angioplasty or atherectomy (PCTA). In addition, cardiac rehabilitation may be indicated for patients who have undergone valvular replacement, cardiac transplantation, and pacemaker implantation (American Association of Cardiovascular and Pulmonary Rehabilitation [AACVPR], 1995).

Cardiac rehabilitation is a comprehensive program designed to promote optimal health and function in a defined population. Although it can vary in form and structure, its cornerstone comprises (1) reduction of cardiac risk factors, (2) exercise and activity guidelines, and (3) patient education.

The goals of cardiac rehabilitation are as follows (Balady, Fletcher, Froelicher, Hartley, Krauss, Oberman, Pollock, & Taylor, 1994):

- To improve functional capacity
- To alleviate or lessen activity-related symptoms
- To reduce disability
- To identify and modify coronary risk factors

Phases of Cardiac Rehabilitation

As cardiac care has evolved, comparable changes have been made in the diversity and the delivery of rehabilitative care. Planning for a traditional rehabilitation program usually begins with the diagnosis of an acute coronary event, such as a myocardial infarction, CABS, or PCTA.

The traditional phases of cardiac rehabilitation are defined as follows:

Phase I: Inpatient. The first phase is the acute inpatient length of stay. The length of stay in acute care continues to decrease as a result of advances in technology, pain management, and treatment. The shorter hospital stay has necessitated an accelerated in-hospital phase of early ambulation and abbreviated education.

Phase II: Immediate Outpatient. The convalescent stage following hospital discharge is the second phase. It typically lasts 8 to 16 weeks and starts immediately after the patient leaves the hospital. This structured, multifactorial outpatient program is usually initiated within 1 to 3 weeks of discharge and lasts a minimum of weeks to 6 months.

Phase III: Intermediate Outpatient. An extended supervised outpatient program, the third phase lasts 3 to 6 months. This phase begins when the patient has stabilized and does not require continuous or frequent intermittent electrocardiographic (ECG) monitoring. Continued emphasis is on endurance exercise and behavioral changes.

Phase IV: Maintenance Phase of Indefinite Length. This fourth phase is critical because the benefits of any exercise that is stopped are lost within a few weeks. A commitment to continued exercise and lifestyle changes is essential to sustain the gains achieved by regular exercise. This may be ultimately the most crucial phase as the patient works to maintain optimal health practices (AACVPR, 1995).

Benefits of Cardiac Rehabilitation

Studies demonstrate that cardiac rehabilitation and efforts targeted at exercise, lipid management, hypertension control, and smoking cessation can have a positive effect for patients with cardiovascular disease. As a result, cardiac rehabilitation is standard care that should be integrated into the overall treatment plan of patients with CHD (Balady et al., 1994). The challenge is to select, develop, and provide appropriate rehabilitative services and to tailor the method of their delivery.

The decision tree shown in Figure 26–4 summarizes the highlights of cardiac rehabilitation. For each component of the decision tree, information is presented within diamonds or rectangles. Diamonds represent yes-no decision points; rectangles represent intervention strategies or other clinical decision making by the provider of the cardiac rehabilitation services. Cardiac rehabilitation is a multifactorial process, and optimal outcomes are achieved when the rehabilitative strategies are combined. The decision tree serves as a pathway for the clinician to address patient categories and aspects of assessment and treatment (Wenger, Froelicher, Smith, et al., 1995).

Cardiac rehabilitation, combined with risk reduction efforts, can achieve the following results (Balady et al., 1994; Wenger et al., 1995):

- Reduce cardiac mortality
- Improve functional capacity
- Improve exercise capacity
- Lower serum lipid levels
- Enhance psychosocial well-being and stress reduction
- Attenuate myocardial ischemia

- Retard the progression and foster reversal of coronary atherosclerosis
- Reduce the risk of further coronary events

Program Components

Cardiac rehabilitation programs should emphasize three areas:

- Risk factor modification
- Exercise training and activity prescription
- Psychosocial and vocational evaluation and counseling

Risk Factor Modification

Despite the emphasis on and greater awareness of risk factor reduction and lifestyle changes, the challenges remain. Some studies suggest that despite individual and community education, the dietary patterns of Americans have shown little modification. The prevalence of obesity among Americans has increased over the past 20 years (St. Jeor, Brownell, & Atkinson, 1993). Trends in cigarette smoking have continued, with increases noted among women, young adults, and members of lower socioeconomic groups. Despite educational efforts and public health campaigns, only one in three patients with coronary artery disease participates in comprehensive secondary risk reduction treatments (American Heart Association Secondary Prevention Panel, 1995).

Nursing diagnoses for patients who require risk factor modification or lifestyle changes are derived after assessment and collection of available data. Common nursing diagnoses for this population are as follows:

1. Knowledge deficit about the disease process, which is manifested by verbal acknowledgment
2. Inaccurate perception of health care status
3. Failure to perform the desired or prescribed health behaviors

Nonadherence to long-term lifestyle modifications manifested by knowledge deficit, inability to follow treatment regimens, lack of social supports, and either lack of active involvement or nonparticipation are often seen in this population.

Table 26–2 lists the known cardiac risk factors, classifying them as reversible (*modifiable*) or irreversible (*nonmodifiable*). Risk factors such as cigarette smoking, hypertension, dietary factors, and sedentary lifestyle are considered modifiable in that they affect the prognosis for a person with CHD. Nonmodifiable risk factors for CHD, which cannot be

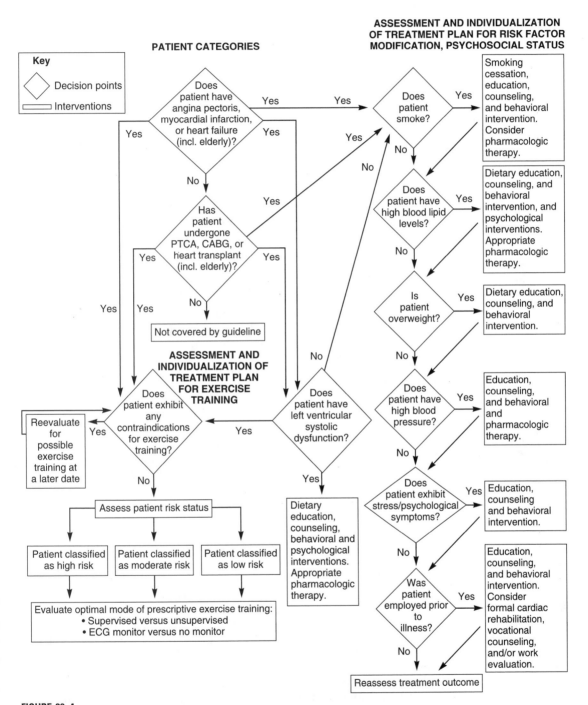

FIGURE 26–4

Decision tree for cardiac rehabilitation services. (Redrawn from Wenger, N. K., Froelicher, E. S., Smith, L. K., et al. [1995]. *Cardiac rehabilitation* [Clinical Practice Guideline No. 17; AHCPR Publication No. 96-0672]. Rockville, MD: Agency for Health Care Policy and Research and National Heart, Lung, and Blood Institute.)

TABLE 26–2 ■ RISK FACTORS FOR CORONARY ARTERY DISEASE (CAD)

Irreversible Risks	Reversible Risks
Male gender	Cigarette smoking
Family history of premature CAD (before age 55 yr in a parent or sibling)	Hypertension
	Low HDL cholesterol [<0.9 mmol/L (35 mg/dL)]
Past history of CAD	Hypercholesterolemia [>5.20 mmol/L (200 mg/dL)]
Past history of occlusive peripheral vascular disease	High lipoprotein A
Past history of cerebrovascular disease	Abdominal obesity
	Hypertriglyceridemia [>2.8 mmol/L (250 mg/dL)]
	Hyperinsulinemia
	Diabetes mellitus
	Sedentary lifestyle

From Braddom, R. L. (1995). *Physical medicine and rehabilitation* (p. 649). Philadelphia: W. B. Saunders.

changed, are age, gender, and personal and family health history.

Cigarette Smoking. CHD risk is increased by the (1) number of cigarettes the person smokes, (2) the total number of years the person has smoked, and (3) the age the person started smoking. Cigarette smoking remains ones of the most preventable causes of CHD. It is estimated that people who stop smoking realize a benefit within 3 years (Froelicher, Berra, Stepp, Saxe, & Deitrich, 1995). All patients require assessment of smoking and should be offered assistance in quitting. Programs are often available in the community, through hospitals, and from organizations such as the American Heart Association and the American Lung Association.

Hypertension. High blood pressure affects nearly 50 million Americans, putting them at risk for CHD, peripheral vascular disease, and stroke. All stages of hypertension are associated with higher risk of nonfatal and fatal cardiovascular disease events. *Mild to moderate hypertension* is defined as systolic blood pressure ranging from 140 to 179 mm Hg and diastolic blood pressure ranging from 90 to 109 mm Hg. Hypertension is predominantly a chronic and lifelong disease that requires awareness, detection, referral, and long-term maintenance of therapy.

Hypertension control begins with detection and requires continued surveillance. Hypertension should not be diagnosed on the basis of a single measurement, and blood pressure should be measured in such a manner that the values obtained are representative of the patient's usual level. The following techniques are recommended:

1. Patients should be seated with the arm bared, supported, and at heart level. They should not have smoked or ingested caffeine within 30 minutes before measurement.
2. Measurement should begin after 5 minutes of rest.
3. The appropriate cuff size must be used to ensure an accurate measurement. The bladder should nearly (at least 80%) or completely encircle the arm.
4. Both systolic and diastolic blood pressure readings should be recorded. The disappearance of sound should be used for the diastolic reading.
5. Two or more readings separated by 2 minutes should be averaged. If the first two readings differ by more than 5 mm Hg, additional readings should be obtained.

Nursing interventions for hypertension should center on behavior modification strategies. Lifestyle modifications for hypertension control include (1) weight control and reduction if needed, (2) limit of alcohol intake to less than 1 oz per day of ethanol (24 oz of beer, 8 oz of wine), (3) regular aerobic exercise, (4) reduction of sodium intake to less than 2.3 g per day, (4) adequate dietary intake of potassium, calcium, and magnesium, (5) smoking cessation, and (6) reduction of dietary intake of saturated fat and cholesterol (Joint National Committee on Detection, Evaluation and Treatment of High Blood Pressure, 1993).

Dietary Factors

Serum Lipids and Lipoproteins. Dyslipidemia is a major risk factor for CHD. Research has continued to affirm that lowering cholesterol reduced recurrent CHD events by 26% and total mortality by 9% (Rossouw, Lewis, & Rifkind, 1990). In a joint statement, the American Heart Association and the National Heart, Lung and Blood Institute have reviewed the evidence for the direct role of cholesterol in the development of atherosclerosis and CHD (American Heart Association, 1990). Numerous studies have demonstrated the positive correlation of elevated serum cholesterol levels with increased CHD risk. Clinical studies have demonstrated that if serum cholesterol is lowered by diet or drugs, the risk of CHD can be lowered (Scandinavian Simvastatin Survival Study Group, 1994).

Nursing Intervention. Efforts aimed at dietary modification of fats, reduction of total body fat, and sufficient exercise are the major components in this risk reduction effort. A 10% reduction in serum cholesterol levels in the population, which should be possible through dietary modification alone, ought to result in a reduction in CHD of approximately 20%.

The ideal serum levels for the general population are as follows:

Total cholesterol <200 mg/dL
Low-density lipoprotein (LDL) cholesterol level <130 mg/dL
Triglyceride levels <200 mg/dL
High-density lipoprotein (HDL) cholesterol level >35 mg/dL

Parameters for patients with coronary disease are listed in Table 26–3.

Outpatient cardiac centers and community health centers have a unique opportunity to establish cost-effective lipid management centers. A successful lipid clinic operation requires comprehensive and aggressive non-pharmacological and pharmacological therapy and compliance strategies. These include dietary instruction about (1) all food groups, (2) use of alcohol, (3) fiber, (4) label reading, (5) portion control, (6) snacking, (7) food preparation, and (8) dining out (Fair & Berra, 1995; La Forge & Thomas, 1996).

Obesity and Weight Change. It is estimated that 61 million American adults weigh 20% or more above their desirable weight. Surveys demonstrate that this change is an increase in prevalence over the last 20 years. Obesity has been determined to be an important risk factor for CHD. It appears to interact with or amplify the effects of other risk factors, although the exact mechanisms are unknown.

Lavie and Milani (1996) studied the effects of cardiac rehabilitation and exercise training in obese patients with cardiac disease, comparing data before and after cardiac rehabilitation in obese and nonobese patients. The data suggest that modest reductions in body mass index, obesity, and severe obesity occurred after cardiac rehabilitation. In addition, obese patients demonstrated significant improvements in most coronary risk factors, although improvements in exercise capacity were greater in nonobese patients.

Dietary Goals. The health impact of diet is generally accepted. The Adult Treatment Panel Guidelines have established desirable levels for serum lipids. A Step 1 diet pattern is recommended for all people who have elevated serum cholesterol levels or known CHD. A Step 2 diet is recommended for people with elevated cholesterol and CHD risk factors in whom 3 months of a Step 1 diet does not achieve a serum LDL cholesterol goal of less than 130 mg/dL. Goals for these diets are shown in Table 26–4 (National Cholesterol Education Program, 1994).

Dietary education that is reinforced with behavioral strategies is required to reduce total cholesterol. Food diaries to examine eating patterns as well as the environments, thoughts, and feelings associated with eating can identify behavioral influences. Once these patterns are recognized, setting goals and making different choices become possible. Review and evaluation of food diaries provides feedback and positive reinforcement (Fair & Berra, 1995).

Effect of Physical Activity on Diet and Myocardial Function. Lack of physical activity is a risk factor for the development of CHD as well as other health issues. Research has demonstrated that a moderate-level activity performed regularly has been shown to increase serum levels of HDL cholesterol and lower those of triglycerides. Higher serum HDL cholesterol seems to afford protection for both men and women against the development of CHD. Exercise appears to reduce the formation of small, dense LDL cholesterol. It also promotes weight loss and control and improves musculoskeletal functioning. When performed in an endurance-type training program for 16 weeks or longer at 65% of functional capacity, exercise also can increase myocardial oxygen supply, decrease myocardial work and oxygen demand, and increase myocardial function (Fair & Berra, 1995).

Diabetes. In the presence of diabetes, the risk of CHD doubles in men and increases five to seven times in women. Dietary recommendations become more complex when hypercholesterolemia, obesity, and diabetes coexist. It is important that a treatment plan be developed to include a comprehensive nutritional evaluation and intervention by a registered dietitian (Froelicher et al., 1995).

Reproductive Hormones. Early age at menopause increases the risk of CHD. Postmenopausal women who experience a natural menopause have a greater risk of CHD because of the unfavorable effect of estrogen

TABLE 26–3 ▪ GUIDE TO COMPREHENSIVE RISK REDUCTION FOR PATIENTS WITH CORONARY AND OTHER VASCULAR DISEASE

Risk Intervention	Recommendations			

Smoking:
  Goal complete
  cessation
	Strongly encourage patient and family to stop smoking.
	Provide counseling, nicotine replacement, and formal cessation programs as appropriate.			

Lipid management:
  Primary goal LDL
  <100 mg/dL
	Start AHA Step II Diet in all patients: ≤30% fat, <7% saturated fat, <200 mg/d cholesterol.
	Assess fasting lipid profile. In post-MI patients, lipid profile may take 4 to 6 weeks to stabilize. Add
	  drug therapy according to the following guide:			

Secondary goals
  HDL >35 mg/dL;
  TG <200 mg/dL
	LDL <100 mg/dL
	
	No drug therapy
		LDL 100 to 130 mg/dL
		
		Consider adding drug therapy
		to diet, as follows:
		
		↘ Suggested drug therapy ↗
		
		<table><tr><td>TG <200 mg/dL</td><td>TG 200 to 400 mg/dL</td><td>TG > 400 mg/dL</td></tr><tr><td>Statin
		Resin
		Niacin</td><td>Statin
		Niacin</td><td>Consider combined drug therapy (niacin, fibrate, statin)</td></tr></table>If LDL goal not achieved, consider combination therapy.
			LDL >130 mg/dL
			
			Add drug therapy to
			diet, as follows:
				HDL <35 mg/dL
				
				Emphasize weight management and physical activity. Advise smoking cessation. If needed to achieve LDL goals, consider niacin, statin, fibrate.

Physical activity:
  Minimum goal 30
  minutes 3 to 4
  times per week
	Assess risk, preferably with exercise test, to guide prescription.
	Encourage minimum of 30 to 60 minutes of moderate-intensity activity 3 or 4 times weekly (walking, jogging, cycling, or other aerobic activity) supplemented by an increase in daily lifestyle activities (eg, walking breaks at work, using stairs, gardening, household work). Maximum benefit 5 to 6 hours a week.
	Advise medically supervised programs for moderate- to high-risk patients.			

Weight management:	Start intensive diet and appropriate physical activity intervention, as outlined above, in patients >120% of ideal weight for height. Particularly emphasize need for weight loss in patients with hypertension, elevated triglycerides, or elevated glucose levels.			
Antiplatelet agents/ **anticoagulants:**	Start aspirin 80 to 325 mg/d if not contraindicated. Manage warfarin to international normalized ratio = 2 to 3.5 for post-MI patients not able to take aspirin.			
ACE inhibitors post- **MI:**	Start early post-MI in stable high-risk patients (anterior MI, previous MI, Killip class II [S_3 gallop, rales, radiographic CHF]). Continue indefinitely for all with LV dysfunction (ejection fraction ≤ 40%) or symptoms of failure. Use as needed to manage blood pressure or symptoms in all other patients.			
Beta-blockers:	Start in high-risk post-MI patients (arrhythmia, LV dysfunction, inducible ischemia) at 5 to 28 days. Continue 6 months minimum. Observe usual contraindications. Use as needed to manage angina rhythm or blood pressure in all other patients.			
Estrogens:	Consider estrogen replacement in all postmenopausal women. Individualize recommendation consistent with other health risks.			

TABLE 26–3 ■ GUIDE TO COMPREHENSIVE RISK REDUCTION FOR PATIENTS WITH CORONARY AND OTHER VASCULAR DISEASE *Continued*

Risk Intervention	Recommendations
Blood pressure control: Goal ≤140/90 mm Hg	Initiate lifestyle modification—weight control, physical activity, alcohol moderation, and moderate sodium restriction—in all patients with blood pressure >140 mm Hg systolic or 90 mm Hg diastolic. Add blood pressure medication, individualized to other patient requirements and characteristics (ie, age, race, need for drugs with specific benefits) **if** blood pressure is not less than 140 mm Hg systolic or 90 mm Hg diastolic in 3 months **or** if *initial* blood pressure is >160 mm Hg systolic or 100 mm Hg diastolic.

ACE, angiotensin-converting enzyme; AHA, American Heart Association; CHF, congestive heart failure; HDL, high-density lipoproteins; LDL, low-density lipoproteins; LV, left ventricular; MI, myocardial infarction; S_3, third heart sound; TG, triglycerides
From American Heart Association Secondary Prevention Panel. (1995). Consensus panel statement: Preventing heart attack and death in patients with coronary disease. *Circulation*, 92, 1–4. By permission of the American Heart Association, Inc.

reduction on lipid metabolism. At menopause, serum HDL cholesterol levels decline and LDL cholesterol levels increase compared with premenopausal values. These unfavorable lipid changes may be modified by hormone therapy, producing a reduced risk of CHD in this population. Research is continuing in this area. Initial studies seem to show a positive effect of hormone therapy, but longer-term study has yet to be completed (Froelicher et al., 1995).

Socioeconomic Status. Lower socioeconomic class is a well-documented risk factor associated with higher mortality in men and women. It also is associated with other risk factors, including hypertension, elevated LDL cholesterol, higher body mass index, and lower HDL cholesterol levels (Luepker, Rosamund, Murphy, et al., 1993).

Lower socioeconomic class may also affect lower participation in cardiac rehabilitation programs. Harlan, Sandler, Lee, Lam, and Mark (1995) found that patients with lower socioeconomic status were disproportionately represented in cardiac rehabilitation pro-

TABLE 26–4 ■ GOALS FOR DIETS TO LOWER BLOOD CHOLESTEROL LEVELS

	Step 1 Diet	Step 2 Diet
Total fat intake (% of calories)	<30	<20
Saturated fat intake (% of calories)	<10	<7
Dietary cholesterol (mg/day)	<300	<200

National Cholesterol Education Program: Second Report of the Expert Panel on Detection, Evaluation, and Treatment of High Blood Cholesterol in Adults (Adult Treatment Panel Part II). Circulation 1994; 89, 1333–1445.

grams. Educational level and income level were strongly related to the decision to enroll in their program, highlighting the need for greater sensitivity about financial barriers faced by lower-income patients.

"Coronary-Prone" Behavior. Often referred to as "type A behavior," "coronary-prone" behavior is characterized by a variety of traits and behaviors, such as competitiveness, a sense of time urgency, and easily provoked hostility. Absence of or a more moderate expression of these characteristics has been labeled "type B behavior" pattern.

Type A behavior was recognized as an independent risk factor for CHD in 1981. Depression, hostility, and anger have also been found to be associated with CHD. The role of these traits is not fully understood. It is recommended, however, that at risk patients undergo a brief screening for depression (Froelicher et al., 1995).

Psychosocial Factors. There is considerable evidence suggesting that psychosocial factors have a strong adverse impact on the prognosis of CHD independent of the severity of disease. Studies suggest that patients who live alone, who are not married, or who lack a confidant are at increased risk for death after myocardial infarction (Case, Moss, Case, McDermott, & Eberly, 1992). Epidemiology studies have demonstrated an increase in mortality related to social isolation. Elderly patients who lack a source of emotional support have twice the risk of death after myocardial infarction.

Clearly, social isolation has negative consequences for survival in patients with heart disease. Assessing patients' sources of social support and helping them identify available sources of support are essential in designing a plan to meet their needs (McCauley, 1995).

Cultural Dimensions. Identifying the cultural factors pertinent to a patient's health can help with one of the most important functions of the provider: developing a successful plan that puts patient teaching in a meaningful context for the patient. Becoming culturally competent is a developmental process for the health care provider, involving self-awareness, understanding others from a cultural frame of reference, and acquiring the skills to provide culturally sensitive practice (Grossman, 1996).

There is an advantage in assessing the cultural factors that influence health and illness, particularly in the home, where the interactions between patients and families are observed as they occur in their natural setting. Cultural influences can be reflected in the following aspects of a patient's life:

- Health beliefs
- Communication style
- Family and kinship structure
- Dietary habits and concepts
- Religion
- Folk practices

These influences can affect the patient's understanding of the disease process and ability to adhere to treatment recommendations.

Health Beliefs. What the patient believes about causation of the disease or symptoms will determine the type of treatment the patient will seek or accept. It is important to assess the patient's health beliefs, particularly as they relate to education in the areas of prevention and risk factor modification.

There are three types of health belief systems, which can be summarized as follows (Geissler, 1994):

Magico-religious: Belief that health and illness are controlled by a god or gods or by supernatural forces
Biomedical: Familiar to most Americans; belief that illness is caused by a disruption in physical or biochemical processes that can be manipulated by humans
Holistic: Belief that health results from a balance or harmony among the elements of nature and that illness is produced by disharmony

For instance, in Russia, biomedical, holistic, and folk practices coexist. A complete medical system that focuses on prevention and cure is available only in the larger cities.

A recent Russian immigrant to the United States may have had no preventive health care nor been exposed to any rehabilitative care and so might require much more teaching of prevention strategies. A Chinese patient may believe in a holistic health paradigm, which might include herbal medicine as a treatment modality. The nurse might consider working with the Chinese herbalist to help the patient with congestive heart failure avoid herbs with high sodium content. The nurse must work with the patient and family to preserve cultural practices that are beneficial, adapt or adjust those that are neutral, and repattern those that have a potentially harmful effect on health (Grossman, 1996).

Exercise and Activity Guidelines

Exercise Training. Many studies of cardiac rehabilitation after myocardial infarction show consistent trends toward survival benefits among patients enrolled in rehabilitation programs. A meta-analysis of randomized trials has demonstrated a 20 to 25% reduction in cardiovascular deaths for patients enrolled in a comprehensive rehabilitation program (Oldridge, Guyatt, Fischer, & Rimm, 1988). Exercise training is an integral component of cardiac rehabilitation. The cardiac response to exercise and the effects of aerobic training are presented here to provide a framework for understanding the exercise component of cardiac rehabilitation (Moldover & Bartels, 1996).

Aerobic capacity is a physiological term describing the work capacity of a person. It is the amount of oxygen consumed per kilogram of body weight per minute. If plotted against workload, the total oxygen consumption ($\dot{V}O_2$) of an exercising person increases in a linear fashion until it levels off in a short plateau (Fig. 26–5). The plateau represents the point at which the $\dot{V}O_2$ cannot increase despite further increase in workload. This is the $\dot{V}O_{2max}$, or aerobic capacity of this person, representing a measure of the increasing metabolic work of the peripheral skeletal muscles. It is a useful measure of the physical work being performed.

Cardiac output (CO) increases with increasing work, as demonstrated in Figure 26–6. Cardiac output has two determinants: heart rate and stroke volume. Heart rate will be shown to increase in a linear manner when plotted against workload such as $\dot{V}O_2$.

The heart rate response to exercise is influenced by the following factors: (1) age, (2) type of activity, (3) body position, (4) fitness level, (5) the presence of heart disease, (6) medications, and (7) blood volume. It is im-

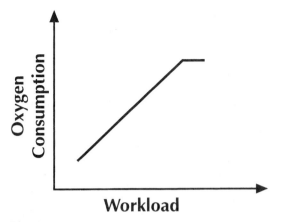

FIGURE 26–5
Relationship between oxygen consumption and intensity of work being performed. (From Braddom, R. L. [1995]. *Physical medicine and rehabilitation* [p. 650]. Philadelphia: W. B. Saunders.)

portant to note that a decline in maximal heart rate occurs with age.

Myocardial oxygen consumption, or $M\dot{V}O_2$, is the actual oxygen consumption of the heart. The *anginal threshold* is defined as the point at which the myocardial demand exceeds the ability of the coronary circulation to meet it. At that threshold, the patient may experience typical anginal chest pain, ischemia, or arrhythmias. It has been demonstrated that heart rate and systolic blood pressure correlate well with the actual myocardial oxygen consumption and can be used as a clinical guide.

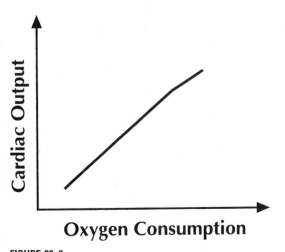

FIGURE 26–6
Relationship between cardiac output and oxygen consumption. (From Braddom, R. L. [1995]. *Physical medicine and rehabilitation* [p. 650]. Philadelphia: W. B. Saunders.)

Aerobic Training. *Aerobic training* refers to an exercise program that involves dynamic exercise with large muscle groups. The four principles that must be considered to alter the cardiopulmonary response to exercise are

- Intensity
- Duration
- Frequency
- Specificity

The *intensity* of aerobic exercise is defined in terms of heart rate response or in terms of exercise intensity (speed or resistance setting). The heart rate range represents an intensity that is generally safe and can produce the cardiopulmonary benefits of aerobic exercise. A typical exercise prescription might be written with a target heart rate to be sustained after an appropriate warm-up period. The target heart rate is usually 85% of age-predicted maximum heart rate, which is determined by a pretraining exercise stress test. If the person is frail or deconditioned or has other limiting factors, an intensity as low as 60% of maximum heart rate can be prescribed as the target rate, and a training effect can still be expected (Moldover & Bartels, 1996).

The *duration* of an aerobic training session is 20 to 30 minutes. This training period is preceded by a warm-up and cool-down phases at a lower intensity.

The *frequency* of exercise is also important. Aerobic training programs usually involve exercise three times a week. In programs involving exercise at lower intensities, exercise should occur five times a week.

Specificity in an exercise training program is an important principle. The changes in cardiac response to exercise apply only to muscles that have been involved in the exercise training. For example, training as a result of a walking or bicycle program does not affect cardiac response to upper extremity work. The design of an exercise program must also take into account the vocational and leisure activities of the person.

Many physicians report that they consider exercise training a component of care for patients with coronary disease. Nevertheless, few patients following acute coronary events (myocardial infarction, revascularization) are referred to supervised cardiac rehabilitation programs in the posthospitalization phase (Leon, Certo, Comoss, et al., 1990).

Resistance Training in Cardiac Rehabilitation. Cardiac rehabilitation programs have traditionally emphasized dynamic, aerobic forms of exercise. However, there is now increasing evidence demonstrating the value of resistance training to improve muscle strength for cardiac patients. In this form of exercise, muscle strength and endurance are enhanced by performing exercise against progressively increasing resistance. Low-weight resistance training should be individualized, and the cardiovascular demands or perceived exertion ratings should be no greater than those of the aerobic component. The use of cardiac monitoring and blood pressure monitoring is recommended. Training measures designed to increase skeletal muscle strength can safely be included in the exercise-based rehabilitation of clinically stable patients with coronary disease, when appropriate instruction and surveillance are provided (AACVPR, 1995; Wenger et al., 1995).

Preparing the Patient to Exercise. Most patients referred to cardiac rehabilitation undergo a comprehensive medical evaluation before beginning an exercise program. This evaluation should include a physical examination and a self-reported history that includes (1) identification of coronary risk factors, (2) symptoms of cardiac ischemia, (3) current medication use, and (4) an exercise history.

The evaluation should also include a maximal or symptom-limited exercise tolerance test (ETT). An ETT is typically performed on a treadmill or stationary bicycle ergometer. It requires patients to be able to exercise gradually at a continually increasing workload to either a maximum or a symptom-limited end point. The purpose of the ETT is to detect abnormalities resulting from the following factors (Fair & Berra, 1995):

- Ischemia (ST depression and symptoms of angina)
- Left ventricular dysfunction
- Heart rate response
- Presence and severity of arrhythmias
- Presence and severity of valvular dysfunction
- Functional capacity
- Limitations of the pulmonary system

After this assessment, initiation, and evaluation of response to activity, patients are ready to proceed with guidelines for home activity and beginning exercise.

Figure 26–7 provides the energy cost in metabolic equivalents (METS) of common activity and exercise. One MET is defined as the energy equivalent for a person at rest in a sitting position. It represents the consumption of 3.5 mL to 4.0 mL of oxygen per kilogram of body weight. This amount of energy (3.5–4.0 METS) is the amount it takes to perform most simple activities of daily living. Patients should be given a gradual conditioning program based on the results of exercise testing. Patients are usually given a METS list to use as a reference for choosing specific exercises and activities. They are shown how to monitor their pulse.

If patients are not able to take a pulse accurately, they are taught about the rating of perceived exertion (RPE) scale (Table 26–5). This scale has proven to be highly correlated with patient's pulse. When given a range of RPE to observe, patients can objectively judge their exercise exertion (Ritchie & Froelicher, 1995).

Psychosocial and Vocational Evaluation and Counseling

Community and Work Reintegration. Participation in activities such as work and driving are important factors in the quality of life for most adults. Patients are commonly concerned about the potential for recovery from myocardial infarction and the ability to resume their previous activities. Unfortunately, cardiac rehabilitation exercise training exerts less influence on rates of return to work than many nonexercise variables, such as employer attitudes, prior employment status, and economic incentives. Exercise training as

TABLE 26–5 ▪ BORG SCALE OF PERCEIVED EXERTION

Score	Perceived Exertion
6	
7	Very very light
8	
9	Very light
10	
11	Fairly light
12	
13	Somewhat hard
14	
15	Hard
16	
17	Very hard
18	
19	Very very hard
20	

From Braddom, R. L. (1996). *Physical medicine and rehabilitation* (p. 665). Philadelphia: W. B. Saunders.

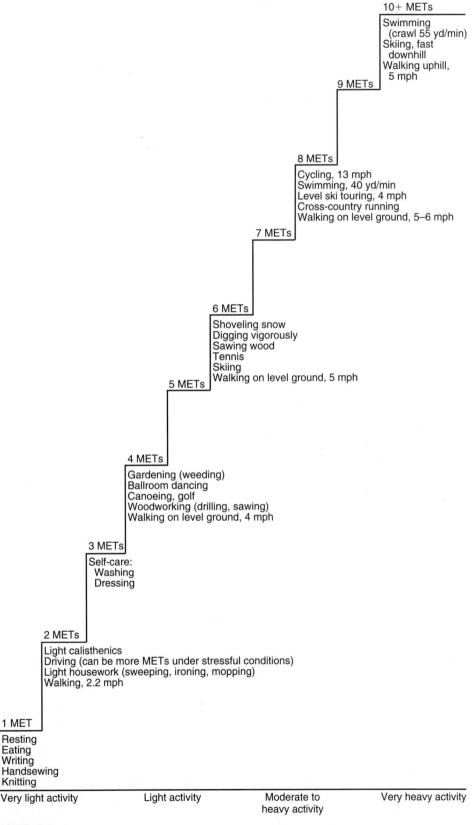

FIGURE 26–7
Energy cost (in METS) of activity and exercise (Redrawn from Woods, S. L., Holpenny, C. J., & Motzer, S. U. [Eds.]. [1995]. *Cardiac nursing* [p. 717]. Philadelphia: Lippincott–Williams & Wilkins.)

a sole intervention does not appear to facilitate return to work (Wenger et al., 1995). Cardiac rehabilitation programs that have a specific vocational counseling component may be more effective in improving the rates of return to work.

Patient Education. Many studies have shown that patients with CHD need structured and easily understood information about their disease. Patients cannot follow treatment recommendations that they do not understand. Patient education is an essential component in the care of the patient with cardiac disease in the hospital as well as in the community setting. It is a cornerstone of treatment in the structured rehabilitation program.

Although patient teaching fulfills an important function, most patients forget much of the information initially presented after they are discharged from the acute hospital phase. Much reinforcement is needed so that patients may be better able to care for themselves after an acute coronary event. Table 26–6 lists common concerns voiced by pa-

tients and spouses after myocardial infarction or CABS. These needs have been identified through counseling and interviewing groups and individuals.

Table 26–7 offers a sample class outline for enrollees in a structured cardiac rehabilitation program. This information can be provided in many different ways. Lindsay, Jennrich, and Biemat et al. (1991), who developed a programmed instruction approach for educating patients after myocardial infarction, found the programmed instruction booklet to be an effective and economical teaching tool. As computers become increasingly available to patients in community and home settings, programmed instruction can be easily adapted for a computer-assisted approach. The Internet also offers a wealth of patient educational materials and other forms of support (e.g., chat rooms) to assist providers in educating the segments of the population they serve.

Stress Management and Intervention. Many medical syndromes are caused or exacerbated by stress. These syndromes include but are not limited to hypertension and coronary artery disease. Stress contributes to the development and intensification of clinical syndromes and therapeutic processes.

Relaxation. The *fight-or-flight stress response* is manifested by such physiological reactions as dilation of pupils, higher blood pressure, and increased respiratory rate resulting from stimulation of the sympathetic nervous system. The *relaxation response* is the physiological opposite to the fight-or-flight response. It has been found to be an effective protective mechanism against stressful stimuli. Eliciting the relaxation response, which is marked by a decrease in pulse, respiratory rate, blood pressure, and metabolism, lessens the harmful effects of stress.

The relaxation response can be elicited through a variety of techniques, such as meditation, imagery, hypnosis, and progressive muscle relaxation (Mandle, Jacobs, Arcari, & Domar, 1996).

Elements of the Psychosocial Evaluation. Many cardiac patients and their families struggle with the adaptive challenges that come with illness and rehabilitation. The psychosocial component of rehabilitation programs should contain at least four elements: (1) assessment, (2) feedback, (3) brief intervention, and (4) referral for specialized intervention. Consideration of the following five

TABLE 26–6 ■ COMMON CONCERNS OF PATIENTS AND SPOUSES AFTER MYOCARDIAL INFARCTION (MI) OR CORONARY ARTERY BYPASS SURGERY (CABS)

MI and CABS
Returning home
Causes of coronary heart disease
Current and future state of health
Resumption of physical activities (including sexual activity)
Exercise guidelines
Dietary guidelines
Physical effects of cigarette smoking
Stress management
Emotional reactions
Family interactions
Changes in how others treat you
Medications
Recurrence and management of chest pain
The healing process
Diagnostic tests
Sleep disturbances
Returning to work or retirement
Emergency preparedness

CABS
Surgical procedure
Wound care
Body image changes and physical sensations
Transient intellectual dysfunction
Potential complications

From Woods, S. L., Froelicher, E. S., Halpenny, C. J., & Motzer, S. U. (Eds.), *Cardiac nursing* (3rd ed., p. 691). Philadelphia: Lippincott-Raven-Williams & Wilkins.

TABLE 26–7 ▪ OUTLINE OF HEART HEALTH CLASSES

Class 1: Anatomy and Physiology of the Heart, Coronary Heart Disease
Objectives
  Describe the circulation of blood throughout the body.
  Describe the process of atherosclerosis.
  Name the coronary arteries.
  Differentiate between angina and myocardial infarction.
  Recognize when to summon help.
Outline
  1. The coronary circulatory system
     a. The blood vessels
     b. The heart
     c. The coronary circulation
  2. Coronary heart disease (CHD)
  3. Angina
     a. Definition
     b. Causes
     c. Symptoms
     d. Things that differentiate it from myocardial infarction (MI)
     e. Things that differentiate it from other aches and pains
     f. Treatment, including medications
     g. When to call for help
  4. Myocardial infarction
     a. Definition
     b. Symptoms and signs
     c. Causes
     d. Diagnosis: electrocardiogram, enzymes, history
     e. Healing

Class 2: Understanding Your Exercise Prescription
Objectives
  List the benefits of exercise.
  Determine target heart rate.
  Describe phases of exercise.
  State slow down precautions.
Outline
  1. Definitions of activity and exercise
  2. Benefits
     a. Physiological
     b. Psychological
  3. Exercise tolerance test
     a. Heart rate responses
     b. Blood pressure responses
     c. Symptoms and signs
  4. Determining a target heart rate
  5. Energy expenditure
     a. Metabolic equivalents (METS): applications to daily activities
     b. Considerations for exercise: graded, interval principle
     c. Energy-saving techniques
  6. General principles for exercise
     a. Dynamic vs. isometric
     b. Warm up, cool down
     c. Exercise period, clothing, when, where
     d. General precautions

Class 3: Risk Factors for Coronary Heart Disease
Objectives
  Assess own risk factor profile.
  Prioritize relative strength of risk factors for them.

  Make a plan for risk factor change.
Outline
  1. Overview of risk factors
     a. Primary, secondary, tertiary prevention
     b. Interactions between risk factors
     c. Modifiable, nonmodifiable risk factors for CHD
     d. Risks related to graft closure in patient with coronary artery bypass surgery (CABS)
  2. Smoking
     a. Physiological effects
     b. Benefits of stopping
     c. Ways of stopping
  3. High blood pressure
     a. Definition
     b. Causes
     c. Physiological effects
     d. Symptoms
     e. Treatment
  4. Obesity
     a. Definition
     b. Risk related to other risk factors
     c. Treatment
  5. Type A behavior pattern
     a. Definition
     b. Treatment options
  6. Sedentary lifestyle
     a. Effects of inactivity
     b. Benefits of regular exercise
  7. Oral contraceptives
  8. Nonmodifiable risk factors
     a. Diabetes
     b. Gender
     c. Age
     d. Family history fo CHD

Class 4: Benefits of Exercise, Sound Exercise Practices
Objectives
  Identify the psychological and physical benefits of exercise.
Outline
  1. Define activity and exercise.
  2. Review psychological benefits of exercise.
     a. Improved self-esteem
  3. Review physiological benefits of exercise.
     a. Improved cardiovascular efficiency
     b. Increased strength
  4. Identify acute and chronic physiological responses to exercise.
     a. Heart rate changes, increased red blood cells, muscle metabolic changes
  5. Energy expenditure
     a. METs: applications to daily activities
     b. Considerations for exercise: graded, interval principle, energy-saving techniques
  6. General principles for exercise
     a. Dynamic vs. isometric
     b. Warm up and cool down
     c. Exercise period: clothing, when, where, climatic considerations
     d. Exercise precautions

Table continued on following page

TABLE 26–7 ■ OUTLINE OF HEART HEALTH CLASSES *Continued*

Class 5: Cardiac Rehabilitation

Objectives

Define the purpose of cardiac rehabilitation.

Identify the components of the cardiac rehabilitation
program.

Outline

1. Overview of the history of cardiac rehabilitation.
2. Discuss the exercise, education, nutrition, and
   psychological support components of the cardiac
   rehabilitation program.
3. Identify the team members and discuss their roles.
4. Review the phases of cardiac rehabilitation and
   expectations and appropriate goals for each phase.
5. Introduce the concepts of goal identification and planning
   for success with behavior change.
6. Discuss gradual graduation of patient from the
   rehabilitation program.
7. Identify potential barriers to long-term compliance with
   behavior changes and how these may be overcome.

Class 6: Emotional Adjustment to CHD

Objectives

Recognize common emotional reactions to CHD.

Discuss own and family's reactions to the diagnosis.

Outline

1. Common reactions to MI, CABS
2. Use of support systems
3. Dealing with co-workers

Class 7: Return to Work, Sexual Activity

Objectives

Recognize options available in making work-related
decisions.

State that sexual activity is safe for patients with CHD.

Understand that CHD does not limit patient's ability to
participate in sexual activity.

Outline

1. Energy expenditure and work
2. Defining work options
3. Physiological responses during sexual activity
4. Medication and sexual performance

Class 8: Treatment of Coronary Heart Disease

Objectives

State purpose of electrocardiogram (ECG), exercise tolerance
test (ETT), echocardiogram, cardiac catheterization,
radionuclide tests.

Recognize role of risk factor reduction in the treatment of
CHD.

Understand use of cardiac medications for CHD.

Describe when percutaneous transluminal coronary
angioplasty may be appropriate.

Understand the purpose of CABS.

Outline

1. Overview of diagnostic tests
   a. ECG
   b. ETT
   c. Echocardiogram
   d. Radionuclide tests
   e. Cardiac catheterization
2. Treatment of CHD
   a. Risk factor modification
   b. Medications of CHD management
      1. Nitrates
      2. Beta blockers
      3. Calcium-channel blockers
      4. Platelet inhibitors
   c. Percutaneous transluminal coronary angioplasty
   d. CABS

**Class 9: Health As a Way of Life . . . Motivation and
Choices**

Objectives

Define priorities related to health practices.

Recognize potential obstacles to successful behavior
change.

Outline

1. Establishing health as a priority, dietary puzzles
2. Barriers to success in exercise and dietary change
   a. Interpersonal barriers
   b. Social barriers, dealing with the holidays
   c. Traveling
3. Planning for obstacles

Class 10: Smoking Cessation

Objectives

Describe physiological effects of cigarette smoking.

Describe physiological effects of sidestream smoke.

List strategies for smoking cessation.

Name smoking cessation programs in the community.

Outline

1. Physiological effects of cigarette smoke
   a. Nicotine
   b. Carbon monoxide
   c. Heart rate and blood pressure responses
   d. Hematological responses
   e. Pulmonary effects
   f. Effects on other organ systems
2. Strategies for giving up smoking

From Woods, S. L., Froelicher, E. S., Halpenny, C. J., & Motzer, S. U. (Eds.), *Cardiac nursing* (3rd ed., pp. 699–700). Philadelphia: Lippincott-Raven-Williams & Wilkins.

questions may be helpful in planning for psychosocial interventions:

■ Is the crisis being caused by illness or entry into rehabilitation that has disrupted the patient's ability to adapt?
■ Does the patient show affective or cognitive impairment of the ability to cope with the demands of illness or those of rehabilitation?
■ Is the patient receiving adequate psychosocial support?
■ Does the patient have any behavioral pattern that warrants immediate intervention (e.g., smoking, substance abuse)?
■ What are the major concerns of the patient and family regarding anticipated psychosocial adjustments?

On the basis of answers to these questions, the cardiac rehabilitation staff can provide support, education, and anticipatory guidance; provide the patient with relaxation training; help the patient identify stress management strategies; and refer the patient to specialized consultation if necessary (AACVPR, 1995).

Rehabilitation of the Patient with Heart Failure

Heart failure affects an estimated 4.6 million Americans and results in average mortality rates of 10% at 1 year and 50% at 5 years. It is a complication frequently associated with CHD and often with myocardial infarction (AHA, 1999).

Heart failure is defined as a condition in which an abnormality of cardiac function is responsible for the failure of the heart to pump blood at a rate adequate to meet the metabolic requirements of the tissues. Heart failure may be characterized by (1) signs and symptoms of intravascular and interstitial volume overload, including shortness of breath, rales, and edema, or (2) manifestations of inadequate tissue perfusion, such as fatigue and poor exercise tolerance. A decrease in pump function leads to an inability to provide adequate cardiac output. The term *heart failure* is used in preference to *congestive heart failure* (CHF), because many patients with heart failure do not manifest pulmonary or systemic congestion (Konstam, Dracup, Baker, et al., 1994).

Symptom Management

Symptoms of heart failure must be monitored and managed so that prompt treatment is obtained and severe deterioration requiring hospitalization is prevented. According to information supplied by the Health Care Financing Administration, Medicare paid $3.6 billion in 1996 in hospital admissions for patients with a principal diagnosis of heart failure (AHA, 1999). Symptoms of heart failure are as follows:

■ Paroxysmal nocturnal dyspnea
■ Orthopnea
■ Dyspnea on exertion
■ Lower extremity edema
■ Decreased exercise tolerance
■ Unexplained confusion, altered mental status, or fatigue in an elderly patient
■ Abdominal symptoms, which may be associated with ascites or hepatic engorgement

Many patients with severe left ventricular dysfunction have no symptoms of heart failure. When clinical heart failure develops, dyspnea on exertion appears to be the earliest symptom (Konstrom et al., 1994).

Activity

Until the past few years, reduced activities and bed rest were considered standard treatment for the patient with heart failure. Later studies have shown, however, that patients with heart failure can exercise safely and that regular exercise may improve functional status and decrease symptoms. The clinical improvement that occurs with exercise training probably results from the effects on skeletal muscle rather than myocardial function. Exercise rehabilitation in patients with heart failure has resulted in reported improvements in peak oxygen uptake and 18 to 34% increases in exercise duration.

Exercise training in patients with heart failure has the following effects (Coats, Adamopoulos, Rodaelli, et al., 1992; Koch, Douard, & Broustet, 1992):

■ Raises anaerobic threshold
■ Reduces resting and submaximal exercise heart rates
■ Reduces exercise minute ventilation
■ Improves peak blood flow to exercising limbs

Regular exercise, such as walking or bicycling, should be encouraged for all patients with stable New York Heart Association class I through III heart failure (Konstrom et al., 1994).

Rehabilitation Program

To date, a specific type of training program or routine use of supervised rehabilitation programs has yet to be determined (what is recognized is that successful management of heart failure requires major lifestyle adjustments for patients and families). Better patient counseling and education are essential for improving outcomes. Table 26–8 lists suggested topics for patient and family education and counseling related to heart failure.

Because of the high prevalence of heart failure and the resulting high cost of caring

---

TABLE 26–8 ■ SUGGESTED TOPICS FOR PATIENT, FAMILY, AND CAREGIVER EDUCATION AND COUNSELING ABOUT HEART FAILURE

General Counseling
 Explanation of heart failure and the reason for symptoms
 Cause or probable cause of heart failure
 Expected symptoms
 Symptoms of worsening heart failure
 What to do if symptoms worsen
 Self-monitoring with daily weights
 Explanation of treatment/care plan
 Clarification of patient's responsibilities
 Importance of cessation of tobacco use
 Role of family members or other caregivers in the
   treatment/care plan
 Availability and value of qualified local support group
 Importance of obtaining vaccinations against influenza and
   pneumococcal disease

Prognosis
 Life expectancy
 Advance directives
 Advice for family members in the event of sudden death

Activity Recommendations
 Recreation, leisure, and work activity
 Exercise
 Sex, sexual difficulties, and coping strategies

Dietary Recommendations
 Sodium restriction
 Avoidance of excessive fluid intake
 Fluid restriction (if required)
 Alcohol restriction

Medications
 Effects of medications on quality of life and survival
 Dosing
 Likely side effects and what to do if they occur
 Coping mechanisms for complicated medical regimens
 Availability of lower cost medications or financial assistance

Importance of Compliance with the Treatment/Care Plan

From Konstan, M., Dracup, K., Baker, D., et al. (1994). Heart failure: Evaluation and care of patients with left-ventricular dysfunction (Clinical Practice Guideline No. 11). (AHCPR Publication No. 94-0612). Rockville, MD: Agency for Health Care Policy and Research.

---

for patients with the disease, many innovative approaches have been developed to address disease and symptom management, self-care skills, exercise training, and patient and family counseling in the heart failure population (Venner & Seelbinder, 1996; Brass-Mynderse, 1996). Undoubtedly, the rehabilitative care of this patient population provides the rehabilitation nurse with many creative opportunities to intervene along the care continuum.

Cardiac Rehabilitation in the Elderly

The benefits of cardiac rehabilitation have largely been defined for the younger and middle-aged patient with coronary disease. Emphasis is now being placed on the benefit of cardiac rehabilitation in elderly patients. This group has largely been underrepresented in formal exercise programs and, therefore, has been less well studied. There are, however, some studies of elderly patients that demonstrate an increase in functional capacity as measured by estimated peak MET levels after 12 weeks of exercise training (Lavie, Milani, & Littman, 1993).

Waldo, Ide, and Thomas (1995) studied the effect of a 6-week exercise program in elderly (mean age 66 years) patients who had experienced a cardiac event. Their results demonstrated a significant conditioning effect, in that mean exercising MET levels doubled by the 6-week measurement point. Oxygen saturation neither increased nor decreased, and there were statistically significant reductions in heart rate, systolic blood pressure, and rate pressure product during exercise over the course of the program.

Gortner, Dirks, and Wolfe (1992) reported on 102 elderly patients who had undergone CABG and received postoperative care consisting of patient education, symptom management, exercise and activity prescriptions, and weekly telephone contact with caregivers. Among the subjects older than 80 years, 79% reported that surgery improved the quality of life, and 67% reported that they had returned to or gone beyond their former activity levels.

Expected Aging Processes

The effects of aging on the elderly are influenced by many variables, such as genetics, lifestyle, exercise, and dietary habits. The impact on the cardiovascular system is summarized by Hellman and Williams (1994) as a decrease in achievable maximum heart rate and decreased cardiac output. Other expected changes associated with aging are (1) reduction in elasticity of peripheral vasculature, (2) decrease in musculoskeletal strength and flexibility, and (3) increasing prevalence of chronic diseases, such as diabetes, and degenerative bone and joint diseases, as well as of malnutrition.

Nursing Implications

Studies have promoted the role of exercise in the elderly and the value of lower-intensity training in patients with heart disease. The cardiac rehabilitation nurse has a unique opportunity to help elderly patients initiate and maintain the healthy behaviors that result from regular exercise. The elderly patient can benefit from formalized cardiac rehabilitation in many settings, from acute and subacute care to outpatient settings and home.

Initial evaluation should include detailed dietary history, including caloric and protein intake as well as calcium and vitamin D intake. Evaluation for sensory deficits, such as hearing and vision, should be made in conjunction with evaluation of comprehension. This is important in identifying potential deficits that impact on a patient's ability to fully participate in cardiac rehabilitation. Neuromuscular limitations, mobility, and self-care abilities should be assessed prior to initiation of an exercise program so that appropriate modifications can be made.

Generally, for elderly patients with heart disease, low-intensity training performed more frequently and for longer duration is recommended; such training can achieve results, though at a slower rate of progression. Because heart rate responses in elderly patients may be altered because of medications or disease processes, ratings of perceived exertion may be useful (Hellman & Williams, 1994).

Cardiac Rehabilitation in the Home

In response to escalating health care costs, medical insurance providers may or may not cover supervised outpatient programs. At the same time, many patients are unable to participate in such programs because of cost, inconvenient class times, or lack of accessibility. Therefore, rehabilitation specialists are being challenged to develop a variety of rehabilitation treatment options.

Traditionally, rehabilitation programs have been conducted in hospital or health care facilities. Attempts to improve patient compliance and participation have begun to include home-based programs. New technology in transtelephonics allows for simultaneous transmission of electrocardiogram (ECG) and voice over a single telephone line. Home-based programs now provide immediate clinical feedback and incorporation of self-management strategies (Sparks, Shaw, Eddy, et al., 1993). Miller, Warren, and Myers (1996) describe a nursing case management model (MULTIFIT) designed to address the challenges in the present health care system that hinder effective delivery of secondary prevention services. The MULTIFIT program offers comprehensive management of risk factors, including behavioral strategies for smoking cessation, lipid management, home exercise training, and stress reduction.

Patient compliance in exercise or other types of behavior modification is not easy to achieve, as evidenced by the low participation rate for patients (particularly women and the elderly) in formal rehabilitation programs. Reaching out into the community and the home may be an alternative for patients who for other reasons are unable to participate in traditional outpatient programs (Gulanick, 1991; Sparks et al., 1993).

Women and Cardiac Rehabilitation

Cardiovascular diseases, especially CHD and cerebrovascular disease, are the leading causes of death in women in the United States. However, women incorrectly perceive their risk of cancer as being much greater their risk of heart diseases or stroke. It is estimated that the onset of CHD occurs 7 to 10 years later in women than in men. By age 65, however, the number of deaths from ischemic heart disease is actually higher for women than for men.

By age 75, the incidence of CHD in women exceeds that in men. Advances in prevention, diagnosis, treatment, and rehabilitation associated with better outcomes have historically been based on research whose sampling has favored male subjects. The literature supports the notion that gender differences exist (Arnstein, Buselli, Renkin, et al., 1996; Lavie & Milani, 1996).

Modifiable Risk Factors

Despite the risks associated with smoking, today more young women smoke than young men. Women who have myocardial infarctions before age 40 years are almost always smokers, and older women who smoke are at five times greater risk for sudden death than women who do not. Women with more body fat, as measured by waist-to-hip ratio, are at greater risk of heart disease. High correlation was found between having upper-body fat and other factors, such as higher blood pressure, elevated cholesterol, anxiety, anger, depression, and smoking. Upper-body fat is also associated with lower serum levels of HDL cholesterol and less perceived social support.

Early in life, women have higher levels of HDL cholesterol and lower levels of LDL cholesterol than men; both factors are strongly associated with a lower risk of heart attacks. At menopause, however, women's serum LDL cholesterol and triglyceride levels generally increase, so that by age 65, these levels exceed those in men. Such increases are strong independent risk factors for the development of CHD (Rich-Edwards, Manson, Hennekens, & Buring, 1995).

The relative risk of having a myocardial infarction as the result of taking oral contraceptives is believed to be insignificant unless a woman also smokes. Use of hormone replacement therapy in the form of estrogen after menopause has been shown to significantly reduce the risk of CHD. Studies suggest that replacement of estrogen increases serum levels of HDL cholesterol and reduces serum levels of LDL cholesterol by as much as 15%, resulting in a 44% reduction in the risk of CHD in women after menopause (Rich-Edwards et al., 1995).

Factors Affecting Rehabilitation

Health care providers must be aggressive in suggesting cardiac rehabilitation activities to women. Only a small percentage of women who have had a myocardial infarction participate in a structured rehabilitation program (Balady et al., 1994). Women who are not socialized to competitive activities or exercising training are frequently uncomfortable with standard rehabilitation services. Differences in socioeconomic status, psychosocial profiles, presenting symptoms, and disease progression as well as a poorer response to treatment suggest that myocardial infarction in women is not fully understood.

Public education strategies and health promotion interventions for women should be geared specifically toward risk identification, awareness, and reduction. Assessment and intervention strategies that take into account the presenting symptoms, female patterns of

variant angina, mobilization of social supports, diagnostic testing, referral, and management of myocardial disease in women require more attention (Arnstein, 1996).

Care Across the Continuum

In the last 10 years, new technology and treatment options, advanced imaging, and new medications for acute and chronic illnesses have appeared regularly. In addition to these new advances and the influences of managed care, the provision of health care has increasingly shifted to subacute facilities and outpatient and home settings. The care of patients and families in the community will require greater coordination and emphasis on health promotion and disease management. The responsibility for providing support during rehabilitation and risk reduction efforts will fall increasingly on the nurse and other care providers in the community, the family, and the social network (Fleury, Peter, & Thomas, 1996).

Some studies have explored new approaches to the delivery of cardiac rehabilitation services, with the goals of increasing availability and decreasing costs while maintaining safety. Case management approaches to exercise training, smoking cessation, dietary and drug management of hyperlipidemia, and provision of emotional support and guidance to patients who rely on telephone contact can be provided to appropriately selected patients with CHD. How these management systems translate to other treatment settings will depend largely on reimbursement status and state regulation. Within each of these settings, managed care programs seeking optimal methods for coronary disease risk factor reduction and exercise rehabilitation may favor case management systems that provide convenient, individualized health care at low cost (Wenger et al., 1995).

PULMONARY REHABILITATION

Chronic obstructive pulmonary disease (COPD) refers to a spectrum of chronic respiratory diseases that result in physiological dysfunction that has severe implications for a patient's level of function and independence. These diseases are characterized by (1) cough, (2) sputum production, (3) dyspnea, (4) air flow limitation, and (5) impairment of gas exchange. Asthma and chronic obstructive disease, which includes chronic bronchitis and emphysema, are the most common obstructive diseases.

COPD is estimated to affect at least 15 million Americans and is the fifth leading cause of death in the United States. Unlike the death rate for cardiovascular disease, the death rate for COPD has risen in the past decade. Trends in COPD and asthma have not affected all ages and races equally. For COPD, recent rate increases have been greater in women than in men and in blacks than in whites. Growth in the total population and an increasing life expectancy will lead to larger numbers of people in need of pulmonary rehabilitation (Higgins, 1993).

Risk Factors for Obstructive Lung Disease

As with cardiovascular disease, a large number of risk factors have been associated with the development of obstructive lung disease. A number of genetic, familial, sociodemographic, behavioral, and environmental factors have been linked with the development of obstructive lung disease. Cigarette smoking remains the number one risk factor in the development of COPD. Eighty percent or more of the cases of COPD in the United States are attributable to cigarette smoking (Higgins, 1993). Quitting smoking is of critical importance for the patient with pulmonary disease and is discussed in further detail later in this chapter.

Physiology of Respiration

In the rehabilitation population, respiratory impairment is noted in patients with chronic respiratory conditions such as COPD as well as in those with neuromuscular disorders, neurological injury, or decreased energy. In order to plan interventions for the patient with pulmonary disease, the nurse must understand the physiology and mechanics of ventilation. A brief review of these subjects is presented.

Respiration is a vital function. The main purposes of respiration are to

- Supply cells of the body with oxygen
- Eliminate excess carbon dioxide produced during oxidation
- Help maintain normal pH of body fluids
- Help eliminate water
- Assist in maintaining normal body temperature

Ventilation is a result of inspiration and expiration. During inspiration, the diaphragm contracts and pulls downward, increasing the vertical length of the thoracic cage. The intercostal muscles pull ribs upward and outward, increasing the lateral and dorsoventral dimensions of the thoracic cage. Pressures in the thoracic cavity become slightly negative. Air is then pulled inward through the airway. During expiration, the diaphragm relaxes and rises, decreasing the volume of the thoracic cavity. The intercostal muscles relax further, decreasing the dimensions of the thoracic cavity. Intrapleural and intrapulmonic pressures rise, and air moves out of the lungs passively (McCourt, 1993).

Respiratory Muscles

The diaphragm is the most important muscle for breathing. It is innervated by the phrenic nerve, which arises from the fourth cervical nerve. Other inspiratory muscles are the external intercostal muscles and accessory muscles, including the trapezius and scalene muscles. The muscles used during the expiratory phase are the internal intercostal and abdominal muscles (McCourt, 1993).

Diseases of respiratory function can be divided into two categories, obstructive and restrictive disease (Table 26–9). *Obstructive* disease is defined as a blockage of air flow through the respiratory system. *Restrictive* disease is the diminution of lung expansion due to muscle weakness and resulting in decreased lung volume and capacity. This discussion is devoted to the discussion of obstructive lung diseases only.

Chronic Obstructive Lung Diseases

Asthma

Asthma is no longer defined as primarily a hyperactive airway disease but rather is regarded as a bronchiolar inflammation with secondary hyperresponsiveness and airway narrowing (Barnes, 1989). It is characterized by a cough, dyspnea, chest tightness, and wheezing. Symptoms can often be worse at night and can be triggered by such stimuli as exercise, cold air, allergens, and airway irritants. Reversible airway obstruction and heightened airway responsiveness can be demonstrated by pulmonary function testing in a patient with asthma.

Treatment of asthma is largely directed at preventing rather than reversing bronchospasm by controlling inflammation (Jacobs,

TABLE 26–9 ■ OVERVIEW OF LUNG DISEASES

Infections	Simple colds
	Bronchiolitis
	Pneumonia
	Human immunodeficiency virus (HIV) and
	acquired immunodeficiency syndrome
	(AIDS)
	Related opportunistic infections
Obstructive	Localized
diseases	Vocal cord paresis
	Laryngeal carcinoma
	Tracheal carcinoma
	Foreign bodies
	Bronchopulmonary dysplasia
	Generalized
	Chronic obstructive pulmonary disease
	Asthma
	Bronchiectasis
	Obliterative bronchiolitis
	Cystic fibrosis
Restrictive	Lung disease
disorders	Extrinsic allergic alveolitis
	Sarcoidosis
	Fibrosing alveolitis
	Asbestosis
	Eosinophilic pneumonia
	Pleural disease
	Pleural effusion
	Pneumothorax
	Chest wall deformity
	Kyphoscoliosis
	Respiratory muscle weakness
	Subdiaphragmatic problems
	Obesity
	Ascites

Modified from National Institutes of Health, National Heart, Lung and Blood Institute. (1995). *Global strategy for asthma management and prevention: NHLBI/WHO workshop.* (Publication No. 95-3659). Bethesda, MD: Author.

1994). *Atopy*, the predisposition for developing an immunoglobulin E–mediated response to common environmental allergens, is the strongest identifiable predisposing factor for the development of asthma (National Institutes of Health [NIH], 1995).

Chronic Bronchitis

Chronic bronchitis is characterized by a cough productive of sputum (not caused by local disease such as pneumonia) on most days for 3 months or longer during 2 or more consecutive years. The pathophysiology results from hypertrophy of bronchial mucous glands and bronchial smooth muscles.

Patients with chronic bronchitis are almost always cigarette smokers. They usually appear to be comfortable and have no significant tachypnea. Common findings are cyanosis, edema, and noisy, rhonchial chest sounds. Symptoms usually are chronic cough (usually without paroxysms), sputum production, recurrent infection, and shortness of breath with activity in later stages. Blood gas determinations typically reveal significant hypoxemia and normal to elevated arterial levels of carbon dioxide ($PaCO_2$) measurements (Jacobs, 1994).

Emphysema

Emphysema is characterized by a distention of the alveoli, an abnormal enlargement of air spaces beyond the terminal bronchiole culminating in permanent destruction of alveolar walls and loss of lung elasticity. Airway collapse or narrowing results from the loss of the protein elastin. Patients with emphysema are usually smokers. A typical patient would be tachypneic and might be seen leaning forward on the arms and using accessory muscles of respiration. Patients are often cachectic and have diminished breath sounds. PaO_2 and $PaCO_2$ (partial pressure of carbon dioxide) readings may be near normal until the later stages of the disease.

Familial emphysema occurs in people with a hereditary deficiency of alpha$_1$-antitrypsin (AAT). It is estimated that 1 to 3% of all cases of emphysema are due to AAT deficiency. The destruction of elastin that occurs in emphysema is believed to result from an imbalance between two proteins in the lung—elastase, which breaks down elastin, and AAT, which inhibits elastase. In the normal person, there is enough AAT to protect elastin, so that abnormal elastin destruction does not occur. When there is a genetic deficiency of AAT, however, the activity of elastase is not inhibited, and the destruction of elastin occurs unchecked.

The exact cause of *nonfamilial emphysema* is unknown, but the destruction of the alveoli is believed to occur as a result of an imbalance between elastin-degrading enzymes and their inhibitors. The elastase–AAT imbalance is thought to result from the effects of smoking. Studies show that tobacco smoke stimulates excess release of elastase from cells normally found in the lung. Oxidants found in cigarette smoke inactivate a significant portion of the elastase inhibitors, thereby decreasing the amount of active antielastase available to protect the lung. Researchers believe that in addition to smoking-related processes, there must be other factors causing emphysema in the general population, because only 15 to 20% of smokers experience emphysema. The nature and role of these other factors in smokers' emphysema are not yet clear (NIH, 1995).

Nursing Diagnoses

Like that of other chronic illness, the general course of COPD is one of steady deterioration marked by exacerbations of pronounced symptoms. There are several nursing diagnoses that commonly affect patients with COPD (Gordon, 1993). Knowledge of the typical problems and how they are managed will help nurses develop the appropriate rehabilitation plan for each patient.

The most obvious characteristic of COPD is obstruction of bronchial air flow during the exhalation phase of the breathing cycle. Emphysema destroys the pulmonary structures, fatigues the diaphragm, and limits the lung's ability to recoil and passively exhale. Chronic bronchitis causes inflammation of the airways, mucosal edema, and excess mucus production, which are thought to be contributing factor(s) in blocking air flow out of the lung.

Ineffective Breathing Patterns

The nursing diagnosis of ineffective breathing patterns related to pathophysiological alterations or airway irritants can be made for any patient in whom the following characteristics are identified:

- Use of accessory muscles, flaring of nostrils
- Dyspnea, cough, pursed-lip breathing, prolonged expiration
- Tachypnea, cyanosis, abnormal blood gas measurements

Nursing Management
During rehabilitation of the patient with obstructive lung disease, breathing patterns should be assessed frequently. The following interventions may be helpful in minimizing the effect of the disease on the patient, particularly in relieving dyspnea:

1. Position patients to maximize ventilation.
2. Assist with coughing and deep breathing.
3. Teach pursed-lip and abdominal-diaphragmatic breathing techniques.
4. Teach relaxation techniques.
5. Promote smoking cessation.
6. Help patient minimize energy demands.
7. Teach proper positioning and body mechanics.

8. Teach patients to pace activities and allow adequate rest between periods of exertion.
9. Administer medications to improve air flow.
10. Teach clients to avoid airway irritants, such as cigarette smoke, smog, aerosols, and various products that produce fumes.

Whether these interventions have been successful for a particular patient can be determined from measurements of adequate oxygenation (pulse oximetry, blood gas results), skin color, and decreases in respiratory rate as well as patient reports of less dyspnea.

Ineffective Airway Clearance

Many patients with COPD who exhibit symptoms primarily related to excess mucus production due to bronchitis may be unable to effectively clear secretions from the respiratory tract. The diagnosis of ineffective airway clearance may be defined by the following characteristics:

- Abnormal breath sounds
- Reduced vital capacity
- Cough, change in rate and depth of respiration
- Dyspnea, tachypnea, cyanosis
- Change in color, amount, or consistency of sputum

Measures to enhance airway clearance may include those previously mentioned. Others are as follows:

1. Teach effective coughing techniques.
2. Perform chest physical therapy.
3. Administer suctioning.
4. Inform the patient about environmental factors and the importance of adequate humidity.

Pulmonary Rehabilitation

Pulmonary rehabilitation has been defined as "an art of medical practice wherein an individually tailored, multidisciplinary program is formulated which through accurate diagnosis, therapy, emotional support, and education, stabilizes or reverses both the physio- and psychopathology of pulmonary diseases and attempts to return the patient to the highest possible functional capacity allowed by his pulmonary handicap and overall life situation" (American Lung Association, 1981, p. 663). Pulmonary rehabilitation has been redefined by an NIH workshop as a "multidisciplinary continuum of services directed to people with pulmonary disease and their families, usually by an interdisciplinary team of specialists, with the goal of achieving and maintaining the individual's maximum level of independence and functioning in the community" (Fishman, 1994, p. 825).

The two principal objectives of pulmonary rehabilitation are (1) to control and alleviate as much as possible the symptoms and pathophysiological complications of respiratory impairment and (2) to teach the patient how to achieve optimal capability for carrying out activities of daily living. Pulmonary rehabilitation has become a well-recognized program of care for patients. A comprehensive program typically consists of education, instruction in respiratory and chest physical therapy techniques, psychosocial support, and exercise training. Table 26–10 lists the common goals and expectations of pulmonary rehabilitation.

Benefits of Pulmonary Rehabilitation

Several studies suggest that pulmonary rehabilitation benefits patients in several ways. Increased exercise tolerance and decreases in total hospital stay and recurrent hospitalizations are cited as common outcomes. Ries, Kaplan, Limberg, & Prewitt (1995) studied the effects of an 8-week comprehensive rehabilitation program with those of education alone on physiological and psychosocial outcomes in patients with COPD. Compared with education alone, pulmonary rehabilitation produced significantly greater improvements in maximal exercise tolerance, maximum oxygen uptake, exercise endurance, reduction of symptoms of perceived breathlessness, and muscle fatigue. Measures of lung function did not differ between the groups that did and did not participate in pulmonary rehabilitation. Other demonstrated benefits of pulmonary rehabilitation are return to work for some patients, greater knowledge about pulmonary disease, and longer survival, which is thought to be associated with supplemental oxygen use (Connors & Hilling, 1993).

Program Components

The essential components of pulmonary rehabilitation are provided by a pulmonary rehabilitation team of health care providers. This team consists of physicians, nurses, respiratory therapists, physical and occupational therapists, exercise physiologists, psycholo-

TABLE 26–10 ■ GOALS AND EXPECTATIONS OF PULMONARY REHABILITATION

Feeling Better
  Less reduced dyspnea
  Greater confidence
  Less depression, anxiety, and panic
  Less frequent insomnia

Greater Activity
  At home
  In the community
  During leisure time

Increased Endurance and Strength
  Muscles of ambulation
  Upper extremities
  Ventilatory muscles

Greater Range of Function
  Self-care
  Care of the home
  Shopping
  Sexual activity
  Leisure activity
  Work (if appropriate)

Self-Control and Self-Management
  Dyspnea
  Living situation
  Clearance of secretions
  Medications
  Oxygen
  Nutrition
  Family matters

Physician-Patient Communication
  More effective visits to the physician, with the understanding that the patient is an extension of the physician

From Casaburi, R., & Petty, T. L. (Eds.) (1993). Principles and practice of pulmonary rehabilitation (p. 303). Philadelphia: W. B. Saunders.

gists, social workers, nutritionists, and vocational counselors. An individualized program of pulmonary rehabilitation designed to meet the specific needs of the patient may or may not involve every member of the team (Connors & Hilling, 1993).

Strijbos, Postma, Van Altena, Gimeno, and Koeter (1996) compared a 3-month rehabilitation program in the home with a standard outpatient program. They reported that the results of the home rehabilitation program were as good as those of the standard program and that patients rehabilitated at home maintained their improvements over an 18-month follow-up. Pulmonary rehabilitation may occur in the outpatient setting, but components of pulmonary rehabilitation may be administered in a home setting, in a subacute care setting, with individual patients, or in groups.

Essential components of a pulmonary rehabilitation are as follows (American Lung Association, 1981):

- Bronchial hygiene, such as effective coughing
- Breathing techniques
- Chest physical therapy, if needed
- Exercise conditioning, including upper extremity strengthening
- Respiratory therapy, such as supplemental oxygen and aerosolized medicine
- Patient and family education

Bronchial Hygiene

For some patients, chronic lung disease predisposes to retained secretions and infection. Such patients may benefit from chest physiotherapy. Postural bronchial drainage, controlled coughing, and chest percussion may help patients clear secretions. These are important techniques for patients with excessive mucus production, particularly during periods of exacerbation of disease.

Chest physiotherapy techniques may also be of benefit when provided on a regular basis as a preventive health care measure, in the patient with a disease such as bronchiectasis or cystic fibrosis. The frequency of treatments must be individualized for the patient according to severity of the disease (Ries, 1990).

Breathing Techniques

Pursed-Lip and Diaphragmatic Breathing. Both pursed-lip and diaphragmatic breathing techniques attempt to alter the breathing pattern of symptomatic patients.

Pursed-lip breathing takes advantage of a maneuver often assumed naturally by patients and results in slower and deeper respirations. The goal is to slow the expiratory phase of expiration and prevent airway collapse by increasing the expiratory airway pressure. In pursed-lip breathing, the patient is instructed as follows:

1. Inhale through the nose, keeping the mouth closed.
2. Exhale slowly for 4 to 6 seconds through pursed lips held in a whistling position, gently contracting the stomach muscles.

This technique has been demonstrated to result in higher oxygen saturation values and lower respiratory rates. During exercise, the shift to pursed-lip breathing decreases dyspnea. This technique should be used by patients when they feel short of breath (Celli, 1995; Ries, 1990).

In *diaphragmatic breathing*, the patient attempts to coordinate abdominal wall expansion with inspiration and to slow expiration by breathing through pursed lips. In this technique, the patient is instructed as follows:

1. Place one hand on the abdomen just below the ribs and the other hand on the upper part of the chest.
2. Breathe in through the nose so that the abdomen moves out against the hand as far as it will go, while keeping the other hand on the chest as still as possible.
3. Exhale slowly and fully through pursed lips.

A review of clinical studies evaluating the effectiveness of breathing training techniques points to the improvement in clinical symptoms such as dyspnea rather than changes in physiological parameters. Most often, these techniques are taught together and are integrated with other components of patient education and support (Ries, 1990).

Exercise Conditioning

Patients with lung disease may have reduced exercise tolerance if, during exercise, (1) they cannot adequately oxygenate the blood or eliminate carbon dioxide or (2) their cardiovascular response is inadequate. Symptoms generally limiting exercise performance in pulmonary patients are exertional dyspnea and fatigue (Wasserman, 1993).

Exercise training is based on the following three physiological principles:

- *Specificity* of training: attributes improvement only in relation to the exercise practiced.
- *Intensity* of training: Only a load higher than baseline will induce a training effect.
- *Reversal* of the training effect: Once training is discontinued, its effect will disappear.

Casaburi (1993) pooled the results of 36 uncontrolled studies evaluating the effect of aerobic training on exercise capacity in patients with COPD. Aerobic training resulted in an increase in exercise endurance. Other findings included improvements in a 12-minute walk distance and oxygen uptake. It is generally accepted that exercise results in both physiological and psychological improvements in patients with COPD. Patients may increase their capacity, endurance, or both for exercise and physical activity, even though their lung function does not usually change. Exercise training also provides an excellent opportunity for patients to learn about their capacity for physical work as well as to practice methods of controlling dyspnea (Ries, 1990; Ries et al., 1995).

The exercise program needs to be safe and appropriate (based on the identified needs of the patient). Walking and bicycling programs are most often selected and can be adapted to the home setting. For patients with advanced COPD, exercise tolerance is typically limited by maximum ventilation and the perception of breathlessness. Some rehabilitation programs tend to define exercise targets and progression during training by symptom tolerance (i.e., breathlessness) rather than by target heart rates. This approach is particularly effective for patients who are elderly or have limited exercise tolerance (Ries, 1990).

Upper Extremity Training. Exercise programs for patients with COPD have typically emphasized lower extremity training such as walking or bicycling. Other types of exercise may have potential benefits for patients with COPD. Many such patients report dyspnea while performing many of the activities of daily living that involve the use of upper extremities, such as bathing and grooming. Upper extremity exercises may therefore be important in the design of a training program for patients with COPD (Ries, 1990).

Respiratory Muscle Training. Respiratory muscle training results in greater strength and capacity of the muscles to endure a respiratory load. There are conflicting results about its benefit on exercise performance or performance in activities of daily living. In some patient populations, there may be a benefit to ventilatory muscle training with the use of a threshold breathing device. The role of respiratory muscle training has not yet been clearly defined (Celli, 1995).

Respiratory Therapy
Oxygen Use. Oxygen should be given at a rate sufficient to produce oxygen saturation at consistently more than 90%. Higher flow rates during exercise or sleep may be required (Jacobs, 1994). The current guideline for long-term oxygen use specifies one of the following parameters in a patient who is breathing room air:

- PaO_2 <55 mm Hg
- SaO_2 (arterial oxygen saturation) <88%

Consideration for the long-term use of oxy-gen is given to some patients with PaO_2 more than 55 mm Hg, such as in those with evidence of factors such as pulmonary hypertension or cor pulmonale.

A variety of oxygen-conserving techniques and delivery and storage devices are available, each with its advantages and disadvantages. Patients who use oxygen need information about (1) safe use, particularly in the home setting, (2) cleaning and maintenance of equipment, and (3) correct phone numbers of resources. This information varies for each piece of equipment and its manufacturer. Such patient information can be obtained directly from the oxygen supplier.

Asthma Management and Prevention. There have been focused initiatives in the management and prevention of asthma. Increasing prevalence, new understanding of the disease process, and a new focus on establishing risk factors for the development of asthma have resulted in a greater focus on identifying appropriate interventions to prevent exacerbation of asthma. Much of this goal is achieved through the patient educational process. The major educational goal of the asthma management and prevention program is to give health care providers strategies designed to keep their patients with asthma well. Such strategies require establishing a management plan with patients that gives them the information and skills necessary to effectively manage their disease. An example of an asthma management plan is shown in Figure 26-8.

Use of an inhaler, nebulizer, or peak flowmeter (Fig. 26-9) for monitoring asthma severity and controlling asthma triggers might be included in the asthma management plan (NIH, 1995).

Patient and Family Education
As with any rehabilitation program, the success of a pulmonary rehabilitation program depends on the active involvement of the patient and family members in learning about the disease and managing the debilitating effects of its symptoms. Patient and family education is an integral part of any pulmonary rehabilitation program. Table 26–11 provides a discharge checklist for patients with COPD. Table 26-12 identifies outcomes and interventions for the nursing diagnosis "knowledge deficit related to onset or exacerbation of COPD."

The following discussion considers common areas of education for patients with pulmonary disease.

TABLE 26–11 ■ DISCHARGE CHECKLIST FOR PATIENTS WITH CHRONIC OBSTRUCTIVE PULMONARY DISEASE (COPD)

Topic	Instruction	Review
1. Disease process		
a. Normal lung function		
b. Pathophysiology of COPD (identify)		
2. Risk factors		
a. Smoking		
b. Environmental irritants		
c. Occupational irritants		
d. Exposure to respiratory infection		
3. Reportable signs and symptoms		
a. Increased dyspnea		
b. Change in sputum		
c. Productive cough		
d. Pain (especially chest)		
e. Upper respiratory infection		
f. Fever, chills		
g. Swelling of hands or legs		
h. Sudden weight gain		
i. Anorexia, nausea, vomiting		
4. Interventions		
a. Medications		
(1) Bronchodilators		
(2) Steroids		
(3) Antibiotics		
(4) Cardiac/antihypertensives		
(5) Diuretics		
(6) Other		
b. Use/care of inhaler(s)		
(1) Without spacer		
(2) With spacer		
c. Use/care of nebulizer(s)		
d. Use/care of oxygen		
e. Use/care of ventilatory equipment		
f. Measures to clear airways		
(1) Drainage		
(2) Percussion		
(3) Effective coughing		
g. Measures to control dyspnea		
(1) Pursed lip/diaphragmatic breathing		
(2) Relaxation techniques		
(3) Planning/pacing of activities		
(4) Energy conservation techniques		
h. Nutrition/hydration		
i. Lifestyle changes		
5. Follow-up care		
a. Outpatient healthcare visit(s)		
b. Outpatient laboratory requirements		
c. Outpatient community services		

From Landis, K. (1993). Discharge teaching for patients with COPD. *Perspectives in Respiratory Nursing, 4*(2), 3–4.

Smoking Cessation. Knowledge about the adverse effects of cigarette smoking has been available for several decades. The prevalence of cigarette smoking has declined in the United States since 1965, although data indicate that this downward trend may have leveled off. Of great concern is that cigarette smoking among younger people remains a major health concern. Each day, 3000 teenagers start to smoke (AHA, 1999). Education about smoking cessation should cover the following three concepts.

TABLE 26–12 ■ OUTCOMES AND INTERVENTIONS FOR THE DIAGNOSIS: KNOWLEDGE DEFICIT RELATED TO ONSET OR EXACERBATION OF COPD

Problem
Knowledge deficit related to onset or exacerbation of COPD

Outcome
The patient will verbalize understanding of chronic obstructive pulmonary disease as evidenced by
  a. Explanation of diagnosis and treatment
  b. Delineation of risk/precipitating factors
  c. Identification of important lifestyle changes

Interventions
1. Provide information (written and/or verbal) about normal lung function and the pathophysiology of the specific chronic obstructive pulmonary disease
  a. Asthma
  b. Bronchiectasis
  c. Chronic bronchitis
  d. Cystic fibrosis
  e. Emphysema
2. Explain the goals of treatment
  a. Management of dyspnea
  b. Bronchodilation
  c. Management of secretions
  d. Maintenance/improvement of functional activities
  e. Compliance with therapy
3. Identify the risk factors that exacerbate the disease(s)
  a. Smoking
  b. Changes in temperature and/or humidity
  c. Exposure to stress/exercise
  e. Exposure to aerosols, fumes, odors
  f. Exposure to others with upper respiratory diseases
  g. Exposure to triggering allergens (environmental or occupational)
4. Make sure the patient understands the signs and symptoms of exacerbations
  a. Increased shortness of breath
  b. Change in amount, color, taste, or consistency of mucus
  c. Development of or change in cough
  d. Occurrence of fever, chills, fatigue, malaise, and chest pain or tightness

From Landis, K. (1993). Discharge teaching for patients with COPD. *Perspectives in Respiratory Nursing,* (2), 4.

ASTHMA CONTROL PLAN FOR _____
(name of patient)

PREPARED BY _____ , M.D.

This plan will help you control your asthma and do the right thing if you have an asthma episode. Keeping your asthma under control will help you:
- Be active without having asthma symptoms. This includes being active in exercise or sports.
- Sleep through the night without having asthma symptoms.
- Prevent asthma episodes (attacks).
- Have the best possible peak flow rate.
- Avoid side effects from medicines.

Here are three ways to control your asthma:

■ Follow your medicine plan (see the next page).
—Follow your Green Zone plan every day to keep most asthma symptoms from starting.
—Recognize your symptoms of an asthma episode. Act quickly to stop them.
—Follow the Yellow Zone plan to stop asthma symptoms and to keep an asthma episode from getting serious.
—Follow the Red Zone plan to take care of a serious episode. This is an emergency plan!

■ Whenever possible, stay away from things that bring on your asthma symptoms. Follow your asthma trigger control plan to reduce the number of things in your home, workplace, or classroom that bother your asthma.

■ See your doctor regularly. Review this plan with your doctor when you visit him or her. Your doctor will write on the plan what you should do.

Your plan has these medicines:

_____

_____

_____

_____

_____

_____

Important Information:

Doctor _____   Hospital _____

Telephone _____   Telephone _____

Address _____   Address _____

_____   _____

Ambulance or Emergency Rescue Squad _____   Friend to Call _____

Telephone _____   Telephone _____

Taxi _____

For more information on Asthma:
National Asthma Education and Prevention Program
Information Center
P.O. Box 30105
Bethesda, MD 20824-0105
(301) 251-1222

Adapted from National Asthma Education Program "Clinician's Guide: Teaching Your Patients About Asthma." National Heart, Lung, and Blood Institute. National Institutes of Health, United States.

FIGURE 26–8
Sample asthma control plan. (Redrawn from National Heart, Lung, and Blood Institute [1995, January]. *Global strategy for asthma management and prevention: NHLBI/WHO workshop report* (Publication No. 95-3659). Bethesda, MD: Author.)

ASTHMA CONTROL PLAN FOR _____

(name of patient)

PREPARED BY _____ , M.D.

Green Zone: All Clear

This is where you should be every day.

Peak flow between _____

(80–100%

of personal best)*

No symptoms of an asthma episode. You are able to do your usual activities and sleep without having symptoms.

The doctor will check which applies to you.

☐ Take these medicines:

Medicine	How much to take	When to take it
_____	_____	_____
_____	_____	_____
_____	_____	_____
_____	_____	_____

☐ Follow your asthma trigger control plan to avoid things that bring on your asthma.

☐ Take _____ before exercise.

(medicine)

Yellow Zone: Caution

This is not where you should be every day. Take action to get your asthma under control.

Peak flow between _____

(60–80%

of personal best)*

You may be coughing, be wheezing, feel short of breath, or feel like your chest is tight. These symptoms may keep you from your usual activities or keep you from sleeping.

☐ *First,* take this medicine:

Medicine	How much to take	When to take it
_____	_____	_____

☐ *Next,* if you feel better in 20 to 60 minutes and your peak flow is over_____ ,

then (70%

of personal best)

☐ Take this medicine:

Medicine	How much to take	When to take it
_____	_____	_____
_____	_____	_____

☐ Keep taking your Green Zone medicine(s)

☐ But, if you DO NOT feel better in 20–60 minutes or your peak flow is under _____ , follow the Red Zone plan.

(70% of personal best)

Let the doctor know if you keep going into the Yellow Zone. Your Green Zone medicine may need to be changed to keep other episodes from starting.

Red Zone: Medical Alert

This is an emergency! Get help.

Peak flow under _____

(60%

of personal best)*

You may be coughing, you may be very short of breath, and/or the skin between your ribs and your neck may be pulled in tight. You may have trouble walking or talking. You may not be wheezing because not enough air can move out of your airways.

☐ *First,* take this medicine:

Medicine	How much to take	When to take it
_____	_____	_____
_____	_____	_____

☐ *Next,* call the doctor to talk about what you should do next.

☐ *But,* see the doctor RIGHT AWAY or go to the hospital if *any* of these things are happening:

–Lips or fingernails are blue.

–You are struggling to breathe.

–You do not feel any better 20 to 30 minutes after taking the extra medicine and your peak flow is still under _____ .

(60% of personal best)

–Six hours after you take the extra medicine, you still need an inhaled $beta_2$-agonist medicine every 1 to 3 hours and your peak flow is under _____ .

(70% of personal best)

*This is a general guideline only. Some people have asthma that gets worse very fast. They may need to have a Yellow Zone at 90–100% of personal best.

FIGURE 26–8 *Continued*

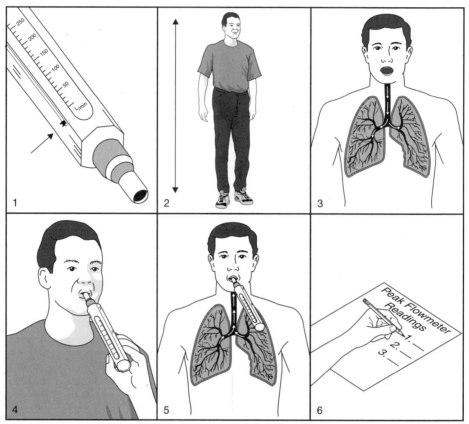

1. Place the indicator at the base of the numbered scale.
2. Stand up.
3. Take a deep breath in until your lungs are as full as possible.
4. Place the PFM in your mouth and close your lips around the mouthpiece. Do not put your tongue inside the hole.
5. Blow out through your mouth in one quick, hard blast.
6. Write down the number you get.
7. Repeat steps 1 through 6 two more times.
8. Mark the highest number you get in your PFM diary.

FIGURE 26–9

Using a peak flowmeter (PFM). Remember: Green = Go; yellow = Slow down; red = Stop. (Redrawn from Dimock Community Health Center. [1997]. *Breathe easier: A guidebook for managing asthma.* Roxbury, MA: Author.)

Cost. Cigarette smoking is costly to both society and the person who smokes. New long-term studies estimate that about half of all regular cigarette smokers will eventually be killed by their habit. Smoking-related illnesses cost the United States about $50 billion annually in medical care. When lost work and productivity are added, the total cost to society is estimated to exceed $97 billion (American Thoracic Society [ATS], 1996).

Cigarette smoking is the principal risk factor for COPD. The exact mechanism by which smoking causes obstructive lung disease has not been firmly established. One proposed mechanism is that smoking allows an imbalance between proteolytic and antiproteolytic activities in the lung, resulting in destruction of alveoli and air flow obstruction. It is estimated that 10 to 15% of all smokers experience clinically significant air flow obstruction (ATS, 1996).

Health Benefits of Quitting. Smoking cessation has immediate health benefits for men and women of all ages. People who quit smoking before they are 50 years old have half the risk of dying over the next 15 years compared with people who continue to smoke. In patients with COPD, the benefits of quitting include a decrease in the amount of mucus formation and a reduction of the risk of respiratory infections such as pneumonia. Patients with asthma who quit smoking may lessen the frequency and severity of asthma.

How to Quit. Withdrawing from nicotine may produce symptoms of withdrawal such as those seen with withdrawal from other highly addictive drugs. Such symptoms include (1) cravings to use nicotine, (2) irritability, (3) anxiety, (4) difficulty concentrating, (5) restlessness, and (6) increased appetite. Addictions are governed by behavioral, psychological, and biological processes; therefore, cigarette smoking presents a challenge to prevent its beginning and promote its cessation. Smokers who have been successful in achieving long-term abstinence report having previously stopped and relapsed multiple times. Therefore, relapse should not be considered a failure.

Many community and scientific resources are dedicated to the efforts to increase the rate of smoking cessation. They include self-help strategies, group programs, nicotine replacement therapy, hypnosis, and worksite and community programs (ATS, 1996). Working with a patient on smoking cessation may be the biggest challenge but also the greatest opportunity for rehabilitation nurses to affect the health of a person.

Treating Tobacco Use and Dependence, a U.S. Public Health Service–sponsored Clinical Practice Guideline (June 2000), offers five key strategies for quitting smoking. Studies have shown that combining all of the following five steps offers the greatest chances of success*:

1. Get ready:
   ■ Set a quit date.
   ■ Rid your home, car, and workplace of cigarettes.
   ■ Once you quit, don't smoke, not even a puff.
2. Get support:
   ■ Tell your family, friends, and coworkers that you are going to quit.
   ■ Get individual group or telephone counseling.
3. Learn new skills:
   ■ Try to distract yourself from urges.
   ■ Change your routines.

■ Do something to reduce your stress.
■ Plan something enjoyable every day.
■ Drink water and other fluids.
4. Get medication:
   ■ The U.S. Food and Drug Administration has approved five medications to help you quit smoking:
   Bupropion SR—available by prescription
   Nicotine gum—available over the counter
   Nicotine inhaler—available by prescription
   Nicotine nasal spray—available by prescription
   Nicotine patch—available by prescription and over the counter
   ■ Ask your health care provider for advice and carefully read the information on the package.
5. Be prepared for relapse:
   ■ Most relapses occur within the first 3 months after quitting. Remember, most people try several times before they finally quit.
   ■ Avoid difficult situations: alcohol, other smokers, weight gain.

Environmental Hazards. Patients with chronic lung disease should be educated in the environmental hazards that might negatively affect their health. Identification of the patient's particular triggers and avoidance of exposure to respiratory irritants are the beginning steps. They are followed by assessment of the patient's smoking history as well as exposure to secondhand smoke, toxic fumes, changes in humidity, and stress within the environment.

It is particularly important to help patients with asthma identify their triggers. Asthma triggers include exposures to factors that have already sensitized the airways of the person with asthma and that cause recurrent asthma exacerbation. Triggers vary with each person. Indoor control measures are just as important as outdoor control measures. Among the wide variety of allergens that occur within human dwellings are domestic mites, animal allergens (from furred animals), cockroach allergen, and fungi. Complete avoidance of these triggers is hard to achieve; however, efforts to help patients identify and recognize their own environmental triggers may prevent exacerbation of their disease (NIH, 1995). A sample patient education tool for identifying asthma triggers is shown in Figure 26–10.

---

*Internet citation: "You can quit smoking." *Consumer Guide,* June 2000. U.S. Public Health Service. http://www.surgeongeneral.gov/tobacco/consquits.htm

Internet Citation: *"Treating Tobacco Use and Dependence."* Summary, June 2000. U.S. Public Health Service. http://www.surgeongeneral.gov/tobacco/smokesum.htm

For each person, asthma flare-ups are caused by different things. To prevent asthma flare-ups, find out which of the triggers listed below make you/your child's symptoms start. These triggers are sometimes hard to see. But even the cleanest home, school room, or office has some of these hidden triggers.

Some of these triggers will be hard to control. You and your family may have to make some changes in the way you live. Please ask your health care provider for advice about resources to help you make these changes—they are very important for good asthma control.

Indoor Triggers

—Cigarette smoke
Ideas for control:

■ There should be no smoking in the home/car/office of anyone who has asthma. Even if the person with asthma is not at home, smoke gets into the curtains and rugs.
■ If anybody in the house smokes, ask them to smoke outside and to ask their doctor about smoking cessation services or nicotine patches.

—Strong fumes in the air from perfume, hair spray, and cleaning solutions
Ideas for control:

■ Don't paint in the house when the person with asthma is home.
■ If you have to use hair sprays, perfumes, or strong-smelling cleaning products, open windows and doors for good air flow.
■ For cleaning, it is better to use mild things like: diluted ammonia for general household cleaning; baking soda for deodorizing room, rug or refrigerator; lemon oil or olive oil for furniture polish; nonchlorine bleaches for laundry; club soda as a spot remover; salt to loosen burned on foods; unscented soap; and vinegar as a household cleaner to remove mold, mineral deposits, and crayon marks.

FIGURE 26–10
Sample patient education tool about identifying asthma triggers. (From Dimock Community Health Center [1997]. *Breathe easier: A guidebook for managing asthma.* Roxbury, MA: Author.)

Prevention and Elimination of Infection. Patients with chronic lung disease should be taught the signs and symptoms of respiratory infections and when to report these changes to the health care provider. Signs and symptoms of infection include (1) the presence of fever and (2) change in the color, consistency, and amount of sputum.

Patients should be reminded to avoid contact with people with respiratory infections. The prevention and early treatment of recurrent or chronic infections are important. Annual vaccination against influenza is recommended for all patients with COPD. Although the benefits of the vaccine are debated, pneumococcal vaccination is recommended as well (Ferguson & Cherniack, 1993).

Nutritional Support. Undernutrition, indicated by a body weight less than 90% of ideal body weight, is estimated to be present in 25% of patients with COPD. Many patients appear to be unable to gain weight even though they are receiving nutritional supplements. These patients cannot maintain an adequate caloric intake, most commonly because their caloric needs have been underestimated. Dyspnea, particularly during acute exacerbations, may limit dietary intake

(Ferguson & Cherniack, 1993). A patient's nutritional status should be assessed and a nutritional plan that meets his or her caloric needs established.

Use of Medications and Inhalers. The use of inhaled medications in patients with chronic lung disease is recognized to be beneficial. The most common mistake in management of such medications is inadequate patient education about the medications and about the techniques for using inhalers. Unfortunately, 25 to 75% of patients using metered-dose inhalers use them incorrectly, and many health care providers do not completely understand their proper use (Interiano & Guntupalli, 1993). Patients should be instructed in the proper technique (Fig. 26–11).

The use of a spacer device with a metered-dose inhaler may decrease deposition of the inhaled medication in the oropharynx and diminish the likelihood of oral candidiasis.

Psychosocial Support

Psychosocial support is an essential component in a comprehensive rehabilitation program. Experts have frequently associated COPD with problems in psychosocial adjustment, specifically anxiety and depression.

HOW TO USE A
METERED-DOSE INHALER

1. Remove the cap and shake the inhaler.
2. Breathe out gently.
3. Put the mouthpiece in the mouth, and at the start of inspiration, which should be slow and deep, press the canister down and continue to inhale deeply.
4. Hold the breath for about 10 seconds.
5. Wait about 30 seconds before taking another inhalation.

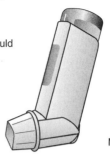

Metered-dose Inhaler

ALWAYS DEMONSTRATE TO THE PATIENT HOW TO USE THE METERED-DOSE INHALER

HOW TO USE A
SPACER DEVICE, e.g., NEBUHALER

Method particularly useful for young children

1. Remove the cap, shake the inhaler, and insert into the device.
2. Place the mouthpiece in the child's mouth (if using the Nebuhaler be careful the child's lips are behind the ring).
3. Seal the child's lips around the mouthpiece by gently placing the fingers of one hand around the lips.
4. Encourage the child to breathe in and out slowly and gently. (This will make a "clicking" sound as the valve opens and closes.) Once the breathing pattern is well established, depress the canister with the free hand and leave the device in the same position as the child continues to breathe (tidal breathing) several more times.
5. Remove the device from the child's mouth.

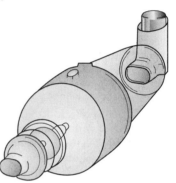

Nebuhaler

ALWAYS DEMONSTRATE TO THE PATIENT HOW TO USE THE NEBUHALER

HOW TO USE AN AUTOHALER

1. Remove the protective mouthpiece by pulling down the lip on back of the cover.
2. Hold the inhaler upright and push the lever up; then shake the inhaler.
3. Breathe out gently. Keep the inhaler upright and put the mouthpiece in the mouth and close the lips around it. (Do not block the air vents at the bottom of the Autohaler.)
4. Breathe in steadily through the mouth. DON'T stop breathing when the inhaler "clicks," and continue taking a really deep breath.
5. Hold the breath for about 10 seconds.
6. While holding Autohaler upright lower the lever. Wait at least 60 seconds before taking another inhalation.

N.B. The lever must be pushed up ("on") before each dose and pushed down again ("off") afterwards. Otherwise it will not operate.

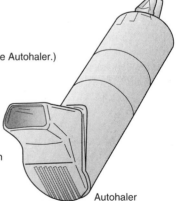

Autohaler

ALWAYS DEMONSTRATE TO THE PATIENT HOW TO USE THE AUTOHALER

Other inhalers are becoming available in addition to those included in this figure. The clinician should demonstrate the use of any device prescribed to the patient, and should have the patient demonstrate back to the clinician.

FIGURE 26–11

How to use inhalers. (Redrawn from National Heart, Lung, and Blood Institute [1995, January]. *Global strategy for asthma management and prevention; NHLBI/WHO workshop report* (Publication No. 95-3659). Bethesda, MD: Author.)

People with COPD frequently have feelings of loss of control of their bodies or their social environment. This response often leaves the person with COPD socially isolated and depressed (Lewis & Bell, 1995). Fortunately, these problems are likely to improve as the patient becomes involved in a pulmonary rehabilitation program. Being able to exercise under the supervision of supportive specialists results in desensitization to dyspnea and fear and regaining of self-control (Celli, 1995).

Dyspnea, the characteristic symptom of respiratory illness, is also a feature of panic attacks. The symptoms of panic attack and pulmonary disease can overlap. Patients with pulmonary disease, particularly with obstructive disease, have a high rate of panic symptoms. Panic may be related to repeated experiences with dyspnea and life-threatening exacerbation of pulmonary dysfunction, hyperventilation, and the stress of coping with chronic disease. Successful treatment of panic in such patients can improve functional status and quality of life by relieving anxiety and dyspnea (Smoller, Pollock, Otto, Rosenbaum, & Kradin, 1996).

Nonpharmacological treatment can be beneficial in controlling panic and anxiety and in reducing stress. The useful properties of relaxation techniques have been well documented. Through relaxation techniques, the patient redirects energy from what cannot be controlled to what can be controlled. Because most relaxation techniques emphasize slow, rhythmical breathing, they may be particularly beneficial for patients with chronic lung disease. Progressive muscle relaxation, visualization, and guided imagery are other relaxation methods often employed to help the patient develop coping strategies, decrease symptoms, and enhance functioning (Jerman & Haggerty, 1993).

Pulmonary Rehabilitation in the Home

Pulmonary rehabilitation as a concept of care applies to the continuum of health care settings: the hospital, the outpatient setting, the community, and the home. *Home health care* of patients with respiratory disease refers to the provision in the home of comprehensive health and support services that help patients achieve and sustain an optimum level of activity, comfort, and independence. These services include (1) nursing, physical, occupational, speech, and respiratory therapies, (2) home health assistance, (3) homemaker ser-

vices, (4) social worker services, (5) medical equipment, (6) transportation, and (7) involvement of nurse practitioners and physicians.

Home care services may be provided as a follow-up to formal inpatient or outpatient pulmonary rehabilitation. Many patients who receive home care are too ill to fit program admission criteria, have declined participation in formal programs, or have no access to such programs. Such patients may benefit from a comprehensive rehabilitative approach to care in the home. The following case study describes a patient who successfully completed rehabilitation in the home setting.

▪ Case 26–1

Mr. Smith is a 72-year-old man with a history of COPD. His past medical history includes repeated admissions for exacerbation of his COPD (emphysema), history of a myocardial infarction, and a 40-year smoking history (quit 8 years ago). He is dyspneic at rest, using accessory muscles of respiration. Recently, he was admitted to a hospital for 5 days of acute care for pneumonia and exacerbation of COPD. He is currently oxygen-dependent. He completed an inpatient pulmonary rehabilitation program 2 years ago. He is very reluctant to go to inpatient rehabilitation again, and would prefer to be home with his wife. He is anxious about leaving her alone. The home program for Mr. Smith will address eight major areas: assessment, medications, bronchial hygiene, physical conditioning, breathing patterns, oxygen use, counseling and support, and case management activities.

Assessment

Assessment for Mr. Smith includes a symptomatic assessment and a cardiopulmonary examination.

Activities of daily living and exercise tolerance, including capability of providing self-care, adequate nourishment, and safety, are assessed. In addition, Mr. Smith's knowledge of medications and their efficacy and of the proper use of inhalers needs to be evaluated.

Mr. Smith's primary concern was his shortness of breath. He was unable to complete activities of daily living without becoming extremely dyspneic. He could ambulate only short distances, requiring many rests. He felt unable to assist his wife in any homemaking activities.

Medications

His understanding of medications and their uses was adequate, but when asked to demonstrate the use of his inhaler, he was unable to correctly administer aerosolized medications. He was given a spacer device and received inhaler instruction until he could adequately perform the correct technique and realize the full benefit of the medication. An updated medication schedule was provided by the nurse and reviewed at each visit. The nurse also arranged for Mr. Smith to receive an influenza vaccine.

Bronchial Hygiene

This is an area that receives considerable attention in home care. Mr. Smith did not require chest physical therapy at this time. Lung sounds revealed markedly diminished breath sounds bilaterally but showed that the lungs were essentially clear. His sputum production was minimal. He was able to cough up small amounts of slightly yellowish sputum. Mr. Smith was instructed in the signs and symptoms of worsening pulmonary infection.

Physical Conditioning

Mr. Smith reported decreased activity tolerance with increased shortness of breath. He had not recovered to his baseline level of function. He felt that the hospital stay "weakened" him. A home program of physical conditioning was designed by the multidisciplinary team. The physical therapist formally evaluated his exercise tolerance and started Mr. Smith on a formal exercise program. He had not been routinely exercising in the last year. His preferred exercise program consisted of a walking program that included warm-up and cool-down exercises. However, the weather was not conducive to walking outdoors. Therefore, until warmer weather returned, he borrowed his son's exercise bike and was given a stationary cycling program that he grew to enjoy. He used the perceived breathlessness scale to gauge his progress. The occupational therapist addressed issues of energy conservation and worked with the patient on bathing and grooming strategies.

Pursed-Lip and Diaphragmatic Breathing

Mr. Smith did not consistently use pursed-lip and diaphragmatic breathing as techniques to control dyspnea. His breathing pattern, particularly during activity, was not always correct. Usually, his breaths were too fast and shallow. With instruction and practice, Mr. Smith was able to incorporate proper breathing techniques and better coordinate breathing with activity, and he reported that it eased his feelings of dyspnea.

Nutritional Support

Mr. Smith reported that he had lost 10 pounds over the last several months. A nutritional evaluation determined that he was 15 pounds underweight. He was instructed to follow a diet low in fat and high in complex carbohydrates. He was initially given liquid dietary supplements, until his caloric intake was sufficient to maintain his weight.

Oxygen Use

Mr. Smith was disappointed that he still required oxygen. This is the first time he had been sent home from the hospital with oxygen. It was overwhelming for him to manage at first, but he soon adjusted to the equipment. His oxygen saturation level was adequate on 1.5 L per minute of oxygen, but Mr. Smith continued to experience desaturation when breathing room air. He was learning how to care for and maintain his equipment.

Case Management Activities

In order for the rehabilitation program to be effective, the care provided needed to be comprehensive and coordinated. Coordination of the home visits was essential because several disciplines were involved in providing direct care. Planned verbal and written communications among the different caregivers occurred frequently.

Mr. Smith was eligible for The Ride, a community transportation service for elders. This enabled him to venture out of the house and not have to depend on his son for all his transportation needs. A homemaker began coming to the house once a week. This relieved Mr. and Mrs. Smith of some of the household chores, which at this point they were unable to accomplish. A home health aide was assigned to Mr. Smith for a short period, until he was better able to manage his bathing and grooming needs. Knowledge of the community resources available to Mr. Smith provided an intensity of support and service that enabled him to function in the home setting.

The Ventilator-Dependent Patient

Patients with chronic respiratory insufficiency may become dependent on a ventilator because of progressive disease or complications of therapy. Ventilator dependence commonly occurs in states of chronic lung disease, kyphoscoliosis, progressive myopathies, and neuropathies.

The usual scenario for ventilator support is acute respiratory failure. A multidisciplinary team is employed to manage the many aspects of care required. Often, major issues confront the nurse in the care of this population of patients. Of great importance in ventilator dependence is malnutrition, particularly during the acute phase. Malnutrition adversely affects respiratory muscle function and lung function itself. This complication has been correlated with development of new infections and ventilator dependence. The presence of a tracheostomy enables the patient to eat.

Profound depression is often evident in ventilator-dependent patients. They often feel trapped, believing that being connected to a ventilator means that they can neither live nor die. External stimuli, friends, and clergy are important during this period, as is contact with the outside world. Activity should be encouraged, with progression from bed to a chair and then to ambulation, as soon as tolerated (Petty, 1993).

Efforts to "wean" a patient from the ventilator continue during the recovery period after respiratory failure. Ventilatory insufficiency that occurs in the setting of progressive or multisystem disease or in primary lung disease that remains active and requires ongoing management is not well suited to long-term use of ventilator. Success in weaning mechanically ventilated patients depends on many variables. If the process of weaning is unsuccessful and long-term ventilation is indicated, movement out of the acute hospital setting to home or another stable environment offers the patient an opportunity to achieve at least some aspects of normal life (Pierson & Kacmarek, 1993).

The key to successful return of a ventilator-dependent patient to his or her home is a well-coordinated discharge plan. The home care team normally consists of the patient, the family, the supplier of the durable medical equipment, home health agencies providing nursing services, physical and occupational therapists, and respiratory therapists.

Patient characteristics that may determine success in home ventilator care have been described as ranging from ideal to unacceptable. *Ideal* candidates are optimistic, motivated, and flexible, with close family and social supports, are educated, and demonstrate an ability to learn. They have adequate personal assets, insurance coverage, stable disease, and significant "free time" off the ventilator. They are able to perform or can direct others in their care.

Patient characteristics that are deemed *unacceptable* for home ventilator care are lack of coping behaviors and lack of social and family supports or financial resources. Patients exhibiting these characteristics are unable to care for themselves or direct others. It is unlikely that home ventilator care will succeed (Pierson & Kacmarek, 1993).

Summary

Pulmonary rehabilitation has evolved over the last several decades. Many studies demonstrate its benefits. As a result, pulmonary rehabilitation has become an essential component in the care of patients with COPD. A comprehensive program that includes patient assessment, patient and family education, exercise, and psychosocial intervention, whether conducted in an inpatient or an outpatient setting, will benefit the patient with COPD. The role of the rehabilitation nurse as part of the multidisciplinary team is essential in helping patients become more knowledgeable about their disease, more actively involved in their own health care, more independent in function, and less dependent on family, health professionals, and expensive medical resources.

REFERENCES

American Association of Cardiovascular and Pulmonary Rehabilitation. (1995). *Guidelines for cardiac rehabilitation programs* (2nd ed.). Champaign, IL: Human Kinetics.

American Heart Association. (1990). *The cholesterol facts: A joint statement by the American Heart Association and the National Heart, Lung, and Blood Institute.* Dallas: Author.

American Heart Association. (1999). *2000 Heart and Stroke Update.* Dallas: Author.

American Heart Association Secondary Prevention Panel (1995). Consensus panel statement: Preventing heart attack and death in patients with coronary disease. *Circulation, 92,* 1–4.

American Lung Association. (1981). American Thoracic Society Official Statement on Pulmonary Rehabilitation. *American Review of Respiratory Disease, 124,* 663–666.

American Thoracic Society. (1996). Official Statement: Cigarette smoking and health. *American Journal of Respiratory Critical Care Medicine, 153,* 861–865.

Arnstein, P. M., Buselli, E., & Renkin, S. (1996). Women and heart attacks: Prevention, diagnosis and care. *Nurse Practitioner, 21*(5), 57–69.

Balady, G., Fletcher, B., Froelicher, E., Hartley, H., Krauss, R., Oberman, A., Pollock, M., & Taylor, C. (1994). Cardiac rehabilitation programs: A statement for healthcare professionals from the American Heart Association. *Circulation, 90*(3), 1602–1610.

Barnes, P. J. (1989). A new approach to the treatment of asthma. *New England Journal of Medicine, 321*(22), 1517–1527.

Brass-Mynderse, N. J. (1996). Disease management of chronic congestive heart failure. *Journal of Cardiovascular Nursing, 11*(1), 54–62.

Casaburi, R. (1993). Exercise training in chronic obstructive lung disease. In R. Casaburi & T. L. Petty (Eds.), *Principles and practice of pulmonary rehabilitation.* Philadelphia: W. B. Saunders.

Case, R. B., Moss, A., Case, N., McDermott, M., & Eberly, S. (1992). Living alone after myocardial infarction. *JAMA, 267,* 515–519.

Celli, B. R. (1995). Pulmonary rehabilitation in patients with COPD. *American Journal of Respiratory and Critical Care Medicine, 152,* 861–864.

Coats, A. J., Adamopoulos, S., Radaelli, A., McCance, A., Myer, T. E., Bernadi, L., Solda, T. L., Davey, P., Omerod, O., & Forfar, C. (1992). Controlled trial of physical training in chronic heart failure: Exercise performance, hemodynamics, ventilation, and autonomic function. *Circulation, 85,* 2119–2131.

Connors, G. and Hilling L. (Eds.). (1993). *Guidelines for pulmonary rehabilitation programs:* American Association of Cardiovascular and Pulmonary Rehabilitation. Champaign, IL: Human Kinetics.

Fair, J., & Berra, K. (1995). Life-style changes and coronary heart disease: The influence of nonpharmacologic intervention. *Journal of Cardiovascular Nursing, 9*(2), 12–24.

Ferguson, G., & Cherniack, R. (1993). Management of chronic obstructive pulmonary disease. *New England Journal of Medicine, 328*(11), 1017–1022.

Fishman, A. (1994). Pulmonary rehabilitation research: NIH workshop summary. *American Journal of Respiratory and Critical Care Medicine, 149,* 825–833.

Fleury, J., Peter, M. A., & Thomas, T. (1996). Health promotion across the continuum: Challenges for the future of cardiovascular nursing. *Journal of Cardiovascular Nursing, 11*(1), 15–26.

Froelicher, E., Berra, K., Stepp, C., Saxe, J., & Deitrich, C. (1995). Risk profile screening. *Journal of Cardiovascular Nursing, 10*(1), 30–50.

Geissler, E. (1994). *Pocket guide to cultural assessment.* St. Louis: Mosby–Year Book.

Gordon, M. (1993). *Manual of nursing diagnosis.* St. Louis: Mosby–Year Book.

Gortner, S., Dirks, J., & Wolfe, M. (1992). The road to recovery for elders after CABG. *American Journal of Nursing, 92*(8), 44–49.

Grossman, D. (1996). Cultural dimensions in home health nursing. *American Journal of Nursing, 96*(7), 33–36.

Gulanick, M. (1991). Is phase 2 cardiac rehabilitation necessary for early recovery of patients with cardiac disease? A randomized, controlled study. *Heart and Lung, 20*(1), 9–15.

Harlan, W., Sandler, S., Lee, K., Lam, L., & Mark, D. (1995). Importance of baseline functional and socioeconomic factors for participation in cardiac rehabilitation. *American Journal of Cardiology, 76,* 36–39.

Hellman, E., & Williams, M. (1994). Outpatient cardiac rehabilitation in elderly patients. *Heart and Lung, 23*(6), 506–512.

Higgins, M. (1993). Epidemiology of obstructive pulmonary disease. In R. Casaburi & T. L. Petty (Eds.), *Principles and practice of pulmonary rehabilitation* (pp. 10–17). Philadelphia: W. B. Saunders.

Interiano, B., & Guntupalli, K. (1993). Metered-dose inhalers: Do health care providers know what to teach? *Archives of Internal Medicine, 153*(1), 81–85.

Jacobs, M. (1994). Maintenance therapy for obstructive lung disease. *Postgraduate Medicine, 95*(8), 87–99.

Jerman, A., & Haggerty, M. (1993). Relaxation and biofeedback: Coping skills training. In R. Casaburi & T. L. Petty (Eds.), *Principles and practice of pulmonary rehabilitation* (pp. 366–374). Philadelphia: W. B. Saunders.

Joint National Committee on Detection, Evaluation and Treatment of High Blood Pressure. (1993). The fifth report of the Joint National Committee on Detection, Evaluation and Treatment of High Blood Pressure. *Archives of Internal Medicine, 153,* 154–183.

Koch, M., Douard, H., & Broustet, J. P. (1992). The benefit of graded physical exercise in chronic heart failure. *Chest, 101*(Suppl. 5), 231S–235S.

Konstam, M., Dracup., K., Baker, D., et al. (1994). *Heart failure: Evaluation and care of patients with left-ventricular dysfunction* (Clinical Practice Guideline No. 11). (AHCPR Publication No. 94-0612). Rockville, MD: Agency for Health Care Policy and Research.

La Forge, R., & Thomas, T. (1996). Outpatient management of lipid disorders. *Journal of Cardiovascular Nursing, 11*(1), 39–53.

Lavie, C., & Milani, R. (1995). Effects of cardiac rehabilitation and exercise training on exercise capacity, coronary risk factors, behavioral characteristics and quality of life in women. *American Journal of Cardiology, 75,* 340–343.

Lavie, C., & Milani, R. (1996). Effects of cardiac rehabilitation and exercise training in obese patients with coronary artery disease. *Chest, 109*(1), 52–56.

Lavie, C., Milani, R., & Littman, A. (1993). The benefits of cardiac rehabilitation and exercise training in secondary coronary prevention in the elderly. *Journal of the American College of Cardiology, 22,* 678–683.

LeDoux, D., & Shinn, J. (1995). Cardiac surgery. In S. L. Woods, E. S. Froelicher, C. J. Halpenny, & S. U. Motzer (Eds.), *Cardiac nursing* (3rd ed., pp. 524–553). Philadelphia: Lippincott–Williams & Wilkins.

Leon, A. S., Certo, C., Comoss, P., et al. (1990). Scientific evidence of the value of cardiac rehabilitation services with emphasis on patients following myocardial infarction: Section 1: Exercise conditioning component [Position Paper]. *Journal of Cardiopulmonary Rehabilitation, 10,* 79–87.

Lewis, D., & Bell, S. (1995). Pulmonary rehabilitation, psychological adjustment and use of healthcare services. *Rehabilitation Nursing, 20*(2), 102–106.

Lindsay, C., Jennrich, J. A., & Biemolt, M. (1991). Programmed instruction booklet for cardiac rehabilitation teaching. *Heart and Lung, 20*(6), 648–653.

Luepker, R. V., Rosamond, W., Murphy, R., Sprafica, J., Folsom, A., McGovern, P., & Blackburn, H. (1993). Socioeconomic status in CHD risk factor trends: The Minnesota Heart Study: Part 1. *Circulation, 93*(88), 2172–2179.

Mandle, C. L., Jacobs, S. C., Arcari, P. M., & Domar, A. D. (1996). The efficacy of relaxation response intervention with adult patients: A review of the literature. *Journal of Cardiovascular Nursing, 10*(3), 4–26.

McCauley, K. (11995). Assessing social support in patients with cardiac disease. *Journal of Cardiovascular Nursing, 10*(1), 73–80.

McCourt, A. E. (Ed.). (1993). *The specialty practice of rehabilitation nursing: A core curriculum* (3rd ed.). Skokie, IL: Rehabilitation Nursing Foundation.

Miller, N. H., Warren, D., & Myers, D. (1996). Home-based cardiac rehabilitation and lifestyle modification:

The MULTIFIT model. *Journal of Cardiovascular Nursing, 11*(1), 76–87.

Moldover, J. R., & Bartels, M. N. (1996). Cardiac rehabilitation. In R. Braddom (Ed.), *Physical medicine and rehabilitation* (pp. 649–670). Philadelphia: W. B. Saunders.

National Cholesterol Education Program (1994). Second Report of the Expert Panel on Detection, Evaluation, and Treatment of High Blood Cholesterol in Adults (Adult Treatment Panel Part I). *Circulation, 89,* 1333–1445.

National Institutes of Health. (1993, November). *Chronic obstructive pulmonary disease.* Bethesda, MD: Author.

National Institutes of Health, National Heart, Lung and Blood Institute. (1995). *Global strategy for asthma management and prevention: NHLBI/WHO workshop.* (Publication No. 95-3659). Bethesda, MD: Author.

Oldridge, N. B., Guyatt, G., Fischer, M., Rimm, A. (1988). Cardiac rehabilitation after myocardial infarction: Combined experience of randomized clinical trials. *JAMA, 260*(7), 945–950.

Osguthorpe, S., & Woods, S. (1995). Myocardial ischemia and infarction. In S. L. Woods, E. S. Froelicher, C. J. Halpenny, & S. U. Motzer (Eds.), *Cardiac nursing* (3rd ed., pp. 461–495). Philadelphia: Lippincott–Williams & Wilkins.

Petty, T. L. (1993). The ventilator-dependent patient. In R. Casaburi & T. L. Petty (Eds.), *Principles and practice of pulmonary rehabilitation* (pp. 468–472). Philadelphia: W. B. Saunders.

Pierson, D., & Kacmarek, R. (1993). Home ventilator care. In R. Casaburi & T. L. Petty (Eds.), *Principles and practice of pulmonary rehabilitation* (pp. 274–282). Philadelphia: W. B. Saunders.

Rich-Edwards, J. W., et al. (1995). The primary prevention of coronary heart disease in women. *New England Journal of Medicine, 332*(26), 1758–66.

Ries, A. L. (1990). Position Paper of the American Association of Cardiovascular and Pulmonary Rehabilitation: Scientific basis of pulmonary rehabilitation. *Journal of Cardiopulmonary Rehabilitation, 10,* 418–441.

Ries, A. L., et al. (1995). Effects of pulmonary rehabilitation on physiologic and psychosocial outcomes in patients with chronic obstructive pulmonary disease. *Annals of Internal Medicine, 122*(11), 823–831.

Ritchie, D. E., & Froelicher, E. S. (1995). Exercise and activity. In S. L. Woods, E. S. Froelicher, C. J. Halpenny, & S. U. Motzer (Eds.), *Cardiac nursing* (3rd ed., pp. 708–724). Philadelphia: Lippincott–Williams & Wilkins.

Rossouw, J. E., Lewis, B., Rifkind, B. M. (1990). The value of lowering cholesterol after myocardial infarction. *New England Journal of Medicine, 323*(16), 1112–1119.

Scandinavian Simvastatin Survival Study Group. (1994). Randomised trial of cholesterol lowering in 4444 patients with coronary heart disease: The Scandinavian Simvastatin Survival Study. *Lancet, 344,* 1383–1389.

Smoller, J. W., Pollock, M., Otto, M., Rosenbaum, J., & Kradin, R. (1996). Panic anxiety, dyspnea, and respiratory disease: Theoretical and clinical considerations. *American Journal of Respiratory and Critical Care Medicine, 154,* 6–17.

Sparks, K., Shaw, D., Eddy, D., Hanigosky, P., & Vantrese, J. (1993). Alternatives for cardiac rehabilitation patients unable to return to a hospital-based program. *Heart and Lung, 22*(4), 298–303.

St. Jeor, S. T., Brownell, K., & Atkinson, R. (1993). AHA prevention conference III: Obesity. *Circulation, 88,* 1392–1398.

Strijbos, J. H., Postma, D., Van Altena, R., Gimeno, F., & Koeter, G. (1996). A comparison between an outpatient hospital-based pulmonary rehabilitation program and a home-care pulmonary rehabilitation program in patients with COPD: A follow-up of 18 months. *Chest, 109*(2), 366–372.

Venner, G. H., & Seelbinder, J. S. (1996). Team management of congestive heart failure across the continuum. *Journal of Cardiovascular Nursing, 10*(2), 71–84.

Waldo, M. J., Ide, B., & Thomas, D. (1995). Postcardiac-event elderly: Effect of exercise on cardiopulmonary function. *Journal of Gerontological Nursing,* February, 12–19.

Wasserman, K. (1993). In R. Casaburi and T. L. Petty (Eds.), *Principles and practice of pulmonary rehabilitation* (pp. 115–122). Philadelphia: W. B. Saunders.

Wenger, N. K., Froelicher, E. S., Smith L. K., et al. (1995). *Cardiac rehabilitation* (Clinical Practice Guideline No. 17). (AHCPR Publication No. 96-0672). Rockville, MD: Agency for Health Care Policy and Research & the National Heart, Lung, and Blood Institute.

Zierler, B. K., & Cowan, M. J. (1995). Pathogenesis of atherosclerosis. In S. L. Woods, E. S. Froelicher, C. J. Halpenny, & S. Motzer (Eds.), *Cardiac nursing* (3rd ed., pp. 187–199). Philadelphia: Lippincott–Williams & Wilkins.

Zimmerman, E., & Horton-La Forge, B. (1996). Detection and prevention of cardiac risk factors: Health risk assessment and targeted follow-up in a managed care population. *Journal of Cardiovascular Nursing, 11*(1), 27–38.

INTERNET CITATIONS

Treating Tobacco Use and Dependence. Summary, June 2000. U.S. Public Health Service. http://www.surgeongeneral.gov/tobacco/smokesum.htm.

You can quit smoking. *Consumer Guide,* June 2000. U.S. Public Health Service. http://www.surgeongeneral.gov/tobacco/consquits.htm.

CHAPTER 27

A Holistic Approach to Burn Rehabilitation

Patricia S. Regojo and Corinne Wright

After World War II, the need for burn nursing grew in response to the popularity of caring for burn patients in a specialty unit. Since then, burn nursing has evolved into a highly specialized profession. In 1982, the American Burn Association developed *Guidelines for Burn Nursing Practice* addressing patient care, research, and prevention (American Burn Association, 1982; Marvin, 1993). In 1989, the Nurse Advisory Council of the Burn Foundation of Philadelphia published the *Standards of Burn Nursing Practice* based on the nursing process in conjunction with education, research, prevention, consultation, administration, infection control, and ethical legal standards. Nursing practice includes the care and treatment necessary to provide comfort; prevent, detect, and treat illness; promote restoration to the highest possible productive capacities; assist individuals in the promotion and maintenance of health; and, when necessary, assist with a dignified death. Burn nursing practice takes into account the interrelatedness of physiological, psychological, and social components of the patient's response or adjustment to the burn injury (American Burn Association, 1982).

Although much has been written regarding the needs of the burn patient during the rehabilitative phase of care, little addresses nursing practice related to the burn patient in a rehabilitative setting. Serious burn injury is a life-threatening stress reaction that requires heroic medical efforts on the part of a variety of medical experts to restore function. Although rehabilitation begins on the first day of injury, interventions in the acute phase relate to survival. Rehabilitation, on the other hand, aims to restore optimal wellness.

The rehabilitation process incorporates ongoing reciprocal learning among and between members of the team, the family, and the patient. Comprehensive rehabilitation of the burn patient encompasses the same team effort as acute care does, although the focus changes from survival to restoration of a purposeful life within the limitation of injury. The team must recognize that what has happened to the patients affects, and will continue to affect, many aspects of their lives extending beyond the body's function. The primary goals of the rehabilitation phase of burn care promote the restoration of function and mobility while maintaining an achieved optimal health (Trofino, 1991).

Rehabilitation nurses have a complex role coordinating numerous facets of the patient's care. While planning daily activity, the nurse anticipates the difficulties the patient will have once he or she leaves the rehabilitation setting, such as returning to work, managing transportation, and conducting daily life at home. A nurse in the rehabilitation unit assumes many roles; the well-organized nurse is flexible and understanding, knowing that the patient must endure long hours of rigorous and painful therapy daily. As a caregiver, the rehabilitation nurse delivers the prescribed treatment modalities and nursing interventions. As an educator, the nurse assesses the patient's readiness to learn and ability to understand the complexities of the injury and recovery. The nurse interprets to the patient what is happening during the course of treatment in a way conducive to the patient's level of understanding. While in a rehabilitation setting, the patient must be prepared to face many life adjustments in a relatively short period of time. Using a systems approach to assess multifaceted needs, the rehabilitation nurse addresses the needs of the burn-injured patient either directly or in collaboration with the patient, the patient's family, and/or other health care professionals.

Using a systems view, Neuman (1989) describes wellness and illness as a continuum. The burn injury acts as a stressor on the client system, which penetrates both the flexible and normal lines of defense of the client system. Disruption of the system creates an energy demand in proportion to the burn injury. The goal of emergent care is to restore the system to equilibrium. Rehabilitation aims at restoring the injured patient to optimal wellness. For the patient to find meaning, value, and a sense of purpose in postinjury life, realistic goals must be set. Rehabilitation nurses, knowledgeable about specific burn care concepts, deliver quality care to their patients. Burn care concepts include knowledge of the burn process, wound care, mobility, function, and care of healed skin. Yet the implications for full recovery extend beyond the physical. The psychological, sociocultural, developmental, and spiritual aspects of a person factor into full recovery or wellness.

The physiological aspects related to the rehabilitation of a burn injury are extensive. Table 27–1 details several physiological concepts related to burn nursing care in the rehabilitation setting.

BURN PROCESS

Although most of the burn repair is complete before the patient enters the rehabilitation facility, there may be a time when further skin grafting or contracture release takes place. Nurses need to be familiar with operative procedures and related care.

According to the American Burn Associa-

TABLE 27–1 ■ PHYSIOLOGICAL CONCEPTS FOR BURN REHABILITATION NURSING CARE

Burn process	Type of burn injury: thermal, electrical, chemical; depth and extent of burn; pathophysiology; pain; related trauma; nutritional status
Wound healing	Wound excision and skin grafting; donor sites; reconstructive surgery
Mobility and function	Range of motion; positioning; mobility and ambulation/gait training; functional capacity
Scarring	Wound contracture; hypertrophic scars and keloids; scar bands
Early complications	Edema; graft loss, cellulitis; deep vein thrombosis, pulmonary embolus
Ongoing complications	Neuromuscular problems; peripheral neuropathy; pruritus; sensory impairment, fragile skin; heterotopic ossification; spontaneous contracture release; reflex sympathetic dystrophy

tion 1990 statistics, over 70,000 persons require hospitalization each year for burn injuries. Seventy percent of the 2 million burns per year are the result of thermal injury (Moy, 1996). Thermal injuries may result from exposure to flame, steam, hot liquids, hot tar, or hot metals or from frostbite. The severity is directly related to the duration and intensity of the exposure. One of the most costly burn injuries is the flame burn resulting from falling asleep while smoking after consuming alcohol (Pruitt & Mason, 1996). Scald burns are prominent in children younger than 5 years, adults older than 65 years, and disabled persons. Burn injuries rank second to motor vehicle accidents as a cause of death in childhood. High morbidity and mortality in elderly persons can be attributed to preexisting problems such as impaired judgment, decreased coordination, or decreased sensation (Moy, 1996).

A contact burn results from contact of a heated substance with the skin. Examples of contact burns include tar burns, burns incurred by children touching a hot stove, and burns from molten metal.

Although electrical burns represent only 6% of all burn injuries (Winkler, DiMola, & Wooten, 1993), they are the most destructive of all burns. Although the trauma to the skin surface can be small, the internal damage can be catastrophic. Electrical burns result from contact with an electrical source. The severity of the injury is directly related to the voltage, type of current, duration of contact, and pathway of the current. Electrical burns typically have small entrance wounds and large exit wounds. Children playing around live wires or electrical outlets, teenagers playing near high-voltage lines, and electrical workers are examples of those who are prone to electrical injury (Haberal, 1986).

Chemical burns result from exposure to strong acids or alkalis. They are commonly seen in toddlers who drink or spill household chemicals or in adults who work with strong industrial agents. Chemical burns are also seen in assault victims. The heat of the chemical reaction causes the initial tissue damage. Subsequent changes result from the chemicals' reacting with skin proteins. Chemical agents continue to cause tissue damage until removed or diluted with water (Moy, 1996). The severity of injury in a chemical burn is directly related to the concentration of the chemical, duration of the exposure, amount, and initial emergency care.

Inhalation injury can occur with or without

surface burns. About 6% of patients admitted to burn centers do not survive because of severe inhalation injuries (Brigham & McLaughlin, 1996).

The depth and extent of the burn injury are important determinants of the course of rehabilitation. The skin is the largest organ of the body and is responsible for various functions. The skin is the first defense against infection and maintains thermoregulation and fluid and electrolyte balance. The skin is closely associated with the identity of the individual and contains important sensory components. Figure 27–1 shows normal histological structures and the corresponding depth of burn injury. The first thin layer of the skin, which is actually composed of six to seven microscopic layers, is the epidermis. Burns involving this layer are relatively minor. The second layer, or dermis, contains hair follicles; nerve endings; sebaceous glands; sweat glands; and the sensory fibers for pain, touch, pressure, and temperature. The dermal layer is thicker than the epidermis, so burns involving this layer can damage either all or some of its structures. The third layer of skin,

composed of connective and adipose tissue, is called the subcutaneous layer. Loss of skin represents loss of function at the corresponding burn depth.

The depth of injury is one of several factors that determine the severity of burn injury. A first-degree injury, or superficial burn, involves the epidermis and is a minor injury that leaves the underlying tissue red and painful. The first-degree injury is not calculated when estimating the total body surface area (TBSA) of a burn injury.

Second-degree, or partial-thickness, burns involve the dermal layer. Often moist and blistered, mottled pink and white, these burns are extremely painful because of the exposed nerve endings. Superficial partial-thickness burns involve fewer dermal appendages. Deep partial-thickness burns can involve dermal appendages as well as areas of subcutaneous tissue. Patients with partial-thickness burns experience rapid heat loss and fluid loss. Deep partial-thickness injuries can take up to a month to heal provided no infection complicates the healing process. Deep partial-thickness burns require grafting to promote faster healing and wound closure. Patients in the rehabilitation setting may need grafting or regrafting procedures even though most of their acute burn care is complete.

Third-degree, or full-thickness, burns occur when all the skin layers are destroyed. Because of the destruction of nerve endings, little pain is experienced. To facilitate healing, full-thickness burns also require skin grafting (Bayley, 1990).

Deep injuries that involve muscle and bone destruction are sometimes referred to as fourth-degree burns. Electrical injuries often result in fourth-degree injury.

The extent of injury is directly related to the severity of injury. The extent of injury is calculated according to the percentage of the patient's body surface, excluding the superficial burns, involved in the injury. The Lund and Browder (1944) method, shown in Figure 27–2, divides the body into specific sections and correlates the body's proportions with the age of the patient. The Rule of Nines, another method, used for its simplicity, divides the body into 11 segments of 9%, with 1% reserved for the perineum (Miller, Richard, & Staley, 1994). Nurses in the rehabilitation setting should be aware of the extent of the original burn injury as well as the wounds that are still open.

Additional factors contribute to determining the severity of injury. The American Burn

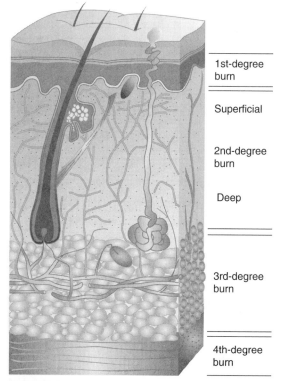

1st-degree burn

Superficial

2nd-degree burn

Deep

3rd-degree burn

4th-degree burn

FIGURE 27–1
Normal skin histological characteristics with the depths of burn injuries indicated.

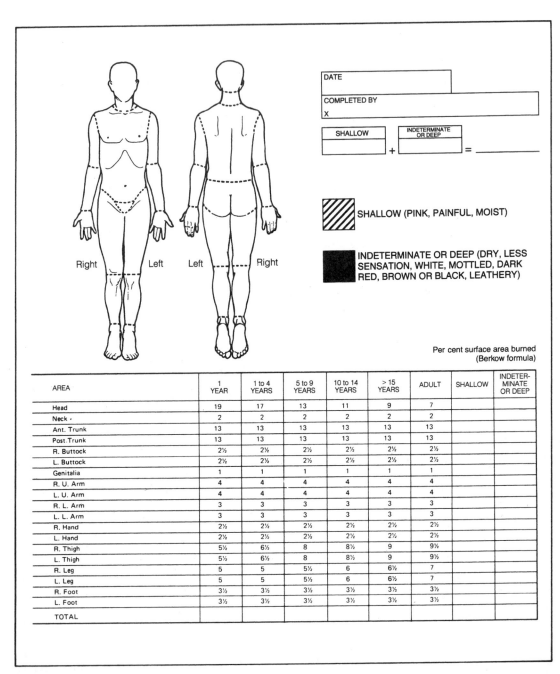

	DATE	
	COMPLETED BY	
	X	

SHALLOW		INDETERMINATE OR DEEP	
	+		= _____

⬛ SHALLOW (PINK, PAINFUL, MOIST)

⬛ INDETERMINATE OR DEEP (DRY, LESS SENSATION, WHITE, MOTTLED, DARK RED, BROWN OR BLACK, LEATHERY)

Right Left Left Right

Per cent surface area burned
(Berkow formula)

AREA	1 YEAR	1 to 4 YEARS	5 to 9 YEARS	10 to 14 YEARS	>15 YEARS	ADULT	SHALLOW	INDETER-MINATE OR DEEP
Head	19	17	13	11	9	7		
Neck ·	2	2	2	2	2	2		
Ant. Trunk	13	13	13	13	13	13		
Post.Trunk	13	13	13	13	13	13		
R. Buttock	2½	2½	2½	2½	2½	2½		
L. Buttock	2½	2½	2½	2½	2½	2½		
Genitalia	1	1	1	1	1	1		
R. U. Arm	4	4	4	4	4	4		
L. U. Arm	4	4	4	4	4	4		
R. L. Arm	3	3	3	3	3	3		
L. L. Arm	3	3	3	3	3	3		
R. Hand	2½	2½	2½	2½	2½	2½		
L. Hand	2½	2½	2½	2½	2½	2½		
R. Thigh	5½	6½	8	8½	9	9½		
L. Thigh	5½	6½	8	8½	9	9½		
R. Leg	5	5	5½	6	6½	7		
L. Leg	5	5	5½	6	6½	7		
R. Foot	3½	3½	3½	3½	3½	3½		
L. Foot	3½	3½	3½	3½	3½	3½		
TOTAL								

FIGURE 27–2
Lund and Browder method of determining skin surface area; the method corrects for differences in the percentage of body surface by age. (From Black, J., & Matassarin-Jacobs, E. [1997]. *Medical-surgical nursing: clinical management for continuity of care* [5th ed, p. 2240]. Philadelphia: W. B. Saunders.)

Association (1990) Classification of Burn Severity (Table 27–2) categorizes the severity of the burn as a mild, moderate, or major injury according to its depth and the percentage of body surface involved, the location and type of the burn, and the age of the patient. Inhalation injuries and burns of the eyes, ears, face, feet, or perineum require hospitalization in a burn treatment center because of the special consideration of wound care, skin grafting, and maintenance of function.

PATHOPHYSIOLOGY OF BURN INJURIES

The body's initial response to burn injury is capillary vasoconstriction. Soon after, vasodilation occurs. Capillary walls become permeable and plasma leaks into the injured site. Within 24 hours, clotting may occur, which decreases or eliminates blood flow, causing further cell death. Because of the ongoing cellular changes, the exact determination of

TABLE 27–2 ■ **AMERICAN BURN ASSOCIATION CLASSIFICATION OF BURN SEVERITY**

Minor burn	15% TBSA partial-thickness burn in an adult
	10% TBSA partial-thickness burn in a child
	2% TBSA full-thickness burn in a child or an adult not involving eyes, ears, face or genitalia
Moderate burn	15–20% TBSA partial-thickness burn in an adult
	10–20% TBSA partial-thickness burn in a child
	2–10% TBSA full-thickness burn in a child or adult not involving eyes, ears, face, or genitalia
Major burn	25% TBSA partial-thickness burn in an adult
	20% TBSA partial-thickness burn in a child
	All full-thickness burns greater than 10% TBSA
	All burns involving hands, face, ears, feet, or genitalia
	All inhalation injuries
	All electrical injuries
	Burn injuries complicated by fractures or other major trauma
	All poor-risk individuals: e.g., preexisting CVA, psychiatric disability, pulmonary or cardiovascular disease, cancer, diabetes

From American Burn Association. (1990). Hospital and prehospital resources for optimal care of patients with burn injury: Guidelines for development and operation of burn centers. *Journal of Burn Care and Rehabilitation, 11,* 98–104.

CVA, cerebrovascular accident; TBSA, total body surface area.

the depth of the burn may not be able to be made until 2 to 3 days after injury. During this time, there is massive fluid loss and elevated metabolism. The integrity of the skin is compromised by the injury, leaving the area prone to infection. If the wound infection is not treated, further tissue destruction occurs. Systemic effects related to major burn injury include hypovolemia, hyperventilation, a marked increase in oxygen consumption, and enormous caloric expenditure. Fluid escaping into the surrounding tissues causing massive edema can progress to the point of interfering with range of motion and circulation. Massive edema associated with serious burn injury can produce compartment syndrome, which results in neurovascular compromise. Compartment syndrome can be avoided by an escharotomy. This procedure, incision through the burned tissue at specific areas, relieves pressure.

Inhalation of soot or noxious gases often leads to pneumonia. In addition, skin destruction that occurs in deep partial- and full-thickness burns causes massive fluid and heat loss through evaporation. Wound sepsis can lead to life-threatening septic shock. Each of these systemic effects can be life-threatening. Patients who survive and progress to rehabilitation are subject to setbacks related to these systemic changes.

PAIN: ASSESSMENT AND MANAGEMENT

Burn patients experience pain in a variety of ways throughout hospitalization and rehabilitation. Some pain can be lifelong. In partial-thickness burns, sensory fibers are damaged but not destroyed; therefore, patients suffering partial-thickness burns experience severe pain. In a full-thickness injury, the sensory nerve endings are destroyed and there is little pain associated with the initial injury. Most persons have injuries that are a combination of partial- and full-thickness burn injury and experience pain (Cromes & Helm, 1993).

Pain assessment scales such as the Visual Analog Scale (Fig. 27–3) or a numerical pain-rating scale (Fig. 27–4) are useful tools to help the patient identify the intensity and management of the pain.

The Visual Analog Scale is used to assess pain intensity. Patients are asked to put an X along the line that best approximates their pain intensity. At one end is "No pain" and at the other end is "Pain is as bad as it could

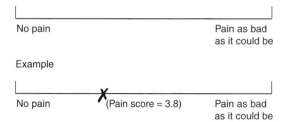

FIGURE 27–3
The Visual Analog Scale. (From Agency for Health Care Policy and Research, Public Health Service, U.S. Department of Health and Human Services. [1992]. *Acute Pain Management: Operative or Medical Procedures and Trauma—Clinical Practice Guideline* [AHCPR Publication No 9200032]. Rockville, MD: Author.)

be." The line is 10 cm long, so the score can be measured as a number from zero to 10.

The Faces Scale is used for children or those who cannot verbalize their feelings. A group of faces ranging from sad and crying to smiling and happy is shown to the patients, who pick out the faces that reflect how they are feeling at the time.

The numerical pain-rating scales require patients to rate their pain using either a 101-point scale or an 11-point scale. They are directed to rate their pain by selecting a number, either from zero to 100 or from zero to 10. Zero represents "no pain," and 100 or 10 represents the "the worst pain ever." Jensen, Karoloy, & Braver (1986) report that numerical rating scales are valid measures of pain intensity and demonstrate sensitivity to treatments aimed at alleviating pain. The Visual Analog Scale may lead to inaccurate measures if the patient has not been given sufficient instruction.

Analgesia is tailored to meet the specific needs of the patient. Many practitioners fear that the patient will acquire a dependency on narcotics. Most patients do not have or acquire a dependency on narcotics unless they have a substance abuse problem before admission. It is not uncommon for patients to build a tolerance to medication after long-term use. Much of the pain a burn patient experiences is a short-lived acute physical pain. The acute pain must be treated. Once the wound is covered with new skin and the donor sites are healed, the pain begins to diminish.

The intensity and type of pain change over time, however. Watkins, Cook, May, & Ehleben (1988) report that burn patients experience several types of pain. During the rehabilitation period, pain is induced through various activities such as stretching and strengthening exercises, range-of-motion exercises, and positioning techniques. Other sources of pain include fatigue, heterotopic ossifications, scar formation, contractures, dressing changes, peripheral neuropathies, and existing medical conditions such as joint disease. Careful pain assessments help the nurse identify patient problems and clarify the type of pain the patient is experiencing.

Procedural pain such as that experienced with a dressing change or range-of-motion exercises must be differentiated from other types of pain. Specific pain medication or sedation can be administered more appropriately when the sources of pain are clarified. Long-acting oral analgesia or patches are popular for treating background pain, whereas short-acting analgesia can be administered before a painful procedure.

Psychological counseling can help reduce pain intensity and provide the patient with coping measures via relaxation techniques. The astute practitioner can identify what the patient is experiencing. Discussions with other team members help identify pain pat-

101 Numeric rating scale

Please indicate on the line below the number between 0 and 100 that best describes your pain. A zero (0) would mean "no pain," and a 100 would mean "as bad as it could be." Please write only one response.

An 11-Point box scale

Zero (0) means "no pain" and 10 means "the worst pain ever." On the 0 to 10 scale below, put an "X" through the number that best pinpoints your level of pain.

0　1　2　3　4　5　6　7　8　9　10

FIGURE 27–4
Numerical pain rating scale.

terns and coping mechanisms. Listening to the patient and working with all members of the rehabilitation team lead to the most effective pain management course for the patient.

The severity of injury is directly related to the depth and extent of the burn itself. In addition to these factors, the patient's past medical history, age, and accompanying trauma also determine the severity of injury. The stress of a burn injury on a person's body can lead to many complications. A major burn injury exacerbates chronic or existing illnesses. Pregnant patients often miscarry. Mortality is highest in burn patients younger than 5 years and older than 65 years. Motor vehicle accidents, explosions, jumps, and falls can result in fractures and multiple trauma for the burn patient. Neurological and musculoskeletal problems often accompany electrical injuries and complicate the recovery and rehabilitation.

Burn injury is a complex injury affecting every system of the body. The rehabilitation team needs to be aware of the many facets of the burn process. Coordinating nursing care with that of other members of the health care team enables the patient to obtain a functional and purposeful life.

NUTRITION

Proper nutrition is essential throughout the rehabilitation process. Good nutrition is essential for wound healing. In the acute phase of care, the dietitian predicts the nutritional requirements based on certain formulas such as the Harris-Benedict formula, the Curreri formula, or indirect calorimetry. Nutritional formulas enable the dietitian to customize the patient's caloric requirements based on height, weight, age, body surface area, and severity of injury (Rodriquez, 1996).

Profound weight loss, a decrease in muscle mass, and weakness in the rehabilitation phase are indications of the hypermetabolic and catabolic states in the acute phase of care (Gottscheich, 1998). A patient suffering from poor nutrition can be identified by monitoring a number of factors including those listed by Flanigan (1997) in Table 27–3.

Although much has been published related to the nutritional needs of patients in the acute phase, little has been published related to the nutritional needs of patients in the restorative phase. It is common practice to supplement the diet with additional protein to promote weight gain and improve muscle strength. As the stress response diminishes, the body's metabolism shifts back to the anabolic state in which proteins are restored at a faster rate than they are being broken down (Demling, 1998). Rehabilitation nurses need to understand that nutrition is an important aspect of healing. Accurate assessment of nutritional status includes monitoring a patient's weight changes, albumin and transferrin levels, total lymphocyte counts, and total calorie intake.

Supplemental feedings via oral or enteral routes are common in the burn population because of the high number of calories required to meet the metabolic needs of the patient. In the rehabilitation setting, the enteral feeds can be given at night so that the patient is able to participate in therapeutic activities during the day. Vitamins and minerals that have specific roles in wound healing include vitamins A, C, and B-complex; zinc; and iron. The protein requirement of 0.8 g/kg of body weight can shift to as high as 2 g of protein per kilogram of body weight for severely stressed patients. Energy from dietary carbohydrates and fats provides fuel for cellular metabolism, meets increased metabolic demands, and prevents protein depletion (Flanigan, 1997).

Wound breakdown, reflected in increased blistering, shearing, or deterioration of the wound, could indicate inadequate nutrition. It is our experience that many patients with burn injuries, especially those with drug- or

TABLE 27–3 ■ INDEXES OF NUTRITIONAL DEPLETION

Index	Mild	Moderate	Severe
Percentage of ideal body weight	80–90	70–80	<70
Percentage of weight loss	5–15	15–25	>25
Albumin (g/dL)	2.8–3.5	2.1–2.7	<2.1
Transferrin (mg/dL)	151–200	100–150	<100
Total lymphocyte count (mm³)	1200–2000	800–1199	<800

From Flanigan, K. H. (1997). Nutritional aspects of wound healing. *Advances in Wound Care, 10,* 48–52.

alcohol-abuse problems, were malnourished before the burn injury. Their entire rehabilitation period can be spent "catching up" on nutritional needs, causing a delay in the healing process.

As burn wound healing proceeds, metabolic demands decrease. Weight gain indicates the shift in dietary demand; however, a well-balanced diet (with fewer calories because of slower metabolism) remains an important part of the rehabilitation phase. As a patient gains weight, custom pressure garments may require refitting to avoid excessive pressure during wear and shear forces with application.

Constipation is another common enteric complication related to inactivity, stress, and pain medication. In most cases, dietary supplements of fruit and vegetable fiber and stool softeners help reduce constipation.

WOUND HEALING

Burn care is divided into three phases: emergent, acute, and rehabilitation. The emergent phase involves providing the patient with lifesaving measures and multisystem stabilization. The acute phase encompasses wound cleaning, wound closure, and infection control. The rehabilitation phase focuses on restoration and function.

It is not unusual for the patient in the rehabilitation or home care setting to have small open wounds that require daily care. The wounds need the attentiveness of those who understand wound healing. Most patients go to a hydrotherapy department for their wound care. Hydrotherapy encompasses the many methods of washing the burn wound or entire patient (Saffle & Schenebly, 1994).

In the rehabilitation phase, a medically stable, ambulatory patient with healing wounds is encouraged to participate in wound care. Strategies may include having the patient use a small tub or shower. Those with smaller wounds or hand wounds can use a basin or sink. Many patients benefit from removing their own dressings and washing their own wounds. Education of the patient is key to the success of these strategies. Patients who remove their own dressings tend to be more careful and take more time than a practitioner would. The supervising therapist can use this time to educate the patient and to examine and record the patient's range of motion and wound healing. Figure 27–5 shows the therapist educating the patient while changing a dressing. Nurses should be familiar with the status of the patient's wounds and the dressings that are used, even though they may never see the wounds without a dressing. Occasionally, the prescribed dressing change is more than once a day. In this case, the nurse must be able to schedule the patient in a manner that enables the patient to receive other necessary therapy and rest. In the rehabilitation phase, it is also possible to overtreat with hydrotherapy. Although overall cleanliness is a goal, the healing wounds need a

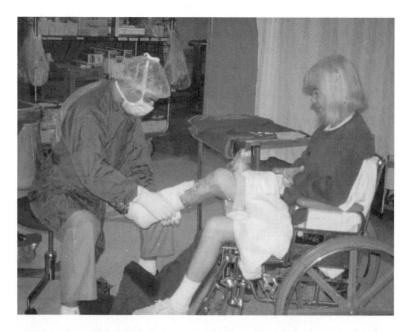

FIGURE 27–5
Involving a patient in wound care.

moist, physiological environment to heal. Daily treatment with bactericidal chemicals can damage the fragile epithelial cells and granulation tissue. This is especially true after surgery. After skin grafting or other surgical procedures, the area should be protected and kept moist with petroleum jelly–impregnated gauze. Cleansing should be done in a sterile field with sterile saline. To eliminate the growth of resistant organisms, antimicrobial topical agents are applied only when there are signs of infection.

Advances in wound care have led to many changes in burn treatment. Early excision and skin grafting allow the physician to débride a wound and cover it with skin long before healing of superficial wounds takes place. By the time patients are ready for rehabilitation, most of their wounds should be covered with new skin; however, some patients require re-grafting because of loss of their original graft. Graft loss can result from infection, shear forces, or inadequate débridement of the burned tissue.

The rehabilitation nurse should not only be familiar with wound care but also be acquainted with skin-grafting procedures and donor site care. On occasion, patients need skin grafting during the rehabilitation phase for contracture release or to cover slow-to-heal areas. Some patients must wait for donor sites to heal before the site can be used again. For whatever reason, the surgical preparation of the patient is vitally important to promote a healthier recovery. Points to emphasize in the preoperative teaching include the explanation of a skin graft, mapping out the donor site, pain management, and donor site and graft care. Although many patients have had multiple surgical procedures, the nurse must treat each surgical episode as the patient's first. Return explanation or mirrored discussion informs the nurse of the patient's understanding of the procedure.

It is important to note the type of skin grafting performed. Burn wounds are generally covered with the patient's own skin, but today new dermal replacements enable surgeons to excise a thinner donor site, thus promoting faster healing with less scarring. The rehabilitation nurse is expected to understand the patient's operative procedure so that postoperative care is risk free and rehabilitation can continue without delay.

The donor site takes from 10 to 14 days to heal. The donor site exudes fluid and must be kept dry to heal. The wound covering chosen by the surgeon has the purpose of preventing infection, promoting healing, and protecting the donor site. Once the covering is removed, the site must be clean, moist, and pliable. Emollients used on the healed donor site reduce pruritus, which may be a problem with both skin grafts and donor sites.

PULMONARY CARE

The surgical procedures for skin grafting usually take place under general anesthesia. Good postoperative pulmonary care promotes adequate ventilation and less risk for complications such as atelectasis or pneumonia. If patients have had an inhalation injury, postoperative recovery could be lengthier. Coughing, deep breathing exercises, and incentive spirometry should be taught to the patient before surgery. Again, return demonstrations are necessary for the nurse to evaluate the patient's level of understanding. Marking preoperative incentive spirometry volumes enables patients to visualize their goal after surgery.

Patients may have restrictive ventilatory problems related to inhalation injuries. Proper postoperative positioning enhances ventilation and respiration. Some patients may also require low-flow oxygen. Unless contraindicated by the location of the graft site, ambulation should begin once the patient is medically stable.

READINESS FOR REHABILITATION

The patient with a burn injury is judged ready for rehabilitation when most of the wounds are either skin-grafted or healing with new skin coverage and when the patient is able to tolerate therapy away from the bedside. Burn patients need extensive rehabilitation for mobility, gait training, activities of daily living, muscle strengthening, scar management, and skin care. Sometimes it can be difficult to get a burn patient into an acute rehabilitation setting. Managed care plays an important role in financing care. Under managed care, a patient must meet certain criteria for an acute rehabilitation stay. A patient who is unable to tolerate a full program is referred to a subacute unit until ready for the extensive rehabilitation program. Patients and their families need to understand these concepts. Case managers help the patient make this transition from one level of care to another.

Not all rehabilitation is done in an inpatient setting. Many patients are able to return home with physical therapy, occupational therapy, and wound care scheduled on an outpatient basis. Careful planning by the burn team includes scheduling appointments with each of the therapies so that the patient receives efficient, appropriate care. When the patient lives a great distance from the burn center, arrangements can be made for outpatient rehabilitation at a center closer to the patient's home. Communication between the burn team and the therapists at the rehabilitation center is important for achieving positive patient outcomes and avoiding complications.

MOBILITY AND FUNCTION

The patient's range of motion is assessed grossly on admission to the burn center to determine the baseline range of motion for all major joints including those that were involved in the burn injury. During the rehabilitation phase, passive range-of-motion exercises can be important in stretching scar bands or as a precursor to splint application. A therapist can perform passive range-of-motion exercises manually or use various types of continuous passive motion devices. Passive range-of-motion exercise is thought to lubricate the joint being moved passively. Patients can warm up with passive range-of-motion exercises, then assist with motion (concentric, active assisted) or resist the direction of pas-

sive motion (eccentric). If the burn crosses joint surfaces, intervention by a therapist and careful attention to positioning is essential to prevent contractures. Figure 27–6 illustrates suggested positioning for all involved joint surfaces to prevent burn contractures.

Early ambulation is a goal for all burn patients relative to the stage, extent of injury, and previous level of patient function. The initial assessment includes the level of function at the time of injury, which helps to set the long-term goals related to the extent of the injury. Ambulation begins in the acute phase of burn care once the patient is hemodynamically stable. A patient who has been on prolonged bed rest due to hemodynamic instabilities is at risk for clot formation. Ambulation must progress gradually from bed mobility, to getting out of bed, to full ambulation. Preexisting or coincident complications such as exposed tendons in the feet, knee, or ankle; cellulitis; orthopedic injuries; neuropathies; strength deficits; or vascular problems can delay or change the goal for ambulation. Mobility and optimal function require the cooperation of all members of the team: the patient, nurses, family, therapists, and physicians. Early ambulation helps to prevent thrombophlebitis and pneumonia; prevent lower extremity contractures; maintain skeletal mass, strength, and endurance; and prevent the decline of mental status (Byl, Cameron, Kloth, & Zellenbach, 1995).

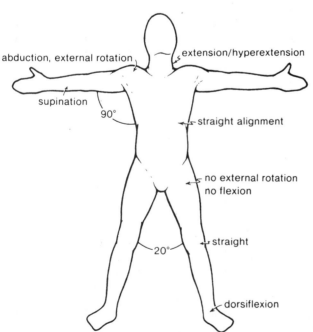

FIGURE 27–6

Suggested positioning guidelines for the prevention of burn contractures. (From Helm, P. A., Kevorkian, C. G., Lushbaugh, M., Pullium, G., Head, M. D., & Cromes, G. F. [1982]. Burn injury: Rehabilitation management in 1982. *Archives of Physical Medicine and Rehabilitation, 63,* 8.)

Progressive mobility is important to healing because it helps reduce edema and venous stasis. Progressive mobility toward ambulation starts with bedside ankle pumps, isometric exercise for the gluteus and quadriceps muscles, and active range-of-motion exercises for the joints of the lower extremities. The timing for beginning of out-of-bed activity must be taken into consideration against the consequences of bed rest. Vital signs of burn patients should be monitored during exercise. Pain should be assessed critically by the therapist and other members of the team (Nothdurft, Smith, & LeMaster, 1984). During ambulation, pain can be related to the generalized pain of the burn injury, edema, burn wound, or venous stasis. Some pain can also be due to thrombophlebitis.

Patients with lower extremity burns, or who are elderly or have compromised circulation, need to have elastic supports applied before ambulation activities. Figure-of-eight wrapping from the base of the foot to the groin including the heel is most effective (Fig. 27–7).

GAIT TRAINING

Gait training is an important part of the rehabilitation of burn patients and requires the specialized skill of a physical therapist as well as the support of all members of the rehabilitation team. Deviations related to pain and the wound itself tend to correct themselves through the course of rehabilitation. Assistive devices should be used only when the patient is unable to bear weight on one of the extremities. Patients in pain with generalized weakness assume a wide base of support and have decreased stride length and loss of rotation in their shoulders and hips. Their entire appearance is guarded. As the injury heals and the patient regains strength and endurance, movement becomes quicker and more confident. Shoulder and hip rotations return gradually as speed and stride length increase. More serious gait deviations can result from scarring to joints—knees, hips, ankles, feet, trunk, and shoulders. Long-term treatment plans always include gait training when there is a burn injury across one or more of these joints. Treatment goals include edema control, normal range of motion for all joints including those affected by the burn injury, normal gait, and normal strength and endurance.

SCARRING AND ONGOING COMPLICATIONS

Assessment of the patient's lifestyle before injury is important to developing a realistic

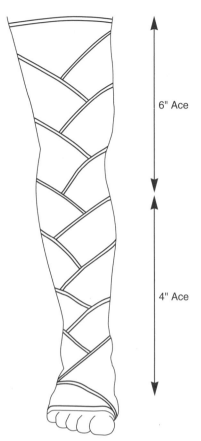

FIGURE 27–7
Figure-of-eight wrap of the lower extremity using Ace bandages. Note: 4-inch Ace wraps for feet and lower legs; 6-inch wraps for upper leg and thigh. Ace wraps are applied before getting out of bed and removed before returning to bed.

6" Ace

4" Ace

plan of care. Patients must learn and practice new strategies to improve outcomes. Daily hygiene, skin lubrication, thermal protection, sun protection, avoidance of temperature changes, and antipruritic measures must be incorporated into the patient's lifestyle (Hegel, Ayllon, & Spiro-Hawkins, 1986). Pruritus can cause severe discomfort. If the pruritus is not treated, scratching can lead to blisters, graft loss, and skin infections. Patients' fingernails should be kept short to discourage scratching. Pressure garments are known to help reduce itching sensations. Systemic antihistamines used in conjunction with topical antipruritic agents can relieve some of the discomfort.

Wounds and skin grafts can have a satisfactory appearance immediately after closure; however, 1 to 3 months later, hypertrophic scars can form from partial- and full-thickness injuries. These scars are characteristically red,

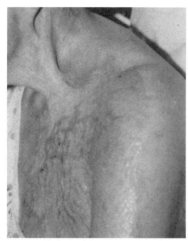

FIGURE 27–8
Early hypertrophic scarring of the neck and axilla in the absence of a pressure sleeve. (From Myers, R. S. [1995]. *Saunders manual of physical therapy practice* [p. 657]. Philadelphia: W. B. Saunders.)

raised, and rigid (Abston, 1987). Figure 27–8 shows a hypertrophic scar forming in the anterior neck, restricting neck motion and potentially distorting the facial appearance. Figure 27–9 shows the application of a mouth splint to prevent a microstomia deformity. Both loss of function and altered appearance are problems that are best addressed by early intervention. Pressure in the form of splints and garments can prevent disfigurement. Pressure has been used since the early 1970s by burn care providers to help minimize the formation of hypertrophic scars. Although the exact physiological mechanism is unknown, clinical observations verify the usefulness of pressure in the form of splints, elastic bandages, and Tubi-Grip and pressure garments (Staley & Richard, 1997). Patient education throughout the course of rehabilitation is essential to ensure compliance after discharge.

Patients having full-thickness burns of the upper extremities of more than 20% TBSA are predisposed to the development of heterotopic ossification (Jay, Saphyakhajon, Scott, Linder, & Grossman, 1981). Once this is diagnosed, only gentle active movement of the involved joint is indicated. Forceful movement of the joint aggravates this painful condition and is therefore contraindicated. Usually heterotopic ossification is first evident as a painful loss in range of motion in the involved joint, with the posterior elbow, the hip, and the shoulder being the most common sites (VanLaeken, 1989). In some cases, nerve entrapment and progressive neurological loss accompany the ossification process.

Neuropathies—mononeuropathy, multiple mononeuropathies, and generalized peripheral neuropathy—are common in persons with serious burn injury. The most common is footdrop related to pressure on the peroneal nerve at the fibular head (Helm, Pandian, & Heck, 1985). Peripheral neuropathies usually are seen in adults with injuries greater than 20% TBSA. The incidence of postburn neuropathy is from 15 to 29% (Fisher & Helm, 1984).

In the recovering burn-injured patient it is important to distinguish between the various

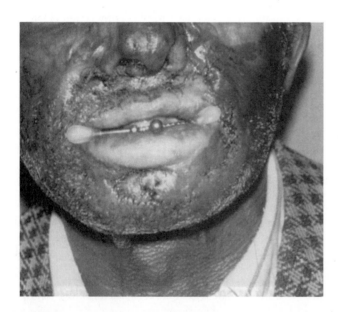

FIGURE 27–9
Microstoma splint used to maintain oral commissure after a facial burn. (From Braddom, R. L. [Ed]. [1996]. *Physical medicine and rehabilitation* [p. 1228]. Philadelphia: W. B. Saunders.)

kinds of pain. Reflex sympathetic dystrophy (RSD) is a painful class of disorders abolished or reduced by sympathetic block (Roberts, 1986). RSD is characterized by painful response to normal touch (allodynia) and increased pain sensitivity. It is believed that trauma, with or without nerve damage, sets off a pain process mediated by the autonomic nervous system. RSD progresses through three stages. In the first stage, the pain is a severe, burning pain near the area of injury. It is sensitive to touch with local edema and stiffness. The early stage can last a few weeks to a few months. In the second stage, the pain becomes more severe and diffuse. Brawny edema, brittle nails, thick joints, and muscle wasting occur. This stage lasts up to 6 months. Severe limb pain, muscle atrophy, and demineralization of the bone accompany the third stage. Nerve blocks have been used successfully to treat RSD. The pain, stiffness, and functional loss can be treated by providing support, pain management, desensitization, weight bearing, motor-planning activities, functional activities, and work reintegration while controlling stress, edema, and stiffness (Stralka, 1994). This progression coincides with rehabilitation strategies for burn rehabilitation, but it is still important to distinguish the pain of RSD from pain from other sources to achieve successful rehabilitation outcomes.

PSYCHOLOGICAL, SOCIOCULTURAL, AND SPIRITUAL ASPECTS OF RECOVERY

The psychological, sociocultural, developmental, and spiritual aspects of a person factor into full recovery or wellness. These aspects often overlap and should be considered interrelated by health professionals. The psychological and spiritual care and support of the burn patient are as important as wound care or therapeutic exercise. Because the injury itself is sensational, that sensation is filled with energy for survival that carries patients and families through the acute period. Quite often, the need for psychological care becomes apparent after the patient is discharged from the hospital. As outpatients, many patients try to "brave out" the experience, projecting to those around them that they are all right and will recover. Because greater attention is given to meeting the physical needs of an acute burn injury, the psychological needs are often ignored in the emer-

gent care setting. Holaday and Yarborough (1996) reported that on discharge from acute care, fewer patients were given referrals for psychological assistance than those who actually demonstrated symptoms of posttraumatic stress disorder and depression. These patients often demonstrate the need for support and psychological counseling by their sleeplessness, flashbacks, and nightmares. These experiences stimulate more sleeplessness, fear of falling asleep, restlessness at night, and long days, and the inability to grasp that something catastrophic has happened to them. Soon the patient becomes too tired to participate in the recovery program and begins to demonstrate progressive apathy, distress, and depression.

Once the need for survival is met, the need to recover begins. According to Morse and Carter (1995), burn survivors have no choice but to endure the consequences of recovery. Endurance is the key. Yet endurance takes all the patients' energy. Once patients are aware that they can no longer endure, suffering begins. When suffering ends, the patients have a new sense of self and a value that they did not possess before their injury. Yet to endure recovery, one must relive the pain of suffering over and over so that one can provide the support that is deserved. Table 27–4 outlines the feelings that take place while the patient endures through burn recovery.

The need for psychological care extends beyond the support a nurse can give, yet patients fail to explore psychological counseling (Holaday & Yarborough, 1996). Cost, time, and inconveniences contribute to a pa-

TABLE 27–4 ■ BURN PATIENT EMOTIONAL EXPERIENCES OF SURVIVAL AND RECOVERY

Guilt, anguish, sleeplessness
Despair, demoralization, fear, regrets
Desperation and pain, dissociation from self
Agony, questioning of religious beliefs, emptiness, altered image
Loss of identity, suffering

Comforting Strategies Used by the Resilient Survivor
1. Enduring to survive: Living through the agony
2. Enduring to live: Protecting the self, refusing to face reality
3. Suffering
4. Reformulating self: Revaluing the experience

Adapted from Morse, J., & Carter, B. (1995). Strategies of enduring and the suffering of loss: Modes of comfort used by a resilient survivor. *Holistic Nursing, 9,* 38–52.

tient's reluctance to seek help. The nurse should advise patients of the long-term benefits of psychotherapy. By acknowledging the patient's feelings as a natural part of recovery, nurses can communicate that it is all right to ask for help. Spiritual distress can be acknowledged and accepted in a similar fashion. Nurses can provide the opportunity to express concerns and allow patients to explore the search for meaning in suffering. Pettigew (1990) states that nursing care that fails to recognize spiritual needs as a vital part of whole-person care, and does not allow these needs to be addressed, becomes disrespectful and unethical.

Spiritual concerns are not religion-specific. Spiritual concerns are similar to the concerns of the psyche. "Why have I survived?" "Why me?" "What does all this suffering mean?" The nurse has the opportunity to create a safe space for the person to ask these questions. Pastoral counselors and chaplains provide support, but survivors of burn injuries need to receive comfort from all members of the team. Interventions include active listening, making a timely referral to a spiritual counselor, using imagery, prayer, or music, and sharing one's own need to find God in life circumstances (Solimine & Hoeman, 1996). People with burn injuries suffer from physical isolation and pain. There is a window of opportunity for caregivers in a rehabilitation environment to "connect" as the person with a serious burn injury passes through "suffering" and "reestablishment of self."

Watkins et al. (1988) portrayed burn survival and recovery as a seven-stage process. Matched with each stage are interventions that members of the burn team can initiate to assist the patient with recovery and adaptation to the injury. Table 27–5 depicts the stage and interventions. In 1996, Watkins, Cook, May, Still, Luterman, & Purvis extended this matrix to include family members' and significant others' adaptation to the burn injury.

Psychological recovery of the burn patient is the responsibility of the entire health care team. Team conferences are a useful time for exchanging ideas, thoughts, and feelings and to plan patient care in an organized, coordinated way. Patients often build trust and confidence with a particular team member. The entrusted team member can assist the patient, staff, and family in identifying issues and developing effective coping strategies during the recovery process.

TABLE 27–5 ■ PSYCHOLOGICAL ADAPTIVE STAGES OF BURN INJURY WITH STAFF INTERVENTION

Adaptive Stage	Intervention
Survival anxiety	Orientation
Problem of pain	Medication
Search for meaning	Validation
Investment in recuperation	Education
Acceptance of losses	Legitimization
Investment of rehabilitation	Commendation
Reintegration of identity	Termination

Adapted from Watkin, P., Cook, E. L., & Ehleben, C. M. (1988). Psychological stages in adaptation following burn injury: A method for facilitating psychological recovery of burn victims. *Journal of Burn Care and Rehabilitation, 9*, 376–383.

AGE-SPECIFIC BURN REHABILITATION

Although generalized wound care and restoration of wellness pertain to the entire burn population, there are specific factors related to patients at either end of the life span.

Children

Some important issues associated with children and burn recovery are mainly psychosocial. Coping with changes, a new body image, awareness of self, and peer acceptance are a few of the challenges that children face (Blakeney, 1996). Emphasis on what the child can do rather than what the child cannot do is a goal for all team members. Parental participation in the care and rehabilitation of the child is of great importance. A supportive environment enhances recovery, whereas factors associated with poor adjustment include a lack of family cohesiveness; prolonged parental stress, guilt, and depression; a lack of sociability; and passive-dependent behavior of the child (Blakeney, 1996).

Communication is vital. Younger children may understand only one-step commands, whereas older children may be able to follow multiple steps. Disruptive behavior must be dealt with immediately to ensure the importance of the therapeutic program. Parents or guardians must also understand the instruction so that they can continue rehabilitation in the home. The rehabilitation team can assist both the child and the parent or guardian in developing strategies that facilitate the child's transition back into society. Yet how well the child functions socially does not predict how well the child feels emotionally. Some problems a child develops, such as nightmares or enuresis, are known only by those intimately acquainted with the child (Blakeney, 1996). It is important for the rehabilitation team to explore all avenues of coping and adjustment to injury.

Therapy is scheduled according to the developmental age and ability of the child. For example, children cannot endure long sessions of exercising owing to their shorter attention spans and pain. Shorter periods of therapy in conjunction with play may obtain the same goals for the younger child (Daugherty, 1996).

For many children, maturation of scars can take up to 2 years. Reconstruction procedures must fit well into the child's developmental phase. In addition, readjustment to pressure garments are done frequently to accommodate the child's rapid growth and development. Pressure garments, if prescribed and used, are available in a variety of styles and colors. Methods of donning the garments also vary according to the age of the child. Garments that open and close in the back are easier for infants and small children who must be dressed by a caretaker. Front-opening pressure garments are more appropriate for older children. The size of the child's hand is used to determine whether the child receives a glove or compression wrap for scar control (Daugherty, 1996).

Children who survive a burn injury may experience difficulty adjusting in both the family and the social setting. School reentry programs are a successful way of incorporating the child back to familiar surroundings. Reentry programs also prepare classmates, teachers, and staff for the return of the student by educating them about burn care, scarring, self-concept, and functional capabilities. Burn camps provide another avenue for social reentry. All participants are burn survivors and have similar needs and desires. The burn camp environment offers safety and security wherein children incorporate functional abilities into daily play and activity (Colt, 1996).

The elderly burn-injured patient presents unique challenges to the restoration of function. Caretakers who are sensitive to the normal changes of aging have better success developing a program for their senior patients. Care goals should be tailored to maximize the patients' potential and assist them in returning to the preinjury activity level. Patient and caretaker communication is essential to the return of optimal health. Fletchall (1996)

observes that geriatric patients have a tendency to spend more energy performing a particular task, rather than distributing their energy to multiple tasks. For example, if the therapeutic exercises are not viewed as equally important as dressing one's self, all the energy will be spent dressing at the expense of the exercise program. It is, therefore, important to include the patient's goals in planning program goals and activities.

Older Persons

Normal visual changes with aging include a slower accommodation reflex and sensitivity to glare. Hearing loss can impair the understanding of instructions. Changes in cognition result in slower processing and reaction time. These changes can make it necessary to pace instructions and repeat directions to enhance new learning. Dressing changes, wound care, skin care, or therapeutic exercises represent new activities that need to be learned in such fashion. Muscle weakness, joint stiffness, and poor endurance can result in taking a longer time to complete tasks.

When hearing loss is a problem, caretakers must face the person directly and speak distinctly and loud enough to be heard. Written instruction and diagrams can assist new learning. Instructions should be written large enough and should be spaced so that the elderly eye can accommodate to read it. Gentle tactile stimulation can also assist in alerting the person to listen (Fletchall, 1996).

Chronic illness, in conjunction with normal aging changes, interferes with burn rehabilitation. Diabetic retinopathy, glaucoma, or cataracts add to visual problems. Arthritis, peripheral vascular disease, and peripheral neuropathies impede mobilization, strengthening, positioning, and performance of activities of daily living. For example, the burn patient with arthritis may find range-of-motion exercises more painful and less tolerable than other patients. Burn patients with peripheral vascular disease or metabolic disease may heal more slowly than expected. Skin changes in elderly persons make them more vulnerable to skin breakdown. Pressure points, especially the heels, should be assessed daily. Emollients should be used to keep the skin supple. Pressure garments and splints may cause skin breakdown if not carefully monitored.

Sleep cycles change in later years. An elderly patient may need to retire earlier and require fewer hours of sleep than a younger patient does. They may benefit from "cat naps" during the day. Environmental changes can contribute to confusion, sleeplessness, and disorientation. Even a change from the burn unit to the rehabilitation unit can cause confusion that delays the rehabilitation process.

The higher than normal metabolic demands of wound healing contribute to fatigue in elderly patients. Schedules of various therapies have to be adjusted to allow for frequent rests that help to restore energy. The reduced metabolic demands and slower digestive patterns in elderly patients result in less food consumption. The elderly patient with a burn injury is not able to consume enough food to meet the caloric demands for wound repair (Turner, 1996). Supplemental feeding should be used to provide nutritional needs.

The rehabilitation team and caretakers need to plan goals and a program to accommodate the individual. Outcomes should be based on patients' priorities and abilities, allowing for the normal and pathological changes related to normal aging and the burn injury.

DISABILITY AND SOCIAL REINTEGRATION

Permanent disability related to the injury is not purely a medical condition. Heat and cold intolerance; sensitivity to sunlight; pain; chemical sensitivity; changes in the sweat glands and sebaceous glands; decreased sensation; decreased coordination; muscle weakness; contractures; and altered physical appearance must be considered within the context of the patient system. Reintegration into the social structures of the family, community, and workplace offer a challenge to the recovering burn-injured individual.

Individuals with chronic disability who are inconvenienced because of sensory limitations are considered to have altered sexual function whether or not the sex organs are affected (Shrey, Kiefer, & Anthony, 1979). The physiological alterations common in survivors of burn injury include impaired physical mobility; increased and/or decreased sensation; pain; and fatigue. Blumenfield and Schoeps (1992) report depression as a major factor as the person realizes the drastic change in appearance, the seemingly endless number of treatments, and the functional implications for the future.

Increasingly, rehabilitation nurses are working in the community as consultants or providing direct services. A great deal of a patient's adjustment to disability occurs after hospitalization. Although the physician is the team member with the ultimate responsibility in deciding when the burn patient is ready to return to work, the physician may need input from nurses and others who have knowledge of the home conditions, working requirements, and other factors related to function (American Medical Association's Council on Scientific Affairs, 1993). Family involvement through rehabilitation is critical to recovery. Moy (1996) suggests three goals:

1. Providing a patient the opportunity to express emotions and encouraging expression of frustrations and concerns
2. Allowing family members to observe wound healing and adjust to changes in the patient's physical appearance and functioning
3. Aiding the family in understanding a patient's day-to-day struggles and offering insight into physical and emotional challenges during rehabilitation

When burn survivors hold positive views about themselves in their family and social roles, they adjust more effectively. A comprehensive medical evaluation by a vocational specialist is required before a patient can resume his or her occupational role. If the burn injury occurred in the work setting, issues such as fear of reinjury, concern about peers, and poor self-confidence can hinder success (Cheng & Rogers, 1989).

DISCHARGE INSTRUCTIONS

The burn survivor's new life begins on discharge from an inpatient environment, whether from an acute care or a rehabilitation setting. Although the patient's needs are changing, support is critical to the patient's readjustment to the environment. Patient education is an important aspect of the support system. Instructions on discharge play a role in how well the patient adjusts. Instructions should be concise and should be easy for the patient to understand and refer to on an as-needed basis. Instruction given to the patient should also be shared with visiting nurses, family members, and/or caretakers.

Often the burn survivor has lost possessions including a home. Social workers play a key role in aiding the patient in obtaining continued health and social services including housing and transportation. Table 27–6 lists nine items that are important for the

TABLE 27–6 ■ DISCHARGE INSTRUCTIONS FOR BURN–INJURED PATIENTS

Skin care including use of soaps for cleansing (high-glycerol, nondrying) and emollients free of perfumes, such as Eutra, cocoa butter, Nivea, Eucerin, and mineral oil

Wound care including topical agents, bandages, frequency of dressing changes, information on where to purchase dressings, follow-up wound care, and appointments

Therapeutic exercises (home program) including frequency and number of repetitions

Restrictions including activities, exposure to sun, and excessive heat and cold

Special instructions related to splints, pressure garments, and positioning

Nutrition including a diet high in protein and vitamin supplements, and monitoring weight gain

Medications and prescriptions, especially pain medication

Information related to return to work or school

Follow-up appointments with physician and therapists, including telephone numbers

---

nurse to include in the discharge instructions. Patients must be given time to absorb oral instructions and should have a written summary. Before the patient leaves the inpatient setting, time must be allowed for the patient to ask questions. Allowing time for questions often prevents patient distress and telephone calls after discharge.

■ CASE STUDY 27–1

MEDICAL HISTORY

Jim, a 40-year-old man, married with two children, sustained a 58% TBSA thermal injury while he was working at a smelting furnace. He had no significant past medical history; the injury was calculated using the Lund and Browder method shown in Figure 27–10.

Transfer to the rehabilitation center followed 4 months in the burn treatment center. During this time Jim underwent 18 surgeries for burn excision and skin grafting. Donor sites included several harvestings of skin from his back, upper chest, and scalp. Repeated grafting procedures to his hip, thigh, legs, and buttocks followed graft loss. Several life-threatening bouts with sepsis complicated his recovery. Despite nutritional support, Jim lost 35% of his body mass during the 4 months after injury. On admission to the rehabilitation center, Jim was medically stable with a hemoglobin level of 9.1, hematocrit of 27.4, and white blood cell count of 8.1. His wounds were covered, and he had completed a course of triple antibiotics. Tube feedings were discontinued, and Jim was beginning to tolerate food. Jim's phosphorus, magnesium, calcium, and potassium levels were normal. The focus for the team approach included communication, nutrition, skin integrity, mobility, activities of daily living, motivation, and pain management. Table 27–7 lists burn injuries related to problems, goals, treatment, and team members addressing the problems.

REHABILITATION

Jim's severe and complex problems required the integrated team approach described in this chapter. Life-threatening bouts with sepsis prevented the consistent early intervention by occupational and physical therapists. In the rehabilitation setting, contractures, weakness, and poor endurance became a challenge for Jim and the entire team. Other problems included poor nutritional status; unhealed wounds; loss of the functional use of his dominant right hand, wrist, and elbow; poor tolerance for treatment; pain; and poor vocalization.

During inpatient rehabilitation, nurses took a lead role in coordinating and prioritizing team efforts. Weekly team conferences and daily rounds were provided to monitor and adjust team goals and set realistic outcomes. For example, the dietitian met with

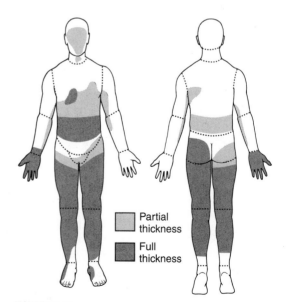

FIGURE 27–10
Lund and Browder determination of the total body surface area of a burn injury: 15% partial-thickness, 43% full-thickness burn injury. (Redrawn from Saint Agnes Burn Center Burn Record. Saint Agnes Medical Center, Philadelphia.)

TABLE 27-7 ■ CASE STUDY: SUMMARY OF PATIENT PROBLEMS, GOALS, AND INTERVENTIONS

Patient Problems	Goal(s)	Interventions(s)	Team Member(s) Responsible
Nutrition		Reintroduce solid food Monitor diet Educate patient and family about nutrition and burn injury	Dietician, physician, nurse, occupational therapist, speech therapist
Albumin level = 2.7 Weight = 122 lb TPN and gastrostomy tube Regurgitation Hiatal hernia Skin integrity	Normal albumin level Normal weight Normal eating patterns, normal electrolyte balance	Reintroduce solid food	Physical therapist, physician/ surgeon, nurse, occupational therapist
Open areas on buttocks and lower extremities	Clean wounds, wound closure, self-care for skin protection and scar management	Hydrotherapy and/or wound care, graft care Patient education Splinting, garments	
Mobility			Physical therapist, occupational therapist, physician/physiatrist, nurse
Contractures	Stretching exercise, active exercise, 2 ×/day, splinting, positioning, joint protection, assistive devices	Physical therapy, occupational therapy	
Both LEs Both UEs Trunk Severe in right elbow, wrist Pins in right thumb and fifth finger			
Poor endurance	Aerobic conditioning, 2 ×/ day	Physical therapy, occupational therapy	
Robot-like gait Weakness Poor balance Balance exercises, education in home program	Gait training Resistive exercises, 2 ×/day		
Communication			Speech therapist, nurse, social worker, physician/ psychiatrist, pastoral counselor
Inability to vocalize	Vocalization improved	Speech therapy, respiratory therapy	
Noncompliance with positioning and treatment	Home visits, family communication, spiritual and psychosocial support	Nursing, social services, pastoral counseling	
ADLs		Occupational therapy, physical therapy	Occupational therapist, physical therapist, nurse, physician
Right thumb and fifth finger	Appropriate assistive devices, patient education to use assistive devices		
Joint instability/pins Splinting Contractures of right elbow and wrist	Joint protection Stretching and active exercises, patient education for self-stretching and exercise		

ADLs, activities of daily living; LE, lower extremity; TPN, total parental nutrition; UE, upper extremity.

Jim to discuss his dietary preferences and to provide information; however, nurses observed the amount of food eaten, and/or regurgitated. Nurses provided the ongoing education to Jim and his family related to good nutrition and wound healing.

The physical losses of mobility, endurance, strength, and functional capacity indicated aggressive physical and occupational therapy; however, the psychosocial impact of the injury demanded goal modification. Jim appeared not to have the motivation or pain tolerance for a challenging program. His inability to vocalize his needs and wishes compounded the problem. Outcomes for Jim had to be determined in consultation with the team and family and with consideration of his perceived motivation and tolerance. From the beginning of the rehabilitation period, it was clear that Jim was determined to go home to his family. His religious beliefs and strong family support provided a will to continue despite his poor tolerance for activity. Associating home visits with physical and functional goals provided a strong incentive to tolerate the therapies and achieve anticipated outcomes. As Jim's ability to vocalize improved, active listening on the part of the rehabilitation team became an important strategy. Team members took on a role of teacher and facilitator and partnered with Jim to achieve weekend passes. Motivational problems gradually decreased, and Jim began to take more responsibility for exercise and activity. Small improvements helped to motivate and encourage him. The contractures, wounds, and pins in his dominant right hand injury delayed activities of daily living. A walker with appliances to accommodate his elbow and hand allowed gait training to begin. At discharge from inpatient rehabilitation, Jim was still using a wheelchair for distances and required help with dressing and other aspects of personal care. Discharge planning from inpatient rehabilitation involved the input of the entire team, including Jim and his family.

REINTEGRATION

After 4 months in the burn center and 4 months in the rehabilitation center, Jim was discharged to outpatient services 5 days a week for wound and skin care, gait training, and occupational therapy. Therapy replaced work as a social structure as Jim reintegrated into his family and church group. Jim's outlook continued to improve, and he continued to make steady improvement in regaining functional activities. The right hand injury was the slowest to improve, but Jim was able to resume gardening and other hobbies within 2 years of his injury. Jim has never considered returning to work. ■

REFERENCES

Abston, S. (1987). Scar reaction after thermal injury and prevention of scars and contractures. In J. A. Wachtel (Ed.), *The Art and science of burn care* (pp. 359–371). Rockville, MD: Aspen.

American Burn Association. (1982). *Guidelines for burn nursing practice.* Chicago.

American Burn Association. (1990). Hospital and prehospital resources for optimal care of patients with burn injury: Guidelines for development and operation of burn centers. *Journal of Burn Care and Rehabilitation, 11,* 98–104.

American Medical Association's Council on Scientific Affairs. (1993). *Guide to evaluation of permanent impairment* (4th ed.). Chicago: American Medical Association.

Bayley, E. W. (1990). Wound healing in the patient with burns. *Nursing Clinics of North America, 25,* 205–222.

Blakeney, P. (1996). The pediatric burn patient considerations. Presented at *Symposium: Burns in the high risk patient,* Nashville, TN: 28th Annual Meeting, American Burn Association.

Blumenfield, M., & Schoeps, M. (1992). Reintegrating the healed burned adult into society. *Clinics in Plastic Surgery, 19,* 599–605.

Brigham, P., & McLaughlin, E. (1996). Burn incidence and medical care use in the United States: Estimates, trends and data sources. *Journal of Burn Care and Rehabilitation, 17,* 95–107.

Byl, N., Cameron, M., Kloth, L. C., & Zellenbach, L. R. (1995). Treatment and prevention: Goal and objectives. In R. S. Myers (Ed.), *Saunders manual of physical therapy practice* (pp. 625–666). Philadelphia: W. B. Saunders.

Cheng, S., & Rogers, J. C. (1989). Changes in occupational role performance after a severe burn: A retrospective study. *American Journal of Occupational Therapy, 43,* 17–24.

Colt, D. (1996). The pediatric burn patient: Nursing considerations. Presented at *Symposium: Burns in the High Risk Patient,* Nashville, TN: 28th Annual Meeting, American Burn Association.

Cromes, G. F., & Helm, P. A. (1993). Burn injuries. In M. G. Eisenberg, R. L. Glueckauf, & H. H. Zaretsky (Eds.), *Medical aspects of disability* (pp. 92–104). New York: Springer.

Daugherty, M. (1996). The pediatric burn patient: Nursing considerations. Presented at *Symposium: Burns in the High Risk Patient,* Nashville, TN: 28th Annual Meeting, American Burn Association.

Demling, R. (1998). Increased protein intake during the recovery phase after severe burns increases body weight and muscle function. *Journal of Burn Care and Rehabilitation, 19,* 161–168.

Fisher, S. V., & Helm, P. A. (Eds.). (1984). *Comprehensive rehabilitation of burns.* Baltimore: Williams & Wilkins.

Flanigan, K. H. (1997). Nutritional aspects of wound healing. *Advances in Wound Care, 10,* 48–52.

Fletchall, S. (1996). Rehabilitation of the geriatric burn client. Presented at *Symposium: Burns in the High Risk Patient,* Nashville, TN: 28th Annual Meeting, American Burn Association.

Gottscheich, M. (1998). Nutrition forum. *Journal of Burn Care and Rehabilitation, 19,* 160.

Haberal, J. (1986). Electrical burns: A five year experience—Evans lecture. *Journal of Trauma, 26,* 103–109.

Hegel, M. T., Ayllon, T., & Spiro-Hawkins, H. (1986). A behavioral procedure for increasing compliance with self-exercise regimen in severely burn injured patients. *Restorative Therapy, 24,* 521–528.

Helm, P. A., Pandian, G., & Heck, E. (1985). Neuromuscular problems in the burn patient: Causes and prevention. *Archives of Physical Medicine and Rehabilitation, 66,* 451–453.

Holaday, M., & Yarborough, J. (1996). Results of a hospital survey to determine the extent and type of psychological services offered to patients with severe burns. *Journal of Burn Care and Rehabilitation, 17,* 280–284.

Jay, M. S., Saphyakhajon, P., Scott, R., Linder, C., & Grossman, B. J. (1981). Bone and joint changes after burn injury. *Clinical Pediatrics, 20,* 724–736.

Jensen, M. P., Karoly, P., & Braver, S. (1986). The measurement of clinical pain intensity: A comparison of six methods. *Pain, 27,* 117–126.

Lund, C. C., & Browder, N. C. (1944). The estimate of areas of burns. *Surgery, Gynecology, and Obstetrics, 79,* 352.

Marvin, J. (1993). Burn nursing history: The history of burn care. *Journal of Burn Care and Rehabilitation, 2,* 252–256.

McLaughlin, J. (1989). *Standards of Burn Nursing Practice.* (1989). Philadelphia: Nurse Advisory Council of the Burn Foundation of Philadelphia.

Miller, S. F., Richard, R. L., & Staley, M. J. (1994). Triage and resuscitation of the burn patient. Burn wound care. In R. L. Richard & M. J. Staley (Eds.), *Burn care and rehabilitation* (pp. 105–118). Philadelphia: F. A. Davis.

Morse, J., & Carter, B. (1995). Strategies of enduring and suffering of loss: Modes of comfort used by resilient survivors. *Holistic Nursing Practice, 9,* 38–53.

Moy, A. (1996). Restorative rehabilitation with burn injuries. In S. P. Hoeman (Ed.), *Rehabilitation Nursing* (2nd ed., pp. 647–659). St Louis: C. V. Mosby.

Neuman, B. (1989). The Neuman Systems Model. In B. M. Neuman (Ed.), *The Neuman Systems Model* (pp. 3–64). East Norwalk, CT: Appleton & Lange.

Nothdurft, D., Smith, P. S., & LeMaster, J. E. (1984). Exercise and treatment modalities. In S. V. Fisher & P. A. Helm (Eds.), *Comprehensive rehabilitation of burns* (pp. 96–147). Baltimore: Williams & Wilkins.

Pettigew, J. (1990). Intensive care nursing: The ministry of presence. *Critical Care Nursing Clinics of North America, 2,* 503–508.

Pruitt, B., & Mason, A. (1996). Epidemiological demographic and outcome characteristics of burn injury. In D. N. Herdon (Ed.), *Total burn care* (pp. 5–15). Philadelphia: W. B. Saunders.

Roberts, W. J. (1986). A hypothesis on the physiological basis for causalgia and related pains. *Pain, 24,* 297–311.

Rodriquez, D. (1996). Nutrition in patients with severe burns: State of the art. *Journal of Burn Care and Rehabilitation, 17,* 62–70.

Saffle, J. R., & Schenebly, W. A. (1994). Burn wound care. In R. L. Richard & M. J. Staley (Eds.), *Burn care and rehabilitation* (pp. 380–418). Philadelphia: F. A. Davis.

Shrey, D. E., Kiefer, J. S., & Anthony, W. A. (1979). Sexual adjustment counseling for persons with severe disabilities: A skill-based approach for rehabilitation professionals. *Journal of Rehabilitation, 45,* 28–33.

Solimine, M. A., & Hoeman, S. P. (1996). Spirituality: A rehabilitation perspective. In S. P. Hoeman (Ed.), *Rehabilitation nursing* (2nd ed., pp. 628–643). St. Louis: C. V. Mosby.

Staley, M. J., & Richard, R. L. (1997). Use of pressure to treat hypertropic burns scars. *Advances in Wound Care, 10,* 44–46.

Stralka, S. (1994). Reflex sympathic dystrophy. Presented at the Pennsylvania Physical Therapy Association Annual Meeting, Philadelphia, PA.

Trofino, R. (1991). *Nursing care of the burn injured patient.* Philadelphia: F. A. Davis.

Turner, D. (1996). The geriatric burn patient: Nursing considerations. Presented at *Symposium: Burns in the High Risk Patient,* Nashville, TN: 28th Annual Meeting, American Burn Association.

VanLaeken, N., Snelling, C. F., Meek, R. N., Warren, R. J., & Foley, B. (1989). Heterotopic bone formation in the patient with burn injuries. A retrospective assessment of contributing factors and methods of investigation. *Journal of Burn Care and Rehabilitation, 10,* 331–335.

Watkins, P., Cook, E. L., May, S. R., & Ehleben, C. M. (1988). Psychological stages in adaptation following burn injury: A method of facilitating psychological recovery of burn victims. *Journal of Burn Care and Rehabilitation, 9,* 376–383.

Watkins, P. N., Cook, E. L., May, S. R., Still, J. M., Luterman, A., & Purvis, R. J. (1996). Postburn psychologic adaptation of family members of patients with burns. *Journal of Burn Care and Rehabilitation 17,* 78–92.

Winkler, J. B., DiMola, M. A., & Wooten, J. A. (1993). Burns. In M. R. Kiney, D. R. Packa, & S. B. Dunbar (Eds.), *Clinical reference for critical-care nursing* (3rd ed, pp. 1195–1231). St. Louis: Mosby–Year Book.

BIBLIOGRAPHY

Bayley, E. W., Carrougher, G. J., Marvin, J. A., Knighton, J., Rutan, R. L., & Weber, B. F. (1992). Research priorities for burn nursing: Rehabilitation, discharge planning, and follow-up care. *Journal of Burn Care and Rehabilitation, 13,* 471–476.

Evans, E. B. (1966). Orthopedic measures in the treatment of severe burns. *Journal of Bone and Joint Surgery. American Volume, 48,* 643–669.

McManus, W. F. (1979). Immediate emergency department care. In C. P. Arzt, J. A. Moncrief, & B. A. Pruitt (Eds.), *Burns: A team approach* (p. 154). Philadelphia: W. B. Saunders.

Staley, M., Richard, R., Warden, G. P., Miller, S. F., Shuster, D. B. (1996). Functional outcomes for the patient with burn injuries. *Journal of Burn Care and Rehabilitation, 17,* 362–367.

CHAPTER 28

Pediatric Rehabilitation Nursing

Patricia A. Edwards

The practice of pediatric rehabilitation nursing, although a relatively newly defined specialty area, has evolved over the years as the special needs of children and their families have changed. The pediatric rehabilitation nurse combines knowledge and skills from the fields of pediatrics and rehabilitation into a blend of roles practiced in a variety of settings. This chapter describes the components of nursing practice at both the basic and the advanced levels and their interrelationship with the principles of pediatric rehabilitation and growth and development. Community-based delivery systems are described as the essential support for services to the child, adolescent, and family. The home, school, and community are the environments that promote normal living patterns, and they are discussed as well as other comprehensive services: basic primary care and specialized secondary and tertiary care.

The assessment and screening of children and adolescents is presented, and specific nursing care related to alterations in health and psychosocial concerns is explained using the nursing process as the organizing framework. Three common conditions affecting children—bronchopulmonary dysplasia, cerebral palsy, and muscular dystrophy—are used as exemplars and are fully described.

PEDIATRIC REHABILITATION NURSING

Description

Pediatric rehabilitation nursing is a dynamic, specialized field of practice, committed to providing a continuum of care for children and adolescents with disabilities or chronic conditions and for their families. This continuum extends far beyond injury and diagnosis to the point of transition to adult services and is aimed at maximizing potential and improving the quality of life. Recognizing the importance of the family in the development of the child, the pediatric rehabilitation nurse advocates for their involvement in the collaborative rehabilitation effort. This includes a systematic use of the nursing process to assess the impact of the disability or chronic condition and, in collaboration with other professionals, to plan, implement, and evaluate an individualized, interdisciplinary plan of care (Association of Rehabilitation Nurses [ARN] Pediatric Special Interest Group, 1992). Table 28–1 shows some of the roles of the pediatric rehabilitation nurse.

Advanced practice nurses in pediatric rehabilitation are an integral part of the health care system and share characteristics and core knowledge with other nurses in similar roles with other populations—clinical nurse specialists and nurse practitioners. Advanced practice nurses' scope of practice includes

- A higher level of autonomy in practice and complexity of decision making
- Nurse-initiated treatment regimens
- Leadership on the interdisciplinary team
- Diagnosing illnesses and prescribing medications
- Skill in managing environments
- Consultation, education, and research
- An ability to integrate various components in managing very complex cases

Advanced practice nurses caring for children and adolescents with disabilities and chronic conditions have a tremendous positive impact on the delivery systems that provide family-centered, community-based care.

Evolution of Pediatric Rehabilitation

Many of today's high-technology rehabilitation hospitals for children had their beginnings in the late 19th and early 20th centuries as "fresh air" summer homes, respite programs for crippled children, camps, or convalescent centers. As medical knowledge and treatment advanced and the possibilities of

TABLE 28–1 ■ ROLES OF THE PEDIATRIC REHABILITATION NURSE

Advocate
  Functions as a child and family advocate
  Facilitates the child's and the family's transition from the hospital to the home and community
  Promotes community and governmental knowledge of pediatric rehabilitation issues
Coordinator
  Works as a valued member of the health care team
  Brings together the expertise of health professionals and integrates that knowledge into the comprehensive continuum of care
  Facilitates the design and implementation of the family's individual plan of care
Leader
  Demonstrates leadership through clinical expertise and delegates responsibilities to other members of the team
  Acts as an agent of change
  Consults with other health professionals
	Teacher
	  Shares knowledge and skills
	  Offers counseling and support to families about the special needs of their children and adolescents with disabilities
	  Teaches other individuals (both in the health care field and in the community) about the special aspects of children's and adolescent's rehabilitation needs
	Team member
	  Works as part of an innovative and creative unit
	  Collaborates in the development of new service delivery models that best meet the needs of young clients and their families
	Primary care provider
	  Implements nursing care based on a sound knowledge base, scientific principles, and a documented therapeutic plan

From Association of Rehabilitation Nurses Pediatric Special Interest Group. (1992). *Pediatric rehabilitation nursing role description.* Skokie, IL: Association of Rehabilitation Nurses.

physical restoration became apparent, greater attention was given to training and educating children with physical disabilities. Efforts involved various types of restorative surgery, specialized bracing of limbs, and other modalities such as heat treatments, massage, exercise, and hydrotherapy.

The early facilities evolved into specialized inpatient rehabilitation hospitals serving children and adolescents with a variety of disabilities and chronic conditions and also serving their families. These facilities are important because children need appropriate medical, nursing, and therapeutic environments to support developmental and educational needs, and their families need professional support and guidance provided with a holistic approach to care. The scope of programs and services continues to change with advances in medicine and technology and the challenge of new populations of children with specialized needs. Some activities involve the establishment of pediatric long-term care units and day hospital facilities, as well as community outreach to schools, day care centers, and ambulatory services. Emphasis will continue to be placed on underscoring the needs and problems of all children and a commitment on the part of specialty hospitals to meet the challenge of caring for children's health in the 21st century is critical. It will become very important to reach out and provide coordination, continuity, and follow-up care by pediatric rehabilitation specialists in

an environment designed "just for kids" (Edwards, 1992, p. 195).

Components of Practice

The pediatric rehabilitation nurse possesses specialized knowledge and skills and uses them as the basis for clinical decision making to meet the individual needs of children and adolescents with disabilities and/or chronic conditions and their families. Components of pediatric rehabilitation nursing practice fully described in the *Pediatric Rehabilitation Nursing Role Description* (ARN Pediatric Special Interest Group, 1992) include

- Using appropriate theory and content
- Maintaining professional practice standards
- Approaching crises systematically
- Collaborating with all members of the team in the plan of care
- Participating in research
- Pursuing professional development
- Providing health education

Growth and development, family and group dynamics, communication, teaching-learning, and leadership are just a few of the theoretical areas that must be part of the body of knowledge applied by the nurse in promoting optimal health and development. Collaboration with other members of the rehabilitation team, including the family, is essential in the development of a comprehensive, individualized plan of care.

Pediatric rehabilitation nurses must also have a commitment to their own professional development and obtain current information about the trends and expertise integral to this specialty nursing practice. Participation in research activities, including the critical analysis of accepted practice, contributes to the field of pediatric rehabilitation nursing and its body of knowledge. The nurse's role in providing health education to children, adolescents, families, consumers, and other health professionals must be implemented to increase their level of knowledge and also to raise awareness of the health needs of children and adolescents with disabilities and chronic conditions.

Standards for Nursing Practice

Standards were developed by rehabilitation nurses to describe and define the elements of quality care and are organized using the American Nurses Association (1991) framework. They consist of standards of care, including assessment, diagnosis, outcome identification, planning, implementation, and evaluation, and standards of professional performance.

Nurses who possess additional skill and knowledge in the practice of pediatric rehabilitation nursing use these standards of rehabilitation nursing care (ARN, 1994) in interactions with children and adolescents with disabilities and chronic conditions and their families. The standards may be integrated differently in various pediatric settings to address specific problems, diagnoses, and/or populations of children. For example, within an acute pediatric rehabilitation setting, the components of a standard of care of the child and family (Nursing Standards Committee, 1994) focus on interventions specific to that environment and identify the problems and needs for each age grouping from neonate through adolescent. Standard components are found in Table 28–2.

The ARN (1996) has finalized standards for advanced practice registered nursing that reflect specific areas of specialization, expansion, and advancement in practice. As stated in the standards, "Advanced practice is based upon graduate nursing education, which provides a greater depth and breadth of knowledge, develops an ability to synthesize data to a greater degree, and develops complexity of skills and interventions." The pediatric rehabilitation nurse in advanced practice applies the standards of care in interactions with children, adolescents, and families, and this includes case management, consultation, health promotion, maintenance and teaching, prescriptive authority, and referral.

Another group of standards organized using the American Nurses Association framework are Standards of Nursing Practice for the Care of Children and Adolescents with Special Health and Developmental Needs (Consensus Committee, 1994). In addition to the components of care and professional performance, these standards include a general structural standard that states, "The delivery of effective health services for children and adolescents with special health and developmental needs requires resources, both human and fiscal, as well as an ongoing commitment to quality care" (Consensus Committee, 1994, p. 24).

When applying standards, the pediatric rehabilitation nurse must individualize the plan and the expected outcomes for the child and family, considering their identified needs. These outcomes derive from nursing diagnoses, are formulated with the child, family, and health care team, and are stated in terms that are realistic in relation to the identified capabilities and available resources. The standards also provide a method for the health care team to assess program quality and show that the interventions work and deliver the desired end result. In this area, pediatric rehabilitation nurses have a challenge to develop comprehensive, discipline-sensitive outcomes that are responsive to the emerging consumer-driven health care system. This enhances recognition of the contribution of nursing care to the efficient, cost-effective provision of rehabilitation services to children and adolescents and their families.

PRINCIPLES OF PEDIATRIC REHABILITATION

Influence of Growth and Development

"Developmental theory is a cornerstone of pediatric rehabilitation nursing" (ARN Pediatric Special Interest Group, 1992). The disruption of life experiences that occurs with injury, disease, or a congenital condition puts the child's growth and development in all domains in jeopardy. Because children are still growing and developing, this creates many physiological differences and changes in relation to their disability or chronic condition. Pediatric rehabilitation nurses must pos-

TABLE 28–2 ■ STANDARD COMPONENTS—CARE OF THE CHILD AND FAMILY

Problem or Need	Intervention
Neonate	
Chronic illness may decrease access to environmental inputs.	Assess adjustment to extrauterine life, and teach parents important signs of illness or problems.
Parental guilt, grief, or anger may interfere with the attachment process.	Encourage parents to express feelings. Give factual information and guide parents in establishing physical and emotional contact.
Infant	
Developing trust depends on having needs met in a consistent manner.	Help families to maintain a constant presence, and facilitate consistent care by others.
Lack of mobility and feeding problems decrease the sense of control.	Encourage parents to give opportunity for exploration and mastery.
Opportunities for exploration and manipulation of objects may be diminished.	Help parents use age-appropriate toys and activities adapted to the child's needs.
Toddler	
Autonomy is aided by opportunities for exploration and independence and experience in making choices, and illness may hamper exploring and using motor skills.	Help parents devise some measurable methods so the child can move independently and can have some opportunities to play independently.
Toddler may not have an opportunity to engage in tasks requiring eye-hand coordination, and assembling and categorizing objects, and some conditions affect the ability to control the bowel and bladder.	Help parents be creative in providing play experiences and using caregiving opportunities effectively. Tasks involving successful toileting should be broken down into small specific behaviors.
Preschooler	
Parents may overprotect, and regression occurs in most children during illness.	Help parents verbalize concerns and encourage independence and self-reliance.
Child may lack exposure to new experiences, and parents may try to buffer interactions with the environment and limit the opportunity to develop coping mechanisms.	Explore possibilities for preschool or other experiences outside the family, encourage play to provide opportunities for risk taking, and explore feelings about illness.
School-aged	
Child may have diminished opportunities for learning and irregular school attendance.	Encourage and facilitate regular school attendance, and educate teachers and healthy peers about chronic illness.
Child may have narrow social and interpersonal relationships.	Encourage enhancing peer relationships through participation in clubs and sports.
Adolescent	
Disease management may make independence difficult, and complying with medical regimen may become a problem.	Encourage families to find areas in adolescents' lives where the adolescents can be independent.
Preoccupation with bodily functions and changes are accentuated for adolescents with chronic illness.	Help adolescents satisfy their need to understand specifics about their condition and treatment and care for their own bodies.
Adolescent may have a decreased opportunity to be part of a peer group.	Encourage participation in activities and initiate friendships.

Adapted from Nursing Standards Committee. (1994). *Care of the child and family* [unpublished standards]. Boston: Spaulding Rehabilitation Hospital.

sess comprehensive knowledge and skills related to growth and development, understand the interaction of the disability or condition and the age-related developmental tasks, and be able to implement plans of care that promote developmental milestones.

In the assessment of the child with a disability or chronic condition, physical growth and human development are equally important. The growth rate is variable, with the most rapid changes occurring during infancy and adolescence. Growth charts can be used to track the growth rate, which is a more sensitive indicator of health than is actual size. The developmental sequence for all children progresses from head to toe and from general to specific, but the rate may vary from child to child. The child with a disability may not lose primitive reflexes and therefore may have difficulty in integrating voluntary movements. As part of a comprehensive assessment, the pediatric rehabilitation nurse must accurately identify the child's mastery of certain developmental milestones to select developmentally based interventions. Screening tools that aid in the detection of delayed development provide a method for examining and grouping children. Several tools to assess development and functional independence (discussed later in this chapter) can be used in a variety of settings. These can be the basis for discussion of the changes a family might anticipate in the development and functional abilities of their child (Burkett, 1989).

Table 28–3 outlines elements of a nursing plan of care related to altered growth and development. It can be used as an outline for planning and documentation but must be individualized to reflect the specific needs and problems of the child and family. Growth and development may be altered because of genetic disorders, trauma, environmental and stimulation deficiencies, congenital deficits, the effects of physical disability, and other factors.

Habilitation/Rehabilitation

Pediatric rehabilitation nursing is practiced in various settings with children who have disabilities that require habilitation and/or rehabilitation. These two approaches are described in the following way:

> Habilitation includes all the activities and interactions that enable an individual with a disability to develop new abilities to achieve his or her maximum potential, whereas rehabilitation is the relearning of previous skills, which often requires an adjustment to altered functional abilities and altered lifestyle (Burkett, 1989, p. 239).

For example, children who are born prematurely or with genetic disorders or fetal development affected by maternal disease, injury, or substance abuse need services that focus on habilitation to achieve new abilities. The child or adolescent who has been developing normally and receives an injury resulting in a disability experiences different consequences depending on the age and developmental level at which it occurred. For this child, there may be a period of relearning skills previously mastered and making alterations in activities based on functional limitations.

General Differences in Rehabilitation Between Children and Adults

Pediatric rehabilitation nursing is based on concepts and assumptions that describe the major differences between the rehabilitation of adults and of children and that provide the basis for services and direct the focus of care. Because children are always developing and maturing, those with disabilities receive some habilitative care as part of the developmental process. The rehabilitation services help to restore skills lost after an injury or disease, and habilitation continues as the child matures both physiologically and psychologically. Children require inclusion of the family, especially parents and siblings, as an integral part of the team.

The complexity of the long-term outlook for services and care is another area in which rehabilitation of children differs from that of adults. In seeking to restore lost function to adults, rehabilitation services are concerned with the consequences of adult development. In the rehabilitation of children, nurses must understand how the child can best function at the current age and stage and must project how the condition and its treatment will impact future development and achievement of age-appropriate abilities and relationships. Children require long-term follow-up to assist them and their families through developmental challenges as their growth and abilities progress.

The physiological differences between children and adults have tremendous implications for rehabilitative nursing care. Immaturity of systems and vital organs leads to difficulties in fluid maintenance, susceptibility to infection and disease, and fluctuations in homeostatic control mechanisms. The dosages of medications and the choices of treatments for conditions such as fractures are all different. Airway management, emergency procedures and equipment, and the size and the replacement schedule of assistive devices and durable medical goods, such as wheelchairs and braces, are also affected, depending on the stage of development. Differences in developmental level must be considered when formulating treatment goals, selecting teaching methods and approaches to the child and family, identifying safety considerations, and stating outcome expectations with regard to a maximal functional level of independence

COMMUNITY, HOME, AND SCHOOL ENVIRONMENTS
Community-Based Delivery Systems

Systems of service delivery are changing very rapidly and will continue to do so in the

TABLE 28–3 ■ NURSING PLAN—ALTERED GROWTH AND DEVELOPMENT

Goal

Recognize deviations as altered growth and development for age (specify) _____ .

Nursing Interventions and Teaching

Perform developmental screening tests appropriate for age (specify) _____ .
Determine the age/stage of growth and development in cooperation with other team members.
Determine preexisting and current knowledge of normal growth and development.
Review information with child/parents/caregivers.
Educate about age-related developmental tasks.
Assist parents/caregivers to understand and cope with developmental issues and "day-to-day" behaviors.

Goal

Maximize potential abilities (specify) _____ .

Nursing Interventions and Teaching

Maintain a safe, structured environment individualized to the child's needs.
Maintain stress precautions for premature infants.
Use a means of communication best suited to needs (specify) _____ .
Provide assistive devices to enhance skills (specify) _____ .
Assist with ADLs but allow as much self-care as possible.
Maximize opportunities for parents/caregivers to participate in care and develop feelings of competency.
Provide adequate rest periods and naps.

Goal

Master developmental tasks appropriate to age and capabilities (specify) _____ .

Nursing Intervention

Provide opportunities for appropriate play experiences.
Manipulate factors influencing mastery to enhance development.

Goal

Integrate age-appropriate skills and tasks (specify) _____ .

Nursing Interventions and Teaching

Integrate age-appropriate skills and tasks into daily activities.
Provide specific information to parents/caregivers.
Contact educational services for identification of the level of learning capabilities.
Help parents use age-appropriate toys and activities adapted to the child's needs.

Goal

Integrate therapeutic goals and activities into the daily routine (specify) _____ .

Nursing Interventions and Teaching

Help parents see and relate to the child as a child.
Select an intervention strategy appropriate to the stage and developmental task.

Expected Outcomes

Client performs motor, social, and/or expressive skills related to the age group and within the scope of present capabilities.
Client performs self-care activities appropriate to age.
Parents/caregivers verbalize their understanding of developmental deviation and the intervention plan.

Adapted from Cervizzi, K., & Edwards, P. (1994). *Care of the child and family.* Poster session presented at the annual meeting of the Association of Rehabilitation Nurses, September, 1994, Orlando, FL.
ADL, activity of daily living.

next decade. The community is viewed as the place where children and families have the right to live, play, and work, so services must be available to them at the local level. This facilitates the promotion of normal living patterns and focuses on the family as equal partners with health care providers in the care of children and adolescents with disabilities and chronic conditions.

The system should serve a broad spectrum of children and adolescents requiring care for health problems that extend beyond the routine and basic modalities. These services should be accessible, flexible, and comprehensive and include basic primary care, secondary specialized care, and highly specialized tertiary care, as well as other social and family support services. It is essential that the delivery system be family-centered, with programs and policies that are coordinated and provide emotional and financial support responsive to family needs. The developmental needs of children and families must be recognized, and appropriate supports must be incorporated into the system.

Comprehensive care requires a range of available and accessible services with linkages between community health professionals and medical centers providing tertiary care. These highly specialized, centralized services are an important component of care but must be linked to the systems providing primary care within the home and community. Components of the community-based service system include

- Early-intervention services
- Educational and vocational services
- Family support and social services
- Mental health services
- Recreation and other leisure activities

Also important are natural supports, or non–service system resources that the families of children and adolescents with disabilities and chronic conditions can draw from to help meet their needs. Examples are church groups, neighbors, children's play groups, public services not disability related, and recreational camps.

Home Environment

Advances in medicine, surgery, and technology have made it possible for children with serious disabilities and conditions to survive and be discharged to home once they are medically stable. This approach developed from a concern about the effects of a prolonged stay in an intensive care unit or acute hospital setting and is consistent with the philosophy of family-centered, community-based care to normalize the child's or adolescent's environment. As parents have assumed a more significant advocacy role for themselves and their children and the cost-effectiveness of home care has been demonstrated, despite the variety of needed services, the goal of returning the child to the family environment is being realized for even the most severely

involved children dependent on technological support.

As the coordinator of care for these children and families, the pediatric rehabilitation nurse assists the family in making an informed and responsible decision and plans for the safe transition to home. The planning process begins with the development of a comprehensive program including the following components:

- Family education
- Funding sources
- Equipment and supplies
- Nonfamily caregivers
- Therapy and rehabilitation services
- Home environment evaluation and modification
- Follow-up plans

An evaluation of the home environment should be made to assess areas essential to facilitating a child's safe and appropriate care at home. These include the residence (house, apartment, trailer) and the neighborhood. It is extremely important to evaluate potential barriers to self-care, the presence of necessary utilities (electricity, water, heat, telephone), and the overall safety and cleanliness of the environment.

A formal evaluation tool that could be used, depending on the age of the child, is the Home Observation for Measurement of the Environment (HOME). There are three inventories: infant/toddler, early childhood, and families of elementary children, each with different subsets. These focus on environmental factors that may foster development and identify certain aspects of the social, emotional, and cognitive supports available to the child in the home. "The HOME can be used in combination with other screening tools to assist parents to solve current problems and prevent development of other problems by providing anticipatory guidance for appropriate parenting" (Caldwell & Bradley, 1994, p. 2182).

A family education plan is another integral part of preparation and should include instruction in daily care; treatments; care, storage, and cleaning of equipment; nutrition and diet; safety; medications; anticipated developmental issues; and available resources (Burkett, 1989; Donar, 1988; Katz, 1992). If the child and the family need specific instruction to manage home care or activities of daily living (ADLs), the nursing diagnosis of "home maintenance management, impaired"

(Carpenito, 1995) may be identified and a plan established as shown in Table 28–4.

School Environment

Pediatric rehabilitation nurses understand the medical and nursing aspects of various disabilities and chronic conditions and the interventions necessary to improve function and enhance the quality of the learning environment for the child and adolescent. They are also aware of the legislation for children's services as shown in Table 28–5 and the provisions related to educational and support services and early intervention.

Beginning with the preschool years, health care issues are increasingly important as young children are introduced to educational services. The nurse, working in coordination with the family, caregivers, and teachers, can be instrumental in developing an individualized plan to meet the identified needs or address specific problems. This can be accomplished through the use of the Individualized Healthcare Plan, a combination of the Individualized Education Plan and a nursing care plan. This plan establishes the health services required by the child to maximize learning in the safest possible environment and includes information about the nature and characteristics of the child's disability or chronic condition. As part of the plan, explanation of the goals is included and recommendations regarding specific activities, techniques, and equipment to address the child's individual needs are incorporated.

As the child makes the transition into the formal school setting or reenters school after an injury or hospitalization, special considerations are undertaken to see that the child participates fully in the total educational process. A disruption in school attendance may occur because of appointments or transportation issues, so adjustments should be negotiated and planning individualized to accommodate the total situation. The child may be excluded from some activities because of unsuitability, so it is important to find creative adaptations or alternatives to allow for the fullest participation. School policies regarding giving medications and self-administration of medications must be understood, and school personnel need an awareness of medication effects and possible adverse reactions. Other needs in the educational setting for these children include special transportation both to and from school and on site; space for wheelchairs in the classroom and bathroom facilities; special equipment to meet the child's individual needs; and new fire drill and safety policies.

Pediatric rehabilitation nurses should initiate contact early in the discharge planning process to discuss the child's needs in school. The school nurse plays a vital role in the educational setting and can assist in the school placement process. Some children require tube feeding and catheterization when discharged, and a school visit by the pediatric rehabilitation nurse and other team members, often coupled with a home visit, "can help to reassure education and school health personnel that this child can be safely and optimally managed in the education setting" (Burkett, 1989, p. 251).

TABLE 28–4 ■ NURSING PLAN—HOME MAINTENANCE MANAGEMENT, IMPAIRED

Goals

Client is able to function in the home environment with the use of available resources and appropriate modification.
Obstacles to self-care in the home are identified.
Client has a environment that is clean, safe, and satisfying and facilitates optimal growth and development.

Interventions

Assess the level of physical functioning as well as cognitive and emotional functioning.
Reduce architectural barriers in as many areas as possible.
Identify learning needs, available support systems, and financial resources. Refer to community agencies.
Support the child or adolescent and the family in their ability to promote a safe environment that promotes and encourages independence. This involves the establishment of a realistic home care plan, including the identification and acquisition of necessary equipment, and structural modifications to facilitate care, considering availability, cost, and durability.
Discuss and plan with the family for opportunities to have respite from care. Allow caregivers opportunity to share problems and feelings.

Adapted from Edwards, P. A., & Posch, C. M. (1990). Impairment of the musculoskeletal system. In P. A. McCoy & W. L. Votroubek (Eds.), *Pediatric home care: A comprehensive approach* (pp. 182–189). Rockville, MD: Aspen.

TABLE 28-5 ■ LEGISLATION FOR CHILDREN'S SERVICES

1970	Developmental Disabilities Act (Pub. L. No. 91-517)	Addressed service gaps; planned for and monitored disability programs.
1970	Education of the Handicapped Act	Defined handicapped children and made funds available for them.
1975	Developmental Disabilities and Bill of Rights Act (Pub. L. No. 94-103)	Provided funds for developmental disabilities programs and special projects. Amendments in 1978 changed the definition of developmental disabilities and in 1984 provided a more functional approach. The 1987 amendment required studies of program effectiveness and customer satisfaction.
1975	Education for All Handicapped Children Act (Pub. L. No. 94-142)	Series of amendments to the 1970 act that required provision of educational and support services for all children older than 3 years, including individual education plans. Amendment in 1984 expanded services.
1981	Omnibus Reconciliation Act	Created Maternal Child Health block grants. Consolidated programs and added sudden infant death syndrome, lead-based poisoning prevention, and hemophilia treatment. Amendment in 1990 broadened state mandates and emphasized the development of community-based systems.
1986	Early Intervention Amendments (Pub. L. No. 99-457) to Education for All Handicapped Children Act	Mandated education and services for 3- to 5-year-olds with a developmental disability in the least restrictive environment. Created or expanded early intervention services for children from birth to 3 years under part H of the statute.
1990	Individuals with Disabilities Education Act (Pub. L. No. 101-476)	Amendment that changed the name of the act and added transition, assistive technology, rehabilitation counseling, and social work to the services that may be provided. Amendment in 1991 emphasized people-first language.

From Edwards, P. (1999). Legislation and public policy. In P. A. Edwards, D. L. Hertzberg, S. R. Hays, & N. M. Youngblood (Eds.), *Pediatric rehabilitation nursing* (p. 45). Philadelphia: W. B. Saunders.

HEALTH PROMOTION/HEALTH MANAGEMENT

Pediatric rehabilitation nurses provide an individualized continuum of care that includes three levels of prevention: primary, secondary, and tertiary. Primary prevention interventions are health promoting and include reducing the incidence of disease, protecting against problems, and encouraging healthy living patterns. Secondary prevention interventions are health supporting and include early identification of illness and prompt intervention and support of the development of new behaviors. Tertiary prevention interventions are health restoring and include surveillance to prevent complications and rehabilitation services to modify or minimize the impact of illness or disease and return the child to the family and community.

Primary interventions, which include the prevention of problems related to the disability or chronic illness, focus on preventing illnesses and educating the child and family about disease transmission and the importance of preventing problems by receiving immunizations and avoiding infectious contacts. Secondary interventions include the early recognition of illness or conditions that lead to disability, the management of the identified problems, and referral for additional services. Tertiary interventions include managing existing disabilities and conditions using ongoing assessments, evaluating progress in growth and development, managing specific procedures and treatments, teaching about and monitoring the administration of medications, and being involved in other areas that evolve from the needs of the individual child and family (Russell & Free, 1994). It is important to remember that children and adolescents have the normal preventive care needs even though they have a disability or chronic condition.

Assessment and Screening

Pediatric rehabilitation nursing includes screening for developmental disabilities as a component of child care and assisting the family to obtain comprehensive assessment and treatment when problems are detected. "Developmental screening of infants aims primarily at detecting sensory deficits and major developmental handicaps associated with central nervous system dysfunction. . . . Other developmental disabilities screened for in the first year of life include cerebral palsy and moderate to severe mental retardation. The nurse can identify infants who are at high risk and monitor the early development of these infants closely" (Marquis, 1991, p. 134).

Children and adolescents with disabilities and chronic conditions should be assessed at regular intervals along the health care and developmental continuums. Assessments can be done in a variety of settings: hospitals, rehabilitation facilities, ambulatory care services, home, preschool, or school. Every pediatric rehabilitation nurse should use assessment, a critical element in the nursing process, as the basis for identifying expected outcomes and planning therapeutic interventions. Assessment should be holistic, encompassing all aspects of the child's life, including the family system; the active involvement of the parents and caregivers in assessment and planning is essential. The process can include interviewing, observation, and/or structuring of a setting. The nurse should enable parents to convey information comfortably and create a climate in which emotions such as anxiety, guilt, or anger can be expressed. Listening to parents and being sensitive to both their spoken and unspoken needs and problems can be a major guide for future interactions with the family and a source of information about the child. Observation, especially of behavior at play and in interactions with others, provides information about the child's growth and development and social skills. The setting in which screening or assessment takes place should be informal and free from stress and should include observations of the parent-child interactions (Meisels & Provence, 1989).

The process and procedures for screening and assessment of children can take many forms: developmental and health screening, diagnostic assessment, and individual program planning. Developmental and health screening involve activities that identify children at high risk for delayed or abnormal development. Diagnostic assessments are used to determine the underlying nature of the delay in development and its cause. From this information intervention strategies are then proposed and implemented. Assessments for individual program planning "are criterion-referenced, focusing on a child's mastery of skills or tasks rather than the child's relative standing in comparison to some normative group" (Meisels & Provence, 1989, p. 14).

Functional Assessment Instruments for Children

"Functional assessment is an effort to systematically describe and measure a child's abilities and limitations when performing the activities of daily living. With this information, professionals can plan and assess rehabilitative and habilitative care. Because the plan of care to promote functional independence evolves directly from the assessment, it is imperative that the tool effectively defines and measures the relevant construct, that is, function rather than development" (McCabe & Granger, 1990, p. 120). This assessment can be accomplished through direct objective testing, review of records, interviews with parents and caregivers, and naturalistic behavioral observations.

The Pediatric Evaluation of Disability Inventory "incorporates four levels of impairment, functional limitations, disability and social role performance as well as developmental and contextual influences" (Coster & Haley, 1992, p. 21) and is appropriate for ages 6 months to 7 years. It includes social outcome measures, ADLs, caregiver assistance, and required modifications. Functional skills content is divided into self-care, mobility, and social function, as shown in Table 28–6. These have broad utility and applicability across home and school contexts for infants and young children. "It is designed to identify the child's functional ability along three scales: (1) typical functional skill level; (2) modifications or adaptive equipment used (i.e., braces, motorized wheelchair); and (3) physical assistance required of the caregiver" (Feldman, Haley, & Coryell, 1990, p. 603). These are depicted in Table 28–7, with the specific rating criteria for each of the measurement scales. This is a useful supplement to other scales because it relates the child's abilities to functional performance. The Pediatric Evaluation of Disability Inventory provides an evaluation tool for pediatric rehabilitation pro-

TABLE 28–6 ■ FUNCTIONAL SKILLS CONTENT OF THE PEDIATRIC EVALUATION OF DISABILITY INVENTORY

Self-Care Domain	Mobility Domain	Social Function Domain
Types of food textures eaten	Toilet transfers	Comprehension of word meanings
Use of utensils	Chair or wheelchair transfers	Comprehension of complex sentences
Use of drinking containers	Car transfers	Functional use of expressive
Tooth brushing	Bed mobility and transfers	communication
Hair brushing	Tub transfers	Complexity of expressive
Nose care	Method of indoor locomotion	communication
Hand washing	Distance or speed indoors	Problem resolution
Washing body and face	Pulling or carrying of objects	Social interactive play
Putting on and removing pullover or	Method of outdoor locomotion	Peer interactions
front-opening garments	Distance or speed outdoors	Self-information
Use of fasteners	Walking on outdoor surfaces	Time orientation
Putting on and removing pants	Walking up stairs	Performance of household chores
Putting on and removing shoes and	Walking down stairs	Self-protection skills
socks		Community function
Performance of toileting tasks		
Management of bladder		
Management of bowel		

Adapted from Haley, S., Coster, W., Ludlow, L., Holtiwanger, J., and Andrellos, P. (1992). *Pediatric Evaluation of Disability Inventory (PEDI) version 1.0 development, standardization and administration manual* (p. 13). Boston: New England Medical Center Hospital.

grams, therapy services, school programs, and community agencies and a uniform mechanism for documenting functional ability for outcome evaluation research and for monitoring change in function over time.

The Functional Independence Measure for Children was developed for use with children aged 6 months to 7 years but can be used for older children under certain circumstances if their condition limits certain behaviors. It is similar to the Functional Independence Measure used for adults, but the components reflect the age-related functional differences seen in children, and it is designed to measure the severity of the disability in relation to the burden of care. It uses a seven-level scale to represent differences in behavior, ranging from 7, independent, to 1, maximal dependence. Eighteen subsets represent six separate domains: self-care, sphincter control, mobility, locomotion, communication, and social cognition. It measures what the child actually does and the type and amount of assistance needed. Scoring can be done by any trained clinician by direct observation or parent report, but the developmental level should be kept in mind to facilitate administration (Lord, Taggart, & Molnar, 1991). Nurses in pediatric rehabilitation settings have adapted its components for use in the documentation of admission assessment and reassessment; in daily patient classification

TABLE 28–7 ■ RATING CRITERIA FOR THE THREE TYPES OF MEASUREMENT SCALES

Part I: Functional Skills	Part II: Caregiver Assistance	Part III: Modifications
197 discrete items of functional skills	20 complex functional activities	20 complex functional activities
Self-care, mobility, social function	Self-care, mobility, social function	Self-care, mobility, social function
0 = unable, or limited in capability, to perform an item in most situations	5 = independent	N = no modifications
1 = capable of performing an item in most situations, or the item has previously been mastered and functional skills have progressed beyond this level	4 = supervise/prompt/monitor	C = child-oriented (nonspecialized)
	3 = minimal assistance	R = rehabilitation equipment
	2 = moderate assistance	E = extensive modifications
	1 = maximal assistance	
	0 = total assistance	

From Haley, S., Coster, W., Ludlow, L., Holtiwanger, J., & Andrellos, P. (1992). *Pediatric Evaluation of Disability Inventory (PEDI) version 1.0 development, standardization and administration manual* (p. 16). Boston: New England Medical Center Hospitals.

and outcome evaluation at both discharge and follow-up; and to measure changes in function over time.

CARE RELATED TO ALTERATIONS IN HEALTH DUE TO DISABILITY AND CHRONIC ILLNESS

Assessment of Family Needs

The pediatric rehabilitation nurse uses the nursing process to assist the family of a child or adolescent with a disability or chronic condition. This begins with the assessment of family structure, relationships, cultural background, and values and beliefs. The problems vary depending on the needs of the family, but certain issues must be considered. Education of the family is of paramount importance so that the members understand the child's condition, understand its short- and long-term implications, and are equipped to make decisions about care needs and treatment goals and plans. Support systems are needed to maintain family strengths and should be identified within the nuclear and extended families and in the natural supports in the community. Parents should also develop relationships with other parents with similar issues or join more formalized groups to obtain support and decrease feelings of isolation. If time away from the child or adolescent can help in relieving stress and preserve psychological well-being, then parents should also consider respite care services in the home or in residential or other types of facilities.

Plans should be initiated to provide assistance, support, and guidance if, in the interactions with the family, the nurse identifies any of the following nursing issues (Carpenito, 1995):

- *Caregiver role strain:* A caregiver is experiencing physical, emotional, social, or financial stressors.
- *Ineffective family coping:* A supportive individual is providing insufficient assistance or encouragement.
- *Parental role conflict:* A parent experiences a change in role because of external factors.
- *Altered family processes:* Previous effective functioning is challenged by stressors.

Culturally Competent Care.   Each child and family is a unique combination of personal characteristics, culture, coping mechanisms, and adaptation skills. Key psychosocial factors determine their success in adapting to and coping with the ongoing life changes in the presence of the disability. The culture and the degree of assimilation into the dominant culture are key factors in adaptation and adjustment to disability. The pediatric rehabilitation nurse must develop cultural competence, accept differences in beliefs and practices, and be sensitive to the needs of children and families from different cultural backgrounds.

Disturbances in Functional Health Patterns

Health and development are intertwined, and a child's state of health influences the ability to participate in and benefit from rehabilitation. The child or adolescent with a disability or chronic condition may have significant disturbances in functional health patterns due to various physiological factors.

Nutritional Needs.   Some conditions place tremendous metabolic and nutritional demands on the body, and the child may be unable to take in enough nutrients to meet energy needs. This significantly affects the child's health, growth, development, and ability to participate in various activities. Analysis of nutrition factors and specific interventions such as supplemental feeding may be necessary to maintain life and facilitate rehabilitation. Table 28–8 outlines a nursing plan for a child receiving less nutrition than body requirements. This problem may be caused by sucking difficulties, impaired swallowing, ineffective feeding patterns, decreased absorption of nutrients, dietary restrictions, fatigue, and other factors. This plan should be individualized to address the specific problems of a child or an adolescent and could also be incorporated into an overall plan of care. An example is provided in the following case study.

▪ CASE STUDY

Jamie is a 2-year-old born with a tracheoesophageal fistula that required several surgical procedures. His nutrition has been provided through gastrostomy feedings, and although he recovered well after the surgical repair, he needed to be taught to feed orally. He was admitted to the pediatric rehabilitation unit for a comprehensive, individualized, highly structured feeding program, implemented by a team consisting of the nurse,

TABLE 28-8 ■ NURSING PLAN—ALTERED NUTRITION: LESS THAN BODY REQUIREMENTS

Goal

Increase oral intake to optimal levels (specify) _____ .

Interventions/Teaching

Determine adequate and realistic caloric requirements. Weigh at least weekly to implement alternative nutrition if needed.
Offer frequent small meals with foods high in calories.
Encourage adequate fluid intake.
Encourage self-feeding with adapted utensils (built-up grips, angled spoons), special cups for drinking, and other devices.
Use and teach safe feeding techniques to promote nutrition and prevent aspiration.
Use appropriate utensils (Teflon-coated spoon), position properly with head upright, and use special adapted seating as required.
Observe the caregivers' ability to feed, including the preparation of equipment and food, positioning of the child. Make additional observations if the child is being fed by tube (nasogastric or gastrostomy) and teach correct techniques.
Note the behavior, response, and tolerance of the dietary regimen. Provide adequate diet teaching, emphasizing the need for food with a high fiber content to facilitate normal elimination.
Note the condition of the teeth and compliance and/or ability to provide an effective oral hygiene program to include flossing and brushing as well as avoidance of cariogenic foods.

Expected Outcomes

Client maintains body weight in relation to the metabolic need while maintaining optimum health.
Client attains desirable body weight with optimum health.

Adapted from Edwards, P. A., & Posch, C. M. (1990). Impairment of the musculoskeletal system. In P. A. McCoy & W. L. Votroubek (Eds.), *Pediatric home care: A comprehensive approach* (pp. 182–189). Rockville, MD: Aspen.

---

dietitian, speech-language pathologist, occupational therapist, social worker, and physician. Initially he refused to put anything in his mouth, even his fingers, and pulled away crying each time an attempt was made at feeding. A behavior modification plan combined with fun activities was developed, and he slowly began to tolerate oral stimulation and then various foods with different tastes and textures. His parents were involved in all aspects of the program, and the pediatric rehabilitation nurse taught and reinforced various components of the plan. They continued it after his discharge, and he is growing into a healthy preschooler and eating normally. ■

Children with disabilities or chronic conditions may have dysfunctions of the oropharynx including persistent tongue thrust, weak or absent suck, swallowing spasms, problems with tongue control, and hyperactive bite and gag reflexes. Proper positioning during feeding, with the head and back upright and arms and feet supported, is essential (Betz, Hunsberger, & Wright, 1994).

Some common conditions that contribute to poor feeding are gastroesophageal reflux, respiratory compromise, constipation, and child responsiveness. In gastroesophageal reflux, stomach contents flow backward into the esophagus, resulting in vomiting, coughing, and respiratory symptoms. Management of gastroesophageal reflux includes (Eicher & Kerwin, 1996)

- Changes in nutrition—formula type, consistency, and volume
- Positioning
- Pharmacological management
- Alternative routes
- Surgery—gastrostomy, gastrojejunostomy, fundoplication

Physical Mobility. The ability to move and explore the environment is crucial to development and provides the necessary basis from which children begin to learn about the world and their role in it. When physical mobility is impaired because of injury, disease, treatment-related devices, strength, or fatigue, specific activities and interventions should be initiated to maximize the possibilities for interaction with the environment. Suggested interventions and teaching are found in Table 28–9.

Self-Care Activities. The earliest learned skills involve meeting basic needs, such as eating, comfort, and protection. These may be delayed or lacking in the child with a disability or chronic condition. The pediatric rehabilitation nurse should work with parents to help them accurately read and interpret the child's cues and determine the right amount of assistance that stimulates the development

TABLE 28–9 ■ NURSING PLAN—IMPAIRED PHYSICAL MOBILITY

Goals

Demonstrate measures that increase mobility and are safe.
Use adaptive devices appropriately to increase mobility.

Intervention/Teaching

Discuss the purposes of mobility, the prevention of disuse phenomena, stimulation and motivation, and the ability to complete activities of daily living.
Promote activity, assist with position changes, and teach correct positioning and therapeutic handling.
Meet the child's safety needs and minimize the potential for injury by providing supervised ambulation, helmets, seat belts, correctly fitting wheelchairs with appropriate safety features, and devices for positioning.
Use assistive devices such as orthoses, splints, and braces to facilitate the protection and stimulation of weak muscles, the relaxation of tight muscles, joint support, functional positioning, and the prevention of contractures.
Establish a home or recreational exercise program.
Teach proper positioning to prevent complications and encourage compliance with the treatment program to delay or prevent complications.
Discuss, teach, and reinforce information about complications with caregivers.

Expected Outcomes

Client maintains independent movement within the environment to the fullest extent possible.
Parents recognize complications of immobility and prevent or treat them.
Client participates in activities within limitations and minimizes the potential for injury.

Adapted from Edwards, P. A., & Posch, C. M. (1990). Impairment of the musculoskeletal system. In P. A. McCoy & W. L. Votroubek (Eds.), *Pediatric home care: A comprehensive approach* (pp. 182–189). Rockville, MD: Aspen.

of necessary self-care skills. Any or all of the following interventions to achieve self-care to the fullest extent possible for the child or adolescent may be needed (Edwards & Posch, 1990, p. 186):

- Identifying barriers and assisting in the provision of necessary adaptations and assistive devices to facilitate self-care activities, and helping with the selection and modification of clothing
- Reviewing/reinforcing instructions from the interdisciplinary team; continually evaluating the care plan with the child and/or family to identify progress and needed modifications
- Continually assessing and evaluating the potential for self-care capabilities and activities and changing daily routines as indicated
- Assessing the child and family response to the level of and/or changes in functioning; providing support and referral to appropriate resources as needed

Skin Alteration. For a variety of reasons—a lack of sensation, immobility, circulatory impairment, and altered nutrition—children and adolescents with disabilities and chronic conditions are at higher risk for skin alterations and must be taught preventive measures. Adequate inspection of the skin, especially bony prominences, is an essential component of daily preventive care, and initiation of treatment immediately on identification of a problem is essential. Table 28–10 outlines a nursing plan if there is a risk for impaired skin integrity.

Bowel and Bladder Function. Children should be on a consistent bladder and bowel program by the time they begin school. The child should be thoroughly evaluated and a program developed that is realistic for the family and that establishes a regular pattern of functioning. Bladder management may be accomplished by

- *Timed programs:* Placing the child on the toilet at scheduled times to encourage urination and then providing positive reinforcement for the desired response
- *Intermittent catheterization:* Inserting a clean or sterile catheter into the bladder four to six times a day to empty it and prevent urinary retention
- *Surgical management:* Artificial urinary sphincter, continent vesicostomy, or ileal conduit

Regardless of the program, the child and family must be taught about the risk of urinary tract infection and how to recognize the signs and symptoms. A urinary tract infection should be thoroughly and promptly treated.

Establishing a regular bowel evacuation program is also essential. The most common

TABLE 28–10 ■ NURSING PLAN—RISK FOR IMPAIRED SKIN INTEGRITY

Goals	Nursing Interventions/Teaching
Identify individual risk factors.	Determine the factors that will impair skin integrity and teach elements of early detection of skin changes and pressure ulcer prevention.
	Understand the child/adolescent/family interpretation of the importance of measures to maintain skin integrity.
Demonstrate behaviors to minimize risk.	Provide optimal nutrition with supplements high in protein as needed.
	Teach hygiene, safety, skin care, and skin inspection techniques, e.g., the use of a mirror to inspect certain areas; teach safety factors for the use of equipment and appliances.
	Reinforce elements of pressure ulcer prevention, e.g., schedule for skin inspection; repositioning schedule; proper fit of clothing; using pushups or a backward tilt if in a wheelchair; and a proper seating system.
	Use appropriate devices such as sheepskin, special wheelchair pads, and mattresses.

Expected Outcomes

Behaviors to prevent skin breakdown are demonstrated by child and/or family. Skin integrity is maintained.

Modified from Edwards, P. (1999). Traumatic injuries. In P. A. Edwards, D. L. Hertzberg, S. R. Hays, & N. M. Youngblood (Eds.), *Pediatric rehabilitation nursing* (p. 514). Philadelphia: W. B. Saunders.

times for toileting are morning and evening, usually after a meal. Interventions to include are (Edwards & Posch, 1990, p. 186)

- Assessing usual or current pattern of elimination
- Evaluating dietary intake
- Determining the use of medications, enemas, or natural laxatives
- Promoting normalization of bowel function with the use of a bowel program including a diet high in fiber and bulk; an adequate amount and type of fluid intake; activity and exercise as tolerated; stool softeners or laxatives; privacy and scheduled times for defecation; and a normal and comfortable position

Communication. Children with disabilities or chronic conditions may have problems in communication—sending, receiving, or processing information. The pediatric rehabilitation nurse must be skilled in assessing these areas and developing strategies so that the child can begin communication interventions early, preventing maladaptive behaviors. Selected strategies for promoting communication include (Morse & Colatarci, 1994)

- Facilitating the use of symbols and educating caregivers to treat all behaviors as language

- Making and using communication boards and other devices
- Using strategies that are interactive and developmentally appropriate
- Providing the use of adapted toys and equipment
- Integrating augmentative and assistive communication devices into the home, school, and community
- Looking at positioning, movement, and mobility to support communication
- Expanding social communication to beyond the family

Vision and Hearing. Children or adolescents with a sensory or perceptual alteration, such as a vision or hearing impairment, need assistance in improving their ability to interact with the environment and respond to it adaptively. Their level of functioning should be periodically assessed through vision and hearing screening, and appropriate interventions should be initiated. Opportunities for self-initiated activities, such as specially adapted toys, should be provided, or stimuli should be individually tailored for the infant or child. The stimuli should present a challenge but within the scope of the child's ability and must capture the child's attention to elicit a response. Environmental safety aspects and the use of assistive devices, including hearing aids and communication devices to promote the acquisition of language skills and/or effective communication patterns, should be taught to family members and caregivers (Edwards & Posch, 1990).

Play. Play is the work of the child and should be integrated into any nursing plan of care. Play and recreational activities vary with the developmental level and abilities of children or adolescents, but these are an essential component of their growth and adaptation in home, school, and community environments. Through play, children gain information about their world, practice new skills, experiment with different roles, and explore options and choices. Children or adolescents with a disability or chronic condition "are often in need of greater and more intense, enriched or varied experiences available through play than other children, but their ability to initiate or sustain play independently may be compromised" (Murphey, 1996, p. 606). Time in the child's day may be filled with physical and medical care and remedial developmental activities, but some time should also be set aside for pleasurable play experiences and opportunities for success in various activities. For the child or adolescent with a physical disability, this may necessitate making special adaptations to play experiences such as modifying the rules, relationships, or environment. Some specific examples are (Murphey, 1996)

- Using puzzles with large pieces and placing them on a dark background
- Attaching play materials, such as a dollhouse, to a firm surface like a table or lapboard
- Making push buttons larger or using plate switches for activating various toys
- Matching a game to the child's or adolescent's ability; computer games appeal to many children
- Adapting instruments and tape or compact disc players and assisting with selection of music
- Demonstrating activities and using symbols and verbal cues

Additional resources for play and recreational activities include toy libraries, athletic activities such as Special Olympics and adaptive sports, and groups such as Girl or Boy Scouts. Some playgrounds and camps have special adaptations, most cultural institutions have special programs, and vacation destinations such as Disney World offer accessibility and safety for leisure activities.

INTERVENTIONS IN COMMON CHRONIC CONDITIONS AFFECTING CHILDREN

The role of the pediatric rehabilitation nurse differs in various settings and with different disabilities or chronic conditions. In this section, the nursing assessment and care of children with three common conditions—bronchopulmonary dysplasia, cerebral palsy, and muscular dystrophy—are discussed. Information previously provided in this chapter and specific to these conditions can also be applied to the care of children and adolescents with similar problems and conditions.

Bronchopulmonary Dysplasia

Bronchopulmonary dysplasia (BPD) is a chronic lung disease that occurs most commonly in babies who have had respiratory problems in the first few days after birth. It is thought to be caused by prolonged oxygen therapy administered by positive-pressure respirators for the treatment of respiratory distress syndrome. BPD is seen primarily in premature infants who have had respiratory distress syndrome and who require oxygen and mechanical ventilation or continuous positive airway pressure to manage their respiratory distress and may also occasionally occur after pneumonia, meconium aspiration syndrome, tracheoesophageal fistula, and congenital heart disease. Eighty percent of BPD infants have a birth weight of 1500 g or less and a gestational age of 32 weeks or less. BPD is diagnosed in infants older than 4 weeks who have persistent lung disease requiring continual supplemental oxygen and who have had abnormal chest radiographs. Symptoms include tachypnea, dyspnea, hypoxemia, and hypercapnia.

Treatment is supportive and includes supplemental oxygen until the therapy goal of continued growth of healthy lung tissue has compensated for the damaged areas. Treatment also includes optimizing nutrition, restricting fluids, and oxygenation. Bronchodilator medications such as theophylline and metaproterenol are often used to open the airways of the lungs by relaxing the muscles around the airways. Anti-inflammatory medications are used long term to reduce airway swelling in more severely ill babies whose wheezing and respiratory distress is occasionally difficult to control with bronchodilators only. Diuretics may also be used in conjunction with this therapy.

BPD infants often require supplemental oxygen continuously to avoid complications, such as heart failure or poor growth and development. Oxygen therapy is essential to decrease the work of breathing, maximize nutrition, and prevent pulmonary hypertension or hasten its resolution. These infants often need hospitalization for respiratory infections because their breathing status and supplemental oxygen requirements change rapidly even with minor infections.

When home care is being considered, one should evaluate the following (Hunsberger & Feenan, 1994):

- *Weight gain:* The weight gain should be steady, and the infant should weigh more than 2 kg.
- *Complexity of care:* The frequency of feedings and the caregivers' ability to feed the infant; number and types of medications; and need for suctioning and chest physical therapy should be considered.
- *Supplemental oxygen requirements during caregiving, feeding, and sleep:* Oximetry with maintenance of oxygen levels at 92% is recommended.

Specifically, the recommended criteria for discharge on low-flow oxygen include the following (Hunsberger & Feenan, 1994, p. 1184):

- Postconceptual age greater than 41 weeks
- Weight above 2000 g and an otherwise medically stable condition
- Absence of any change in FiO_2 or medications (diuretics) during the few days before discharge
- Absence of high pulmonary arterial blood pressure
- Acceptance by parents
- Community support system (physician and community health nurse)
- Satisfactory home assessment by a health care professional
- Presence of more than one adult in the home

Figures 28–1 and 28–2 show the use of the cannula for low-flow oxygen therapy in an infant and a 4-year-old child. A cap is used for the older child to secure the cannula, which is positioned below the nares in both pictures.

The pediatric rehabilitation nurse as the coordinator of care for the child and family interacts in a variety of settings with other

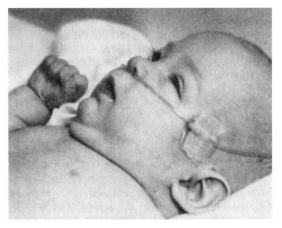

FIGURE 28–1
Use of cannula for low-flow oxygen in an infant. (From Betz, C. L., Hunsberger, H., & Wright, S. [1994]. *Family-centered nursing care* [2nd ed.]. Philadelphia: W. B. Saunders.)

nurses and health professionals. The critical-thinking skills inherent in the nursing process are essential in the provision of quality care that meets the needs of the child and family and obtains desired outcomes. Many nursing

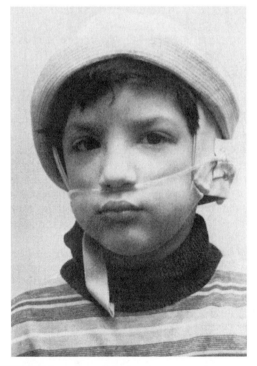

FIGURE 28–2
Use of cannula for low-flow oxygen in an older child. (From Betz, C. L., Hunsberger, H., & Wright, S. [1994]. *Family-centered nursing care* [2nd ed.]. Philadelphia: W. B. Saunders.)

diagnostic statements and collaborative problems are applicable to the complex care of children with BPD. Age, the developmental level, and associated problems greatly affect the priorities in nursing assessment.

A health history and nursing and functional assessment are essential. They focus on prenatal and birth information and complications; a systems review including current problems and preexisting conditions; a list of medications and known allergies; and a personal history focusing on diet, sleep patterns, activity, and parents' psychosocial issues. These are important initial elements in determining the needs and problems of the child and family. Assessment of the infant's respiratory status is important, and changes in the infant's clinical presentation are evaluated in relation to other diagnostic findings, such as chest radiographs and blood gas levels.

Nursing assessment must focus on the following areas:

- *Respiratory:* Vital signs, respirations, and heart rate; breathing pattern; signs of respiratory distress and infection; reaction to stress, exercise, and activity
- *General:* Fatigue; feeding difficulties; family response to child (e.g., overprotection); family support systems; sleep and rest patterns; caregiver knowledge about the condition and treatment regimen
- *Nutrition:* Caloric and fluid intake
- *Visual impairment*
- *Growth and development:* Progression in developmental tasks

After a thorough, individualized assessment of the child and family, a list of problems is developed and nursing diagnoses and a plan of nursing care identified. The main problems that might be identified depend on the age of the child, the severity of the condition, and identified issues that are specific to the nurses' clinical practice setting (e.g., rehabilitation unit, day care, home). Some possible nursing problems and interventions are outlined in Table 28–11. The plan that is developed must be specifically tailored to the age, abilities, and needs of the child and family.

The overall expected outcomes for the child include

- Adequate oxygenation
- Gradual growth with improved respiratory status and progression through developmental milestones as appropriate

- Freedom from oral feeding aversions
- Appropriate ratio of fluid intake and urine output
- Freedom from signs of respiratory distress
- No untoward side effects from diuretics or electrolyte supplements
- Clear skin; no rashes, breakdown, or infection

The overall expected outcomes for the family include

- Family verbalizes and demonstrates understanding of the disease process and the treatment regimen
- Family demonstrates decreased anxiety and stress, increased ability to care for the child, and a trusting relationship with care providers
- Family uses healthy, appropriate coping mechanisms
- Mealtime is a positive experience for the child and family

An interdisciplinary team composed of nurses; physicians; nutritionists; social workers; respiratory, physical, and occupational therapists; and speech-language pathologists is involved with the infant and family beginning with the initial diagnosis and continuing through the various levels of interventions. For home care and management of the child, family-centered teaching, as outlined in Table 28–12, is very important. This includes specific information on maintaining fluid and nutritional balance, preventing infection, maintaining oxygenation, and encouraging family coping and the use of support systems.

Cerebral Palsy

The most frequent childhood disability is cerebral palsy, a term used to describe a nonprogressive abnormality of muscle coordination, balance, and purposeful movement caused at some time during the child's development by one of the conditions in Table 28–13. The immature brain is damaged in some way, and the specific area is associated with different clinical signs. The main manifestation is motor dysfunction, especially tone changes and difficulty with balance, coordination, and purposeful movement.

The terms used to describe cerebral palsy refer to extremity involvement as follows:

- *Monoplegia:* One extremity
- *Diplegia:* Lower extremities
- *Hemiplegia:* Upper and lower extremities on the same side
- *Quadriplegia:* All four extremities

TABLE 28–11 ■ ACTUAL OR POTENTIAL PROBLEMS AND NURSING INTERVENTIONS, BRONCHOPULMONARY DYSPLASIA

Problems	Nursing Interventions
Impaired gas exchange	Carefully assess for signs of respiratory distress; closely monitor blood gases; maintain body temperature; oxygen may need to be increased during stress (feeding, crying, suctioning, procedures).
Risk for infection	Teach the parents to avoid proximity with known respiratory infections; seek early treatment for signs of respiratory distress; consider influenza vaccinations.
Altered nutrition: less than body requirements	Monitor the caloric intake; balance the calorie and fluid intake and feeding behaviors; feeding difficulties and intolerances may require specific interventions.
Fluid volume excess	Monitor the fluid intake and output; weigh the child daily; use the lowest volume of fluids to meet the caloric requirements; assess for respiratory changes indicating difficulty and possible pulmonary edema.
Activity intolerance related to altered cardiac output	Exercise and stress are poorly tolerated; organize care and procedures to reduce interruptions to sleep and rest.
Altered growth and development	Encourage the parents to touch, hold, and talk to the infant; discuss the effects of bronchopulmonary dysplasia on growth and development and the importance of adequate nutrition.
Ineffective family coping: compromised	Involve the parents in care early; provide ongoing teaching about the nature of the problem; assess the parents' ability to care for the child and their level of comfort.
Impaired home maintenance management	Inform the parents about their infant and his or her care needs; teach the assessment of growth and weight; encourage the voicing of concerns about growth and development, management, and stresses on family functioning.

A child with mild cerebral palsy may have some muscle spasticity and appear to be clumsy but have no significant impairments and require very little treatment. Children with a more severe form may have speech and feeding problems, seizures, and learning disability and in some cases immobility, vision and hearing impairments, and mental retardation. Associated problems include spasticity as well as joint contractures, hip dislocation, and orthopedic deformities. Every child is different, and the assessment, which is a continuous process, needs to be highly individualized and reflect the child's age, degree of involvement, and additional problems.

Preventive measures include good maternal health care during childbearing years, especially control of diabetes, anemia, and high blood pressure; immunizations; proper nutrition; avoiding unnecessary drugs, medications, and radiographs; and protecting infants and toddlers from injuries.

The diagnosis is made based on a history indicating high risk stemming from the previously mentioned causes of cerebral palsy; physical signs and symptoms including tone and reflex abnormalities, abnormal posture, and abnormal gait; abnormalities in vision, communication, and swallowing; persistence of primitive reflexes (startle, tonic neck, parachute); and delayed development and abnormal motor behavior. Early diagnosis and intervention is important so that symptoms can be treated and complications prevented. Referral to appropriate services for any infant or child suspected of having neurological abnormalities should be the expected practice.

Although cerebral palsy is nonprogressive, physical deformities and functional limitations may occur because of persistent postural reflexes and abnormal tone. Although the neurological condition is stable, there may be additional problems and symptoms as the child grows and develops. The ultimate level of function and independence varies with the severity of associated conditions and deficits in motor control. "Sitting by the age of 2 years is a good prognostic sign for walking. Eventual independence depends on intellect, upper extremity function and availability of appropriate assistive devices" (Molnar et al., 1989, p. S167).

An interdisciplinary approach to the care of the child and family should include collaboration of many areas: nursing, physical therapy, occupational therapy, medicine, nutrition, social work, speech therapy, orthotics,

TABLE 28–12 ■ FAMILY-CENTERED TEACHING: HOME CARE MANAGEMENT OF CHILD WITH BRONCHOPULMONARY DYSPLASIA

Maintaining Fluid and Nutritional Balance

Oxygen administration during feeding is usually necessary because of the work of breathing and sucking.

Infants with cardiac involvement may require fluid restriction.

Sometimes the use of medium-chain triglycerides or 24- or 30-cal/oz formulas is required to meet caloric needs for growth.

Occasional gavage feedings may be necessary if the baby is especially tired; therefore, parents may need to learn this type of feeding.

Gastrostomy tube may be necessary if adequate weight gain is not accomplished with oral or gavage methods.

Preventing Infection

The usual preventive measures appropriate for a child with a chronic respiratory problem must be stressed: the avoidance of smoking near the infant, the avoidance of close proximity with those known to have a respiratory infection, and early treatment of signs of respiratory illness.

Careful feeding techniques to avoid aspiration are taught to parents as a way to reduce the risk of infection.

Chest physical therapy and suctioning need to be increased for the removal of secretions from the lungs to prevent lower respiratory infections.

Bronchodilators (by inhalation) for wheezing may be required, especially during respiratory infections. Parents must be helped to secure the equipment from a supply company and be taught its proper administration.

Maintaining Oxygenation

The oxygen-dependent infant or child usually can tolerate a cannula for oxygen administration. It can be taped to a stoma-adhesive patch. This needs to be changed only once a week and protects the skin. A nasopharyngeal catheter is used for an oxygen concentration of 35% or greater.

Oxygen for home care is supplied by concentrates, tanks, or liquid oxygen systems. Of these, the concentrates seem to be preferred because no tank changing is necessary. However, the availability of liquid oxygen enables portability.

Financial considerations may limit availability, as equipment is very costly.

Chest physical therapy and suctioning may be required three to four times a day. Parents must have had supervised practice and demonstrate the necessary skills.

Maintaining Family Coping

If there is a lack of an identified support system, the family should be encouraged to find a few support people to help them during this period of adjustment.

The interruption of family life may sometimes lead to marital stress. A competent baby sitter should be taught how to care for the infant to allow parents to have time together and to themselves.

Parents should have an understanding about the illness, recognizing that respiratory infections may require readmission to the hospital, but this does not mean they have failed.

From Hunsberger, M., & Feenan, L. (1994). Altered respiratory function. In C. Betz, M. Hunsberger, & S. Wright (Eds.), *Family-centered nursing care of children* (2nd ed., p. 1257). Philadelphia: W. B. Saunders.

and various support systems (dental, vision). The goal of the team is to recognize the child's intellectual and physical abilities and to coordinate a plan of care that maximizes the child's potential and includes management of motor deficits, parent education and training, and provision of developmentally appropriate experiences to enrich the child's quality of life.

The pediatric rehabilitation nurse functions in many settings as the coordinator of care and enables the child and family to achieve independence and lead normal lives. Management involves all aspects of physical, mental, social, and emotional growth and development and focuses on specific problems such as alterations in skin integrity, elimination, and nutrition. Corrective positioning and therapeutic handling techniques are important components of the plan of care.

Expectations for the child and family include

TABLE 28–13 ■ CAUSES OF CEREBRAL PALSY

Prenatal	Perinatal	Postnatal
Prenatal trauma	Premature birth	Chemical poisoning
Viral infection	Birth trauma	Trauma: falls, motor vehicle
Poor health and diet	Prolonged or precipitous labor	accidents, swimming
Blood incompatibilities	Interference with the	Child abuse
	umbilical cord	Infections (meningitis,
	Untreated jaundice	encephalitis)
	Anoxia	

- Maximal independence in mobility, self-care, and communication
- Minimal effects from associated conditions such as spasticity, seizures, and contractures
- A supportive environment including education, psychosocial systems, and coordination of resources

Significant advances in surgical procedures to release contractures and correct deformities and assistive technology have contributed to improving the child's mobility, communication, and control of the environment. Available programs and services include special education, vocational training, leisure activities, transportation, and independent living arrangements that allow access to and participation in the home, school, and community environments.

As the coordinator of care for the child and family, the pediatric rehabilitation nurse interacts in a variety of settings with other nurses and health professionals. The critical-thinking skills inherent in the nursing process are essential in the provision of quality care that meets the needs of the child and family and obtains desired outcomes. Many nursing diagnostic statements and collaborative problems are applicable to the complex care of children with cerebral palsy. Age, the developmental level, the severity of the condition, and associated problems greatly affect the priorities in nursing assessment.

A health history and nursing and functional assessment, focusing on information about the condition and associated problems; a systems review including current problems and preexisting conditions; and a personal history focusing on diet, medications and known allergies, sleep and elimination patterns, mobility and activity, and psychosocial status are important initial elements in determining the needs and problems of the child and family.

In the area of mobility it is important to assess the following:

- The degree of functional impairment and functional abilities, including activity intolerance, coordination, strength, endurance, the level of discomfort, the joint range of motion, and risk factors for injury
- The effects of cognitive and perceptual impairment
- Complications of immobility, especially skin breakdown, infection, decreased vital capacity, weakness, contractures, elimination problems, and continence

- Psychosocial areas related to attitude, self-esteem, and socialization

An individualized plan for impaired physical mobility can be formulated, as shown in Table 28–9, if this problem exists for the child or adolescent.

Because of feeding difficulties and high energy levels with insufficient adequate caloric intake, these children and adolescents must have their nutritional needs carefully monitored. The pediatric rehabilitation nurse should assess for

- Consumption of adequate fluids and calories, including the use of assistive devices for feeding or eating
- Effectiveness of swallowing-facilitation techniques, including the use of verbal cuing, modification of food type and/or consistency, and positioning
- Hydration status, including a review of the pattern of weight gain, intake versus output, skin turgor, and the condition of mucous membranes
- Caregiver knowledge of common feeding problems such as aspiration, vomiting, abdominal cramping, and diarrhea

An individualized plan for altered nutrition can be formulated, as shown in Table 28–8, if this is found to be a problem.

These children and adolescents are at high risk for body image disturbance and low self-esteem, which can lead to altered role performance. The pediatric rehabilitation nurse should assess the level of knowledge about the present condition and diagnosis and the child's response, as well as that of the family, to changes in function. Important interventions include providing information; reinforcing explanations and referring the child and/or family to support groups or counseling; encouraging positive attitudes and effective communication patterns; and acknowledging and accepting adaptation responses while setting limits on inappropriate behavior. With the help of caring professionals in a variety of settings, the child or adolescent can verbalize understanding of body differences and acceptance of self and can recognize and incorporate changes into the self-concept in an accurate manner with preservation of self-esteem (Edwards & Posch, 1990).

For the child or adolescent with impaired communication, it is important to use language appropriate to the client's developmental stage, assist with the provision of a communication system, and allow adequate time for response to questions and requests. The use of a communication board with pictures and words can be an important intervention.

The nursing plan described previously for altered growth and development (Table 28–3) should be used as appropriate because these children and adolescents are at high risk for delays. The family should be assessed for parenting problems, and education and emotional support should be provided as indicated. For the child experiencing seizures, the information contained in Table 28–14 should be incorporated into the plan of care.

Muscular Dystrophy

The muscular dystrophies are a group of hereditary disorders characterized by progressive muscle weakness and loss of muscle tissue and distinguished by the type of inheritance, age when symptoms appear, and the types of symptoms that develop. The most common types are shown in Table 28–15.

Individuals with a family history of muscular dystrophy are at risk for having children with this condition, so genetic counseling is advised. The condition can be detected with about 95% accuracy by genetic studies performed during pregnancy. The symptoms include

- Muscle weakness that is progressive; frequent falls; delayed walking; waddling gait; difficulty using a muscle group; eyelid drooping; drooling
- Hypotonia
- Skeletal deformities
- Clawfoot or clawhand

Some of the signs are a loss of muscle mass, muscle contractures, cardiomyopathy, and arrhythmias. The diagnosis is made based on the clinical examination and an abnormal muscle biopsy. Important areas of the clinical examination include observation of gait, testing of muscle strength, the ability to rise from a sitting position off the floor (Gower maneuver—affected children walk their hands up their legs until they assume a standing position), and sensory testing. Tests include a muscle biopsy; blood tests for creatinine phosphokinase levels, which are elevated early in the disease; and an electromyogram to confirm weakness.

There is no known cure or treatment for the underlying defect, so managing symptoms and maintaining functional abilities and the quality of life are the main foci. Activity is encouraged, and therapies are prescribed to maintain muscle strength and function and to prevent contractures. Gait training and practicing safe transfers are also part of the plan. Adaptive equipment, such as splints and braces, may be employed to facilitate self-care, and special wheelchairs may be used to enhance mobility. Figure 28–3 shows the use of a motorized wheelchair with seat cushion and trunk support.

Complications include deformities; permanent, progressive disability with decreased mobility and ability for self-care; cardiomyopathy; and respiratory failure, which can cause death. Surgery may be beneficial to release contractures, and limited spinal instrumentation and fusion may be done for scoliosis.

A multidisciplinary approach must be used to facilitate maximal wellness for the child or adolescent. This must be family-centered with collaborative goal setting and evaluation by a team consisting of neurologists,

---

TABLE 28–14 ▪ TEACHING TOPIC: SEIZURE PRECAUTIONS AND MANAGEMENT, IMPORTANT AREAS

Remain calm and stay with the child
    Speak softly
    Reassure
Protect from injury
    Do not restrain or restrict movement
    Move harmful objects away
    Assist the child to lie down
    Place soft material under the head
    Loosen restrictive clothing
Provide time for recovery
    Turn the child to side-lying position
    Give nothing to eat or drink
Reassure and provide support
    Answer questions
Call for emergency help if
    Breathing does not resume; then begin mouth-to-mouth resuscitation
    Seizure lasts more than 5 min
    Seizures continue without a return to consciousness in between
    There are serious injuries
    It is the child's first seizure
Safety considerations
    Helmets
    Chairs with arms
    Evaluation of the environment, especially the sleeping area
    Activities of daily living with supervision

From Edwards, P. (1999). Traumatic injuries. In P. A. Edwards, D. L. Hertzberg, S. R. Hays, & N. M. Youngblood (Eds.), *Pediatric rehabilitation nursing* (p. 522). Philadelphia: W. B. Saunders.

TABLE 28–15 ■ MUSCULAR DYSTROPHIES

Type	Onset	Clinical Manifestations	Progression
Duchenne's	Early childhood to about 2–6 yr	Generalized weakness and muscle wasting affecting limb and trunk muscles first; calves often enlarged	Disease progresses slowly, with survival rate beyond late 20s
Becker's	2–16 yr	Almost identical to Duchenne's but less severe	Slower and more variable than Duchenne's
Limb-girdle	Late childhood to middle age	Weakness and wasting affecting shoulder and pelvic girdle first	Usually progresses slowly, with cardiopulmonary complications often occurring in later stages of disease
Fascioscapulohumeral	Childhood to early adulthood	Facial muscle weakness with weakness and wasting of shoulders and upper arms	Progresses slowly with some periods of rapid deterioration; may span decades

Adapted from Mason, K., & Wright, S. (1994). Altered musculoskeletal function. In C. Betz, M. Hunsberger, S. Wright (Eds.), *Family-centered nursing care of children* (2nd ed., p. 1843). Philadelphia: W. B. Saunders.

orthopedists, nurses, physical and occupational therapists, educators, social workers, genetic counselors, psychiatrists, and orthotists. The plan varies depending on the symptoms and prognosis, but the overall goals are to

- Maintain a reasonable lifestyle for the child and family, including school and recreation
- Maintain functional skills
- Prevent complications (contractures, scoliosis, respiratory infections)
- Instruct the family in the care of the child at home

Many nursing diagnostic statements and collaborative problems are applicable to the complex care of children with muscular dystrophy. The age, developmental level, severity of the condition, and associated problems greatly affect the priorities in nursing assessment. A health history and nursing and functional assessment, focusing on information about the condition and associated problems; a systems review including current problems and preexisting conditions; information about medications and known allergies; and a personal history focusing on diet, sleep, and elimination patterns, mobility and activity, and psychosocial status are important initial elements in determining the needs and problems of the child and family. Other important areas of assessment are

- Developmental level
- Muscle strength and range of motion
- ADLs
- Family concerns
- Respiratory function
- Disease progression
- Mobility
- Use of equipment

In the area of self-care, it is important to

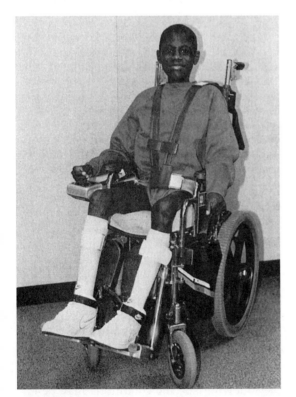

FIGURE 28–3
Power wheelchair with seat cushion and truck support. A firm back and seat insert are needed to provide midline trunk and pelvic positioning. (From Campbell, S. K. [1994]. *Physical therapy for children*. Philadelphia: W. B. Saunders.)

assess capabilities and activities and the response of the child or adolescent and family to the current level of functioning and changes in abilities. Then an individualized plan can be formulated to deal with identified self-care deficits, specifying the areas of intervention for feeding, bathing, hygiene, dressing, grooming, and toileting. It is important to identify barriers and assist in the provision of necessary adaptations and assistive devices to facilitate self-care activities and help with the selection and modification of clothing. Instructions from the interdisciplinary team should be reviewed and reinforced, daily routines changed as indicated, and the plan of care evaluated with the child or adolescent and family to identify progress and needed modifications. Achieving self-care and participation in ADLs to the fullest extent possible within the current limits of the situation is the expected outcome.

As the condition progresses, opportunities for positive interactions may begin to decrease and the adolescent may experience a sense of powerlessness. It is important for the pediatric rehabilitation nurse to

- Explore the options for possible activities given the current strengths and abilities
- Stimulate involvement in identifying needs and planning both physical and mental activities
- Acknowledge the reality of the situation and explore the adolescent's and family's perceptions and concerns and assist in dealing with feelings of hopelessness and anger
- Continue school, socialization, and diversional activities as long as possible
- Support the adolescent and family in making treatment choices (e.g., opting for ventilator-assisted living)

The goal of the nursing interventions is for the adolescent to (Edwards & Posch, 1990, p. 187)

- Engage in meaningful activities appropriate for tolerance and abilities
- Initiate coping actions appropriate for identified problems
- Maintain an appropriate level of social interaction

Another area of nursing intervention is anticipatory grieving. The pediatric rehabilitation nurse assesses current needs and behaviors involving the child or adolescent and family, noting family interaction patterns and alterations imposed by the condition, and gives information, identifies strengths, and makes referrals to other resources as appropriate (e.g., counseling, support groups, spiritual resources). Assistance is provided to the child or adolescent in expressing feelings and dealing with changes in familiar patterns, and the nurse incorporates the family and significant others into the support structure.

Other general areas of intervention that may be included in the nursing plan at various points in time are

- Encouraging and facilitating a maximal level of ability
- Helping the family learn how to use adaptive equipment
- Encouraging frequent position changes and ensuring proper body alignment
- Teaching skin inspection and protective measures
- Teaching and encouraging coughing, deep breathing, and the use of an incentive spirometer
- Assessing the adequacy of fluid intake
- Monitoring elimination patterns and habits
- Providing emotional support and clear, concise information to the family, whose needs will change as the disease progresses

The nurse's participation is essential during times of increased stress for the child or adolescent and family, especially during transition periods, such as a change in mobility (from walking to using a wheelchair); identification of a need for special equipment or modifications; surgery; leaving school; and entering the terminal stages. Support groups may be beneficial to both the child and the family.

PEDIATRIC REHABILITATION POPULATION

It is impossible to cover the entire scope of pediatric rehabilitation nursing within a single chapter, so the nursing assessment and plan of care for three common conditions have been described. However, there are other serious health problems, such as injuries and genetic and congenital conditions, that are increasing in frequency and result in limitation of activity and long-term disability in children and adolescents. Children with the following specific conditions may be encountered in pediatric rehabilitation nursing practice in a variety of settings:

- Traumatic brain injury
- Spinal cord injury
- Burns

TABLE 28–16 ■ RESOURCES

American Lung Association
(800) 586-4872
If Your Baby Has BPD: A Guide for Parents
Web site: www.lungusa.org

United Cerebral Palsy Association Inc.
1660 L Street NW, Suite 700
Washington, DC 20036
(800) USA-5UCP

Muscular Dystrophy Association
3300 E. Sunrise
Tucson, AZ 85718
(602) 529-2000

National Easter Seal Society
70 East Lake Street
Chicago, IL 60601
(312) 726-6200

National Association for Rare Disorders
(800) 999-667
Web site: www.nord-rdd.com/~orphan

Exceptional Parent
Dept. EP
Denville, NJ 07834-9919
(800) 562-1973

Spina Bifida Association of America
4590 MacArthur Boulevard NW
Suite 250
Washington, DC 20007-4226
(800) 621-3141

Pediatric Evaluation of Disability Inventory (PEDI)
Available from
NEMC Hospitals Inc.
PEDI Research Group
750 Washington Street
Boston, MA 02111
(617) 956-5031

Guide for the Uniform Data Set for Medical
  Rehabilitation for Children (WeeFIM)
Available from
SUNY at Buffalo
232 Parker Hall
SUNY South Campus
3435 Main Street
Buffalo, NY 14214

- Spina bifida
- Developmental disabilities
- Other neurological or orthopedic problems
- Behavior problems

For extensive information about these problems, the pediatric rehabilitation nurse should consult a more comprehensive text, but the nursing plans and teaching tools within this chapter can be applied across a variety of conditions. After completion of the initial assessment, the nurse can incorporate some of the previously described plans into one individualized to meet the specific needs of the child or adolescent in the setting in which care is provided. References provided at the end of the chapter as well as the additional resources listed in Table 28–16 can be used to supplement and amplify the content presented in the chapter.

SUMMARY

Numerous suggestions have been made for improving care and preventing health problems in childhood. As we look to the future, specific actions must be taken to represent children's needs and invest in their health and well-being. Pediatric rehabilitation nurses at all levels of practice can provide a strong body of representation to influence child health policy and make a difference in the quality of children's lives. Collaboration with families, consumers, and other service providers is imperative to make systems accessible, well-coordinated, and operating in a manner such that the child's developmental progress is fostered.

REFERENCES

American Nurses Association. (1991). *Standards of Clinical Nursing Practice*. Washington, DC: Author.

Association of Rehabilitation Nurses. (1996). *Scope and standards of advanced clinical practice in rehabilitation nursing*. Glenview, IL: Author.

Association of Rehabilitation Nurses. (1994). *Standards and scope of rehabilitation nursing practice* (3rd ed.). Skokie, IL: Author.

Association of Rehabilitation Nurses Pediatric Special Interest Group. (1992). *Pediatric rehabilitation nursing role description*. Skokie, IL: Association of Rehabilitation Nurses

Betz, C., Hunsberger, M., & Wright, S. (1994). *Family-centered nursing care of children* (2nd ed.). Philadelphia: W. B. Saunders.

Burkett, K. (1989). Trends in pediatric rehabilitation. *Nursing Clinics of North America, 24*(1), 239–255.

Caldwell, B., & Bradley, R. (1994). Home observation for measurement of the environment. In C. Betz, M. Hunsberger, & S. Wright (Eds.), *Family-centered nursing care of children* (2nd ed., pp. 2182–2190). Philadelphia: W. B. Saunders.

Carpenito, L. (1995). *Handbook of nursing diagnosis* (6th ed.). Philadelphia: J. B. Lippincott.

Consensus Committee. (1994). *Standards of nursing prac-*

tice for the care of children and adolescents with special health and developmental needs. Lexington, KY: University of Kentucky Chandler Medical Center College of Nursing.

Coster, W. & Haley, S. (1992). Conceptualization and measurement of disablement in infants and young children. *Infants and Young Children, 4*(4), 11–22.

Donar, M. (1988). Community care: Pediatric home mechanical ventilation. *Holistic Nursing Practice, 2*(2), 68–80.

Edwards, P. (1992). The evolution of rehabilitation facilities for children. *Rehabilitation Nursing, 17,* 191–195.

Edwards, P. A., & Posch, C. M. (1990). Impairment of the musculoskeletal system. In P. A. McCoy & W. L. Votroubek (Eds.), *Pediatric home care: A comprehensive approach* (pp. 182–189). Rockville, MD: Aspen.

Eicher, P., & Kerwin, M. (1996). Feeding and nutritional concerns. In L. Kurtz, P. Dowrich, S. Levy, & M. Batshaw (Eds.), *Handbook of developmental disabilities resources for interdisciplinary care* (pp. 327–341). Gaithersburg, MD: Aspen.

Feldman, A., Haley, S., & Coryell, J. (1990). Concurrent and construct validity of the pediatric evaluation of disability inventory. *Physical Therapy, 70,* 602–610.

Hunsberger, M., & Feenan, L. (1994). Altered respiratory function. In C. Betz, M. Hunsberger, & S. Wright (Eds.), *Family-centered nursing care of children* (2nd ed., pp. 1167–1275). Philadelphia: W. B. Saunders.

Katz, K. (1992). Trends in management of chronically ill children. In K. Katz (Ed.), *Headed home: Developmental interventions for hospitalized infants and their families* (pp. 1-6). Palo Alto, CA: Vort.

Lord, J., Taggart, P., & Molnar, G. (1991). Assessment instruments for evaluation of motor skills in children. *Physical Medicine and Rehabilitation: State of the Art Reviews, 5,* 389–402.

Marquis, P. (1991). Developmental disabilities in primary care. In A. Capute & P. Accardo (Eds.), *Developmental disabilities in infancy and childhood* (pp. 133–137). Baltimore: Paul H. Brookes.

McCabe, M., & Granger, C. (1990). Content validity of a pediatric functional independence measure. *Applied Nursing Research, 3(3):*120–122.

Meisels, S., & Provence, S. (1989). *Screening and assessment: Guidelines for identifying young disabled and developmentally vulnerable children and families,* Washington, DC: National Center for Clinical Infant Programs.

Molnar, G., Easton, J., Badell, A., Binder, H., Dykstra, D., Matthews, D., Noll, S., & Perrin, J. (1989). Pediatric rehabilitation: 2. Brain damage causing disability. *Archives of Physical Medicine and Rehabilitation, 70,* S166–S169.

Morse, J., & Colatarci, S. (1994). The impact of technology. In S. Roth & J. Morse (Eds.), *A life-span approach to nursing care for individuals with developmental disabilities* (pp. 351–383). Baltimore: Paul H. Brookes.

Murphey, K. (1996). Play and recreation. In L. Kurtz, P. Dowrick, S. Levy, & M. Batshaw (Eds.), *Handbook of developmental disabilities resources for interdisciplinary care* (pp. 605–617). Gaithersburg, MD: Aspen.

Nursing Standards Committee. (1994). *Care of the child and family* [unpublished standard]. Boston: Spaulding Rehabilitation Hospital.

Russell, F., & Free, T. (1994). The nurse's role in rehabilitation. In S. Roth & J. Morse (Eds.), *A life-span approach to nursing care for individuals with developmental disabilities.* Baltimore: Paul H. Brookes.

BIBLIOGRAPHY

American Lung Association. (1997). *American Lung Association fact sheet—Bronchopulmonary dysplasia* [On-line]. Available: www.lungusa.org

A national goal: Building service delivery systems for children with special health care needs and their families. (1987). Rockville, MD: National Maternal Child Health Resource Center.

Cervizzi, K., & Edwards, P. (1994). *Care of the child and family.* Poster session presented at the annual meeting of the Association of Rehabilitation Nurses, September, 1994, Orlando, FL.

DuPont Hospital for Children Child Health Talk. (1996). *Service coordination is key to cerebral palsy program* [On-line]. Available: kidshealth.org/ai/cht/edition.o/service_coord_key

Grindley, J. (1988). The handicapped child in school: Considerations for health care. *Holistic Nursing Practice, 2*(2), 11–19.

Mason, K., & Wright, S. (1994). Altered musculoskeletal function. In C. Betz, M. Hunsberger, & S. Wright (Eds.), *Family-centered nursing care of children* (2nd ed., pp. 1815–1873). Philadelphia: W. B. Saunders.

Muscular dystrophy. Applied Medical Informatics Inc. [On-line]. (1996). Available: www.housecall.com/databases/ami/convert/001190.html

National Easter Seal Society. (1996). *Understanding cerebral palsy* [On-line]. Available: seals.com/publish/understanding/ucp.html

Selekman, J. (1991). Pediatric rehabilitation: From concepts to practice. *Pediatric Nursing, 17,* 11–14.

Shelton, T., & Stepanek, J. (1994). *Family-centered care for children needing specialized health and developmental services* (3rd ed.). Bethesda, MD: Association for the Care of Children's Health.

Stuberg, W. (1994). Muscular dystrophy and spinal muscle atrophy. In S. K. Campbell (Ed.), *Physical therapy for children* (pp. 295–323). Philadelphia: W. B. Saunders.

CHAPTER 29

Gerontological Rehabilitation Nursing

Kristen L. Easton

This chapter discusses some of the roles and practice settings for nurses working with elderly clients in rehabilitation. Aging is common to all living things, yet individuals age in unique ways depending on a variety of factors such as the influence of culture, health practices, social support, and access to resources. Several functional changes associated with aging are also presented. Special issues related to gerontological rehabilitation nursing such as abuse of elders, safety, fall prevention, community reintegration, access to resources, and social support are discussed.

THE AGING POPULATION

The world's population is aging as never before with the increase in the number of people living to reach old age. People older than 65 years account for more than 12% of the U.S. population, or about 32.8 million individuals (Fowles, 1994). One out of every eight Americans is elderly (U.S. Department of Commerce, Economics and Statistics Administration, Bureau of the Census, and U.S. Department of Health and Human Services, National Institutes of Health, National Institute on Aging [USDC, USDHHS], 1991). By the year 2050, one in five Americans will be older than 65 years (Goldstein & Damon, 1993). The world's elderly population is also increasing. By 2025, the total number of persons aged 60 years and older is expected to reach about 1.1 billion worldwide (United Nations, Department of International Economic and Social Affairs, 1991).

Presently, the majority of older adults in the United States are white, but elderly ethnic minority groups are the fastest-growing subgroup of the elderly population (Espino, 1995). The concept of double jeopardy has been used to characterize aging in minorities. That is, as age increases, so does the incidence of chronic illness and disability, often more so among ethnic minorities. Kart & Engler (1994,

p. 301) stated that "negative effects of aging are compounded among minority group members." This can be complicated by the fact that certain ethnic groups use social and health-related resources differently than others do. Minority elders, such as African Americans, Hispanics, and Native Americans, have been shown to be at increased risk of morbidity and mortality due to socioeconomic as well as health status factors. Yet these groups may use health services less often than those in a white majority group (Ries, 1990), often relying on folk cures or folk medicine before, in place of, or in conjunction with more formal health services. This has serious implications for nurses, who will need to be knowledgeable about cultural and ethnic variations in health beliefs and practices in order to provide culturally competent care. Additionally, nurses may need to take rehabilitation into the community instead of relying on individuals to come to a traditional health care setting. Such will be the trends for the future in gerontological rehabilitation.

DOMAINS OF GERONTOLOGICAL REHABILITATION NURSING

Rehabilitation nurses working in gerontology face particular challenges. This specialty area requires knowledge in the areas of both rehabilitation and gerontology. The gerontological rehabilitation nurse (GRN) may work in a variety of settings. These include acute care hospitals, rehabilitation units, subacute care facilities, nursing homes, extended care facilities, and home- or community-based facilities. Within long-term-care facilities, several different levels of care may be required. These are usually termed *skilled*, *intermediate*, and *residential*, representing increasing levels of independence. Persons requiring skilled care, such as frequent suctioning, dressing changes, or tube feedings, are placed on a unit that is staffed around the clock by a registered nurse. Those in intermediate care facilities require less nursing care and can usually perform many activities of daily living with some assistance or direction but may need additional help with things such as taking medications or bathing. Persons in residential care levels are basically independent or require only minimal supervision with medications or activities of daily living. Some of those in residential care are unable to live alone merely because of a history of falls or lack of social support. Residential care is often provided as part of a larger extended care community in which persons reside in separate homes within a complex and can come to a dining room for meals or have staff check on them daily. This is similar to senior housing but may be considered a separate part of a convalescent center or nursing home. Some extended care facilities have a residential section within the main building. Home- and community-based programs include group homes program, adult day care, assisted living, senior housing projects, hospices, and home health care. Although a wide range of care and services is represented in these settings, GRNs may work effectively in any of these areas to promote independence of self-care of elderly clients, provided rehabilitation principles are applied.

The roles of the GRN include caregiver, teacher, leader, mediator, consultant, and researcher. The nurse includes some aspect of each of these roles in the care of the older adult. However, the amount of time devoted to each role varies depending on the client's diagnosis, situation, and setting. Most GRNs concentrate their efforts on caregiving, teaching, and mediating. The amount and type of nursing care required depend on the individual's cognitive and physical limitations. Regardless, the nurse not only uses nursing skills but also applies rehabilitation knowledge to the care of the client. Assessment and communication skills are essential in this specialty area, and quality nursing care cannot be provided without them.

The educational component of nursing in this field often takes on greater significance than in other areas of nursing. This is because clients have to learn to adjust to and cope with life-changing physical alterations. The GRN should be able to apply adult learning principles to rehabilitative care and teaching. Family members may require in-depth instruction if they are to assist with the care of a loved one with a long-term disorder. For example, the elderly stroke patient with hemiplegia, aphasia, and dysphagia may need assistance with ambulation and communication and may even require long-term use of a percutaneous endoscopic gastrostomy tube, all skills that the caregiver, who may also be elderly, needs to be taught.

The GRN may also need to act as an advocate, or mediator, for the client and the family. *Mediator* may be a more reflective term than *advocate*, as all team members should be client advocates, but the nurse is most likely to mediate between the disciplines. Again, this requires excellent communication skills.

Areas in which the GRN should have specialized knowledge and skills include those that have particular implications for older adults. For instance, prevention of skin breakdown is more of a challenge when the client has fragile skin and uses adaptive equipment. Wound healing may be slower and require aggressive nursing interventions. Sensory/perceptual deficits, as well as a higher pain threshold, can delay reporting of pain until infection is present. Nutritional needs may not be met if resources are inadequate, further contributing to slow bone and wound healing. Mobility is also affected by aging, and impairments can lead to falls, further complicating independence. The nurse needs to be aware of the effects of normal aging, as well as how these impact rehabilitation.

GENERALITIES AND DIVERSITY IN AGING

All persons age somewhat differently, based on a variety of factors. Aging can be influenced by such things as culture, heredity, socioeconomic status, educational level, environmental factors, and social support. Life expectancy differs with regard to race and gender, with women living longer than men and with whites living longer than blacks (USDC, USDHHS, 1993). Multiple life changes also occur with aging, including changes in living arrangements, marital status, and income (USDC, USDHHS, 1993).

The aging process, common to all living things, does have many predictable effects that can alter a person's health and sense of well-being. However, because of the variations seen in the group labeled *elderly*, sociologists have divided the "aged" into three groups: the young-old (aged 65 to 74 years), middle-old (aged 75 to 84 years), and oldest-old (aged 85 and over), often called the *frail elderly*. There is great variance of functional abilities and limitations among these sub-groups. For example, in 1990, 25% of the oldest-old lived in nursing homes, compared with 1.4% of the young-old (Goldstein & Damon, 1993). Once the age of 85 years is reached, more pronounced changes are seen in functional capacity, even in healthy elderly people.

Generally, as age increases, so does the likelihood of disease and disability. Almost all elders report having at least one chronic problem (Zarle, 1989). Arthritis is the most commonly reported complaint, followed by hypertension (which is especially prevalent among African Americans). About half of frail elderly people experience some hearing loss. Other common chronic conditions include heart conditions, chronic sinusitis, visual disturbances, orthopedic problems, respiratory conditions, cancer, diabetes, and varicose veins. However, the nurse should not assume that the presence of multiple chronic conditions automatically indicates a serious loss of function or decreased independence, as this is highly variable (Hills & Bernstein, 1997).

Some cultural or ethnic differences among elderly people are of particular importance to note. Puerto Rican and Mexican Americans experience a higher incidence of diabetes (25%) than the general population (Bassford, 1995). Native Americans constitute one of the most poverty-stricken groups in the United States. Over a quarter of this population has diabetes, and many suffer from stress-related disorders. Alcoholism, tuberculosis, diabetes, and pneumonia are major causes of death in Native Americans. Elderly African Americans are more likely to have functional loss compared with other groups, and more than half experience hypertension (Brangman, 1995; Gillies, 1991), which contributes to a higher incidence of stroke. Ethnic minority elders may also experience socioeconomic disadvantage and may have less access to the health care system. Despite cultural diversity, however, the leading causes of death among the elderly population seem to remain constant. These include heart disease, stroke, and cancer.

AGE-RELATED FUNCTIONAL CHANGES AND REHABILITATION

The normal effects of aging can complicate or contribute to existing health problems in older adults. Even apart from disease, aging

TABLE 29–1 ■ COMMON PRIMARY ADMITTING DIAGNOSES OF ELDERLY REHABILITATION CLIENTS

Stroke
Hip fracture (often with a prosthesis)
Knee replacement (may be bilateral)
Other orthopedic disorders
Parkinson's disease
Amputation
Functional debility
Multiple trauma (usually a result of an accident or fall)

is often accompanied by increased frailty and a decrease in the ability to care for oneself (Boult et al., 1994; Hasselkus, 1989; Jopp, Carroll, & Waters, 1993; Mulrow et al., 1994). Common problems such as arthritis contribute to joint deformities and pain, affecting an individual's functional capabilities. Hypertension is the number one risk factor for stroke, which can seriously affect cognitive, emotional, and physical abilities. The seventh leading cause of death in elderly people is diabetes, a disease with multiple long-term implications.

Not only can the effects of aging contribute to serious long-term health alterations, but they can also complicate problems that occur. Examples of common medical diagnoses for which elders are admitted to rehabilitation appear in Table 29–1. A crisis such as a stroke may be attributed to hypertension and then complicated by hypertension and other problems such as those listed in Tables 29–2 and 29–3. Each year approximately 350,000 Americans survive a stroke, leaving many with residual disabilities. Even some modifiable risk factors of stroke, such as hyperten-

TABLE 29–2 ■ COMMON CONCOMITANT HEALTH ALTERATIONS IN THE GERIATRIC REHABILITATION CLIENT

Arthritis
Hypertension
Diabetes
Hearing deficits
Visual deficits (especially cataracts and glaucoma)
Heart disease
Chronic obstructive pulmonary diseases (such as emphysema, chronic bronchitis)
Cancer
Peripheral vascular disease
Chronic sinusitis
Congestive heart failure

TABLE 29–3 ■ SECONDARY COMPLICATIONS THAT MAY SLOW REHABILITATION PROGRESS

Neurogenic bowel or bladder with incontinence
Pressure ulcers
Spasticity, contractures
Deep vein thrombosis
Acute confusion
Effects of polypharmacy
Immobility, unsteady gait, weakness, dizziness
Infections
Other postoperative complications

sion or cardiovascular disease, are often associated with aging. Many of the long-term health problems listed contribute to immobility and increased dependence for older adults. Rehabilitation nurses attempt to assist and educate clients in ways that will promote self-care and independence. Not all elderly people will be able to achieve complete independence after a serious illness or accident. This requires the rehabilitation nurse to be flexible and able to adapt care and teaching to a wide variety of settings and situations. The nurse working with the gerontological client has additional considerations. Table 29–4 provides a summary of age-related changes and their impact on functional capacity.

There appears to be a strong relationship between age and the need for assistance. About 45% of persons in the community older than 85 years need help with activities of daily living (Goldstein & Damon, 1993; USDA, USDHHS, 1991). Between 4.4 and 6.7 million noninstitutionalized elderly people have functional dependencies (Tauber, 1993). In 2000, an estimated 7.3 million elders will require some type of assistance to remain independent. This figure may nearly double by the year 2050 (Zarle, 1989).

The premise of gerontological rehabilitation is that elderly people with functional deficits can increase their ability to perform self-care (Gill & Balsano, 1994; Gregor, McCarthy, Chwirchak, Meluch, & Mion, 1986; Heacock, Walton, Beck, & Mercer, 1991; Kalra, 1994). Whatever the person's admitting diagnoses, rehabilitation generally promotes positive outcomes and independence of elderly patients. Exercise and activity programs have been shown to increase functional capacity (Bohannon & Cooper, 1993; Lyngberg, Harreby, Bentzen, Frost, & Danneskiold-Samsoe, 1994; Mills, 1994; Nugent, Schurr, & Adams, 1994). Elderly people with orthopedic problems such as hip fracture, knee arthroplasty, arthritis, or amputation show improved functional status with rehabilitation (Bohannon & Cooper, 1993; Fisher et al., 1993; Montgomery

TABLE 29–4 ■ AGE-RELATED CHANGES AND THE IMPACT ON REHABILITATION

System	Changes	Impact on Rehabilitation
Integumentary	Skin dry, less flexible, less elastic	Prone to breakdown, skin tears, pressure ulcers
	Less perspiration	Altered body temperature control
	Fatty distribution to trunk	Less fat on arms and legs, resulting in cooler extremities
Musculoskeletal	Joint stiffness, arthritis	Decreased ROM, pain
	Decreased muscle mass	Less muscle strength
	Bone demineralization	More prone to fractures
Neurological	Slower reflexes	Response time increased
	Decreased ability to respond to multiple stimuli	May need more time to perform tasks
Genitourinary	Increased incidence of incontinence, especially urge and stress; frequency and nocturia	Prone to UTIs
		Uncontrolled incontinence is major cause of institutionalization; prior problems complicated by neurogenic bladder
Gastrointestinal	Decrease in digestive enzymes; esophageal peristalsis and gut motility slows	More difficulty swallowing
		Constipation, impaction
	Dentures	Ill-fitting dentures from weight loss can result in poorer appetite, further weight loss
Circulatory	Less cardiovascular reserve; heart pumps less effectively	Heart less able to meet demands placed on it
	Increased incidence of hypertension and cardiac dysrhythmias	Medications to control blood pressure or pulse may cause orthostatic hypotension or other side effects
Respiratory	Increased airway resistance and decreased amount of useful oxygen with each breath	More SOB with exertion; may require supplemental oxygen in case of COPD

COPD, chronic obstructive pulmonary disease; ROM, range of motion; SOB, shortness of breath; UTI, urinary tract infection.

Orr & Bratton, 1992). Most stroke patients continue to improve even after discharge home if they have participated in rehabilitation (Davidoff, Keren, Ring, & Solzi, 1991; Easton, Rawl, Zemen, Kwiatkowski, & Burczyk, 1995). Cognitively impaired elderly people also benefit from care with a self-care focus (Heacock et al., 1991).

Nurses can also positively influence client outcomes. Easton et al. (1995) found that clients who received additional follow-up from a rehabilitation nurse after discharge used more positive coping strategies than those who did not. Other outcomes that may be affected by nursing interventions include the length of hospital stay, improvement in functional status including mobility skills, the use of positive coping mechanisms, and the increased likelihood of a home discharge destination (Folden, 1993; Gill & Ursic, 1994; Heafey, Golden-Baker, & Mahoney, 1994; Lichtenstein, Semaan, & Marmar, 1993).

Considerations in gerontological rehabilitation nursing include the process of aging with a disability. Before the development of antibiotics and technological advancements, people with service-related injuries, spinal cord injuries, or stroke rarely lived to reach old age. Now, the average life span for a teenager who experienced a spinal cord injury and received prompt and proper medical care is nearing that of the general population. However, aging with functional limitations has other serious implications for practice. For example, those with paraplegia experience a greater incidence of arthritis and shoulder problems owing to the increased stress placed on the upper body. The shoulder was not designed to be a weight-bearing joint and thus ages prematurely. Amputation is another example. Those missing a lower limb but ambulating with a prosthesis have been found to have arthritis in the nonaffected leg more often. Arthritic changes can eventually lead to the need for joint replacement, a much more complex problem for a person who already has a severe functional deficit.

SPECIAL ISSUES IN GERONTOLOGICAL REHABILITATION NURSING

Abuse

Abuse of the aged by caregivers or others can take several forms (Table 29–5). Often, more than one type of abuse is present (Decalmer & Glendenning, 1993). The most commonly rec-

TABLE 29–5 ▪ TYPES OF ELDER ABUSE

Physical
  Involves bodily injury
  May include misuse of medications, withholding food, pushing, hitting, slapping, punching, squeezing, kicking, biting, choking, suffocating, burning, sexually assaulting, murder
  Can result in bruises, skin tears, lacerations, burns, fractures, internal bleeding, starving, coma, death
Psychological/emotional
  Involves verbal insults, threats of harm, humiliation, verbal degradation, harassment, screaming, yelling, shouting, throwing things
  Can lead to feelings of isolation, helplessness, hopelessness, unworthiness, fearfulness, anxiety, suicidal thoughts, or behaviors such as rocking, thumb sucking, withdrawal, cowering, sleep deprivation or nightmares, isolation, agitation, acting out
Neglect
  Involves physical isolation, lack of needed supervision, inadequate nutrition, lack of privacy, unfit living environment, abandonment
  Can result in dehydration, malnutrition, feelings of hopelessness, bodily sores from urine or feces, lice, animal bites, death from caregiver's complete abandonment of a physically or mentally impaired person
Financial
  Involves theft or extortion of property, money, medications, social security or pension checks, material possessions, or home; fraud; deceit through ingratiating of the abuser to an isolated elder who needs assistance
  Can result in forced servitude or blackmail of the elder, misuse of authority or power of attorney, change in the elder's will, bankruptcy of the victim, and even murder to acquire possessions

ognized type is physical. This may occur as a result of a combination of factors. However, one particular risk factor of note that can contribute to abuse of dependent elders is caregiver burnout (Eliopoulos, 1997). In many instances, caregivers are middle-aged daughters, whose other responsibilities may compound feelings of being overwhelmed and helpless. When such feelings create resentment and hostility, a potentially abusive situation is present.

The most important fact for GRNs to remember is that elder abuse crosses all social and cultural classes and can occur anywhere. Dependent and functionally impaired elders, especially women who are socially isolated, are at high risk for abuse and mistreatment. It is especially important to note that although many generalities about typical profiles of victims and perpetrators can be stated, the research on many factors such as the age and gender of abusers is conflicting. However, victims often live alone or with one other person (Sengstock & Barrett, 1993). Family members are often the perpetrators, and alcohol or other substance abuse by the caregiver is associated with the mistreatment of elders (Pritchard, 1995). Nurses should be alert to signs of abuse of elders such as unexplained bruises, burns, or lacerations; frequent broken bones; perineal tears, rashes, or bruising; hair loss; poor hygiene; and the emergence of infantile habits or behaviors (such as thumb sucking, biting, rocking, destructive patterns, or sleep disorders).

Physical abuse involves bodily harm inflicted on the elder from another in the form of violence such as pushing, hitting, kicking, beating, unnecessary use of restraints, or sexual abuse. Sometimes this occurs between spouses. Negligence is probably a more common form of abuse but should be recognized by the nurse. Caregivers who neglect elders may withhold or limit food, give poor attention to the elders' hygiene, speak harshly or threateningly to the elders, isolate them, or ignore in other ways. Elders who are victims of negligence are made to feel like a burden and usually exhibit weight loss, social isolation, depression, and low self-esteem.

Other forms of abuse may be more subtle. Children who frequently take advantage of their retired elderly parents' bank account, or compel them to cosign for loans that they do not pay, are committing financial abuse. Psychological abuse may accompany any other types of abuse or neglect. Elders may be made to feel unloved, unworthy, guilty, and burdensome. Caregivers may take advantage of the frail aged by stealing items, money, or medications. Such situations contribute to the elders' sense of helplessness. Threats of physical harm to the person or the family may prevent them from sharing information about the abuse with someone who could help.

Nurses must be constantly aware of the potential for abuse in any setting where the caregiver may experience burnout. Direct questions should be asked of the suspected victim, but the nurse should realize that elders may be reluctant to reveal abuse because of fears of retaliation from the abuser and helplessness over the situation. Assessment tools and plans for action should be in place. Prevention is the best solution, but this takes careful planning and education of the client, family, and community.

Respite care and support group information should be provided for and planned before discharge from rehabilitation, as social support can act as a buffer to stress. For those already in the community, the nurse is legally and morally bound to report any suspicions of abuse that might occur in the home. Nurses themselves can be held liable for failing to report such a case, misusing safety devices, or handling another person's property in an unprofessional manner. Most states require a criminal background check to be done on any person providing care within the home.

The facility protocol for documenting the use of safety devices should be followed. Unnecessarily restraining an individual can result in charges of battery or aggravated assault. Safety devices such as vest restraints or lap belts should be used only to keep the patient safe, not for the convenience of the staff. Because elderly rehabilitation patients are particularly at risk for physical injury because of functional limitations, GRNs should be especially careful to use appropriate safety measures, but the least restrictive means possible. Proper documentation of the use of safety devices is required by law. This is for the protection of both the patient and the staff.

Safety

Falls are the second leading cause of accidental death in the elderly population (Brady et al., 1993). Falls can have numerous damaging effects on the persons involved, including injury; decreased confidence; insecurity; increased dependence; extended length of stays because of complications; greater expense to the hospital and patient; increased provider liability; increased mortality (Ross, 1991); and potential lawsuits. Falls occur more often on the rehabilitation unit than on other medical units and are often associated with a downward spiral of health and increased mortality in elderly persons. Most people who fracture a hip during a fall never fully recover. In rehabilitation, clients who fall most often are those with a diagnosis of stroke or head injury.

Because falls tend to occur more frequently in the older population, fall risk assessment and teaching related to prevention are relevant nursing issues. Fall risk factor studies are abundant, with the majority of research being done with older long-term-care residents. In 1991, falls were ranked as the second leading cause of accidental death in the United States. It is estimated that about half of all nursing home patients have fallen at

TABLE 29–6 ■ FALL RISK FACTORS IN ELDERLY PERSONS

Age over 65 years

Diagnosis of stroke or head injury

Medications that affect fluid balance, behavior, or sensorium (such as tranquilizers, sedatives, hypnotics, hypotensives, diuretics, laxatives)

Impaired physical mobility

Altered mental state (such as confusion, memory loss, Alzheimer's disease, seizures)

Prior history of falls

Weakness, dizziness

Sensory deficits (such as blindness, visual disturbances, neuropathy, presbycusis)

Bowel or bladder incontinence

Psychosocial factors (such as not using call light, denying falls, removing safety devices)

least once (Ross, 1991; Tinetti, 1986). Table 29–6 lists fall risk factors identified in the health literature.

Nurses can reduce a patient's risk of falling by being alert to risk factors particular to the setting and unit in which they work and by implementing appropriate strategies. Unit-specific fall risk tools may be of greater benefit than standardized tools and encourage thorough assessment of the patient's abilities, limitations, and needs. In addition to implementing usual safety precautions, the nurse can help promote patient safety in several ways. Items at the bedside or in the patient's room should be arranged to maximize the performance of self-care activities. That is, if the person has left hemiplegia, items should be placed on the stronger side, the right, so as not to cause further limitations to the person. The exception to this is when the caregiver or therapist is working with the individual to promote the use of the affected extremity, which should be done often. However, in view of safety issues, forcing the patient with a functional deficit to be unable to use his or her strengths is setting the person up for failure and additional safety risks. Drug therapy should also be evaluated for its possible contributions to patients' unsteadiness or risk of falls. Cognitive deficits and the level of alertness should be continually noted.

The environment should be kept free from clutter so that equipment does not pose a hazard. Because older persons require more light to see because of changes in the lens and accommodation, adequate night-lights should be left on throughout the night. Some patients experience unilateral neglect. That is, they may be unaware of their hemiplegic arm or leg, predisposing them to injury. A person can easily let the weak arm dangle, contributing to painful shoulder subluxation, or catch the fingers in the spokes of the wheelchair without realizing it. A lack of safety awareness, combined with impulsiveness, is especially common in males with right hemisphere stroke. In such situations, the nurse must take extra care to protect the affected extremity while encouraging the person to take charge of his own safety. Those with neglect may need frequent safety reminders. This is done through verbal and tactile cues such as, "Where is your left arm now?" or "Look where your leg is" (while touching the affected leg). Signs posted at the bedside as well as other reminders to call for assistance are indicated.

Community Reintegration

Community reintegration is an important issue in gerontological rehabilitation. One of the objectives of rehabilitation is to assist individuals and families so that clients can reenter society at their maximal functional level. This poses a challenge for those with disabilities in terms of accessibility and fear of how they are perceived by others. Participating in activities in the community requires much more planning than it did before a disability. Most rehabilitation units take the client and family on at least one community outing before discharge to guide them through the process of planning; making telephone calls ahead; and checking for wheelchair or walker access, the presence of stairs, and menu preparation for those with special dietary needs. Many seniors deem the extra expenditure of energy required to reenter society not worth the positive feedback from doing so. This contributes to social isolation and depression.

One community option for older adults is termed *adult care*, also known as *adult day care*. There are over 3000 such programs in the United States (Eliopoulos, 1997). This form of comprehensive care was developed for those who live at home with a family member but cannot be left unsupervised throughout the day. Adult care is flexible, providing a variety of services for older adults from supervision to intense care. Many centers provide transportation and meals. The staffing requirements for adult care facilities, whether free-standing or hospital based, are set by the state. The nurse is an essential staff member, sometimes serving as director for the center. Social workers, therapists, aides, secretarial help, activity directors, physicians, and consultants are other common team members. A variety of treatment modalities may be used including pets, art, music, or horticultural therapy. Individual client goals are set and care plans developed in order to promote positive outcomes unique to each client.

For many families, community adult care allows them an alternative to institutionalization (Masson, 1986). Adult care can be used on a full- or part-time basis but is open only during daytime hours. Participants can interact with others, promoting socialization skills. Activities and trips are often planned, with adequate trained personnel to assist.

Requirements for admission to adult care usually include freedom from communicable disease, the ability to participate in group activities, and the capacity to walk independently or with an assistive device. Eligibility is determined by criteria established by each individual program, and Medicare and Medicaid provide monies for support. Adult care centers have a rehabilitation focus. The program is designed to maximize independence while preventing deterioration in a supportive environment (Mehlferber, 1990). This type of care merges traditional health, social, and therapeutic services to promote positive outcomes.

Intergenerational care is a model being used at several facilities. These centers combine adult care with child care in the same center. Although they provide separate facilities for adults and children, activities are planned that promote interaction between these age groups. This is thought to help older adults participate in socialization activities in a different way and provide a sense of well-being, purpose, and belonging. The children can learn and grow from the experience and wisdom of the elderly clients. This concept has been used with success and appears to be a future trend in care.

Access to Community Resources

Accessibility to resources is a common issue in gerontology. Elders may not be able to access needed health care because of physical limitations. This is especially complicated when the individual has a long-term disability that requires the use of a wheelchair. A lack of transportation or distance from the facility may decrease the use of needed services. People in ethnic minority groups often require more health services because of an increased incidence in functional limitations

and poorer health but have less access to the health care system (Damron-Rodriguez, Wallace, & Kington, 1994). People often use informal services such as the advice of friends and folk cures before and in addition to seeking medical help.

GRNs should be aware of the services provided in their community for elders with functional limitations. Rehabilitation facilities have begun to develop their own home health care programs to meet these clients' special needs. Postdischarge follow-up of patients by a rehabilitation nurse has been shown to decrease anxiety and promote the use of more positive coping strategies (Easton et al., 1995).

Mobile health care units are another attempt to bring the needed services to the community. Taking medical and nursing personnel, along with supplies, to the areas in which care is needed promotes the use of services. Providing culturally competent care also promotes the use of the health care system. Clients begin to develop a trust and rapport with the staff. Information can also be provided that links the client and the family with available supports of which they might not have been aware.

The role of the nurse practitioner was initially designed to bring care to rural areas where physician care was unavailable. Advanced practice nurses now have a variety of ways in which to practice. Nurse-managed clinics are becoming more popular, particularly in areas where the need is great but service utilization is poor. Bringing care into the community thus remains one of the best uses of the skills of the advanced practice nurse.

Mental Health and Social Support

As a person ages, some minimal changes in short-term memory are expected. However, when memory loss interferes with the person's ability to perform activities of daily living or self-care, additional assessments must be made. An assessment of basic cognitive function includes orientation, memory, three-stage commands (simple), situational judgment, and calculations or sequencing. Characteristics of cognitive impairment include memory loss; an inability to concentrate; a poor attention span; agitation; changes in personality or behavior; lethargy; disorientation; sequencing difficulties; trouble initiating tasks; an inability to process commands involving three or more steps; decreased decision-making ability; and the inability to correct one's own mistakes. Nursing interventions include controlling the environment; allowing more time for processing information; speaking in simple sentences; and using a variety of stimuli when working with the client, such as verbal, tactile, and visual (demonstration) cues.

Of particular importance is the recognition of differences between depression, confusion (or delirium), and dementia. Many elders in long-term-care facilities experience confusion that is not recognized, diagnosed, or treated. This has serious implications for rehabilitation in this setting, as those elders who are thought to be cognitively impaired are usually not targeted for rehabilitative interventions by long-term-care staff. The cause of any cognitive or behavioral deficits must be explored. Confusion is characterized by an acute onset and disorientation. This can be caused by infection, anemia, electrolyte imbalances, hypoxia, malnutrition, or hypotension. It can also be related to changes in surroundings, such as entering the hospital. The unfamiliarity of the environment is a common contributor to acute confusion. The cause of confusion is often treatable. Confusion is acute by nature and should be dealt with as such.

Dementia, on the other hand, has a chronic progression with expected deterioration. Dementia can be caused by alcoholism, multi-infarcts, parkinsonism, organic brain syndrome, or Alzheimer's disease. The risk of having Alzheimer's disease increases with age. This common type of dementia affects about one in five of those older than 75 years and one in two of those older than 85 years. Only definitively diagnosed through autopsy, Alzheimer's disease results in a progressive forgetfulness and eventual deterioration of mental and physical functions. This results in a great burden on the caregiver, for whom support groups are an important coping mechanism. Research has newly identified two genes associated with Alzheimer's in younger persons (aged 40 to 60 years) (Alzheimer's Association, 1996).

Depression is another condition often experienced by elderly persons and is sometimes misinterpreted as dementia or confusion. Depression coincides with life changes such as the death of a loved one or the loss of a job. The person who is depressed may exhibit a selective memory but score higher on mini–mental status examinations than those with confusion or dementia. A thorough history and physical examination are essential. Social isolation and diminished support systems are significant risk factors that should be considered. Medications can also contribute to depression in the elderly person. These include a wide variety of drugs such as antihypertensives, hormones, sedatives, tranquilizers, sleeping pills, alcohol, levodopa, and cimetidine (Tagamet). Depression is largely treatable with counseling, therapy, and antidepressants if needed.

Coping is learned early in life, and older adults tend to use coping strategies that may have worked for them in the past. However, sometimes old age brings on new problems, and new coping mechanisms must be developed for individuals to positively adapt. Elders who are cognitively intact display and use the same processes as younger adults do (Costa & McCrae, 1993). This means they can benefit from similar therapeutic interventions, many of which can be provided in the rehabilitation setting. Those with mental status changes are at increased risk of maladaptive coping, including the use of alcohol and drugs.

Social support has been shown to affect outcomes in elderly persons. This is particularly true in rehabilitation. A supportive spouse or significant other has a positive influence on functional and psychological outcomes of the elderly rehabilitation client (Baker, 1993; Folden, 1993; Watson, 1986). Cummings et al. (1988) found that elderly patients with a greater number of social supports recovered more completely after a hip fracture. The coping strategies of patients, as well as their caregivers, can also positively influence the rehabilitation process. However, a lack of social support can negatively affect the long-term-care situation (Evans, Bishop, & Haselkorn, 1991; Periard & Ames, 1993).

The effectiveness of nursing interventions in long-term care and rehabilitation is an area where further research is needed. Discharge planning is a critical component to the nursing role, receiving increased attention in the literature (Haddock, 1991; Neal, 1995; Shiell, Kenny, & Farnworth, 1993). Supportive-educative nursing interventions have been influential in helping clients and family members to cope with long-term health alterations.

FUTURE DIRECTIONS

The field of gerontological nursing is quickly expanding. The exponential growth of the elderly population and the aging of the "baby boomers" bring issues of long-term care for the aged to the forefront of health care. More persons are living to see old age and are having to adapt to life with chronic diseases and functional limitations. Care of the older adult with long-term illnesses cannot be adequately separated from the principles and concepts of rehabilitation. Rehabilitation nurses must be able to emphasize the importance of self-care for older adults in order to promote their independence. This will become more essential as the number of persons needing care may outnumber the available caregivers in the future.

The future of health care is uncertain, but there will likely be an increased need for health care professionals who can adapt and care for aged persons in a wide variety of settings outside the hospital. A nurse trained in the principles of rehabilitation, with sufficient knowledge of the aging process, will be able to meet the future challenges of the complex elderly population. New roles for health professionals may emerge, and families will likely play a more crucial part in the care of aged persons than ever before. The nurse will also need to be aware of cultural differences as communities become more culturally diverse. It is essential to provide culturally competent care for the older adult if self-care is to be taught and maintained.

If "socialized" medicine becomes a reality in the United States, the quality of care for elderly persons will deteriorate. More aged adults will be cared for in the home by unprepared family caregivers. The home health industry is already understaffed and underfunded, and managers realize that something else is needed, that there is a missing link to long-term care. Additional resources for nurses will be needed to guide us into the future and provide direction for those seeking answers to the question: What is the key to quality care for our elderly patients and clients? The answer lies in the marriage between rehabilitation concepts and gerontological nursing. This has given rise to the emerging specialty of gerontological rehabilitation nursing.

REFERENCES

Alzheimer's Association (1996). *Newsletter.* Chicago, IL: Author.

Baker, A. (1993). The spouse's positive effect on the stroke patient's recovery. *Rehabilitation Nursing, 18*(1), 30–33.

Bassford, T. (1995). Health status of Hispanic elders. *Clinics in Geriatric Medicine: Ethnogeriatrics, 11*, 25–38.

Bohannon, R. W., & Cooper, J. (1993). Total knee arthroplasty: Evaluation of an acute care rehabilitation program. *Archives of Physical Medicine and Rehabilitation, 74*, 1091–1094.

Boult, C., Boult, L., Murphy, C., Ebbitt, B., Luptak, M., & Kane, R. L. (1994). A controlled trial of outpatient geriatric evaluation and management. *Journal of the American Geriatrics Society, 42*, 465–470.

Brady, R., Chester, F. R., Pierce, L. L., Salter, J. P., Schreck, S., & Radziewicz, R. (1993). Geriatric falls: Prevention strategies for the staff. *Journal of Gerontological Nursing, 19*(9), 26–32.

Brangman, S. A. (1995). African American elders: Implications for health care providers. *Clinics in Geriatric Medicine: Ethnogeriatrics, 11*, 15–24.

Costa, P., & McCrae, R. R. (1993). Psychological stress and coping in old age. In L. Goldberger & S. Breznitz (Eds.), *Handbook of Stress* (pp. 403–412). New York: Free Press.

Cummings, S. R., Phillips, S. L., Wheat, M. E., Black, D., Gossby, E., Wlodarczyk, D., Trafton, P., Jergesen, H., Hunter Winograd, C., & Hulley, S. B. (1988). Recovery of function after hip fractures: The role of social supports. *Journal of the American Geriatrics Society, 36*, 801–806.

Damron-Rodriguez, J., Wallace, S., & Kington, R. (1994). Service utilization and minority elderly: Appropriateness, accessibility and acceptability. *Gerontology and Geriatrics Education, 15*, 45–62.

Davidoff, G. N., Keren, O., Ring, H., & Solzi, P. (1991). Acute stroke patients: Long-term effects of rehabilitation and maintenance of gains. *Archives of Physical Medicine and Rehabilitation, 72*, 869–873.

Decalmer, P., & Glendenning, F. (Eds.). (1993). *The mistreatment of the elderly people.* London: Sage.

Easton, K. L., Rawl, S. M., Zemen, D., Kwiatkowski, S., & Burczyk, B. (1995). The effects of nursing follow-up on the coping strategies used by rehabilitation patients after discharge. *Rehabilitation Nursing Research, 4*, 119–127.

Eliopoulos, C. (1997). *Gerontological nursing.* Philadelphia: J. B. Lippincott.

Espino, D. V. (Volume Ed.) (1995). *Clinics in Geriatric Medicine: Ethnogeriatrics, 11*(1), xi.

Evans, R. L., Bishop, D. S., & Haselkorn, J. K. (1991). Factors predicting satisfactory home care after stroke. *Archives of Physical Medicine and Rehabilitation, 72*, 144–147.

Fisher, N. W., Gresham, G. E., Abrams, M., Hicks, J., Horrigan, D., Pendergast, D. R. (1993). Quantitative effects of physical therapy on muscular and functional performance in subjects with osteoarthritis of the knees. *Archives of Physical Medicine and Rehabilitation, 74*, 840–847.

Folden, S. L. (1993). Effect of a supportive-educative nursing intervention on older adults' perceptions of self-care after a stroke. *Rehabilitation Nursing, 18*(3), 162–166.

Fowles, D. G. (1994). *A profile of older Americans.* Washington, DC: American Association of Retired Persons and Administration on Aging, U.S. Department of Health and Human Services.

Gill, H. S., & Balsano, A. E. (1994). The move toward subacute care. *Nursing Homes, 43*(4), 6–7, 9–11.

Gill, K. P., & Ursic, P. (1994). The impact of continuing education on patient outcomes in the elderly hip fracture population. *The Journal of Continuing Education in Nursing, 25*, 181–185.

Gillies, D. A. (1991). Content and significance of minority aging curriculum guide. *MAIN Dimensions, 2*(9), 1–4.

Goldstein, A. & Damon, B. (U.S. Department of Commerce, Economics and Statistics Administration, Bureau of the Census). (1993). *We the American elderly.* Washington, DC: U.S. Government Printing Office.

Gregor, S., McCarthy, K., Chwirchak, D., Meluch, M., & Mion, L. C. (1986). Characteristics and functional outcomes of elderly rehabilitation patients. *Rehabilitation Nursing, 11*(3), 10–14.

Haddock, K. S. (1991). Characteristics of effective discharge planning programs for the frail elderly. *Journal of Gerontological Nursing, 17*(7), 10–13.

Hasselkus, B. R., (1989). Occupational and physical therapy in geriatric rehabilitation. *Physical and Occupational Therapy in Geriatrics, 7*(3), 3–20.

Heacock, P., Walton, C., Beck, C., & Mercer, S. (1991). Caring for the cognitively impaired: Reconceptualizing disability and rehabilitation. *Journal of Gerontological Nursing, 17*(3), 23–25.

Heafey, M. L., Golden-Baker, S. B., Mahoney, D. W. (1994). Using nursing diagnoses and intervention in an inpatient amputee program. *Rehabilitation Nursing 19*(3), 163–168.

Hills, G. A., & Bernstein, S. R. (1997). Assessment of elders and caregivers. In J. Deusen & D. Brunt (Eds.), *Assessment in occupational therapy and physical therapy* (pp. 401–413). Philadelphia: W. B. Saunders.

Jopp, M., Carroll, M. C., Waters, L. (1993). Using self-care theory to guide nursing management of the older adult after hospitalization. *Rehabilitation Nursing, 18*(2), 91–94.

Kalra, L. (1994). The influence of stroke unit rehabilitation on functional recovery from stroke. *Stroke, 25,* 821–825.

Kart, C. S., & Engler, C.A. (1994). Predisposition to self-health care: Who does what for themselves and why? *Journal of Gerontological Nursing, 49,* S301–308.

Lichtenstein, R., Semaan, S., Marmar, E. C. (1993). Development and impact of a hospital-based perioperative patient education program in a joint replacement center. *Orthopaedic Nursing, 12*(6), 17–23.

Lyngberg, K. K., Harreby, M., Bentzen, H., Frost, B., Danneskiold-Samsoe, B. (1994). Elderly rheumatoid arthritis patients on steroid treatment tolerate physical training without an increase in disease activity. *Archives of Physical Medicine and Rehabilitation, 75,* 1189–1195.

Masson, V. (1986, January/February). How nursing happens in adult day care. *Geriatric Nursing,* 18--21.

Mehlferber, K. (1990). In C. Eliopoulos (Ed.), *Caring for the elderly in diverse care settings* (pp. 284–289). Philadelphia: J. B. Lippinncott.

Mills, E. M. (1994). The effect of low-intensity aerobic exercise on muscle strength, flexibility, and balance among sedentary elderly persons. *Nursing Research, 43,* 207–211.

Montgomery Orr, P., & Bratton, G. N. (1992). The effect of an inpatient arthritis rehabilitation program on self-assessed functional ability. *Rehabilitation Nursing, 17,* 306–310.

Mulrow, C. D., Gerety, M. B., Kanten, D., Cornell, J. E., DeNino, L. A., Chidod, L., Aguilar, C., O'Niel, M. B.,

Rosenberg, J., Solis, R. M. (1994). *Journal of the American Medical Association, 271,* 519–524.

Neal, L. J. (1995). The rehabilitation nursing team in the home healthcare setting. *Rehabilitation Nursing, 20*(1), 32–36.

Nugent, J. A., Schurr, K. A., & Adams, R. D. (1994). A dose response relationship between amount of weight bearing exercise and walking outcome following cerebrovascular accident. *Archives of Physical Medicine and Rehabilitation, 75,* 399–402.

Periard, M. E., & Ames, B. (1993). Lifestyle changes and coping patterns among caregivers of stroke survivors. *Public Health Nursing, 10*(4), 252–256.

Pritchard, J. (1995). *The abuse of older people: A training manual for detection and prevention.* London: Jessica Kingsley.

Ries, P. (1990). Vital and health statistics: Health of black and white Americans, 1985–1987. National Center for Health Statistics. *Vital Health Statistics, 10*(171).

Ross, J. E. R. (1991). Iatrogenesis in the elderly: Contributors to falls. *Journal of Gerontological Nursing, 17*(9), 19–23.

Sengstock, M. C., & Barrett, S. A. (1993). Abuse and neglect of the elderly in family settings. In J. Campbell & J. Humphreys (Eds.), *Nursing care of survivors of family violence* (pp. 173–208). St. Louis: C. V. Mosby.

Shiell, A., Kenny, P., & Farnworth, M. S. (1993). The role of the clinical nurse co-ordinator in the provision of cost-effective orthopaedic services for elderly people. *Journal of Advanced Nursing, 18,* 1424–1428.

Taeuber, C. (1993). Sixty-five plus in America (pp. 3, 11–16) [Brochure]. Washington, DC: U.S. Department of Commerce, Economics and Statistics Administration, Bureau of the Census.

Tinetti, M. E. (1986). Performance-oriented assessment of mobility problems in elderly patients. *Journal of the American Geriatrics Society, 34*(2), 119–126.

United Nations, Department of International Economic and Social Affairs. (1991). *Aging and urbanization.* Proceeding of the United Nations International Conference on Ageing Populations in the Context of Urbanization. New York: United Nations.

U.S. Department of Commerce, Economics and Statistics Administration, Bureau of the Census, & U.S. Department of Health and Human Services, National Institutes of Health, National Institute on Aging. (1991). *Profiles of America's elderly: Growth of America's elderly in the 1980's.* Washington, DC: U.S. Government Printing Office.

U.S. Department of Commerce, Economics and Statistics Administration, Bureau of the Census, & U.S. Department of Health and Human Services, National Institutes of Health, National Institute on Aging. (1993). *Profiles of America's elderly: Living arrangements of the elderly.* Washington, DC: U.S. Government Printing Office.

Watson, P. G. (1986). Stroke in the family: Theoretical considerations. *Rehabilitation Nursing, 11*(5), 15–17.

Zarle, N. S. (1989). Continuity of care: Balancing care of elders between health care settings. *Nursing Clinics of North America, 24,* 697–705.

PART **IV**

Rehabilitation Nursing Issues of the 21st Century

CHAPTER 30

Health Care Financing and Reimbursement

Barbara A. Marte

Reimbursement in health care has evolved from too little to what some consider too much. For the first time, however, nurses are adversely affected by the reimbursement system, which is currently driving health care decisions. Reported cutbacks of nursing staff in hospitals became headline news during the mid 1990s in many parts of the country. This chapter describes how health care has been and will be reimbursed. Nurses can meet and conquer the challenges of the current health care reimbursement system when there is a knowledge base for understanding the systems that drive the decisions.

HISTORICAL BACKGROUND OF HEALTH CARE REFORM

To understand where nurses need to position themselves in the constantly changing health care environment, it is valuable to understand what led to the current situation. Our country has not operated and does not operate within a coordinated health care system. Health insurance was designed to pay for treating illness. Within a capitalistic society, such a system provides financial incentive to the provider organization for maintaining sick care services.

Before the Depression in the 1930s, community-based hospitals and physicians delivered health care. Although fees were based on what the individual could afford, only the very wealthy sought professional, routine health care. Providers believed that people could and should be able to save for any excessive health care need. However, when the Depression wiped out the savings of most people, hospitals began to feel the effects of treating those who could not pay their bills.

Hospitals needed to find an alternative source of payment. During this period, groups of hospitals began to join together to offer guaranteed hospital care in exchange for a small monthly payment by groups of individuals in the communities they served. This idea originated in the Baylor Hospital System in Texas to serve schoolteachers and evolved into what we now know as the Blue Cross plans. It is important to note that these plans were developed, funded, and directed by the hospitals that developed them.

Similarly, Blue Shield plans were created to ensure physicians' payment from those who could not afford additional charges associated with the hospital stays covered by the emerging insurance plans. The origins of these hospital and physician plans laid the groundwork for our current system of health care financing and its provider orientation (Merrill, 1994).

The regional Blue Cross plans offered Americans an opportunity for protection against the prospect of high hospital costs. This was done through enrollment in a prepayment plan that was usually open to everyone at a uniform, community-rated premium. This private, nonprofit health insurance system underwent rapid growth during World War II when the federal government agreed unions could bargain for health care benefits without violating the prevailing wage freeze. (During the years the United States was involved in World War II, all available resources were dedicated to the war effort. One of the strategies used to reallocate resources was to freeze wages of the workers who remained in the private sector.) Federal tax codes also contributed to this expansion of the health insurance system. Employer premium payments for health insurance benefits were treated as a nontaxable business expense, and the value of employee benefits was exempted from income tax liability.

Besides the employer and employee tax advantages, further tax incentives were provided when the government supported hospital building programs. These policies are the essential reason why today hospitals are the central element of the health care system, constituting the single largest category of national health expenditures. Hospital expenditures per day and per stay in the United States are the highest among industrialized countries.

In the 1950s, commercial health insurance programs began competing with the Blue Cross plans by offering employers lower premiums based on experience rating rather than a community rate.

> *Experience-rated premium* is a premium calculation method that takes into account the actual utilization of the group rather than the combined utilization of all groups. The purpose is to more closely match a group's premiums to its costs.

> *Community rating* is a method of determining a premium structure that is not influenced by the expected level of benefit utilization by specific groups, but by expected utilization of the population as a whole. Everyone in a specified community would pay the same premium for the same package of benefits regardless of age, sex, medical history, lifestyle or place of residence (Trans-Century's Managed Care Glossary).

Competitive pressures in Texas led Blue Cross to also offer employers experience-rated premiums.

Private health insurance was founded on employment: a benefit added to workers' wages. Those who stopped working because of age or disability were no longer covered, just at the point in life when they had an increasing need for health care. Elderly people, chronically ill people, and other high-risk groups all encounter difficulty obtaining health insurance at a price they can afford (Ginzberg, 1994).

In 1993, President William Clinton made national health care reform a major issue for his first presidential term. This stimulated many debates and received much media exposure. However, national health care as a presidential issue did not originate with President Clinton. Since 1912, presidents have thought about introducing legislation to provide access to and payment for health care on a national basis. When John F. Kennedy ran for the presidency in 1960, one plank of his platform was the early enactment of Medicare. He met unyielding resistance from the American Medical Association, which called it "socialized medicine," and was unable to persuade fiscal conservatives in Congress to act on his proposal. In 1965, President Lyndon B. Johnson benefited from his overwhelming popular and electoral victory over Barry Goldwater by convincing Congress to enact Medicare (Title 18) as an entitlement program funded by tax dollars for virtually all individuals reaching the age of 65. Medicaid (Title 19) was enacted at the same time. The focus of these legislations was to ensure the availability of health care to seniors and individuals with disabling conditions (Medicare) as well as federally designated categories of the poor, principally women and children (Medicaid), who could not access the employer-based health insurance plans that covered most other Americans. These programs are financed through the Health Care Financing Administration (HCFA), an agency of the Department of Health and Human Services. Both federal and state governments fund Medicaid through a system in which federal funds match state revenue budget allocations. Income and resources determine eligibility.

To ensure that services provided to Medicare beneficiaries are effective, Medicare is designated a *cost-based* reimbursement program. Statistical data are evaluated to determine reasonable and customary charges. The provider of services to this population is required to submit a cost report at the end of each fiscal year to determine if charges were adequately reimbursed. Lower-than-anticipated costs demand that the provider pay back the Medicare fund. A provider whose costs exceed those assigned by HCFA is compensated for the additional costs if the costs can be validated as legitimate to the provision of services. This type of system encourages cost escalation. Through the "most-favored-nation" clause, the Medicare regulations stipulate that no payer can be charged less than the Medicare system. Therefore, providers who escalated their costs to ensure that Medicare beneficiaries received the "best" care are obligated to submit at least the same charges to the private insurers.

In 1983, after it was recognized how health care costs were escalating, the *prospective payment system* for Medicare-funded hospital services was initiated. This system was based on the determination of costs for *diagnosis-related groups* (DRGs), and hospitals were paid a set fee for each discharge based on the DRG classification. Although this system succeeded in reducing lengths of stay in hospitals for most categories, the real outcome of the system was cost shifting, not cost reduction. Hospitals discharged individuals "quicker and sicker" into a community-based service that remained in the *fee-for-service and cost-reim-bursed* system for payment. In effect, the costs to the Medicare system continued to escalate by shifting from one cost center to another.

During this period, there existed an opportunity for rehabilitation hospitals to enjoy growth and recognition because they remained exempt from the DRG system. Medicare regulations did, however, provide definite diagnoses and criteria for reimbursement for Medicare recipients in a rehabilitation hospital.

Incentives built into this system allow each provider to initiate treatment without any effort to coordinate with other services being delivered. Specialist providers, general practitioners, hospitals, and ancillary service centers all develop charges for their services, which are submitted to the payer in a fragmented manner. The claims are paid as submitted as long as the clinical criteria of the Medicare benefit or the health plan benefit are met. With both Medicare and the employer-based, experience-rated system, the health insurer has no incentive to monitor utilization because the increase in cost to the plan is passed on to the taxpayer and the employer.

In 1973, President Richard Nixon signed into law the Federal Health Maintenance Organization (HMO) Act. This legislation allowed the use of HMOs to encourage more cost-effective treatment.

> Health Maintenance Organizations (HMOs) offer prepaid, comprehensive health coverage for both hospital and physicians' services. An HMO contracts with health care providers, such as physicians, hospitals, and other health professionals, and members are required to use participating providers for all health services. Members are enrolled for a specified period of time. Model types include staff, group practice, network and Independent Practice Association (IPA). (The Texas Medical Association, 1998.)

This plan did not gain momentum until the early 1990s, when employers began crying for relief. They were no longer able to bear the ever-increasing costs of health insurance premiums. Employees had come to expect benefits that included fully paid health insurance and resented the financial contributions they were now being asked to bear to cover a portion of the premium. This is when managed care entered the system as a major player.

The managed care organizations, primarily HMOs, offered the employer lower premiums and increased services (such as covered physician office visits, annual physical examinations, immunizations, and well-child care).

The sale of traditional health insurance plans involved the negotiation of premiums with purchasing groups, primarily employers. In exchange for a specified dollar amount, the group received services that were defined by the number of visits to a provider, number of hospital days, and/or lifetime maximums on services. The number of enrollees determined the richness of the benefits and the number of people over which to spread the risk and the amount of premium the group purchaser was willing or able to pay.

Managed care organizations, on the other hand, negotiate contracts with the providers. The providers agree to service a population of members for a predetermined fee that is frequently an all-inclusive, per-member, per-month or per-day amount. Incentives are built into the provider's agreement that encourage efficient or limited utilization of resources. Managed care organizations have the management of care built into the system. It is either a primary care physician who is the gatekeeper of the system or a sophisticated case management program. After negotiating the cost of services, the HMO then presents a package of these services to a purchasing group at a premium significantly less than that of the health insurance company.

Our current health insurance system was developed to benefit the insurance company and providers of care rather than the consumer. The predominant risk is assumed by the consumer, who may or may not receive coverage for needed services in case of illness or accident. Both the health care provider and the insurer spread the risk over a defined population and then calculate carefully the element of risk imposed by that population. Rates are based on these actuarial calculations. Managed care plans are challenging the providers to assume more risk than they have ever allowed themselves to be exposed to in the past. Although this adds one more element to the risk sharing, it is still the consumer who may not receive coverage for needed services and therefore carries the greatest risk.

By the early 1990s, the focus of the health care crisis expanded to include access to care. In 1998, 44 million (16.3%) U.S. citizens had no health care coverage (U.S. Bureau of the Census, 1998). Because of the cycle of cost shifting and the growth of small businesses, some employers could not afford to provide health insurance. The uninsured encompassed a large number of employed middle-class citizens, who joined the voices advocating reform of the health care system and the need for universal access. It was no longer simply an issue for those on welfare or who were unemployed.

In the competition for the health care dollar through employer and other group purchasers, Medicare has continued to use resources at an ever-increasing rate. This gave rise to the health care reform effort by the Clinton administration in 1993–1994.

Although the anticipated global governmental reform did not take place, the incentive to improve the health care system has been unleashed. There is a plethora of changes taking place that offer exciting opportunities for nurses, especially rehabilitation nurses, whose primary focus has always been to improve function and promote wellness behaviors for all individuals. Throughout this chapter, these opportunities and responsibilities are evaluated. Initially, however, it is necessary to evaluate some dilemmas being faced by the rehabilitation client in the midst of the evolving reform.

DILEMMAS: HEALTH CARE FINANCING FOR THE REHABILITATION CLIENT

Efforts at resolving the health care crisis remain focused on reducing the costs of hospital services. DRGs did not affect freestanding rehabilitation hospitals, long-term care facilities, or home health services. In fact, these organizations enjoyed some of the advantages derived from cost shifting during the initial phase of the cost-cutting era. During this time, individuals requiring rehabilitation enjoyed the benefit of participating in fully-cost-reimbursed programs. However, as more and more of the health care financing was derived from the managed care model, the rehabilitation hospitals experienced the effects of reduced levels of reimbursement. Nursing was among the hospital's highest cost driver and therefore became a prime target for reductions. This fact had a dramatic effect on the type and level of services provided to individuals rehabilitating themselves from a major illness, injury, or exacerbation of a chronic condition.

Reimbursement for the rehabilitating client has always posed special concerns. As previously discussed, health care financing has been directed to those individuals who have incurred an illness or acute injury. By definition, rehabilitation is

> . . . the restoration of normal form and function after illness or injury, or the restoration of the ill or injured patient to optimal functional level in all areas of activity (*Dorland's Pocket Medical Dictionary,* 1995).

Rather than treating illness, rehabilitation services help those who are not achieving independent function to the highest degree of their capacity. The present and evolving system of health care financing separates the medical model and the social model into separate and distinct entities. Individuals who are not able to function at their highest capacity and who do not fit the definition of having illness or acute injury are assigned to the social model of services. These services tend to provide basic necessities such as food, clothing, and shelter but do not have an element that manages and monitors physiology, physical capacity, and independent function.

Through 1998, most health plans covered well-defined rehabilitation services, commonly including designated numbers of visits by a physical therapist. Occupational therapy, speech therapy, and psychosocial and nutritional services may or may not be covered, and when covered, they are usually delivered in conjunction with or incidental to nursing and/or physical therapy. The place in which these services are delivered also dictates the type of service covered through any health plan. The rehabilitation industry has made significant progress, however. Through education of the payer groups and the consumer groups, there has evolved a better understanding of the benefits of durable outcomes achieved through rehabilitation services. By the middle 1990s, managed care organizations were judged by the level of customer satisfaction as well as cost-effectiveness. It became important to maintain a satisfied customer, and outcomes that maintained the individual in a higher state of wellness and improved function were considered cost-effective. Rehabilitation professionals have become vocal in educating decision makers about the value of "the right service at the right time by the right professional" to genuinely achieve cost savings and improved health outcomes.

The question of how to communicate the value of ongoing intervention by rehabilitation professionals to sustain maximal function for an individual with a chronic disabling condition remains a dilemma. The individual who has attained an improved independent function secondary to rehabilitation should be evaluated periodically to ensure that physiological and psychological function remain stable to sustain the desired durable outcome.

The following factors influence a lack of compliance with follow-up evaluations:

- The health insurance will not cover the follow-up evaluations.
- The insurance plan has changed.
- The insurance plan has been discontinued.
- The individual is no longer employed or has changed employers and is no longer eligible for benefits under the plan.
- The individual without benefits usually chooses not to pursue additional services until such a time that a small problem has exacerbated into a major problem requiring intense services to regain independent function.

The following section reviews how the various insurances respond to the needs of the individual requiring rehabilitation services.

THIRD-PARTY PAYERS

To acquire a better comprehension of the various mechanisms for health care financing, basic tenets of the most common methods will be reviewed.

Public

Medicare

Medicare is a federally funded program designed to provide health care to seniors (65 years and older) and those who qualify for Disability. The disability must have occurred at least 24 months before the initiation of benefits, and an approved physician has to determine the extent of the disability. Specific regulations govern the administration of the program and the licensing of providers who may participate in the program. As of 1996, HCFA continued to administer the program as a cost-reimbursed/fee-for-service program except for those services covered under the prospective payment system part of the program. Managed care has entered the Medicare program by agreeing to be capitated by HCFA for up to 95% of the premium based on the geographical service area of the beneficiary. Managed care organizations are obligated to provide the same benefits to Medicare beneficiaries as defined by Federal law.

Medicare, prior to the Balanced Budget Act (BBA) of 1997 (Pub. L. No. 105-33), was a cost-reimbursed program, Some HMOs received larger capitation allotments than others, based on the cost of services in designated areas of the country. These HMOs had the distinct advantage of being able to offer a much richer benefit to individuals who joined their plans. All the rules changed with the implementation of the BBA.

Balanced Budget Act of 1997

The BBA was signed into law by President Clinton in August 1997. This legislation enacts the most significant changes to the Medicare and Medicaid programs since their inception 30 years age. In addition, it expands the services provided by HCFA through the new Child Health Insurance Program (Title XXI).

The anticipated result of this legislation is to

- Extend the life of the Medicare Trust Fund and reduce Medicare spending
- Increase health care options available to America's seniors
- Improve benefits for staying healthy
- Fight Medicare fraud and abuses
- Look at ways to help Medicare work well in the future (HCFA Web Page)

As of this writing, the actual outcomes remain to be determined. The financial stability of the large-chain nursing homes has become tenuous. For the nursing home providers, the BBA means changing from a cost-reimbursed system to a prospective payment system (PPS), as with the DRGs for hospital care. Providers claim that they can no longer afford to care for the frail elderly within the limited reimbursements provided under the BBA.

It is evident that the Medicare system must change to ensure continued services. When the methods of paying for health care services change, the means of providing the services change also. Nurses must be aware of the changes and be prepared to monitor practice patterns to ensure that persons receiving services are not adversely affected. At the same time, it is important to manage the business of health care in a manner that allows providers to remain solvent.

Medicaid

Medicaid is a state-funded program that is subsidized by the federal government with matching funds. Those states that have more funds allocated to health care of the poor receive more funds from the federal government. States are not motivated to provide too rich a plan, however, because that would encourage the entry of more poor people into their states. HMOs are gaining access to Medicaid programs to encourage more wellness programs and control the escalating costs to the state governments. Each state determines how its Medicaid monies will be distributed. Some are implementing case management programs and promoting home-based services that prevent health-related problems. Many states fund their programs on a cost-based allocation, others determine a case mix allocation, and still others use a form of DRG/prospective payment system.

Private

Health and Accident Insurance

Health and accident insurance is primarily an indemnity insurance plan. Health care services are financed based on contract language with no specific criteria for outcomes or characteristics of conditions treated. These plans are provided year to year for a premium payment. Until recently, the people paying the claims were interested only in meeting the criteria outlined in the contract for services that would or would not be paid. There was no incentive to evaluate long-term benefits of services delivered. Claims adjusters operated under the principle that there is no relevancy to how much the recommended noncontractual services save in 5 years, or over a lifetime, because the limits of the policy will be reached before the saved dollars are realized.

As competition from managed care increased, most of these indemnity plans changed their approach and, subsequently, their way of doing business. The managed indemnity plans in which case managers determine the value of "out-of-contract" services to achieve improved outcomes were developed in an attempt to bring together the best of all models. In fact, several hybrids are emerging from this product line that may establish how health care will be financed for many of the larger groups.

Managed Care

Managed care is a generic term that refers to health care delivery that has a component that focuses on results and outcomes of services delivered. The system integrates financial criteria with clinical outcomes. Managed care can be as small as a group practice of physicians, or as large as a national network that services millions of members in multiple states.

Casualty Insurance

Casualty insurance covers incidents that occur through accident or negligence. Workers' compensation, medical bills resulting from automobile accidents, and liability from personal injury are examples of medical claims on casualty insurance. These products vary in levels of medical coverage, again based on the purchaser's decision about the degree of liability assumed and purchased. Some automobile insurance and all workers' compensation plans have minimal requirements dictated by public policy. Primarily, the goal of the casualty claim is to resolve the condition and close the file. In actuality, it was the causality insurance industry that initiated managed care. Workers' compensation carriers learned early that the degree to which an injured worker recovered sufficient function to allow a return to work and closure on the claim could be significantly influenced by the assignment of a case manager to manage the services. The case manager sought to provide a continuum of uninterrupted care to ensure maximal recovery. These plans frequently cover the medical and rehabilitation services for as long as required to attain the highest level of independent function possible as determined by a qualified physician.

Casualty insurance plans have also experienced consistent increases in costs and utilization and are moving to a more structured managed care model. It is apparent that some form of care that manages resource utilization will govern health care financing. It is uncertain exactly when and to what extent Medicare will become a managed care product. Certain trends are sure to move this payment mechanism to a more managed environment as evidenced by the following:

- 86% of elderly persons (persons older than 75 years) suffer from some form of chronic illness (Gill, 1996).
- Baby boomers will be elders by 2020 (Gill, 1996).
- Elders will account for more than 40% of all hospital days early in the 21st century (Gill, 1996).
- Hospital services will need to shift from acute care to chronic care model (Dixon & Trenchard, 1996).

In summary, we have a changing structure for financing health care. No one can predict the outcome of this evolution, but one thing is certain: nurses will and must be active in the change process.

NURSING IMPLICATIONS

Historically, neither providers nor consumers have been accountable for overall costs. Decisions about care have been made by physicians whose individual fortunes rose or fell according to the volume of services provided rather than the efficiency or efficacy of services provided (Taylor & Lessin, 1996). Financially, providers should increasingly expect health plans to demand risk sharing, not risk shifting. It is also imperative that the success formula demand factors that include member satisfaction. Until the late 1990s, HMOs paid physicians on a fee-schedule or modified fee-for-service basis, and hospitals were paid at charges or a discount from charges. The HMOs sought to control their costs primarily through controls on utilization. This approach did not take into account any of the conditions affecting the individual receiving services such as the level of acuteness, comorbidity, or culture. It assumed that the providers of health care were arbitrarily overtreating and overutilizing resources. Although many of these managed care plans brought nurses into the picture as utilization review professionals, the nurses had to answer to the financial aspects of care more than the clinical aspects. They frequently made decisions without conferring with the treating professionals or seeing the clients. The actuarial data provided the only source for decision making. The past tense is used here because this system is gradually being recognized as inadequate and failing to accomplish the goals of cost reduction with quality outcomes. The system is moving away from the first wave of managed care companies that were designed to minimize excessive or unnecessary care through restrictive utilization review and preauthorization mandates on individual discounted fee-for-service providers. In more mature managed care markets, the focus is shifting from this tactical, short-term, cost-focused approach toward the strategic and thoughtful application of an accountability philosophy designed to restructure the way provider systems deliver care. That philosophy is grounded in prepayment to risk-bearing delivery systems.

The change in American health care that is occurring is the largest change effort to be managed by an industry since deregulation transformed the transportation and telecommunication industries in the 1980s. It is a people-intensive transformation. In the health care industry, which accounts for 14% of the gross domestic product, approximately 65% of the total expenditures are people related (Spiker, Miron, Lesser, & Jackson, 1994).

Attorney Carol Schaffer (1996) defined three stages of managed care as follows:

> *Stage 1:* Providers use a fee-for-service approach with price compression and fierce competition.
> *Stage 2:* Service providers begin to affiliate, looking at episodes of care.
> *Stage 3:* The insurance market becomes controlled by managed care plans. This eliminates providers who cannot remain financially viable.

The stage of managed care that is evolving as the market matures is described as follows (Taylor & Lessin, 1996):

> *Stage 4:* There is prepayment to risk-sharing delivery systems (with strong case management and information management systems to serve communities or populations) with strategic and thoughtful application of an accountability philosophy.

In the coordinated health care system that is emerging, services will be delivered more efficiently and the emphasis will be more on quality than on cost. It becomes the provider's or practitioner's responsibility to manage costs within designated financial resources.

Employers remain the drivers of the process because (as a society) we continue to function in an employer-based health insurance system. Employers are realizing that they are being challenged to choose a product with no basis for comparative shopping. In other words, employers have only the information presented by the salesperson of each health insurance product to define its value. The demand for missing performance information has been heard and responded to by entrepreneurs. Health service research is developing methods to attempt to establish standards of performance for the health plans. There are several accrediting bodies for health insurance organizations. In each case, along with cost-effectiveness, there is a drive to evaluate customer satisfaction and outcomes of services. More and more, the system is focusing on clinical outcomes, prevention, and wellness programs. In order to achieve this goal, the up-front cost to a health plan in securing new members is significant. The promotion of healthy behaviors requires education, evaluation, printed literature, and follow-up. It is therefore propitious for the health care system to retain members as long as possible to achieve a return on the investment.

As the managed health care system moves forward, there are four constituents whose needs must be met to achieve success:

- The consumer
- The provider
- The payer
- The employer and group purchaser

The successful delivery system must efficiently meet and coordinate the needs of each constituent.

As the model that no longer focuses only on the acute care services develops, the number of covered lives will be more important than patient days. The majority of health care resource utilization will be in an integrated chronic care continuum. In this continuum the health care system will need to

- Minimize the progression of pathophysiological changes
- Prevent and/or minimize the progression of the disability
- Maximize socialization
- Recognize that decreased function and isolation are major predictors of resource consumption

An increasingly demanding well-informed purchaser of health care services will focus on outcomes of the service. The system will evaluate what services delivered to what population in what environment have the most potential to effect positive outcomes.

Currently, DRGs are based on a patient's principal diagnosis rather than on demographic factors such as race and age. For the same diagnosis, hospitals may use more resources on patients who are older and of minority origin than is recognized through data on which DRGs are based (Shi, 1996). As the move continues into a more integrated delivery system, more sophisticated data will be required to appropriately manage the population. Critical factors in the success of the integrated health care delivery system include

Physician, nurse, ancillary professional, and paraprofessional selection criteria: Roles will be redefined and functions changed. The measurement of group and individual success will be defined based on the efficiency and efficacy of the services provided.

Practice guidelines: Looking at conditions with potential for high resource use, clinical guidelines and standards of practice will have to be defined in a manner that allows consistent follow-through and the measurement of deviations from the expected outcomes. Today, this is usually identified as a clinical pathway. The clinical pathways required by an integrated delivery system will need to encompass the entire disease cycle from the onset of acute disease to rehabilitation, stability, instability, deterioration, and end-stage disease.

Financial controls: The clinicians will have to work in concert with those who control the scarce resources to ensure efficient utilization.

Case management: The case manager in the evolving integrated health care delivery system will have an ever-expanding role. The case manager will function as the hub of the wheel and ensure that all elements of the wheel function smoothly—for example, that the clinical, financial, consumer, and public needs are being met in a manner that meets the majority of needs.

Continuous performance improvement: Data collected will be consolidated into formats that provide knowledge that leads to improved efficiencies and efficacies.

Larry Gamm (1996) states, "Accountability of health services organizations is defined here as taking into account and responding to *political, commercial, community and clinical/patient interests and expectations.*" In this case, the key words for nurses are *accountability to clinical/patient interests and expectations.* Today and for the future, the challenges to all who work within the health care system will revolve around the triple tensions of access, cost, and quality. Nurses must be accountable to all the stakeholders in the health care system to ensure availability, affordability, and the effectiveness of outcomes while balancing the issues of ethics with business objectives.

As complex issues are addressed, it should be noted that although health care is increasingly interdisciplinary, nursing is the one profession that delivers, manages, and coordinates the care across the disciplines. The ability of nurses to practice within multiple settings positions them to become a keystone of the integrated delivery systems. The integrated delivery systems must be prepared to participate in outcome assessment and to demonstrate the quality of care and concurrently collect data that accurately reflect the cost of each element of the care. This cost must compare with the clinical outcomes. It will also be crucial to account for the education provided to individuals receiving services and to their families, to their primary caregivers, to professionals who treat them, to paraprofessional staff, and to the community. Outcomes of the educational programs will also need to be measured and priced effectively to allow this critical element of the formula to be included in the cost of providing comprehensive services. It has been the philosophy of rehabilitation nurses since the onset of the designation of a specialty practice that education is key to successful rehabilitation outcomes. The integrated health care delivery systems will also need to adopt this philosophy to ensure success.

Another essential element of a successful health care delivery system will be to demonstrate linkage to other provider organizations. Having multiple institutions in the same area competing for the same customer base must be recognized as inefficient, costly, and counterproductive. In an integrated health care delivery system, the community needs will be assessed, services will be designed and delivered to ensure access, and services will be managed centrally through comprehensive case management.

Outcomes that result in improved health with reduced utilization of scarce resources will be sought. Through research, nurses must demonstrate the value of the primary nurse's interventions as a vital element of the integrated health care delivery system. As the public evolves through the changing paradigm, wellness will be the focus of the system, and services will no longer originate with hospitals and physicians.

IMPLICATIONS OF NURSING RESEARCH ON HEALTH CARE FINANCING

The evolution of traditional health care services into an integrated health care delivery system provides nurses with the greatest opportunity since the beginning of the profession to assume a role of leadership in this emerging process. Within the framework of research, nurses must document the contribution the nursing profession makes to the delivery, management, and coordination of care.

Rehabilitation nurses have been functioning in the role of case managers since the early days of workers' compensation "medical managers." The case manager of tomorrow will be coordinating services and facilitating improved independent function in much the same manner, but with improved technological resources and a more diverse team of professionals, paraprofessionals, community resources, and family resources. Nurses will coordinate services throughout the continuum of health care services and throughout a lifetime. Nursing is the profession to lead this research through decisions based on scientific knowledge and accurate information accrued from comprehensive data. Anecdotal data support the theory that nursing involvement in the coordination of services; consumer, customer, and community education; and collaborative professional practice has a positive impact on health care outcomes. Without credible, validated data, these views will not be valued or supported in the restructuring of the system that delivers health and wellness services.

NURSING'S INVOLVEMENT IN PUBLIC POLICY TO AFFECT HEALTH CARE FINANCING

Nurses are the bedrock of the health care system but have not generally used that influence to promote the public good. We have been exploring the evolving health care delivery system. It is necessary to emphasize that much of the actual service delivery system originates through public policy.

The voice of nursing in public policy development has been a mere whisper. If we are to influence decision making, we must be willing to be heard. The most effective way to achieve this goal is to join forces with our peers and have our voices heard in unity. It is the responsibility of professional nurses to participate in their organizations. Likewise, it is critical that the professional nursing organizations support a common mission that will empower the professional nurse to influence and provide vision for the future direction of health care. This is an opportunity that must be seized. Nurses have the perspective of health and wellness. They must use that knowledge and professional value system to evaluate health policy issues, most of which are cost dominated. Nurses must assist the policymakers to understand the quality-of-life issues that drive healthful behaviors. These factors will allow prevention and health-oriented services to be the focus of America's health care reform.

REFERENCES

Dixon, R., Trenchard, P. M. (1996). Theoretical evaluation of the role of precision and quality in clinical costings. *Health Care Management Review, 21*, 7–15.

Dorland's Pocket Medical Dictionary (25th ed.). (1995). Philadelphia: W. B. Saunders.

Gamm, L. D. (1996). Dimensions of accountability for not-for-profit hospitals and health systems. *Health Care Management Review, 21*, 74–86.

Gill, H. (1996, June). Managing post acute care services under Medicare capitation. *Post Acute Care Strategy Report, 1*.

Ginzberg, E., Ostow, M. (1994). *The road to reform: The future of health care in America* (pp. 8, 9, 60–86). New York: Free Press.

Merrill, J. C. (1994). *The road to health care reform: Designing a system that works* (pp. 7–65). New York: Plenum Press.

Schaffer, C. (1996, March). Integration, contracting to change case management. *Continuing Care, 15*(3), 29.

Shi, L. (1996). Patient and hospital characteristics associated with average length of stay. *Health Care Management Review, 21*, 46–61.

Spiker, B. K., Miron, D. K., Lesser, E., & Jackson, D. H. (1994). Managing change in the healthcare industry. *Marsh & McLennan Companies Quarterly, 23*.

Taylor, R., Lessin, L. (1996). Restructuring the health care delivery system in the United States. *Journal of Healthcare Finance, 22*(4), 33–60.

Trans-Century's Managed Care Glossary. www.trancent.com/glos.htm15-Sept.-98.

U.S. Bureau of the Census. (1998). www.census.gov/hhes/hlthins/hlthin98/h.98 + 8.htm

BIBLIOGRAPHY

Coile, R. (1997, April). Millennium management, strategies for managing 21st century health care organizations. *Health Trends, 9*(6).

Huber, D. (1996). *Leadership and nursing care management.* Philadelphia: W. B. Saunders.

Milstein, A. (1994). Health Care in America: An industry in transition. *The Marsh & McLennan Companies Quarterly, 23*.

Strauss, A., Corbin, J. M. (1988). *Shaping a new health care system* (pp. 5, 143, 144). San Francisco: Jossey-Bass.

Wiggins, S. R. (1996). Commentary on capitation. *Journal of Healthcare Finance, 22*, 10–14.

CHAPTER 31

Rehabilitation Nursing in Vietnam: A Prototype for Bringing Rehabilitation Nursing to a Third World Nation

Jill B. Derstine

A review of the literature shows little evidence of the establishment of rehabilitation nursing in developing countries. As an example, in the Socialist Republic of Vietnam during the early 1990s, the word *rehabilitation* was usually associated with the work done by physical therapists. Nurses took no part in the rehabilitative process, and it was unheard of for a nurse to suggest even such a commonplace activity as passive or active exercises. Nurses in most settings still assumed the role of handmaiden to the physicians, and it was difficult to ascertain the role of nurses, as it seemed they only administered medications and completed treatments. Feeding, bathing, toileting, and ambulating activities were performed by a selected family member who slept at the patient's bedside. Rehabilitation as a medical specialty was in its infancy, and nurses were not even aware that they should be included in the field. The introduction of rehabilitation nursing to this Third World country presented challenges that required skillful teaching and negotiating skills. This chapter describes the process of introducing rehabilitation nursing concepts, principles, and procedures to a Third World or developing country using an experience in Vietnam as a prototype.

REVIEW OF THE LITERATURE

Leininger (1991), the founder of transcultural nursing, stressed that the modern nurse must be able to assess, understand, and work effectively with people of many different cultures. Adapting to a new or different way of helping clients while valuing their cultural differences and needs is a challenge in the practice setting where the clients speak a different language, have different health practices, and have different values. Transcultural nursing has become a vehicle for helping nurses move from traditional practice to more flexible, innovative, and meaningful practice. When working in a developing country, the foreign nurse is in the minority and must have insight as to why people of specific cultures behave as they do when there is an ill or disabled family member. The definition of transcultural nursing by Leininger (1991, p. 60), a "humanistic and scientific area of formal study and practice in nursing which is focused upon differences and similarities among cultures with respect to human care, health (or well being), and illness based upon the people's cultural beliefs, and practices, and to use this knowledge to provide cultural specific or culturally congruent nursing care to people," can be used as the foundation for any nursing effort in a Third World country. Before one can hope to help a people of a different culture, one must become aware of personal bias and be willing to learn and understand the culture and its care needs.

Others have introduced Western-oriented nursing to developing countries; however, Hertzberg (1993) reported the only project related to rehabilitation in her article that described an undertaking in the Republic of Armenia after the earthquake of 1988. A member of an interdisciplinary team, she was able to bring a view of the role of the rehabilitation nurse to the health care personnel in Armenia. She writes of cultural differences, conflict because of the bureaucratic structure, and psychological, physical, and emotional factors. Misunderstandings owing to language problems, difficult living conditions, and tension from the conflict of ongoing border difficulties emerged as barriers to the completion of objectives.

In a Canadian-Chinese exchange program, Chamberlain, Fothergill-Bourbonnais, Li, and Song (1995) found the biggest challenge to be integrating Western methods of nursing care while continuing to value Chinese traditions. "It would be unfortunate if, in our zeal to help, we eradicated the established traditional Chinese ways for methods that have not necessarily been shown to be the best for clients in the West" (Chamberlain et al., 1995, p. 146).

DeSantis's (1995) model for counterparts in international nursing suggested that in order for programs to be successful and ongoing, personnel in the developing country who can carry on the work after the training group leaves must be trained. Under the auspices of project HOPE, DeSantis participated in an instructor preparation program at Xi'an University in the People's Republic of China. She stated that the two main impediments to the project were the lack of nurses prepared at a level considered appropriate for teachers and a lack of understanding of the nursing content. If the program is to be successful, the author suggested that certain tasks be accomplished by the donor and the host group and their respective counterparts, the most important one being the agreement between both groups regarding roles, responsibilities, and qualifications of the participants (DeSantis, p. 201.)

Others have participated in foreign exchange programs in general nursing involving faculty and/or students (Frisch, 1990; Mmtli & Mossieman, 1995; Rosenkoetter, Reynolds, Cummings, & Zakutney, 1993; Toyoshima, 1994); however, when the literature is examined as a whole, there is little or no reference to rehabilitation nursing.

ASSESSMENT

Before rehabilitation nursing is introduced to a developing country, it is necessary to conduct an in-depth assessment of the number and nature of resources available. For the Vietnam experience, an interdisciplinary group from the sponsoring volunteer organization made a preparatory visit to the country to explore facilities, accommodations, and transportation and to make contacts with appropriate personnel (O'Toole, Melli, Moore, & Derstine, 1996). The team consisted of a nurse, a physician, a physical therapist, and the executive director of the sponsoring volunteer organization, Health Volunteers Over-

seas (Coby, date unknown). After a series of visits to various hospitals in all parts of the country, the site assessment team realized that rehabilitation practice was scant or not present at all, and that the candidates for rehabilitation care, especially head trauma patients, were strongly evident in all settings.

During the site assessment, the nurse member of the team noted a great deal of role conflict among the nurses. "The nurses in Vietnam recognized that something vital was missing from the care administered to individuals, and they sensed that they could fill this void" (O'Toole et al., 1996, p. 39). The rehabilitation team concept was also missing; rehabilitation in Vietnam implied that patients would spend a bit of time in a very primitive gymnasium or learn to walk with a homemade wooden cane (Fig. 31–1).

In a developing country, conditions may appear so primitive that at first glance the helping professional is stunned into inaction. For example, in Vietnam, "hospital wards are large and crowded, sometimes making it nec-

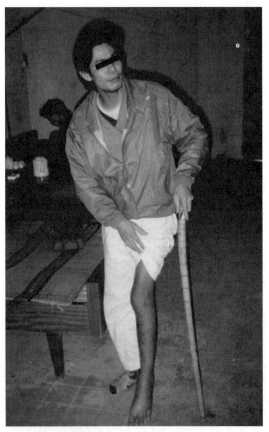

FIGURE 31–1
Patient using a homemade cane.

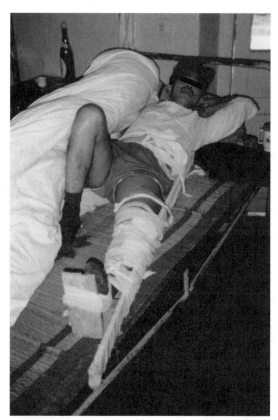

FIGURE 31–2
Patient in bed with only a thin straw mat as a mattress.

essary for two patients to one bed, sleeping head to foot. Most beds have no mattresses or sheets, only a thin straw mat [Fig. 31–2]. Family members are responsible for the care of the patient, attending to all activities of daily living" (Poremba, 1995, p. 121). The assessment team found numerous family members with each patient, but the family members had little knowledge of how to assist their relative. When a seemingly hopeless situation is first encountered by the health professional, a sense of powerlessness may be the immediate reaction. Prior exposure to the conditions in an underdeveloped country either by sensitivity training or by actual experiences can help with this problem. The helping professional should strive to observe practices, traditions, and beliefs in order to be able to complete a comprehensive assessment so that the intervention is culturally sensitive.

PLANNING

After the in-depth assessment, a plan of action that will effectively establish rehabilitation nursing in the country is necessary. Every step of the plan should be sensitive to the social and cultural differences inherent in the host country. Culturally competent care is of the utmost importance in this situation because the persons introducing the changes in nursing and health care are usually of a different culture than those with whom they are working.

In the Vietnam experience, the site assessment team decided that a series of workshops focusing on collaborative rehabilitation care would be a logical first step. This would meet the initial need of defining interdisciplinary rehabilitation practice and also serve as a demonstration of how to implement the specialty. The team designed six workshops that covered a variety of common rehabilitation diagnoses and would be presented at various sites in the country including the northern, central, and southern areas. Each workshop would be conducted by a different team consisting of at least a physiatrist, a nurse, and a physical therapist, with other team members as appropriate. The workshops were designed to present didactic material and provide hands-on clinical experience. The attendees, which included persons from each discipline, would attend all of the lectures at a given workshop (regardless of discipline) and then break into discipline-specific groups that would work with patients. It was planned to offer the workshops to those who would be teaching other health professionals throughout the country. The topics that were requested by the Vietnamese health care workers included amputations, arthritis, cerebral palsy, cerebrovascular accidents, spinal cord injury, and trauma. The workshops were spaced over a 2-year period, and the site assessment team members were responsible for recruiting and orienting the prospective team members (O'Toole et al., 1996). After the interdisciplinary workshops, each discipline would take the data generated and plan to implement discipline-specific rehabilitation workshops, continuing training as long as resources were available. Rehabilitation nursing definitely emerged as an area in need of development.

IMPLEMENTATION

When any type of international work is proposed, a certain amount of groundwork must be done to be certain of protocol in the host country. If there is a ministry of health, the proper officials must be contacted and in-country support established. The ideal support is an English-speaking citizen of the host country who not only can translate but can ease the way with everyday tasks. At the very least, a good translator is of the utmost importance.

To implement a project in a developing country, the plan should call for an in-depth orientation of the prospective volunteers. A knowledge of what to expect in the way of living conditions, climate, and health care facilities is an essential prerequisite to beginning any kind of work with health care personnel. Face-to-face meetings, conference calls, or e-mail communications can be scheduled for orientation and to plan the teaching responsibilities. These can be directed by a coordinator, a person who has experienced the country in some way, either as a volunteer or in a working situation.

In the Vietnam experience, six 5-day teaching workshops took place over a period of 2 years. The standard format was for each team to present two identical workshops in two different locales, usually one in the northern part of the country and one in the southern part of the country. The workshop format consisted of 2 days of lecture and 3 days of clinical demonstration and practice. Much of the practice consisted of return demonstrations including a demonstration of an interdisciplinary team evaluating a real patient. Because the Vietnamese did not speak English, all teaching and learning had to be done through translators. This required that lectures be planned within a time span that included enough time for the translation of every word. To practice for this "double timing," the lecturer can deliver the lectures into a tape recorder and then double the time spent on each topic. The lecturer needs to be aware that the translator may not be familiar with certain idioms used by Americans and should stick to using language that does not include slang.

EVALUATION

Evaluation activities should provide immediate and long-term feedback on the effectiveness of the program. Immediate feedback can be obtained with end-of-course evaluations. Because those in the host country are often very eager to please their teachers, this feedback will probably be positive, regardless of the quality of the teaching. Here again, a knowledge of the culture of the country is desirable. The Vietnamese people, for example, value respect and harmony above all, and the desire for harmony may take precedence over truth (Giger & Davidhizar, 1995, p. 446). Therefore, when questioned about the value of the workshop or teaching session, the response may be positive so as not to cause disharmony with the teachers who have come such a long distance to help the people in their country.

If at all possible, the value of the teaching should be assessed by specifying the desired outcomes before the workshops and then setting up observation sessions that will determine whether the effects are lasting and whether the attendees are teaching the newly learned material to others in their country. On subsequent visits to the host country, the nurse educator can determine if there are any changes in behavior by observing the host country faculty interacting with their students and patients.

Implementing a specific program under the auspices of a sponsor is merely the first step in bringing the specialty of rehabilitation nursing to a developing country. It is necessary for the nurses of the host country to understand the philosophy of rehabilitation nursing and how it can be integrated within their present method of health and nursing care delivery. Perhaps the most important step is to ensure that the visiting nurse educators understand the cultural norms of the host country and that they prepare their lectures and demonstrations to include sensitivity to the everyday practices of living. Skill in intercultural communication is essential. "Framing communication experiences in the health context provides a background useful for international nursing" (May & Meleis, 1987, p. 39). A knowledge of the language of the host country provides the ideal background for understanding the health care experiences of the country. If this is not possible, the nurse educator should be willing to use words and phrases in the host's language. A good preparation for teaching in a developing country is to meet with recent immigrants or visitors from that country before the teaching experience.

To continue the work in Vietnam, the nurse educators returned to the country to conduct a 2-week curriculum workshop on rehabilitation nursing that was attended by nurses from almost every nursing school in Vietnam. Five nurse educators taught various sections of a curriculum that included teaching and learning methods and rehabilitation nursing content. The content included nursing care related to head injury and stroke, spinal cord injury, amputations, and cerebral palsy. The role of the rehabilitation nurse was covered in detail, emphasizing empowerment, which in some cases meant merely speaking up in a team conference. Role playing was used extensively, using situations that included nurse-patient and teacher-student interactions. To demonstrate the concept of the rehabilitation team, mock team conferences were held. The Vietnamese nurses felt uncomfortable speaking up at a team conference if there were physicians present until it was emphasized that within the body of nursing knowledge there were important issues that would add to the total care of the patient. The nurses were encouraged to introduce concepts including bowel and bladder training, nutrition and feeding techniques, and sexuality at team conferences.

COLLABORATIVE AGREEMENTS

The goal of a collaborative relationship is to develop the host country to the point at which their own teachers can carry on the work. To attain ongoing viability of the rehabilitation nursing project in Vietnam, the next step was to forge linkages with three nursing programs in the country located strategically in the northern, central, and southern areas. Each of the three nursing schools in Vietnam was linked with a nursing program in the United States. An agreement was worked out with each school with the goal of developing a reservoir of nurse educators in Vietnam. In working out the individual agreements for continued association, the goals included fostering understanding of each other's cultures while helping the host school by offering lectures and supplies if possible. Often the host country professionals perceive the visitors as having vast supplies of resources including money and supplies that can be given to the host country. For example, the nurse educators in the host country were very eager to be funded for trips to the United States to observe teaching methods; but with their limited command of English, information exchange would be greatly diminished. They were advised to provide English lessons for their faculty as a first step toward this goal, a realistic one in that English is a desired language in Vietnam and there are English teachers available.

Rehabilitation nursing concepts that nurses in the United States take for granted may have been unheard of in a developing country. An example of this is bowel and bladder training, an idea that when first explained brought incredulous looks from the Vietnamese nurses. They expressed verbally that such a technique could not be successful. By the end of 2 weeks, they were familiar with the term and were prescribing it for their patients in team conferences. Sexuality was another taboo subject, and the nurses from the United States were told in no uncertain terms that it was a private thing and nothing to be discussed between patient and nurse. Despite all efforts, this attitude prevailed until one day when one of the nurse educators was demonstrating taking a history from a spinal cord patient, a young man of about 18, and his father, who was standing nearby, asked, "But will my son be able to have children?" What a wonderful example to demonstrate this point! This provided the perfect lead into sexuality teaching.

CONCLUSION

It is evident that many factors need to be taken into account when rehabilitation nursing is introduced into a developing country. The nurses from the outside must have not only an understanding of rehabilitation techniques and principles but also a deeper understanding of the country and the culture of the host country. Culturally sensitive teaching that includes an emphasis on culturally competent care must be adhered to at all times.

Giger and Davidhizar (1995, p. 10) suggest a transcultural assessment model that examines six cultural phenomena: (1) communication, (2) space), (3) social organization, (4) time, (5) environmental control, and (6) biological variations. Stauffer (in Giger & Davidhizar, 1995, pp. 441–471) provides a detailed discussion of Vietnamese traits under each of these six phenomena:

1. *Communication:* A distinct feature of Vietnamese culture related to the language is that emphasis is placed on moderation and caution, and people are taught to wait and think before speaking. The word *yes* is used in Vietnam as being respectful and is used often as an answer to queries. It does not necessarily mean agreement.
2. *Space:* Touching, such as backslapping or hugging, is limited. Even those who are to be married do not touch in public. Touching the head is not accepted, and social exchanges usually consist of handshakes.
3. *Social organization:* Families live in close quarters; therefore, it is not unusual to see

a crowd of family members around a patient's bed and even in bed with the patient. A high value is place on filial piety.

4. *Time*: Time is thought of in terms of cycles, events, or occurrences, and there is less emphasis on being on time. Being early or late is perfectly acceptable.

5. *Environmental control:* Belief in folk medicine is widespread, and lately, practices incorporating Chinese medicine with traditional medicine are common.

6. *Biological variations*: Vietnamese people are usually small, with average body weight for their height. They recognize two possible causes of mental illness: one in which the nerves of the brain are damaged and the second in which behavior is attributed to causes such as sin or disobedience.

Giger and Davidhizar (1995) provide information on a variety of cultures that would be helpful to health care professionals establishing projects in these countries.

Rehabilitation nursing pioneers in the United States stressed that the goal of rehabilitation is to return the patient to the community as a useful citizen. That goal was modified over the years to include ensuring that the patient achieves an acceptable quality of life and achieves maximal independence in activities of daily living. The goal of introducing rehabilitation nursing to a developing country can be similar, but it must be congruent with the country's level of development. The rehabilitation nurse should first assess the level of general nursing care in the country and plan the teaching of rehabilitation skills accordingly. It takes astute communication skills and excellent assessment skills to plan a teaching project in a country that is several years behind the United States in health care. The nurse is advised to move slowly and cautiously and take advantage of the work of others who have been in the same situation. The principles of rehabilitation nursing remain the same, regardless of the setting.

REFERENCES

Chamberlain, M., Fothergill-Bourbonnais, F., Li, Y., & Song, J. (1995). Cultural differences in Canadian-Chinese nursing. *International Nursing Review, 42,* 143–149.

Coby, J. C., & Kelly, N. A. *A guide to volunteering overseas* (3rd ed.). Washington, DC: Health Volunteers Overseas.

DeSantis, L. (1995). A model for counterparts in international nursing. *International Journal of Nursing Studies, 32,* 198–209.

Frisch, N. C. (1990). An international nursing student exchange program: An educational experience that enhanced student cognitive development. *Journal of Nursing Education, 29,* 10–12.

Giger, J. N., & Davidhizar, R. E. (1995). *Transcultural nursing: Assessment and intervention* (2nd ed.). St, Louis: Mosby–Year Book.

Hertzberg, D. L. (1993). The interdisciplinary team: The experience in the Armenia pediatric rehabilitation program. *Holistic Nurse Practitioner, 7,* 42–48.

Leininger, M. (1991, April–May). Transcultural nursing: The study and practice field. *Journal of National Student Nurses Association,* pp. 55–66. Imprint.

May, K. M., & Meleis, A. (1987). International nursing: Guidelines for core content. *Nurse Educator, 12,* 36–40.

Mmtli, K., & Mossieman, D. S. (1995). A model of distance education for nurses: The Botswana experience. *Nursing and Health Care: Perspectives on Community, 16,* 221–224.

O'Toole, M. T., Melli, S. O., Moore, M. N., & Derstine, J. B. (1996). Global gladiators: A model for international nursing education. *Nurse Educator, 21,* 38–41.

Poremba, B. A. (1995). An American nurse visits Vietnam. *Nursing and Health Care: Perspectives on Community, 16,* 118–124.

Rosenkoetter, M. M., Reynolds, B. J., Cummings, H., & Zakutney, M. (1993). The Barbados project: An experience in collaboration and mutuality. *Nursing and Health Care, 14,* 528–532.

Toyoshima, E. (1994). Continuing education for nursing staff development through technical cooperation of southeast Asia countries. *The Journal of Continuing Education in Nursing, 25,* 67–70.

CHAPTER 32

Research in Rehabilitation Nursing

Audrey Nelson

Nurses, as part of their everyday clinical practice, make many decisions and solve complex problems. Pause for a minute and consider the basis on which you answer clinical questions. Each nurse brings unique knowledge, experience, and skills to his or her practice in rehabilitation nursing. There are several ways nurses "know how" to respond to clinical practice dilemmas. Nurses can use trial and error combined with common sense to answer many issues that arise in practice; they can follow authority (policy and/or procedures) or tradition embedded in the setting in which they are employed; and they can solve problems through either intuition or logical reasoning. Complementing these approaches is the knowledge gleaned over time through research. Research provides nurses with a scientific approach to describe, explain, or predict nursing practice and clients' responses to interventions.

Findings from research can be applied to practice to (1) improve the access, quality, and satisfaction of rehabilitation services; (2) improve the quality of life of persons with disabilities; and (3) decrease the cost in rehabilitation settings. Rehabilitation settings with active research efforts facilitate professional growth and enhance clinical skills of their staff while garnering credibility with consumers. Research can foster collegial relationships among disciplines and create an intellectually stimulating and innovative environment.

The purpose of this chapter is to first provide a historical overview of research in rehabilitation and identify research goals for professional practice. Next, the role of the rehabilitation nurse in research is described. A historical overview of published rehabilitation nursing research from 1986 is 1996 is provided. Last, research-based practice guidelines, rehabilitation research priorities, and future directions for research in rehabilitation nursing are discussed.

HISTORICAL OVERVIEW OF THE CONTRIBUTIONS OF RESEARCH IN REHABILITATION

Before the 1940s, the primary goal of research in rehabilitation was to improve the survival of trauma victims and identify medications to combat infections (DeJong & Batavia, 1991). Research in acute rehabilitation was virtually nonexistent in the literature until the 1950s. The primary goal for acute care rehabilitation at that time was to enhance recovery, reduce secondary complications, and maximize function and independence (DeLisa, 1992). Many tools for assessing functional levels and the severity of disability did not exist until the 1970s, when the Injury Severity Scale and Revised Trauma Score were developed and tested. The independent living movement in the 1970s also prompted research related to rehabilitation (DeJong & Batavia, 1991).

Research was instrumental in advancing technology. In the 1980s, technology exploded with knowledge and clinical equipment for careful monitoring—for example, renal scanning, ultrasonography, urodynamic tests, and lithotripsy (DeLisa, 1992). Intrathecal catheters and pumps allow the administration of neuroactive and possibly neurotropic agents directly into the spinal cord for the treatment of spasticity and pain (DeLisa, 1992; Paice & Magolan, 1991). Wheelchair sports led to the design of lighter, stronger wheelchairs, with an increased focus on esthetics. Other equipment and devices for persons with disabilities include one-handed joystick-controlled drive cams; voice-controlled wheelchairs and beds; environmental control systems; articulated prone carts; bowel care chairs; and standing and walking aids. Therapeutic and functional standing could be achieved in a greater number of individuals using existing technology; however, barriers that prevent the equipment from being more widely used still exist (Jaeger, Yarkony, & Roth, 1989).

GOALS FOR NURSING RESEARCH IN REHABILITATION

Research goals can be as diverse as the clinical services, delivery systems, and practice settings in which rehabilitation is provided. Rehabilitation nursing research goals include the following:

- To examine the effect of the organization, financing, and management of health care on the delivery of, quality of, cost of, and access to health care and on health outcomes
- To develop or design devices or equipment to improve nursing practice and the quality of life for persons with disabilities
- To advance knowledge leading to improvements in the prevention, assessment, and interventions of nursing diagnoses or client care problems
- To identify, develop, and evaluate ways to improve the quality of care

NURSES' ROLES RELATED TO RESEARCH

Rehabilitation nurses have many options for becoming involved in research, including being consumers of research, conducting and disseminating research, and applying research to practice. Figure 32–1 depicts the three overlapping research roles for the rehabilitation nurse. Nurses frequently participate in all three research-related roles to varied degrees.

Being a Consumer of Research

By virtue of education and experience, most nurses possess a number of skills and the knowledge necessary to become "consumers" of research. These skills include basic knowledge of research design and methods as well as a basic understanding of data analysis pro-

cedures. A rehabilitation nurse can participate in research in several ways. First, the nurse observes nursing practice and the responses of clients to that care. This places the nurse in an optimal position to identify questions and problems to be studied. Second, to enhance clinical knowledge and skills, the nurse needs to keep abreast of the literature and evaluate research in the appropriate field.

Conducting and Disseminating Research

Professional practice, by definition, requires that the discipline develop a knowledge base that is grounded in research. Nurses with special training in research methodology can make a significant contribution to rehabilitation nursing through the conducting of research. Specifically, nurses can be involved as principal investigators responsible for designing a study and providing leadership throughout the research process, or as coinvestigators participating on the research team. Novice nurse researchers can participate as site coordinators for a multisite study or assist an established researcher with data collection.

Research has little value in practice unless the findings are shared with others (LoBiondo-Wood & Haber, 1986). Findings from research can be disseminated through presentations both within and outside the profession; through publications, including professional journals and books as well as lay publications targeted at the consumer; and through the development of products, such as teaching guides, models of care delivery, staffing guidelines, and clinical practice guidelines.

Using Research

Research utilization is defined as the process of analyzing and synthesizing research findings with the goal of implementing and refining a change in practice (Horsley, Crane, Crabtree, & Wood, 1983). Nurses can develop specific expertise in the application of research findings to practice. Research utilization involves the use of research outcomes, research methods, and planned change processes (Horsley et al., 1983). Additionally, national clinical practice guidelines provide nurses with a unique opportunity to apply scientifically based knowledge to their practice. In this ever-changing technology-driven society, the quick and effective application of research findings is critical to the establish-

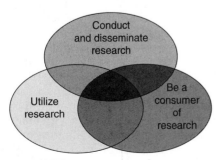

FIGURE 32–1
Nurses' roles related to reasearch.

ment of the nursing profession as a research-based practice. Research utilization has implications for improved client outcomes, nursing standards, policies and procedures, quality improvement, and care delivery systems.

The research utilization process involves several steps. First, a problem is identified for which extensive research has been conducted. Next, a comprehensive review of the literature is conducted. Each study is carefully reviewed and evaluated, with consideration given to the sample, design, methods, and scientific merit. As a whole, the set of studies is carefully analyzed and synthesized, and an innovation is selected. Administrative support is obtained to implement the innovation, carefully including all levels of staff in the change process. The innovation is pilot tested and refined and, if successful, implemented on a wider scale. Table 32–1 compares the process of conducting research with the process for applying research to practice.

One example of a research utilization project related to rehabilitation nursing is a hypothetical project titled "Uncovering Nursing Rituals in Acute Rehabilitation Nursing Practice." This project would question practice issues grounded in tradition that are time-consuming or have questionable merit. Several staff members could be involved in identifying potential rituals, and an extensive

review of the literature would be initiated on priority practice issues. With the use of published research studies, the goal would be to explore a possible rationale to support the existing practice or a rationale to support a practice change. Involving staff at all levels makes implementation of practice innovations easier.

Other examples of research utilization projects might include (1) strategies to promote oral hydration for clients at risk for aspiration, (2) effective interventions for managing combative behavior of clients with dementia, (3) strategies to promote mobility in frail elderly persons, and (4) strategies to prevent client falls in a restraint-free environment. It is important to keep in mind that the research utilization process necessitates that there be an adequate number of sound scientific studies on the topic selected and that the studies can be generalized to the client population in the nurse's setting.

REHABILITATION NURSING RESEARCH 1986–1996

Using the Cumulative Index to Nursing and Allied Health Literature (CINAHL) database, a search of nursing research related to rehabilitation nursing over the past 10 years was conducted. Rehabilitation was entered as a

TABLE 32–1 ■ PROCESSES FOR THE CONDUCT AND APPLICATION OF RESEARCH

Process for Conducting Research	Process for Applying Research to Practice
Identify the problem, puzzle, or phenomenon to be investigated.	Identify the problem, puzzle, or phenomenon to be investigated.
Explicate the linkage of the research questions or problems to a theoretical framework. Select a quantitative and/or a qualitative approach. Conduct a review of the literature.	Conduct a comprehensive review of the literature to capture research that has been completed on the topic.
Design the study. For a quantitative study, formulate testable research questions or hypotheses for the study; refine research questions/hypotheses and measurement instruments for data collection; conduct a pilot study if needed; specify the sample to be studied; and plan data management.	Carefully review and evaluate each study, considering the sample, design, methods, and scientific merit.
For a qualitative study, determine research questions, identify data collection methods, identify data collection methods, and plan data management and analysis techniques.	
Collect the data.	Carefully analyze and synthesize the set of studies as a whole, and select an innovation.
Analyze the data and interpret the findings. Identify the conclusions and recommendations from the findings.	Obtain administrative support to implement the innovation, carefully including all levels of staff in the change process.
Disseminate the findings.	Pilot-test, refine, and, if successful, implement the innovation on a wider scale.

floating heading, and the search was limited to nursing journals or dissertations. The search was further delimited to exclude studies related to substance abuse, learning disabilities, mental retardation, and mental disorders. A total of 132 studies was identified. These 132 studies are briefly summarized, providing a 10-year overview of the state of the science of rehabilitation nursing research. Specifically, the discussion focuses on (1) clinical areas researched, (2) research designs, (3) samples, (4) setting, (5) variables, and (6) measurement tools commonly used.

The clinical areas most frequently studied were cardiac rehabilitation (29%), stroke (23%), and spinal cord injury/neurological deficits (18%). Less studied clinical areas included pulmonary rehabilitation (6%), orthopedic rehabilitation (6%), traumatic brain injury (5%), cancer rehabilitation (5%), and trauma (4%). Other clinical areas included pain, renal conditions, human immunodeficiency virus infection/acquired immunodeficiency disease, and fatigue (total, fewer than 6%).

Of the 132 studies identified, 78% were quantitative, 20% were qualitative, and fewer than 3% used a combination of quantitative and qualitative methods. The most commonly used design for research in rehabilitation nursing was correlational (34%), followed by experimental/quasi-experimental (29%), descriptive (17%), ethnographic (7%), grounded theory (3%), tool development (3%), phenomenology (2%), case study (2%), and longitudinal (2%).

Excluding case studies, sample sizes ranged from 12 to 248. The majority of studies included persons with disabilities as the subjects, but a moderate number of studies included spouses, caregivers, and health care providers as well. The samples were predominantly adult (55%) and elderly (35%), with pediatric/adolescent age groups represented in fewer than 11% of the studies.

The settings included inpatient rehabilitation units, intensive care units, long-term care units, and community-based settings. A significant number of studies measured variables at different points along the continuum of care. Over the full 10-year period, 39% of the studies were conducted in inpatient rehabilitation units, 37% were community based, 21% were conducted across the care continuum, and fewer than 3% were conducted in either long-term care facilities or intensive care units. A definite trend was noted in the research settings over time. Between 1986 and 1991, the majority of the studies were conducted on inpatient rehabilitation units (51%), and fewer than 27% were community-based. After 1992, fewer than 26% were conducted in inpatient settings, and the majority were either community based (47%) or across the continuum of care (26%) (Keith, 1988).

Variables

Researchers in rehabilitation have studied a wide variety of variables. These variables include biophysical, psychosocial, resource-re-

TABLE 32–2 ■ VARIABLES STUDIED IN REHABILITATION NURSING RESEARCH 1986–1996

Activity	Coping	Immobility	Range of motion
Adaptation/adjustment	Costs	Intention	Reading skills
Age	Cultures	Knowledge	Rehabilitation outcomes
Attitudes	Disabilities	Lengths of stay	Resource utilization
Behavior	Discharge disposition	Levels of nursing care	Risk factors
Beliefs	Dyspnea	Life satisfaction	Roles
Biophysical measures	Endurance	Marital status	Satisfaction
Body changes	Environments	Medication use	Self-care/self-efficacy
Body images	Exercise	Memory	Self-concepts
Caregiving skills	Facial disfigurement	Mental status	Self-medication
Caring	Fatigue	Mobility	Sexuality
Case outcomes	Feeding	Muscle tone	Sleep
Cognitive functioning	Feelings	Nursing interventions	Social functioning
Coma	Fitness	Nutrition	Social supports
Communication	Functional status	Pain	Torque
Compliance	Gait	Physical functioning	Types of nursing
Conditioning levels	Gender	Psychosocial skills	Word recognition
Continence	Goal attainment	Quality of care/services	Wound healing
Contractures	Hemodynamic function	Quality of life	

lated, and health-related variables for a wide range of clinical areas and settings. Most of the intervention studies evaluated strategies to enhance knowledge, self-care, adjustment, and support. Some studies explored interventions to decrease symptoms, complications, and setbacks. Table 32–2 outlines some of the variables related to rehabilitation nursing research.

Measurement Tools Commonly Used

A variety of measurement tools were identified by researchers. Most frequently, these tools were related to the assessment of (1) function, disability, or activities of daily liv-

ing; (2) cognition; (3) the quality of life; (4) health; (5) family or caregiver functioning; (6) pain; (7) satisfaction; (8) knowledge; and (9) mental status. Other measures included biophysical measures, access to care, resource utilization, and cost. Table 32–3 depicts measurement tools used in rehabilitation nursing research between 1986 and 1996.

RESEARCH-BASED PRACTICE GUIDELINES

Research-based practice is facilitated through the development of clinical practice guidelines. Clinical practice guidelines are defined as systematically developed statements to assist the practitioner and client in making deci-

---

TABLE 32–3 ■ COMMONLY USED MEASUREMENT TOOLS IN REHABILITATION NURSING RESEARCH

Activity Summary Questionnaire
Amsterdam/Nijmegen Everyday Language Test
Barrett's Power-as-Knowing–Participation-in-Change Tool
Barthel Functional Index
Baseline and Transition Dyspnea Index
Basic Cardiac Knowledge Scale
Beck Depression Inventory
Body Image Visual Analogue Scale
Cantril Ladder Scale
Cardiac Health Knowledge Questionnaire
Cardiac Lifestyle Knowledge Scale
Cardiac Misconception Scale
Center for Epidemiologic Studies Depression Scale
Chronic Pain Modifier Questionnaire
Clifton Assessment Procedure for the Elderly
COPD Self-Care Action Scale
Coronary Artery Bypass Grafting Patient Learning Needs
   Inventory
Duke Activity Status Index
Dyspnea Visual Analog Scale
Exercise of Self-Care Agency Scale
Family Crisis Oriented Personal Evaluation Scales
Ference Human Field Motion Tool
Functional Independence Measure
HAQ Disability Index
Health Assessment Questionnaire
Hollingshead Index
Home Pass Assessment Form
Hospital Anxiety and Depression Scale
Human Activity Profile
Index of Well-Being
Industrial Injury Management Outcome Tool
Instrumental Activities of Daily Living Scale
Jenkins Activity Checklist
Jenkins Self-Efficacy Expectation Scales
Karnofsky Performance Status Scale
Katz Index of Activities of Daily Living
Knowledge Test
List of Outcome Variables
Marital Interactions Coding System

McGill Pain Questionnaire
Mini–Mental Status Examination
Modified Borg Scale
Motor Assessment Scale
Multidimensional Health Locus of Control Scale
Neurobehavioral Rating Scale
N.Y. Heart Association Functional Classification of Heart Disease
Nottingham Health Profile
Numerical Rating Scale for Pain
Pain Reception Scale
Patient Satisfaction with Quality of Care Questionnaire
Patient Wound Assessment
Patterson Sargent Functional Scale
Perception of Home Management Planning
Personal Resource Questionnaire
Psychosocial Adjustment to Illness Scale
Pulmonary Functional Status and Dyspnea Questionnaire
Quality of Life Index
Quality of Well-Being Scale
Quick Test
Rancho Los Amigos Coma Recovery Scale
Rancho Los Amigos Levels of Cognitive Function Scale
Ratio Property Category Scale
Reason for Activity Survey
Rehab Success Scale
Rosenberg Self-Esteem Scale
Self Care Resource Inventory
Self-Efficacy for Walking
Self-Efficacy Scale
Self-Esteem Inventory
Shortness of Breath Questionnaire
Sickness Impact Profile
Social Support Questionnaire
Sunnaas Index of ADL
Symptom Assessment Scales
Symptom Checklist
Symptom Inventory
Tennessee Self-Concept Scale
WHO Questionnaire
Wolfer-Davis Recovery Inventory

TABLE 32–4 ■ CLINICAL PRACTICE GUIDELINES PUBLISHED BY THE AGENCY FOR HEALTH CARE POLICY AND RESEARCH

Acute Pain Management: Operative or Medical Procedures and Trauma	Benign Prostatic Hyperplasia: Diagnosis and Treatment
Urinary Incontinence in Adults	Management of Cancer Pain
Pressure Ulcers in Adults: Prediction and Prevention	Unstable Angina: Diagnosis and Management
Cataract in Adults: Management of Functional Impairment	Heart Failure: Evaluation and Care of Patients with Left Ventricular Systolic Dysfunction
Depression in Primary Care: Vol. 1. Detection and Diagnosis	Otitis Media with Effusion in Young Children
Depression in Primary Care: Vol. 2. Treatment of Major Depression	Quality Determinants of Mammography
	Acute Low Back Problems
	Treatment of Pressure Ulcers
Sickle Cell Disease: Screening, Diagnosis and Management	Post-Stroke Rehabilitation
	Cardiac Rehabilitation
	Smoking Cessation
Evaluation and Management of Early HIV Infection	

sions about appropriate health care for specific clinical circumstances (Agency for Health Care Policy and Research, 1993). Guidelines have the potential to reduce unnecessary and inappropriate care, control geographical variations in practice patterns, and make more effective use of health care resources (Woolf, 1990).

Several guidelines applicable to rehabilitation have been published since 1995. The Agency for Health Care Policy and Research has published guidelines on urinary incontinence and pressure ulcers (Table 32–4 outlines the AHCPR practice guidelines published to date). The Paralyzed Veterans of America has established a consortium of interdisciplinary experts to guide the development of practice guidelines pertinent to spinal cord injuries and disorders, including topics such as neurogenic bowel. The American Association of Spinal Cord Injury Nurses published practice guidelines on dysreflexia in 1995. Clinicians can benefit from these concise presentations of research findings.

NATIONAL RESEARCH PRIORITIES

Priority areas for future research have been delineated by several professional organizations, including the Association of Rehabilitation Nurses (ARN), the American Association

of Spinal Cord Injury Nurses, the National Institute of Disability Rehabilitation Research, and the National Institute of Neurological Disorders and Stroke.

Association of Rehabilitation Nurses

The ARN established its first research agenda in 1996 through the use of interactive computer technology. The following five research priorities were identified:

1. Health promotion, primary prevention, and secondary prevention to facilitate the management of self-care and independence for persons with or at risk for chronic illness and/or disability
2. Interventions and symptom management for persons with disability to maximize function
3. A community context of care for persons at risk for illness or injury or with a chronic illness and/or disability and their quality of life
4. Rehabilitation nurse–sensitive outcomes and costs in the continuum of care and in an interdisciplinary setting or settings
5. Rehabilitation practice and roles in the changing health care system

American Association of Spinal Cord Injury Nurses

The American Association of Spinal Cord Injury Nurses research priorities were identified through a Delphi study. Results were published in *SCI Nursing* and include the following:

■ The effectiveness of home care programs, outpatient programs, or other community-based programs
■ The effectiveness of teaching programs for spinal cord injury (SCI) clients and/or significant others
■ Aging in SCI and quality-of-life issues
■ The effectiveness of discharge planning
■ Defining and promoting community reentry
■ The effectiveness of rehabilitation after discharge
■ Defining and promoting the quality of life after discharge
■ The effectiveness of teaching programs for SCI nurses
■ Attributes of SCI centers with quality client outcomes

- Nursing's contribution to SCI clients' success at home
- Attendant care or caregiver strain and/or problems
- Rehabilitation outcomes
- Defining and fostering community independence
- The home management of pressure sores
- Nursing interventions to decrease depression and self-neglect
- The prevention and/or treatment of pressure sores
- Wellness/fitness programs for SCI clients
- Nursing interventions to humanize hospital routines on SCI units
- The effectiveness of interdisciplinary team collaboration and the role of nurses
- The prediction of outcomes in SCI nursing interventions
- The impact of health care policy reform on SCI nursing practice and client care

National Institute of Disability Rehabilitation Research

The National Institute of Disability Rehabilitation Research has identified six areas for outcome research: community reintegration, vocational rehabilitation, empowerment and independence, employment, human functioning, and the translation of knowledge into practice (Graves, 1993). Furthermore, the institute identified six crosscutting issues, common to each of the six outcome areas previously identified: (1) promoting positive attitudes toward persons with disabilities, (2) promoting environmental access, (3) promoting policy and financial access, (4) improving the skills of persons with disabilities, (5) improving support for and capacities of family members, and (6) improving the functioning of the service system (Graves, 1993).

A Consensus Validation Conference on Prevention and Management of Urinary Tract Infections Among People with Spinal Cord Injuries was held in January 1992, sponsored by the National Institute of Disability Rehabilitation Research. Some of the research priorities identified include the following:

- Identification of the best methods for teaching people with spinal cord injures to observe, monitor, and respond quickly to warning signs that urinary tract infections may be developing
- Determination of strategies to integrate the expertise of the professional as well as the consumer to improve bladder management

techniques and reduce medical complications of the neurogenic bladder

- Assessment of the impact of peer counseling on the management of the neurogenic bladder and on reducing the incidence of urinary tract infections
- The extent to which esthetic issues influence adherence to bladder management techniques that minimize urinary tract infections
- The advantages and disadvantages of various bladder management methods on fertility and sexual pleasure
- Determination of the results of the treatment of symptomatic and asymptomatic infection more than 6 months after injury
- Determination of the psychosocial impact of a neurogenic bladder in childhood and the impact of incontinence on social skills development, on the emotional response of the child to the disability, and on family stress
- Determination of methods to prevent leakage of urine in women
- Identification of ways in which optimal bladder management may differ between women and men
- Study of the use of intermittent catheterization in women to determine its medical and social advantages/disadvantages as well as its cost/benefit ratio
- Determination of the frequency of incontinence across various types of bladder management
- Comparison of urinary tract infection methods across the lifetime of people with SCIs for the prevention of future problems and increasing longevity
- Study of the impact of bladder management procedures on the quality of life of people with SCIs

National Institute of Neurological Disorders and Stroke

The National Institute of Neurological Disorders and Stroke developed an implementation plan for the Decade of the Brain (1990s). Within this plan, several research priorities were identified (National Institute of Neurological Disorders and Stroke, 1993, p. 321), including the following:

- Initiation of new efforts to define the long-term impact of SCI and fostering of the new field of restorative neurology, so that new therapies will be devised to alleviate long-term consequences and improve the quality of life

▪ Evaluating effectiveness of collaborative efforts with citizen organizations to educate health professionals and the general public about injury prevention and treatment

FUTURE DIRECTIONS FOR RESEARCH IN REHABILITATION NURSING

There is little doubt that research has played a significant role in advancing knowledge in the field of rehabilitation. The future holds many opportunities for nurses to conduct studies and apply research to practice. Research provides the key for providing cost-effective nursing care delivery; high-quality services; access to services and care; technology; and improved health outcomes for the clients served.

REFERENCES

Agency for Health Care Policy and Research. (1993). *AHCPR program note: Clinical practice guideline develop-ment* (AHCPR Publication No. 93-0023). Rockville, MD: U.S. Department of Health and Human Services.

DeJong, G., & Batavia, A. (1991). Toward a health services research capacity in spinal cord injury. *Paraplegia, 29*(6), 373–389.

DeLisa, J. (1992). Clinical rehabilitation research advances in spinal cord injury. *Paraplegia, 30*(1), 73–74.

Graves, W. H. (1993). NIDRR plans for the future. *Assistive Technology, 5*, 3–6.

Horsley, J., Crane, J., Crabtree, M. K., & Wood, D. J. (1983). *Using research to improve nursing practice: A guide CURN Project.* New York: Grune & Stratton.

Jaeger, R., Yarkony, G., & Roth, E. (1989). Rehabilitation technology for standing and walking after a spinal cord injury. *American Journal of Physical Medicine and Rehabilitation, 68*(3) 128–133.

Keith, R. (1988). Observations in the rehabilitation hospital: Twenty years of research. *Archives of Physical Medicine and Rehabilitation, 69*(8), 625–631.

LoBiondo-Wood, G., & Haber, J. (1986). *Nursing research: Critical appraisal and utilization.* St. Louis: C. V. Mosby.

National Institute of Neurological Disorders and Stroke. (1993). Progress and promise 1992: A status report on the NINDS Implementation Plan for the Decade of the Brain. *Annals of Neurology, 33*(3), 320–324.

Woolf, S. H. (1990). Practice guidelines: A new reality in medicine: I. Recent developments. *Archives of Internal Medicine, 150*, 1811–1818.

Appendices

Resources for Persons Needing Rehabilitation Services

Acquired Immunodeficiency Syndrome

National AIDS Hotline
c/o American Social Health Association
PO Box 13827
Research Triangle Park, NC 27709
(800) 342-AIDS

Aging

Alzheimer's Disease and Related Disorders
    Association
70 Lake Street
Suite 600
Chicago, IL 60601
(312) 853-3060

American Aging Association
110 Chesley Dr
Media, PA
(610) 627-2626

Arthritis

American Juvenile Arthritis Organization
1314 Spring Street, NW
Atlanta, GA 30309
(404) 872-7100

American Rheumatism Association
17 Executive Drive, NE
Suite 280480
Atlanta, GA 30329
(404) 633-2377

Arthritis Foundation
1314 Spring Street, NW
Atlanta, GA 30309
(404) 872-7100

Cancer

American Cancer Society
1599 Clifford Road, NE
Atlanta, GA 30329
(800) 227-2345

Disability Services

Clearinghouse on Disability Information
U.S. Department of Education
Switzer Building, Room 3132
330 C Street S.W.
Washington, DC 20202
(202) 731-1241

Independent Living for the Handicapped
1301 Belmont Street NW
Washington, DC 20009
(202) 797-9803

Information Center for Individuals with
    Disabilities
Fort Point Place, First Floor
27–43 Wormwood Street
Boston, MA 02210
(617) 727-5540

Library of Congress National Library Ser-
    vice for the Blind and Physically Handi-
    capped
1291 Taylor Street NW
Washington, DC 20542
(202) 707-5100 *or* (800) 424-9100

Mainstream, Inc.
1030 15th Street NW, Suite 1010
Washington, DC 20005
(202) 898-0202

National Council on Disability
800 Independence Avenue SW,
    Suite 808
Washington, DC 20591
(202) 267-3846
TDD: (202) 267-3232

Easter Seal
230 West Monroe Street, Suite 1800
Chicago, IL 60606
(800) 221-6827

National Foundation March of Dimes
1275 Mamaroneck Avenue
White Plains, NY 10605
(914) 428-7100

National Rehabilitation Information Center
8455 Colesville Road
Silver Spring, MD 20910
(800) 346-2742 *or* (301) 588-9284

Federal Agencies

Agency for Health Care Policy and Research
Executive Office Center, Suite 501
2101 Jefferson Street
Rockville, MD 20890
(301) 495-3453

National Institute on Disability and Rehabilitation Research
U.S. Department of Education
400 Maryland Avenue SW, Room 3060
Washington, DC 20202
(202) 732-1134

Rehabilitation Services Administration
Department of Human Services
605 G Street NW, Room 101M
Washington, DC 20001
(202) 727-3211

U.S. Department of Health and Human Services
Office of Disease Prevention and Health Promotion
Switzer Building, Room 2132
330 C Street SW
Washington, DC 20201

Head Injury

National Head Injury Foundation
1776 Massachusetts Avenue NW, Suite 100
Washington, DC 20036
(202) 842-4444

Health Care Facilities and Commissions

American Health Care Association
1202 L Street NW
Washington, DC 20005
(202) 842-4444

American Hospital Association
840 North Lake Shore Drive
Chicago, IL 60611
(312) 280-4444

Commission on Accreditation of Rehabilitation Facilities (CARF)
101 North Wilmot Road, Suite 500
Tucson, AZ 85711
(602) 748-1212

Joint Commission on Accreditation of Healthcare Organizations (JCAHO)
One Renaissance Boulevard
Oakbrook Terrace, IL 60181
(708) 916-5600

National Association of Rehabilitation Facilities (NARF)
PO Box 17675
Washington, DC 20041
(800) 368-3513

Incontinence

Continence Restored
785 Park Avenue
New York, NY 10021
(212) 879-3131

Help for Incontinent People Organization
PO Box 544
Union, SC 29379
(803) 579-7900

Simon Foundation
PO Box 835X
Wilmette, IL 60091
(800) 237-4666

Neuromuscular Conditions

Amyotrophic Lateral Sclerosis Association
21021 Ventura Boulevard, Suite 321
Woodland Hills, CA 91364
(818) 990-2151

Epilepsy Foundation of America
4351 Garden City Drive
Landover, MD 20785
(301) 459-3700

Guillain-Barré Syndrome Foundation International
PO Box 262
Wynnewood, PA 19096
(215) 667-0131

Muscular Dystrophy Association
810 7th Avenue
New York, NY 10019
(212) 586-0808

Myasthenia Gravis Foundation, Inc.
53 West Jackson Boulevard
Chicago, IL 60604
(312) 427-6252

National Ataxia Foundation
15500 Wayzata Boulevard, Suite 750
Wayzata, MN 55391
(612) 473-7666

National Multiple Sclerosis Society
205 42nd Street
New York, NY 10017
(800) 624-8236

National Parkinson's Disease Foundation,
Inc.
1501 Ninth Avenue NW
Miami, FL 33136
(305) 547-6666

Parkinson's Disease Foundation
William Black Medical Research Building
Columbia Presbyterian Medical Center
650 West 168th Street
New York, NY 10032
(800) 457-6676

United Cerebral Palsy Foundation Association
7 Penn Plaza, Suite 804
New York, NY 10001
(212) 268-6655

Professional Associations

American Academy of Physical Medicine
and Rehabilitation
122 South Michigan Avenue, Suite 1300
Chicago, IL 60603
(312) 922-9366

American Association of Neuroscience
Nurses
224 Des Plaines Street, Suite 601
Chicago, IL 60661
(312) 993-0043

American Association of Spinal Cord Injury Nurses
75–20 Astoria Boulevard
Jackson Heights, NY 11370
(718) 803-3782

American Congress of Rehabilitation Medicine
5700 Old Orchard Road, First Floor
Skokie, IL 60077
(708) 966-0095

American Occupational Therapy Association
1383 Piccard Drive, Suite 301
Rockville, MD 20850
(301) 948-9626

American Physical Therapy Association
111 North Fairfax Street
Alexandria, VA 22314
(703) 684-2782

American Speech-Language-Hearing Association
10801 Rockville Pike
Rockville, MD 20852
(301) 897-5700

Association of Rehabilitation Nurses
5700 Old Orchard Road, First Floor
Skokie, IL 60077
(708) 966-3433

National Rehabilitation Association
633 South Washington Street
Alexandria, VA 22314
(703) 836-7677

National Therapeutic Recreation Society
3101 Park Center Drive, 12th Floor
Alexandria, VA 22302
(703) 820-4940

Respiratory Nursing Society
5700 Old Orchard Road, First Floor
Skokie, IL 60067
(708) 966-8673

Respiratory Conditions

American Lung Association
1740 Broadway
New York, NY 10019

Sexuality

Sex Information and Education Council of
the U.S.
130 West 42nd Street, Suite 2500
New York, NY 10036
(212) 819-9770

Spinal Cord Injury

American Spinal Injury Association
250 E Superior Street, Room 619
Chicago, IL 60611
(312) 908-3425

National Spinal Injury Association
600 Cummings Park, Suite 2000
Woburn, MA 01801
(617) 935-2722

Paralyzed Veterans of America
801 18th Street NW
Washington, DC 20006
(202) 872-1300

Sports

National Handicapped Sports and Recreation Association
445 East-West Highway, Suite 603
Bethesda, MD 20814
(301) 652-7505

Special Olympics International
1350 New York Avenue NW, Suite 610
New York, NY 10016
(212) 447-7248

Stroke

National Institute of Neurological and Communicative Disorders and Stroke
Building 31, Room 8A52
9000 Rockville Pike
Bethesda, MD 20892
(301) 496-9746

National Stroke Association
300 East Hampden Avenue, Suite 240
Englewood, CO 80110
(303) 762-9922

Stroke Clubs International
805 12th Street
Galveston, TX 77550
(409) 762-1022

Common Rehabilitation Acronyms

ADA	Americans with Disabilities Act
ADLs	Activities of daily living
AFDC	Aid to Families with Dependent Children
AHASRHP	American Hospital Association Section for Rehabilitation Hospitals and Programs
AIDS	Acquired immunodeficiency syndrome
AKA	Above-the-knee amputation
ANA	American Nurses Association
ARN	Association of Rehabilitation Nursing
ASCIA	American Spinal Cord Injury Association
BKA	Below-the-knee amputation
CARF	Commission on Accreditation of Rehabilitation Facilities
CRRN	Certified Registered Rehabilitation Nurse
CSF	Cerebrospinal fluid
CVA	Cerebrovascular accident
CVP	Central venous pressure
DAI	Diffuse axonal injury
DDST	Denver II Developmental Screening Test
DI	Diabetes insipidus
DJD	Degenerative joint disease
DVT	Deep vein thrombosis
FIM	Functional Independence Measure
GOAT	Galveston Orientation and Amnesia Test
HO	Heterotopic ossification
ICIDH	International Classification of Impairments, Disabilities, and Handicaps
ICP	Intracranial pressure

ILC	Independent living center
LMN	Lower motor neuron
MMSE	Mini-mental state examination
NHIF	National Head Injury Foundation
NRC	National Rehabilitation Caucus
OA	Osteoarthritis
OBRA	Omnibus Budget Reconciliation Act
OVR	Office of Vocational Rehabilitation
PEDI	Pediatric Evaluation of Disability Inventory
PM&R	Physical medicine and rehabilitation
PTA	Posttraumatic amnesia
QI	Quality improvement
RA	Rheumatoid arthritis
RIND	Reversible ischemic neurological deficit
RNF	Rehabilitation Nursing Foundation
ROM	Range of motion
SAH	Subarachnoid hemorrhage
SCI	Spinal cord injury
SIADH	Syndrome of inappropriate antidiuretic hormone (secretion)
SNF	Skilled nursing facility
SSDI	Social Security Disability Income
SSI	Supplemental Security Income
TBI	Traumatic brain injury
THR	Total hip replacement
TIA	Transient ischemic attack
UMN	Upper motor neuron
VNA	Visiting Nurses Association
WMS-R	Wechsler Memory Scale—Revised

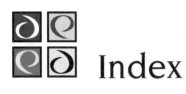

Index

Note: Page numbers in *italics* refer to illustrations; page numbers followed by t refer to tables.

ISBN 0-7216-6977-8

90038
9 780721 669779